TRENDS IN CANCER

INCIDENCE AND MORTALITY

WORLD HEALTH ORGANIZATION
INTERNATIONAL AGENCY FOR RESEARCH ON CANCER

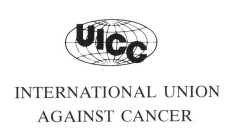

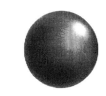

INTERNATIONAL UNION
AGAINST CANCER

INTERNATIONAL ASSOCIATION
OF CANCER REGISTRIES

TRENDS IN CANCER INCIDENCE AND MORTALITY

Michel P. Coleman, Jacques Estève, Philippe Damiecki

Annie Arslan, Hélène Renard

IARC Scientific Publications No. 121

International Agency for Research on Cancer
Lyon 1993

INTERNATIONAL AGENCY FOR RESEARCH ON CANCER

The International Agency for Research on Cancer (IARC) was established in 1965 by the World Health Assembly, as an independently financed organization within the framework of the World Health Organization. The headquarters of the Agency are at Lyon, France.

The Agency conducts a programme of research concentrating particularly on the epidemiology of cancer and the study of potential carcinogens in the human environment. Its field studies are supplemented by biological and chemical research carried out in the Agency's laboratories in Lyon and, through collaborative research agreements, in national research institutions in many countries. The Agency also conducts a programme for the education and training of personnel for cancer research.

The publications of the Agency are intended to contribute to the dissemination of authoritative information on different aspects of cancer research. A complete list is printed at the back of this book.

INTERNATIONAL UNION AGAINST CANCER

The International Union Against Cancer (UICC) is devoted exclusively to all aspects of the worldwide fight against cancer. Its objectives are to advance scientific and medical knowledge in research, diagnosis, treatment and prevention of cancer and to promote all other aspects of the campaign against cancer throughout the world. Founded in 1933, the UICC is a non-governmental, independent association of more than 250 member organizations in about 80 countries. Members are voluntary cancer leagues and societies, cancer research and/or treatment centres and, in some countries, ministries of health. The UICC is non-profit and non-sectarian, and its headquarters are in Geneva, Switzerland.

INTERNATIONAL ASSOCIATION OF CANCER REGISTRIES

The International Association of Cancer Registries (IACR) was created following a decision taken during the Ninth International Cancer Congress held in Tokyo, Japan, in 1966. The Association is a voluntary non-governmental organization in official relations with WHO, representing the scientific and professional interests of cancer registries, with members interested in the development and application of cancer registration and morbidity survey techniques to studies of well-defined populations.

The constitution provides for a Governing Body composed of a President, General Secretary, Deputy Secretary and eight regional representatives. From 1973 the IARC has provided a secretariat for the Association with the primary functions of organizing meetings and coordinating scientific studies.

CONTENTS

Foreword vii

Acknowledgements viii

1   Introduction 1
2   Material 5
3   Method 27
4   Presentation of results.. 39
5   Lip (males) 43
6   Tongue 65
7   Mouth 97
8   Pharynx 129
9   Oesophagus 161
10   Stomach 193
11   Colon and rectum 225
12   Pancreas 257
13   Larynx (males) 289
14   Lung 311
15   Bone 343
16   Melanoma of the skin 379
17   Breast (females) 411
18   Cervix uteri 433
19   Corpus uteri 455
20   Ovary 477
21   Prostate 499
22   Testis 521
23   Bladder 543
24   Kidney 577
25   Thyroid 609
26   Non-Hodgkin lymphoma 641
27   Hodgkin's disease 673
28   Myeloma 705
29   Leukaemia 737
30   Childhood cancer 769
31   Summary 787

References 795

Published by the International Agency for Research on Cancer,

150 cours Albert Thomas, 69372 Lyon Cédex 08, France

Distributed by Oxford University Press, Walton Street, Oxford OX2 6DP, UK

Distributed in the USA by Oxford University Press, New York

The International Agency for Research on Cancer welcomes requests for permission
to reproduce or translate its publications, in part or in full. Applications
and enquiries should be addressed to the Editorial & Publications Service,
International Agency for Research on Cancer, Lyon, France, which will be glad to provide
the latest information on any changes made to the text, plans for new editions,
and reprints and translations already available.

ISBN 92 832 2121 4

ISSN 0300 5085

Printed in France

FOREWORD

Changes in cancer patterns with the passage of time are of vital interest in cancer control. Cancer trends offer clues as to the underlying causes of the disease and the wide variation in its frequency around the world, and they are the basic elements of information from which to judge how successful we have been in reducing the burden of cancer. Further, because the recent past is our best guide to what is likely to happen in the near future, cancer trends provide a sketch map of future cancer patterns, for the guidance of public health policy-makers.

Data on cancer incidence from population-based cancer registries around the world have been published first by UICC and later by the Agency in six successive volumes of *Cancer Incidence in Five Continents* between 1966 and 1993, covering the period 1950-87, and national cancer mortality data have been collected by WHO for periods from 1955 to 1988. These data have already provided a wealth of information on geographical variation in cancer risk by personal characteristics such as age, sex and racial or ethnic group. Time, the third element in the classic triad of epidemiological descriptors — person, place and time — is the central interest of this book, in which these data sets are used to provide the first comprehensive analysis of changes in cancer incidence and mortality around the world over the past 30 or so years. The analyses cover 60 populations in 29 countries for cancer incidence and 36 national data sets for cancer mortality, covering 42 countries in all.

Information is presented on time trends by year of diagnosis or death and by year of birth, for each of 25 major cancers in adults and for leukaemia and all cancer in children.

Special algorithms were developed to ensure that the 4000 and more data sets were each analysed according to explicit and standard criteria, and these are fully described. A particular effort has been made to present the many tables and graphics containing the results of the analyses as clearly as possible, in order to simplify their interpretation; further material is presented in a companion volume, *Trends in Cancer Incidence and Mortality: Detailed Tables by Region and Country* (IARC Technical Report No. 17, IARC, Lyon, 1993).

It is hoped that the production of this first volume on world-wide trends in cancer incidence and mortality will provide valuable new information, stimulate fruitful new lines of enquiry and prompt critical review of progress in cancer control as we approach the end of the century.

L. Tomatis, M. D.
Director, IARC

vii

ACKNOWLEDGEMENTS

This work would not have been possible without the sustained effort over many years of many cancer registry staff, too numerous to mention individually, and the staff of vital statistics offices in many countries, including those from which data have not been included but which considerably widened the choice of representative material for analysis. We trust that they will see this work as one of the many valuable uses to which the data they have collected can be put.

The editors of volumes I to VI of *Cancer Incidence in Five Continents* have coordinated a world-wide data set of immense value in the fight against cancer. Their systematic and painstaking attention to the quality and validity of the data over the years represents a collective effort which it would have been impossible for us to replicate from the raw data, and to the extent that the analyses presented here are of interest, it is largely because most of the available data sets have been brought up to a comparable standard of excellence.

The mortality data from the World Health Organisation data bank in Geneva were provided by Dr Alan Lopez, supplemented by data from the USA supplied by Dr Susan Devesa of the US National Cancer Institute. Dr Roger Black provided additional incidence data for Scotland.

Planning of the project was greatly assisted by a meeting of expert advisers, held in Lyon in April 1987. The participants were David Clayton (UK), Susan Devesa (USA), Alan Lopez (WHO), Clive Osmond (UK), Timo Hakulinen (Finland), Eugène Schifflers (Belgium), Max Parkin, Peter Boyle, Michel Smans and Florence Casset (IARC).

Professor Eugène Schifflers, Alain de Coninck and Michel Smans originally created the database of incidence and mortality which was used as the basis for the analyses reported in this book. In addition, Professor Schifflers played a major role in the design and development of the analytic approach during a short-term consultancy at IARC. We are indebted to him for a number of ideas which have been incorporated in the statistical methodology.

We are most grateful to Lynda Burkitt (Thames Cancer Registry), Annick Rivoire (IARC) and Bill Noble (Vardas, Bristol) for assistance in preparation of the manuscript.

viii

Chapter 1

INTRODUCTION

Examination of how both cancer incidence and cancer mortality have been changing over time is of interest for several reasons. These may be summarised in the form of three questions: how has cancer risk been changing, why, and what is likely to happen in the future? From these questions a fourth naturally arises, namely, what can be done to reduce the likely future burden of cancer? The material in this book, and in the companion technical report[60], is mainly intended to contribute to answering the first question, by providing a coherent set of analyses of selected cancer incidence and mortality data from around the world as a source of reference for researchers in cancer, public health and health care planning. The results should also be of some relevance for understanding why these changes have occurred, and what cancer trends are likely to occur in the near future.

There are four introductory chapters. The data sets are described in detail in Chapter 2, the analytic approach in Chapter 3, and the presentation of the results for each cancer in Chapter 4. The body of the book is taken up with 26 chapters describing the trends in incidence and mortality for each selected cancer, with a final summary chapter. The brief commentary on the results for each cancer, in Chapters 5-30, is intended to help the reader evaluate the results in the context of the method of analysis and of known or possible problems with the quality of the data.

The question of why a given cancer has been increasing or declining in frequency, often with different temporal patterns by age and sex between various populations, requires a more complete understanding of the causes of cancer, and of how human exposure to these causes has been changing over time, than is currently available for most cancers. Quantitative descriptions of trends in cancer risk may, however, give rise to aetiological hypotheses which can be tested in other studies, as for example with cancer of the stomach[134,195]. Analyses of cancer trends may also provide support for the plausibility of a hypothesis based on other types of evidence, as for example with the trends in lung cancer incidence, which reflect time-lagged trends in exposure to tobacco smoke[76,83], or with the trends in endometrial carcinoma in the USA, which reflect the temporal pattern of prescribing of non-contraceptive oral oestrogens for menopausal symptoms[177].

To some extent, the question of what is likely to happen in the future is implicit in any attempt to analyse cancer trends, since the methods incorporate an assumption that the relationship between cancer risk by age and either calendar time or year of birth has a particular form, the nature of which is not likely to change suddenly. This is so whether or not statistical models are explicitly used to describe the data. For example, many investigators have used the percentage change in age-standardised rates as a measure of trend: this approach implies an underlying age-period model (see Chapter 3). Since risk at older ages for those who are young today has not yet been observed, the relationship between age, cancer risk and time is assumed to continue to apply in the near future for the purposes of estimating lifetime cancer risk for people born recently. Similarly, the same relationship is assumed to have applied in the more distant past for the purposes of estimating the risk at younger ages of those who are now elderly, and for whom reliable data are only rarely available before 1940. In these analyses, all the data relate to the period since 1950.

A more useful answer to the question about future trends in cancer risk requires projections of cancer incidence or mortality rates, or of the numbers of cases or deaths likely to arise each year in a given population, or of the rate of change in risk over time. The choice of measure will depend on whether the information is to be used for planning the provision of health care facilities[255], or for evaluating the priorities for cancer prevention, screening[21] or research[117,118,257]. The extra uncertainties in making projections of cancer risk into the future, and the constraints on interpretation imposed by the underlying assumptions, such as the accuracy of population projections, will also vary accordingly. The information provided here can be used as the basis for making cancer projections.

An additional reason for carrying out these analyses has been the desire to make best use of a very long time-series of cancer incidence and mortality data: in effect, to transform a series of cross-sectional snap-shots of cancer occurrence into a coherent longitudinal sequence, enabling additional information to be derived from the data. The Nordic group of cancer registries, for example, has provided comparable trend analyses for 23 cancer sites, from five countries with effi-

1

cient national cancer registration systems which have covered a total population of some 25 million people for more than 30 years, and was able to make use of data on trends in the consumption of alcohol, tobacco and various foods over similar periods of time as an informal aid to interpretation of the data[116]. Population census data available for each country also provided a complete and regular set of denominators for the calculation of rates.

Systematic analysis of trends in cancer risk for most major cancers, and for many populations, was also expected to provoke a range of additional questions. Quantitative comparison of trends for different cancer sites may prompt a further search for common risk factors, and comparison of trends between populations, whether on a geographical or ethnic basis, may enable the plausible impact of strategies for prevention, screening or treatment to be evaluated. Equally, the effect of not implementing proven strategies of primary prevention can also be estimated[234].

Comparison of the observed temporal trends in both incidence and mortality was also expected to sharpen the assessment of the likely underlying patterns of change, to highlight issues of the quality of the data, and to provide the basis for an evaluation of the population impact of recent advances in treatment. Major improvements have taken place in the treatment of several cancers in the last 20 years, notably for childhood leukaemia, Hodgkin's disease, melanoma of the skin and cancers of the testis, yet there is relatively little published information on trends in survival from these or other malignancies in the population as a whole[3,27,46,159,194,239,275]. Similarly, in the absence of any major advance in the treatment of a given malignancy, when there has been little change in survival, the relationship between incidence and mortality in a given population should be stable[239]. Where trends in incidence and mortality diverge in the absence of major therapeutic advances, this may indicate a change in the biological spectrum of disease diagnosed or registered as malignant, as for example with cancers of the prostate, the stomach (especially in Japan) and the breast.

Time trends in cancer incidence or mortality have been examined recently for most major cancers in a number of areas or countries, particularly Connecticut (USA)[252], Henan province (China)[169], Singapore[153,154], France[128], the five Nordic countries[116], Switzerland[160,164], England and Wales[212,213], Europe[145-149] and various other countries[198]. Long-term trends in both incidence and mortality in the USA have been examined[77]. Many authors have examined trends in incidence or mortality for selected cancer sites, particularly those for which large changes are known to have occurred, e.g. cancers of the lung, stomach, cervix and testis[190] and melanoma of the skin.

Interpretation

The question of whether the observed trends in cancer incidence and mortality can safely be interpreted at all, given the problems of data quality, and if so, whether trends in cancer occurrence, especially cancer mortality, should be interpreted as society 'losing the war against cancer'[14] or, alternatively, 'clearly winning the war'[83], has sustained a vigorous debate in recent years[2,15,24,36,45,62,63,71,79,91,100,104,113,127,129,175,250,266,276,280,292,305], mainly based on data from the USA, Sweden and western European countries. That such diametrically opposed views could be derived by distinguished scientists from just a few data sets is a measure of the difficulty in interpreting cancer trends, and of the lack of consensus over which measures of trend are most appropriate in reaching a judgement. The presentation here of trends in cancer incidence and mortality from many populations should help broaden the debate. This is not just an academic issue: major decisions on the funding of cancer prevention and treatment programmes, and of cancer research, are made in the light of how these trends are evaluated, not to mention the intrinsic importance of deciding whether any progress is being made against the public health challenge with which cancer confronts society.

References

Frequent reference was made during preparation of this book to a number of standard works or major articles, particularly for the introductory section of each chapter of results. These works will in general not be explicitly cited in later chapters. They include the six published volumes of *Cancer Incidence in Five Continents*[86,87,202,221,298,299]; several different types of overview of the data presented in *Cancer Incidence in Five Continents* have also been published[199,274,300]. Other major works include *Cancer: Causes, Occurrence and Control*[286]; *Cancer Epidemiology and Prevention*[259], and several key publications on the frequency of cancer world-wide[219] and on trends in incidence and mortality in the USA[76,77], incidence in the Nordic countries[116] and mortality in the UK[213] and in various developed countries[61].

The literature on cancer trends has been selectively rather than exhaustively cited in each chapter, generally where it was felt to provide important corroboration — or contradiction — of the results in this book, or to offer an interpretation of the observed trends likely to have application beyond the region or country from which the report originated. Whilst acknowledging that 'interpretation of the trends for specific cancers is hazardous without personal knowledge of local circumstances'[83], we have nevertheless felt it possible in some cases to make an additional comment of our own, relying on the breadth provided by comparable analyses of many data sets for the same cancer, on the coherence which was often found between trends in incidence and mortality, and on further detailed exploration of individual data sets to pinpoint anomalies.

The bibliography is provided as a list of references at the end of the book, in alphabetical order, rather than as a separate list of references at the end of each chapter.

Chapter 2
MATERIAL

The availability at IARC of cancer incidence and mortality data for periods of up to 35 years has enabled the systematic examination of time trends in cancer risk for most major cancers, and for different countries and regions of the world, using the same methodological approach for all cancers and for incidence and mortality data. The aim of the project was to bring together much of the available data of adequate quality on time trends in cancer incidence and mortality, and to provide a consistent set of analyses and commentary on most major cancers in a single volume. The intention was to provide a stimulus for further research, and to enable other workers to pursue their own interpretation of the data.

This volume represents the most extensive compilation so far of data and analyses on global trends in cancer incidence and mortality. It is hoped that the results will contribute useful information on cancer trends, prompting new avenues of aetiological research, allowing improved forecasts of cancer incidence and mortality, and providing better data on which to assess priorities for the longer-term commitment of cancer prevention.

Cancer sites

The analyses cover 25 of the most frequent cancers in adults (Table 2.1). Twenty cancers arising in both sexes are examined, although cancers of the lip and larynx in females and cancers of the breast in males were excluded as being too infrequent for satisfactory analysis. Five sex-specific cancers are examined (cervix, body of uterus, ovary, prostate and testis).

The scope of the project precludes detailed analyses by anatomical sub-site, for example of trends in cancer incidence in different parts of the colon, or of shifts over time in the anatomical distribution of melanoma of the skin. Such analyses are better done on smaller, more homogeneous data sets. Cancers of the colon and rectum have in fact been combined in these analyses, in order to avoid the problems of interpretation of observed trends that might arise from varying misclassification of tumours close to the rectosigmoid junction.

No attempt has been made to examine trends for particular morphological types of cancer at any site (other than for melanoma of the skin, which has a separate three-digit topographic code in the seventh to ninth revisions of the International Classification of Diseases [ICD-7 to ICD-9]). This is because most of the incidence data sets included in the first four volumes of the series *Cancer Incidence in Five Continents* were submitted in the form of tables of the numbers of cases by age, sex and site, without breakdown by morphology. Data in the form of anonymised case records, containing morphology data for each case, were submitted by some registries for volumes V and VI, and while these data sets will eventually permit separate examination of trends in, say, adenocarcinoma and small cell carcinoma of the lung, there were not enough data sets with sufficient time coverage to make such an analysis practicable at this stage. Tumours of liver and brain were not included. Variability in coding practice of secondary tumours of the liver and benign tumours of the CNS between countries and registries was judged too great to permit satisfactory international comparison of trends, and local or national analyses would probably be more informative.

Analyses have been restricted to the age range 30-74 years for most cancers. Malignancy in childhood (0-14 years) accounts for less than 0.5% of all malignancies in most populations, and trends are also presented separately for all childhood malignancies combined and for childhood leukaemia, which often accounts for more than a third of all malignancies in this age group. Data for persons aged 75 or over are not presented, partly because of the conventional wisdom that the accuracy of death certification is lower in the very elderly, and partly because cancer trends in very elderly persons usually reflect changes in exposure affecting older generations, and are likely to be less relevant for evaluating present-day priorities for aetiological research and primary prevention. Further, incidence data were sometimes available only for the open-ended age group 75 years or over (75+), rather than for groups such as 75-79 and 80-84 years. With a few exceptions, the great majority of malignant neoplasms in adults arises after the age of 30 years, and most analyses were therefore restricted to the age-range 30-74 years. Cancers of the testis and Hodgkin's disease are exceptions to the general rule, in that both are common in the age range 15-29 years. For cancer of the testis, the age range presented is for 15-64 years, and for Hodgkin's disease, 15-74 years.

Table 2.1 Cancer sites and site groups analysed, ages 30-74 years

Site	ICD-7	ICD-8	ICD-9
Lip (males)	140	140	140
Tongue	141	141	141
Mouth	143-144	143-145	143-145
Pharynx [a]	145-148	146-149	146-149
Oesophagus	150	150	150
Stomach	151	151	151
Colorectal cancer	153-154	153-154	153-154
Pancreas	157	157	157
Larynx (males)	161	161	161
Lung	162-163	162	162
Bone	196	170	170
Melanoma of skin	190	172	172
Breast (females)	170	174	174
Cervix uteri	171	180	180
Corpus uteri	172	182	179, 182
Ovary	175	183	183
Prostate	177	185	185
Testis [b]	178	186	186
Bladder	181.0	188	188
Kidney, other urinary organs	180	189	189
Thyroid	194	193	193
Non-Hodgkin lymphoma	200, 202, 205	200, 202	200, 202
Hodgkin's disease [c]	201	201	201
Multiple myeloma [d]	203	203	203
Leukaemia [e]	204	204-207	204-208

[a]   ICD-9 146-148 for incidence, i.e. excluding ill-defined sites within lip, oral cavity and pharynx. For mortality in the Americas, ICD-9 140-149, except USA, data for which exclude major salivary glands (ICD-9 142)

[b]   15-64 years

[c]   15-74 years

[d]   Excludes solitary plasmacytoma in ICD-9 (238.6)

[e]   Results also presented for children (0-14 years)

Table 2.2   Cancer incidence and mortality data sets

	INCIDENCE DATA			MORTALITY DATA	INCIDENCE and/or MORTALITY DATA
	Populations	Registries	Countries	Countries	Countries
Europe	23	22	16	22	23
Asia and Oceania	18	11	7	6	8
Americas	19	15	6	8	11
Total	60	48	29	36	42

Incidence data

Incidence data from 60 populations were analysed, covering periods from as early as 1953 up to 1987. The data were reported from 48 cancer registries in 29 countries in Europe, Asia, Oceania, and North and South America (Table 2.2).

Details of the incidence data sets used in the analyses are given in Table 2.3, including the calendar period spanned from the first to the last year of available data and the number of years within that calendar span for which data were actually available (data years). The data spanned calendar periods ranging from 10 to 35 (median 21) years up to the end of 1987, covering a minimum of three and up to seven separate data sets from each registry. Individual data sets covered periods from one to seven years, while the total data years available from a given registry represented between three and 34 years of actual data. The longest sequence of data was from Denmark, covering 34 years of the 35-year period 1953-87, while the data from São Paulo (Brazil), consisted of data for the three single years 1969, 1973 and 1978 in a calendar span of 10 years.

Some registries could provide population-based data for earlier periods than those published in *Cancer Incidence in Five Continents*. These data were not requested, since it was considered important for the purposes of international comparison to retain the advantage of each data set having been reviewed contemporaneously under the same criteria as other data sets for the period.

No African data were suitable for analysis, since the only data covering three time periods, those from Ibadan (Nigeria), consisted of data sets which completely overlapped in time and showed signs of declining completeness. Data for Kingston and St Andrew (Jamaica) were available for the 20-year period 1958-77 (volumes I-IV), but despite their intrinsic interest, these data were considered too old to provide useful information on recent trends: some information on trends up to 1987 has been published[42]. The earliest data sets from Hawaii (USA), New Zealand and Cali (Colombia) were discarded because they were also included in the next data set in the series. Data for Chinese in Singapore for the period 1950-61 (volume I) were excluded because the 12-year period covered by this single data set was too long to provide useful additional information on trends. In the San Francisco Bay Area (USA), data sets for the first two calendar periods overlapped by one year (1973). The numbers of cases in this year were estimated by age, sex and site and subtracted from the numbers of cases in the first period.

Iceland is one of the few countries in the world with long-standing national cancer registration of high quality, and can present data from 1955. Trends for Iceland were analysed, but are not presented here because they add little information. The trends were often similar to those in the other Nordic countries, and have been published in some detail[116]. The population aged 30-74 years in Iceland is small (about 90 000) and trends were often unstable because of small numbers of cases.

Data for the period 1978-87 for blacks and whites in Connecticut (USA) were combined to enable comparison with previous data, which had been reported without separation by race. Data from the five regional registries in Scotland were combined for 1973-87 and supplemented for earlier periods by the Information and Statistics Division, Edinburgh.

Although Hawaii is a state of the USA, its incidence data have been presented with those of

Table 2.3   Cancer incidence data: populations and calendar periods

	I	II	III	IV	V	VI	Calendar period (years)	Data period (years)
			Cancer Incidence in Five Continents volume					

EUROPE (except European Community)

	I	II	III	IV	V	VI	Calendar period (years)	Data period (years)
Finland	59-61	62-65	66-70	71-76	77-81	82-86	28	28
Hungary								
County Vas	-	62-66	68-72	73-77	78-82	83-87	26	25
Szabolcs-Szatmar	-	62-66	69-71	73-77	78-82	83-87	26	23
Israel								
All Jews	-	60-66	67-71	72-76	77-81	82-86	27	27
Non-Jews	-	60-66	67-71	72-76	77-81	82-86	27	27
Norway	59-61	64-66	68-72	73-77	78-82	83-87	29	26
Poland								
Warsaw City	-	65-66	68-72	73-77	78-82	83-87	23	22
Romania								
County Cluj	-	-	-	74-78	79-82	83-87	14	14
Sweden	59-61	62-65	66-70	71-75	78-82	83-87	29	27
Switzerland								
Geneva	-	-	70-72	73-77	79-82	83-87	18	17
Yugoslavia								
Slovenia	56-60	61-65	68-72	73-76	78-81	82-87	31	28

EUROPE (European Community)

	I	II	III	IV	V	VI	Calendar period (years)	Data period (years)
Denmark	53-57	58-62	63-67	68-72 73-76	78-82	83-87	35	34
France								
Bas-Rhin	-	-	-	75-77	78-81	83-87	13	12
Doubs	-	-	-	77-77	78-82	83-87	11	11
Germany (FRG)								
Hamburg	60-62	63-66	69-72	73-77	78-79	-	20	18
Saarland	-	-	68-72	73-77	78-82	83-87	20	20
Germany (ex-GDR)	-	64-66	68-72	73-77	78-82	83-87	24	23
Italy								
Varese	-	-	-	76-77	78-81	83-87	12	11
Spain								
Navarra	-	-	-	73-77	78-82	83-86	14	14
Zaragoza	-	-	68-72	73-77	78-82	83-85	18	18
UK								
Birmingham	60-62	63-66	68-72	73-76	79-82	83-86	27	24
Scotland [a]	-	63-66	70-72	73-77	78-82	83-87	25	22
South Thames [b]	60-62	-	63-66 67-71	73-77	78-82	83-87	28	27

Table 2.3 (cont.):   Cancer incidence data: populations and calendar periods

	Cancer Incidence in Five Continents volume						Calendar period (years)	Data period (years)
	I	II	III	IV	V	VI		
ASIA								
China								
Shanghai [b]	-	-	-	75-75	78-82	83-87	13	11
Hong Kong	-	-	-	74-77	78-82	83-87	14	14
India								
Bombay	-	64-66	68-72	73-77	78-82	83-87	24	23
Japan								
Miyagi	59-60	62-64	68-71	73-77	78-81	83-87	29	23
Nagasaki	-	-	-	73-77	78-82	83-87	15	15
Osaka	-	-	70-71	73-77	79-82	83-87	18	16
Singapore								
Chinese	-	-	68-72	73-77	78-82	83-87	20	20
Indian	-	-	68-72	73-77	78-82	83-87	20	20
Malay	-	-	68-72	73-77	78-82	83-87	20	20
OCEANIA								
Australia								
New South Wales	-	-	-	73-77	78-82	83-87	15	15
South Australia	-	-	-	77-77	78-82	83-87	11	11
Hawaii								
Caucasian [c]	-	60-64	68-72	73-77	78-82	83-87	28	25
Chinese	-	60-64	68-72	73-77	78-82	83-87	28	25
Filipino	-	60-64	68-72	73-77	78-82	83-87	28	25
Hawaiian [c]	-	60-64	68-72	73-77	78-82	83-87	28	25
Japanese [c]	-	60-64	68-72	73-77	78-82	83-87	28	25
New Zealand [c]								
Maori	-	62-66	68-71	72-76	78-82	83-87	26	24
Non-Maori	-	62-66	68-71	72-76	78-82	83-87	26	24

Table 2.3 (cont.): Cancer incidence data: populations and calendar periods

	Cancer Incidence in Five Continents volume						Calendar period (years)	Data period (years)
	I	II	III	IV	V	VI		
AMERICAS (except USA)								
Brazil								
São Paulo	-	-	69-69	73-73	78-78	-	10	3
Canada								
Alberta	60-62	63-66	69-72	73-77	78-82	83-87	28	26
British Columbia	-	-	69-72	73-77	78-82	83-87	19	19
Maritime Provinces [d]		-	69-72	73-77	78-82	83-87	19	19
Newfoundland	60-62	63-66	69-72	73-77	78-82	83-87	28	26
Quebec	-	63-66	69-72	73-77	78-81	83-87	24	22
Colombia								
Cali [c]	-	62-66	67-71	72-76	77-81	82-86	25	25
Cuba	-	-	68-72	73-77	-	86-86	19	11
Puerto Rico	62-63	64-66	68-72	73-77	78-82	83-87	26	25
AMERICAS (USA)								
Bay Area, Black [c]	-	-	69-73	73-77	78-82	83-87	19	19
Bay Area, Chinese [c]	-	-	69-73	73-77	78-82	-	14	14
Bay Area, White [c]	-	-	69-73	73-77	78-82	83-87	19	19
Connecticut [e]	60-62	63-65	68-72	73-77	78-82	83-87	28	26
Detroit, Black	-	-	69-71	73-77	78-82	83-87	19	18
Detroit, White	-	-	69-71	73-77	78-82	83-87	19	18
Iowa	-	-	69-71	73-77	78-82	83-87	19	18
New Orleans, Black	-	-	-	74-77	78-82	83-87	14	14
New Orleans, White	-	-	-	74-77	78-82	83-87	14	14
Seattle	-	-	-	74-77	78-82	83-87	14	14

[a] Data for 1970-72 and 1973-77 complemented by Information Statistics Division, Edinburgh.

[b] Boundary changes in 1974 (S Thames) and 1983 (Shanghai).

[c] Some data periods overlap. **Hawaii** (Caucasian, Hawaiian, Japanese): data from vol. I (1960-63) not used; in each case, these data were also included in vol. II. **New Zealand**: vol. I data not used: data for Maori and non-Maori not presented separately, and time period (1960-62) overlapped with data in vol. II. **Colombia, Cali**: data from vol. I (1962-64) also included in volume II: not used. **San Francisco Bay Area**: 1969-73 data reduced by one year - see text.

[d] Nova Scotia, New Brunswick, Prince Edward Island.

[e] Data combined for blacks and whites for 1978-82, 1983-87, for consistency with earlier data sets.

Oceania for reasons of geographic and ethnic proximity, even though separate mortality data were not available to assist in the comparison with other populations in the region. Similarly, data for Israel have been presented with those for Europe (except European Community). Data for the former German Democratic Republic have been presented with those for the European Community, in order to facilitate comparison with data from the Federal Republic of Germany. Incidence data for Slovenia, until recently a republic of Yugoslavia, have been presented as such, whilst its mortality data are included in those for the former Yugoslavia.

Data from 29 populations in Europe (11) and North America (18), for which data of adequate quality and time coverage were also available, were not included in the analyses (Table 2.4), either because it appeared unlikely they would present significant additional features to those of neighbouring registries, or because there were too few cases to permit satisfactory analyses for rarer cancers, or for clarity of presentation in graphs and tables. Sometimes, more than one consideration applied.

Quality of cancer incidence and mortality data

Improvement over time in the quality of incidence data from cancer registries has been cited as a general argument for preferring mortality data for the examination of patterns and trends in cancer risk[83]. Mortality (strictly, death certification) data are certainly available for a wider range of countries and, in most but not all countries, for longer time periods than cancer incidence data. Medical certification of death is very widespread, often statutory, and the routine recording of death is a relatively simple procedure to implement. The accuracy of the death certification and coding processes which underpin routine cancer mortality data has been reviewed[5,125,135,227-229,247]. It is often high, and the errors are not always such as to bias interpretation of the data, but these surveys are sporadic rather than systematic. There has been a steady expansion of cancer registration in many parts of the world for the last 30 years, and many cancer registries have now been producing incidence data sets of a quality sufficient to meet the rigorous editorial standards for inclusion in *Cancer Incidence in Five Continents* for 20 years or more. The argument for generally preferring mortality data to incidence data must now be considered weaker than in the past[84].

The completeness of cancer registration is likely to be lower than that of death certification in most regions, but compared to mortality data, cancer incidence (strictly, cancer registration) data have several inherent advantages, both procedural and biological, for the study of time trends in cancer risk. The data items recorded for each incident cancer are usually checked for internal coherence by expert cancer registry staff at the point of registration, when errors and omissions can still be corrected by reference to the medical record. Most registries also carry out regular quality control measures on their data as a whole. Prior to inclusion in *Cancer Incidence in Five Continents*, the entire data set is again reviewed, both on the basis of specific quality indices and for coherence with any previous data from the same registry. Data sets submitted as anonymised case listings are also examined case by case with validity control programs, and registries are given an opportunity to correct faulty data[102]. The overall validity of cancer incidence data supplied by cancer registries is certainly better than that of cancer mortality data for these reasons. Further, there is no equivalent for mortality data of the indices of quality which have been available for many years as an aid to the interpretation of cancer incidence data.

From the biological viewpoint, the date of diagnosis of cancer is evidently closer in time to the causal exposure(s) than the date of death, particularly for the less rapidly fatal cancers. Incidence may be affected by screening programmes or improved diagnostic methods, but not by changes in treatment and survival. Trends in mortality are often more complex to interpret, since they are affected by changes in both incidence and survival. For cancers with relatively good survival, mortality trends may completely fail to reveal sharp trends in incidence, as with the increase in endometrial carcinoma among middle-aged US females associated with the use of oestrogen replacement therapy in the 1970s[76,198]. For many cancers, therefore, incidence data are more relevant for understanding aetiology and for determining the priorities for cancer prevention. The parallel analysis of incidence and mortality for many of the data sets reported here often broadens the interpretation which would be possible from analysing either type of data without the other[30,76,77,84].

Chief among the indices of quality for cancer incidence data is the proportion of all cases registered for which there is microscopic evidence to confirm the diagnosis of cancer. It is usually expressed as the percentage of cases which were histologically verified. Table 2.5 gives the figures for histological verification for all cancers (except non-melanoma skin cancer) for all the populations reported here, by sex and broad age-group

Table 2.4   Cancer incidence data sets: calendar period and geographical region

| | Cancer Incidence in Five Continents volume | | | | | | |
	I	II	III	IV	V	VI	
Region							
Period (approx.)	**1960**	**1965**	**1970**	**1975**	**1980**	**1985**	**Overall**
Europe (except EC) [a]	4	9	10	11	11	11	11
Europe (EC) [b]	4	6	8	12	12	11	12
Africa	-	-	-	-	-	-	-
Asia	1	2	6	9	9	9	9
Oceania [c]	-	7	7	9	9	9	9
Americas (except USA) [d]	3	5	9	9	8	8	9
Americas (USA) [e]	1	1	7	10	10	9	10
Total	**13**	**30**	**47**	**60**	**59**	**57**	**60**

[a]   Including Israel (2 populations): All Jews (three subgroups by place of birth not analysed) and non-Jews.
[b]   Including German Democratic Republic; S Thames (UK) data for 1963-66 in volume III; Hamburg (FRG) not in volume VI.
[c]   Including Hawaii (5 populations).
[d]   Cuba not in volume V; São Paulo (Brazil) not in volume VI.
[e]   Chinese, San Francisco Bay Area not in volume VI; Connecticut data for blacks and whites treated as single population for volumes V and VI, for consistency with earlier data sets.

Populations not included:

Europe (except European Community), 6 populations: Iceland (volumes I, III, V, VI); Poland: Cracow (II-VI), Nowy Sacz (III-VI) and Warsaw, Rural (II-IV, VI); Switzerland: Neuchâtel (IV-VI) and Vaud (IV-VI).

Europe (European Community), 5 populations: UK: Mersey (volumes I-VI), South Western (I-III, V-VI), Oxford (II-VI), Trent (II-VI) and North Western (IV-VI).

Americas (except USA), 4 populations: Canada: Manitoba (volumes I-VI), Ontario (IV-VI), Saskatchewan (I-VI) and Northwest Territories and Yukon (IV-VI).

Americas (USA), 14 populations: California, Alameda County (2 populations) (volumes II-VI), New York State (I, III-VI), Los Angeles County (5) (IV-VI), Atlanta (2) (IV-VI), New Mexico (3) (III-V) and Utah (III-VI).

(35-64, 65-74 years), for the data in each of the last three volumes of *Cancer Incidence in Five Continents*. This provides a broad and comparable overview for each population of the degree to which the incidence data may be considered reliable. The term 'histological verification' is not interpreted in the same way by all registries[201,220] but it is taken here to mean confirmation of diagnosis by pathological evidence from biopsy, autopsy, cytology or haematology, unless otherwise indicated in the Table. More detailed information is provided in some of the chapters to assist in the interpretation of incidence trends for specific cancers. The successive volumes of *Cancer Incidence in Five Continents* should be consulted for further details.

Cancer registrations based only on death certificates are included by most cancer registries[220]. The data from Hong Kong for the most recent period, 1983-87, include for the first time cancer registrations established solely on the basis of a death certificate: such information was unavailable before 1980. This gives rise to an overall increase of about 9% in the number of registrations compared to the preceding period, and should be taken into account in the interpretation of the results. In Birmingham (UK), where a similar change occurred, the increase was only 2.7%.

Completeness of cancer registration and other aspects of data quality are major problems to be overcome in the initial phase of operation of a cancer registry. New registries often exclude data for the early years of registration from trend analyses for these reasons. The registries for which the third data set required for inclusion in the analyses only appeared in volume VI of *Cancer Incidence in Five Continents* were not all newly established when their first data sets were published in the series, however: while those from Europe, Australia and the USA were established in the 1970s, the cancer registries of Cuba, Hong Kong, Nagasaki (Japan) and Shanghai (China) had all been producing population-based data for four years (Cuba) or more (9-15 years for the other three registries) by the time the data analysed here were collected. All the data sets included in volume IV of the series were also subjected to rigorous quality control procedures. It would nevertheless be prudent to give less weight in the international comparison of trends in cancer incidence to data from more recently established cancer registries, or those for which only three data sets are available, than to data from the more long-established cancer registries.

Populations

There was a range greater than 100-fold in the size around 1980 of the populations included in the analyses, in the age range 30-74 years, from less than 50 000 in some ethnic groups to over four million in Sweden and in Osaka (Japan), and over seven million in the German Democratic Republic (Table 2.6). By contrast, the Chinese population aged 30-74 years in Hawaii was only about 15 000 in each sex. The three main ethnic groups in Singapore are Chinese (77% of the population), Malay (15%) and Indian (6%)[154], the last group including only 57 000 people in the age range 30-74 years.

The proportion of the total population covered by the registry that was actually included in the analyses — i.e. persons aged 30-74 years — ranged from little more than a quarter in young populations such as New Zealand Maoris (28%) to about half in many of the populations in developed countries. These variations in population size are reflected in the numbers of cases or deaths, and for some of the smaller populations, particularly the ethnic sub-groups, estimates of trend for the rarer neoplasms are more or less uninterpretable, since there are so few cases or deaths. Ethnic variation in cancer risk is often considerable, however, and these populations have nevertheless been retained for the intrinsic interest of the whole data set, rather than make a separate selection of populations for analysis of each of the less common malignancies.

The precision of population denominators is not controlled by cancer registries, and it can vary with time in industrialised countries as well as in developing countries[201]. Many of the countries included here carry out a decennial census at the beginning of each decade, so the population data for these countries around 1970 (volume III) and 1980 (volume V) are likely to be more precise than those for volumes IV and VI, which were often based on projections from the previous census. To some extent, however, such fluctuations in the quality of population estimates will have been reduced in these analyses by the process of interpolating the population data by birth cohort to obtain the population density for each sex, age group and time period, before the estimation of age-specific rates (see Chapter 3).

Additional problems arise for registries covering several ethnic groups, such as Hawaii, when the definition of ethnic group used in the census may change, and may not coincide with that used in the hospitals for classifying cancer patients[201], and when the ethnic classification of children whose parents are of different ethnic group may be somewhat arbitrary. This may lead to bias in incidence rates, and for small populations and the less common cancers the effect may be appreciable. Census populations may also be incomplete if there is substantial avoidance of enumeration by illegal immigrants or for other reasons, and this may give rise to over-estimation of incidence.

Changes in population coverage

The population covered by some registries has changed substantially during the period covered by the analyses, either by natural growth or by administrative change in the registry's territory. These changes may affect the examination of cancer trends. Rapid demographic growth in developing countries produces a population that is both larger and has a younger age structure, and the precision of inter-censal estimates may be lower (see example in Chapter 3). Administrative change may alter not only the size of the population but also its cancer risk profile, if there is substantial variation in cancer risk within the territory covered by the registry.

For example, the population covered by the registry in South Thames (UK) was reduced by some 30% to 6.5 million in 1974 as a result of administrative changes in the health care system. Cancer risk in South Thames is broadly comparable to that in the territory no longer covered. Both the populations and the numbers of cases in the data analysed reflect this change; as a result, the number of cases tabulated for a given rate in 1985 is substantially lower than the number for a similar rate in 1970. Similarly, the urban area covered by the cancer registry in Shanghai (China) increased in the early 1980s, and the total population covered rose by 16.2% to 6.9 million. The population aged 30-74 increased by 21.8% to 3.5 million, and from 48.6% to 50.9% of the total population.

The estimated population of Cali (Colombia) was 22% higher in 1979 than in 1974, an extremely rapid demographic change. The 1979 population, used for calculating the incidence rates reported in Volume V, was estimated by linear projection from censuses in 1964 and 1973, and despite the large estimated increase, was considered to have been an under-estimate. The population for 1984, used for calculating the rates for 1982-86, had risen a further 19% in five years, but is considered likely to have been more accurate, since it was based on back-interpolation from a census in 1985. The population denominators for Cali were re-estimated by cohort interpolation for the analyses (see Chapter 3).

Mortality data

National mortality data were taken from the WHO data bank for 36 countries in Europe, Africa, Asia, Oceania, the Caribbean and North and South America (Table 2.7). These data sets do not provide breakdowns by race or ethnic group. Data from the UK are presented for two of the three constituent countries under which it reports mortality to WHO (England and Wales, and Scotland). Trends for Northern Ireland were analysed, but were either very similar to those of neighbouring countries or unstable because of small numbers. Some data on mortality trends in Northern Ireland have been published[224]. Mortality data for Luxembourg were also analysed, and excluded for the same reasons.

Data were taken for single years from 1955 up to the last year for which data were available, usually 1988 (see Table 2.7). The data take the form of the numbers of deaths by five-year age group, cause and sex, and the populations by age and sex, for each quinary age-group. The upper age group available varied from 65+ to 85+ years. The data were grouped into standard five-year calendar periods where possible. For some countries, information on some cancers was available only for a shorter time period than others, or with gaps in the time sequence, or not at all: some trend statistics were not calculated if there was missing information for any period in the last 15 years. For other countries, the data for some cancers were available only for broader site groups (e.g. ICD-9 140-149: all lip, oral and pharyngeal cancers): these data have been examined and commented upon where relevant, but are not reported in detail here.

Some of the known changes in coding practices affect the interpretation of time trends in cancer mortality[211]. In Sweden up to 1980, cancer was often coded as the underlying cause of death for mortality statistics even if certified as a contributory cause, whereas from 1981 cancer certified as a contributory cause was only coded as the underlying cause of death if the underlying cause of death on the death certificate was judged insufficient[253]. This led to an artefactual dip in some cancer mortality rates. In Germany (FRG), introduction of the ninth revision of the ICD in 1979 led to an artefactual drop in mortality from multiple myeloma (ICD-9 203) because solitary or monostotic plasmacytoma, coded with myeloma in the eighth revision, was coded to a different rubric (238.6) in the ninth revision[64].

Deaths assigned to uterus, not otherwise specified (NOS) (ICD-9 179) constitute a substantial proportion of all deaths from cancer of the uterus, and this proportion varies widely between countries and over time. The value of mortality data coded to cancer of the cervix or corpus uteri for geographical comparison of time trends is therefore limited. Whilst it is possible to make suitable adjustments for some countries at a given point in time, however, by age-specific redistribution to the cervix and corpus uteri of deaths assigned to uterus NOS[137], it is impractical to make similar corrections for many countries over long time periods and in different ICD revisions. Mortality data for cancers of the body and cervix of the uterus have therefore been examined separately here, with the preceding caveat in mind; together with the incidence trends, some interpretation of the mortality trends is still possible.

Correspondence between incidence and mortality data

In all, 42 countries were represented in the analyses by data sets on cancer incidence (29 countries) or cancer mortality (36 countries), or both (Table 2.8). For 23 countries, there were both incidence data and national mortality data. In nine of these countries (*Europe*: Denmark, Finland, Norway, Sweden and Scotland; *Asia and Oceania*: Hong Kong, Singapore and New Zealand; *Americas*: Puerto Rico), both incidence and mortality data sets covered the entire national population. In the other 14 countries for which national mortality data were available, the one or more registries providing the incidence data analysed here covered between less than 5% and more than 50% of the national population. For six countries (*Europe*: Israel; *Asia and Oceania*: China and India; *Americas*: Brazil, Colombia and Cuba), only incidence data were used, although for Israel and Cuba the cancer registries cover the entire national population. For the remaining 13 countries, national mortality data were available, but there were no suitable incidence data.

The incidence data for the former German Democratic Republic (1964-87) were collected on a national basis, before reunification of the two German states: corresponding mortality data were not available for the GDR before 1975. Data for Slovenia were collected for the same territory now covered by the new republic of Slovenia when it was still a constituent republic of the former Yugoslavia. The mortality data reported here for Yugoslavia include those for Slovenia. Throughout the book, the names of countries are used to imply the geographical areas represented by those countries during the period for which data are analysed.

The map (Figure 2.1) identifies each country from which either incidence or mortality data, or both, have been used. Sub-national regions from which incidence data were used are also identified.

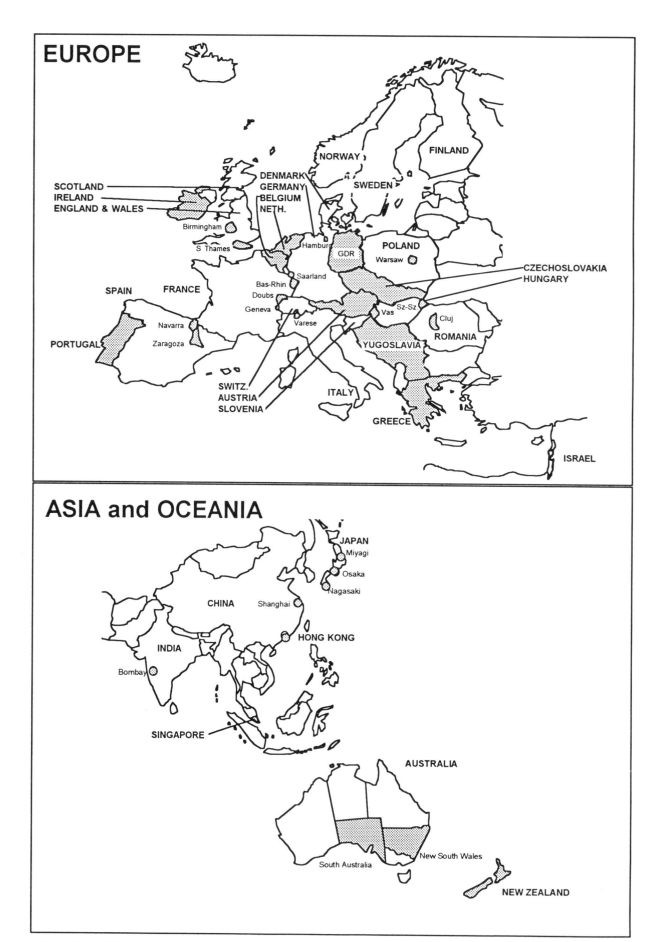

Figure 2.1.   Map showing regions and countries from which incidence and/or mortality data were analysed. Mauritius not shown.

AMERICAS

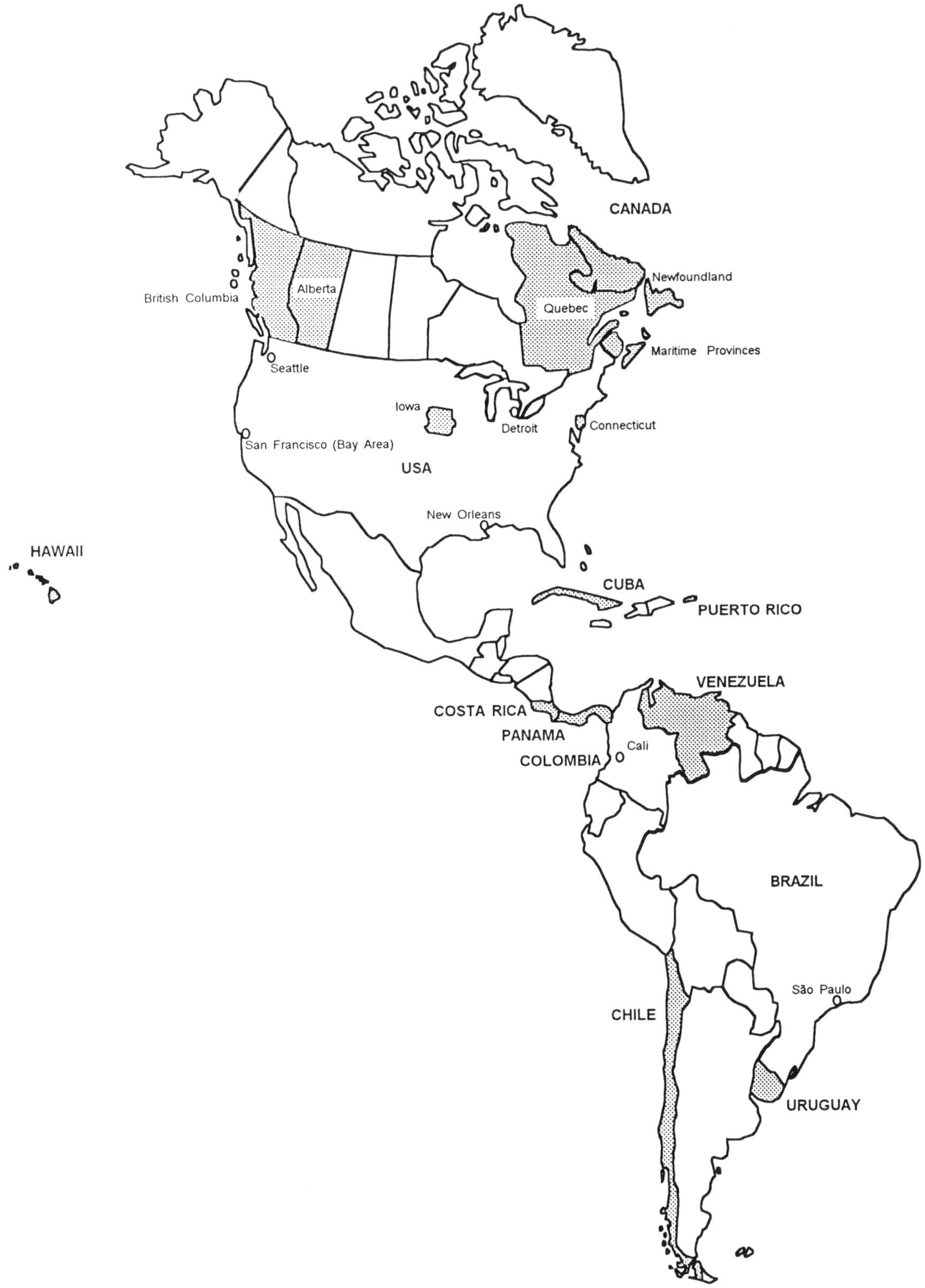

CANADA

British Columbia

Alberta

Newfoundland

Quebec

Seattle

Maritime Provinces

Iowa

Detroit

Connecticut

San Francisco (Bay Area)

USA

New Orleans

HAWAII

CUBA

PUERTO RICO

VENEZUELA

COSTA RICA

Cali

PANAMA

COLOMBIA

BRAZIL

São Paulo

CHILE

URUGUAY

Table 2.5 Percentage of all tumours (except non-melanoma skin) histologically verified: sex, age group and registry: Cancer Incidence in Five Continents, volumes IV-VI

	Males						Females					
	35-64			65-74			35-64			65-74		
	IV	V	VI	IV	V	VI	IV	V	VI	IV	V	VI
EUROPE (except European Community)												
Finland [a]	87	90	97	78	82	95	96	97	98	89	92	95
Hungary												
County Vas [a]	85	79	81	75	67	80	90	87	86	81	72	78
Szabolcs-Szatmar [b]	75	81	79	65	76	78	83	87	90	66	81	84
Israel												
All Jews	87	92	92	81	87	87	91	94	95	81	89	89
Non-Jews	81	88	83	66	82	75	85	90	90	69	75	77
Norway [a]	92	95	97	87	91	95	96	98	98	91	93	96
Poland												
Warsaw City [a,b]	64	61	68	47	45	54	78	72	79	60	53	63
Romania												
County Cluj	52	55	49	35	39	36	69	68	65	44	51	43
Sweden [a]	84	97	98	77	96	97	92	98	99	88	96	97
Switzerland												
Geneva	97	98	98	95	96	97	98	99	99	96	95	97
Yugoslavia												
Slovenia	73	74	92	60	62	83	80	86	95	67	71	87
EUROPE (European Community)												
Denmark	84	95	95	82	92	91	89	97	97	84	94	93
France												
Bas-Rhin [a]	88	93	96	82	89	92	78	91	97	77	87	95
Doubs	92	95	95	90	93	93	92	96	96	91	92	94
Germany (FRG)												
Hamburg [a]	73	69	..	61	55	..	84	81	..	70	67	..
Saarland	*	86	92	*	76	84	*	91	95	*	82	89
Germany (GDR) [a,b]	87	89	91	77	79	83	93	95	95	84	86	88
Italy												
Varese [a]	69	76	92	58	63	85	84	90	95	74	77	89
Spain												
Navarra [a,b]	64	84	91	52	77	85	74	87	94	53	74	83
Zaragoza [a]	80	77	91	72	70	83	81	90	83	71	81	71
United Kingdom												
Birmingham [a,b]	72	77	80	60	67	71	84	88	84	73	77	75
Scotland [c]	77	77	82	87	69	74	70	85	87	79	76	76
South Thames [a]	80	88	76	70	81	66	87	92	82	76	84	69

Table 2.5 (cont.): Percentage of all tumours (except non-melanoma skin) histologically verified: sex, age group and registry: Cancer Incidence in Five Continents, volumes IV-VI

	Males						Females					
	35-64			65-74			35-64			65-74		
	IV	V	VI	IV	V	VI	IV	V	VI	IV	V	VI
ASIA												
China												
Shanghai	50	49	55	43	37	43	61	63	68	46	38	43
Hong Kong [a,b]	58	65	64	53	62	60	61	67	70	53	61	62
India												
Bombay [a]	67	68	73	51	54	63	70	70	76	50	55	64
Japan												
Miyagi [a,b]	70	78	81	56	65	74	75	81	86	58	65	72
Nagasaki [b]	66	70	80	65	68	80	74	77	90	63	62	80
Osaka [a]	50	64	74	39	58	71	61	75	83	40	58	70
Singapore												
Chinese [a]	72	81	84	60	71	77	85	92	94	67	76	82
Indian [a]	76	80	87	67	77	79	82	91	94	73	73	93
Malay [a]	61	72	77	57	64	72	76	84	85	57	71	69
OCEANIA												
Australia												
New South Wales [a]	91	95	91	84	89	86	96	97	94	89	92	88
South Australia [a]	*	*	*	*	*	*	*	*	*	*	*	*
Hawaii												
Caucasian [a]	99	96	99	97	94	97	99	98	99	99	97	97
Chinese [a]	99	98	99	99	94	97	98	99	99	99	93	98
Filipino [a]	99	96	99	97	96	97	99	98	99	98	90	96
Hawaiian [a]	98	93	97	96	91	95	99	97	98	95	96	93
Japanese [a]	99	97	98	96	96	97	99	99	99	97	95	98
New Zealand												
Maori	*	80	85	*	66	75	*	89	91	*	74	80
Non-Maori	*	82	94	*	81	89	*	77	96	*	89	91

Table 2.5 (cont.): Percentage of all tumours (except non-melanoma skin) histologically verified: sex, age group and registry: Cancer Incidence in Five Continents, volumes IV-VI

| | Males | | | | | | Females | | | | | |
| | 35-64 | | | 65-74 | | | 35-64 | | | 65-74 | | |
	IV	V	VI	IV	V	VI	IV	V	VI	IV	V	VI
AMERICAS (except USA)												
Brazil												
São Paulo [a]	73	63	..	63	54	..	75	66	..	71	54	..
Canada												
Alberta [a]	96	90	95	93	86	97	97	95	91	96	89	93
British Columbia [a]	93	82	92	88	77	89	96	90	94	92	81	90
Maritime Provinces	92	89	94	89	84	92	96	95	96	90	89	92
Newfoundland	94	91	95	92	88	90	97	97	98	94	91	94
Quebec [a]	89	79	72	88	76	69	93	84	77	90	80	71
Colombia												
Cali [a,b]	80	76	76	70	68	69	87	82	85	77	70	69
Cuba [a]	59	..	59	48	..	52	71	..	77	55	..	60
Puerto Rico [a]	89	91	94	85	88	92	94	95	97	87	88	92
AMERICAS (USA)												
Bay Area, Black	96	93	97	92	89	97	97	95	96	91	90	95
Bay Area, Chinese	95	91	..	90	84	..	99	95	..	93	90	..
Bay Area, White	97	95	97	94	92	96	98	91	98	95	89	96
Connecticut [d]	95	95	97	92	92	95	98	97	98	94	94	96
Detroit, Black [a]	94	93	96	91	89	95	96	96	98	91	88	94
Detroit, White [a]	95	94	97	91	91	96	98	97	98	94	93	96
Iowa [a]	94	95	98	89	91	99	97	98	96	93	94	96
New Orleans, Black [a]	94	87	95	86	83	93	93	92	96	84	86	91
New Orleans, White [a]	93	91	97	88	87	95	96	94	98	90	90	94
Seattle	96	96	98	94	93	97	98	98	99	95	95	97

[a] For volume IV, cytological diagnoses are **not** included with histologically verified tumours for this population
[b] For volumes V and VI, cytological diagnoses are **not** included with histologically verified tumours for this population
[c] Overall figure for Scotland not available for volume IV; figures in table are averages of HV% for the five regional registries
[d] Figures for whites only (about 90% of population) in volumes V and VI. Figures for blacks are within 2% of those for whites in each age-sex group, however.

.. : Incidence data not presented in this volume
* : Histological verification figures not reported
99 : 99% or more

Table 2.6   Population (thousands) covered by each cancer registry around 1980: age and sex

	Males			Females		
	All ages	30-74	%	All ages	30-74	%
EUROPE (except European Community)						
Finland	2309	1143	49.5	2466	1280	51.9
Hungary						
County Vas	139	70	49.9	146	76	52.1
Szabolcs-Szatmar	308	135	44.0	313	148	47.1
Israel						
All Jews	1585	627	39.5	1594	668	41.9
Non-Jews	308	69	22.4	299	72	24.1
Norway	2025	994	49.1	2061	1019	49.5
Poland						
Warsaw City	724	375	51.9	830	457	55.0
Romania						
County Cluj	365	174	47.7	372	184	49.4
Sweden	4115	2199	53.4	4190	2237	53.4
Switzerland						
Geneva	165	92	55.6	184	102	55.7
Yugoslavia						
Slovenia	916	434	47.4	970	485	49.9
EUROPE (European Community)						
Denmark	2528	1284	50.8	2592	1332	51.4
France						
Bas-Rhin	440	201	45.7	461	215	46.7
Doubs	236	111	47.1	241	112	46.2
Germany (FRG)						
Hamburg	772	435	56.5	892	515	57.8
Saarland	506	260	51.4	562	307	54.6
Germany (GDR)	7845	3749	47.8	8890	4631	52.1
Italy						
Varese	380	196	51.6	407	217	53.3
Spain						
Navarra	252	120	47.8	255	123	48.3
Zaragoza	406	202	49.8	422	220	52.0
United Kingdom						
Birmingham	2513	1282	51.0	2586	1321	51.1
Scotland	2495	1220	48.9	2685	1351	50.3
South Thames	3108	1624	52.3	3394	1784	52.6

	Males			Females		
	All ages	30-74	%	All ages	30-74	%
ASIA						
China						
Shanghai	2955	1458	49.3	2882	1439	49.9
Hong Kong	2626	1069	40.7	2412	947	39.3
India						
Bombay	4537	1718	37.9	3491	1156	33.1
Japan						
Miyagi	1025	510	49.7	1056	549	52.0
Nagasaki	211	103	48.6	236	120	51.0
Osaka	4198	2110	50.3	4267	2217	52.0
Singapore						
Chinese	900	332	36.8	888	344	38.8
Indian	80	36	44.4	63	21	33.5
Malay	167	52	31.2	161	50	31.3
OCEANIA						
Australia						
New South Wales	2577	1202	46.7	2595	1215	46.8
South Australia	655	305	46.6	665	312	47.1
Hawaii						
Caucasian	154	69	45.0	127	61	47.7
Chinese	28	14	49.0	29	15	50.0
Filipino	70	29	41.4	66	26	40.3
Hawaiian	88	27	30.7	87	29	32.6
Japanese	120	63	52.8	127	70	55.0
New Zealand						
Maori	140	39	27.9	139	40	28.6
Non-Maori	1439	648	45.1	1457	665	45.6

	Males			Females		
	All ages	30-74	%	All ages	30-74	%
AMERICAS (except USA)						
Brazil						
São Paulo	3336	1273	38.2	3512	1419	40.4
Canada						
Alberta	1143	465	40.7	1094	450	41.1
British Columbia	1365	647	47.4	1379	657	47.7
Maritime Provinces	826	360	43.6	840	371	44.2
Newfoundland	285	112	39.3	282	110	38.9
Quebec	3149	1418	45.0	3237	1507	46.6
Colombia						
Cali	523	153	29.3	598	180	30.2
Cuba [a]	4765	1750	36.7	4567	1666	36.5
Puerto Rico	1559	593	38.0	1643	658	40.0
AMERICAS (USA)						
Bay Area, Black	192	81	42.0	205	89	43.5
Bay Area, Chinese	71	34	48.2	73	36	49.6
Bay Area, White	1232	630	51.1	1279	658	51.4
Connecticut	1490	711	45.1	1600	788	49.2
Detroit, Black	416	160	38.4	470	193	41.1
Detroit, White	1504	701	46.6	1581	761	48.1
Iowa	1418	620	43.8	1498	670	44.7
New Orleans, Black	174	59	34.2	201	77	38.0
New Orleans, White	334	156	46.7	354	170	48.0
Seattle	1362	623	45.7	1377	642	46.7

Source: *Cancer Incidence in Five Continents* volume V

[a] Not included in volume V: population figures from volume IV (1975)

Table 2.7   Cancer mortality data: country and calendar period [a]

Period (approx.)	1955-	1960-	1965-	1970-	1975-	1980-	1985-
EUROPE (except European Community)							
Austria	55-59	60-64	65-69	70-74	75-79	80-84	85-88
Czechoslovakia	55-59	60-64	65-69	70-74	75-79	80-84	85-88
Finland	55-59	60-64	65-69	70-74	75-79	80-84	85-87
Hungary	55-59	60-64	65-69	70-74	75-79	80-84	85-88
Norway	55-59	60-64	65-69	70-74	75-79	80-84	85-87
Poland	-	60-64	65-69	70-74	75-79	80-84	85-88
Romania	-	60-64	65-69	70-74	75-79	80-84	-
Sweden	55-59	60-64	65-69	70-74	75-79	80-84	85-87
Switzerland	55-59	60-64	65-69	70-74	75-79	80-84	85-88
Yugoslavia		60-64	65-69	70-74	75-79	80-84	85-87
EUROPE (European Community)							
Belgium	55-59	60-64	65-69	70-74	75-79	80-84	85-86
Denmark	55-59	60-64	65-69	70-74	75-79	80-84	85-88
France	55-59	60-64	65-69	70-74	75-79	80-84	85-88
Germany (FRG)	55-59	60-64	65-69	70-74	75-79	80-84	85-88
Greece	-	61-65	66-70	71-75	76-80	81-85	86-87
Ireland	55-59	60-64	65-69	70-74	75-79	80-84	85-87
Italy	55-59	60-64	65-69	70-74	75-79	80-84	85-87
Netherlands	55-59	60-64	65-69	70-74	75-79	80-84	85-87
Portugal	55-59	60-64	65-69	70-74	75-79	80-84	85-88
Spain	55-59	60-64	65-69	70-74	75-79	80-84	85-85
UK England & Wales	55-59	60-64	65-69	70-74	75-79	80-84	85-88
UK Scotland	55-59	60-64	65-69	70-74	75-79	80-84	85-88
ASIA AND OCEANIA							
Australia	55-59	60-64	65-69	70-74	75-79	80-84	85-88
Hong Kong	-	61-65	66-70	71-75	76-80	81-85	86-87
Japan	55-59	60-64	65-69	70-74	75-79	80-84	85-88
Mauritius	-	61-65	66-70	71-75	76-80	81-85	86-87
New Zealand	55-59	60-64	65-69	70-74	75-79	80-84	85-87
Singapore	-	-	63-67	68-72	73-77	78-82	83-87
AMERICAS							
Canada	55-59	60-64	65-69	70-74	75-79	80-84	85-87
Chile	55-59	60-64	65-69	70-74	75-79	80-84	85-87
Costa Rica	-	-	63-67	68-72	73-77	78-82	83-87
Panama	55-59	60-64	65-69	70-74	75-79	80-84	85-87
Puerto Rico	-	-	63-67	68-72	73-77	78-82	83-86
Uruguay	55-59	60-64	65-69	70-74	75-79	80-84	85-86
USA	55-59	60-64	65-69	70-74	75-79	80-84	85-87
Venezuela	55-59	60-64	65-69	70-74	75-79	80-83	-

[a]   Some data sequences are defective for certain cancer sites: either no data at all, or data for only some of the years covered by the national data as a whole.

24

Table 2.8 Correspondence between incidence and mortality data sets

COUNTRY	MORTALITY	INCIDENCE Registry	Population coverage (%) [a]
EUROPE (except European Community)			
Austria	Yes	-	-
Czechoslovakia	Yes	-	-
Finland	Yes	National	100
Hungary	Yes	Szabolcs-Szatmar	5.8
		County Vas	2.7
Israel	-	National	100
Norway	Yes	National	100
Poland	Yes	Warsaw City	4.3
Romania	Yes	County Cluj	3.2
Sweden	Yes	National	100
Switzerland	Yes	Geneva	5.5
Yugoslavia	Yes	Slovenia	8.2
EUROPE (European Community)			
Belgium	Yes	-	-
Denmark	Yes	National	100
France	Yes	Bas-Rhin	1.7
		Doubs	0.9
Germany (FRG)	Yes	Hamburg	2.7
		Saarland	1.7
Germany (GDR)	-	National	100
Greece	Yes	-	-
Ireland	Yes	-	-
Italy	Yes	Varese	1.4
Netherlands	Yes	-	-
Portugal	Yes	-	-
Spain	Yes	Navarra	1.3
		Zaragoza	2.3
UK England & Wales	Yes	Birmingham	10.3
		S Thames	13.1
UK Scotland	Yes	National	100

Table 2.8 (cont.):   Correspondence between incidence and mortality data sets

COUNTRY	MORTALITY	INCIDENCE Registry	Population coverage (%) [a]
ASIA and OCEANIA			
Australia	Yes	New South Wales	34.2
		South Australia	8.7
China	-	Shanghai	0.6
Hawaii	(USA)	Hawaii	100
Hong Kong	Yes	National	100
India	-	Bombay	1.2
Japan	Yes	Miyagi	1.8
		Nagasaki	0.4
		Osaka	7.2
Mauritius	Yes	-	-
New Zealand	Yes	National	100
Singapore	Yes	National	100
AMERICAS			
Brazil	-	São Paulo	5.6
Canada	Yes	Alberta	9.1
		British Columbia	11.2
		Maritime Provinces	6.8
		Newfoundland	2.3
		Quebec	26.0
Chile	Yes	-	-
Colombia	-	Cali	4.3
Costa Rica	Yes	-	-
Cuba	-	National	100
Panama	Yes	-	-
Puerto Rico	Yes	National	100
Uruguay	Yes	-	-
USA	Yes	San Francisco Bay Area	1.4
		Connecticut	1.3
		Detroit	1.7
		Iowa	1.3
		New Orleans	0.5
		Seattle	1.2
Venezuela	Yes	-	-

[a]   Percentage of national population (around 1980) covered by the registry

Chapter 3

METHOD

Previous studies of trends in cancer incidence and mortality have used various analytic approaches and measures of trend, including graphical display[62,64,65,74,77,116,145,146] and the overall or mean annual percentage rate of change in age-standardised[13,80,128,136,152,154,164,198] or age-specific[77,83,85,190] rates, as well as modelling of age, period and cohort effects[3,154,213,252,293]. Time trends in age-standardised rates, however, are strictly interpretable only when the effect of calendar time on cancer risk is multiplicative, i.e. when the age-incidence or age-mortality curves for successive calendar periods are parallel on a logarithmic scale. Trends observed in age-standardised rates may be misleading when the time trends in different age-groups are significantly different from one another[83,94,131].

In these circumstances, the evolution of cancer risk with time is more readily understood by examination of trends in the age-specific rates. Such an approach can be satisfactory for the detailed examination of a single data set[190] or of a small number of homogeneous data sets. Examination of age-specific rates alone can suggest the existence of a cohort effect, for example with a rapid increase in risk at younger ages, and progressively smaller rates of increase, or even decline, in successively older age groups. When the age-specific trends are summarised only by rates of increase, however, much useful information is ignored; further, the estimates of age-specific trend are carried out independently of each other, using only that portion of the data corresponding to the relevant age group. For analysis of the large number of heterogeneous data sets presented here, detailed presentation of age-specific trends for all populations at each cancer site was impractical, and a more synoptic presentation was necessary.

A good graphical display of trends is invaluable; as the sole means for comparing trends between many countries or regions, however, graphical display is inadequate. Statistical models can supplement graphical displays considerably, by providing quantitative and comparable estimates of trend, based on objective criteria for selecting the best description of the data, and significance tests of whether the observed trends are real or random[94,131]. In most cases, fitting an age-period-cohort model will provide a succinct and interpretable summary of the data[55,56,95,130,258], and this approach formed the basis for the analyses.

The statistical principles of the analysis of time trends are straightforward, but their practical application may become quite complex when the database to be examined is extremely large, and when the overall purpose of the analysis is to compare and interpret thousands of statistics of varying precision derived from data of variable quality. In this situation, compromises are necessary, and the final approach adopted for this book was driven by practical as well as theoretical considerations. Three basic decisions were taken before choosing the methods of analysis:

(i) given the high random variability, some form of smoothing would be essential;

(ii) modelling would be done independently *within* each registry or country (i.e. no information was to be borrowed from other countries or regions to carry out the smoothing of data for any given region); and

(iii) several different statistical and graphical presentations of the data would be provided to aid interpretation.

Independent analyses

Borrowing information from other countries or geographical regions to assist in statistical modelling of time trends in a given region or country is, in principle, attractive[22,70]. It seems reasonable to believe that cancer trends in various regions of the same country or in adjacent countries of similar cultural background should be similar, and it would be helpful to be able to use this *a priori* belief to improve the estimates of trend in individual populations, and in particular to provide a more reliable estimate of trends which are not statistically significant simply because they lack precision. It would avoid undue emphasis being placed on the lack of statistical significance of the trend in individual populations, and a more coherent pattern of trends would emerge from the use of a collective estimate based on all the data sets in a particular region. This approach has not been adopted, however, because there is no widely accepted method of incorporating *a priori* information of this type into the modelling process. In addition, there were few geographical regions or countries represented in the available data for which such a technique could be implemented. It might also be considered that the results for each population would not be independent of the results for neighbouring populations, thus undermining the utility of the results for comparative purposes.

In the analyses presented here, data from each population have been examined independently. The same procedures and the same criteria have been used in fitting the statistical models to each data set. Comparison and interpretation of the results is a matter of overall judgement; it may need to take into account external information, for example about changes in cancer registration and death certification, which is generally too qualitative to be incorporated into statistical models.

Modelling strategy

The method of smoothing was based on age-period-cohort modelling. This choice was motivated by the desire to provide both trends in the age-standardised rates with calendar period and trends in the cumulative risk with year of birth. Polynomial functions were used to obtain effective smoothing of the age, period and cohort effects. Efficient smoothing is especially important for the study of cohort effects[39], since the calculation of the cumulative risk for the oldest and youngest generations represented in the data implies a considerable degree of extrapolation (see Table 3.1). This approach provides the advantage of a simple and efficient description of time trends when the data may be described by a smooth function, which implies that the data are well fitted by polynomials of low degree with only slight curvature, but it may produce spurious results when the data are markedly irregular. Under these circumstances, any extrapolation beyond the range of the observed data may be grossly misleading (an example is given later in the chapter). In order to avoid these problems, the degree of the polynomial used in each model was kept low unless there was a strong argument to the contrary, and extrapolation beyond the range of the observed data was kept to a minimum. It is worth noting that when this modelling strategy produced high-order polynomials and sharply irregular curves, it enabled a number of errors in the raw data to be detected in incidence, mortality and population data. Errors in incidence and population data have been corrected where possible. The practical application of the modelling strategy is described more fully below.

The polynomial models were fitted as generalised linear models with Poisson-distributed errors and logarithmic link[95]. In other words, the number of events (cases or deaths), k_{xt}, in a

given age and time interval of centre x and t, respectively, was considered to follow a Poisson distribution for which the logarithm of the mean was a polynomial function of age (x), period (t), and year of birth ($u = t - x$). We shall now describe this approach more precisely for each class of model.

1. The age-period model

This model implies that the age-specific incidence at age x in period t, denoted by λ_{xt}, is proportional to the age-specific incidence in a baseline period t_0. In other words, the age-incidence curves in *successive calendar periods* are parallel on a logarithmic scale. In this class of model, the expectation of the number of events (cases or deaths), k_{xt}, is defined by the following equations (3.1 and 3.2):

$$E\left(k_{xt}\right) = \lambda_{xt} m_{xt} \qquad (3.1)$$

$$Log\, \lambda_{xt} = a\left(\frac{x - x_0}{\Delta x}\right) + p\left(\frac{t - t_0}{\Delta t}\right) \qquad (3.2)$$

where m_{xt} is the number of person-years accumulated in the corresponding age-period interval, and a and p are polynomials of degree l and m, respectively. Such a model will be denoted by $A_l P_m$. For example, model $A_2 P_3$ will be written (expression 3.3):

$$Log\, \lambda_{xt} = \alpha_0 + \alpha_1\left(\frac{x - x_0}{\Delta x}\right) + \alpha_2\left(\frac{x - x_0}{\Delta x}\right)^2$$

$$+ \beta_1\left(\frac{t - t_0}{\Delta t}\right) + \beta_2\left(\frac{t - t_0}{\Delta t}\right)^2 + \beta_3\left(\frac{t - t_0}{\Delta t}\right)^3 \qquad (3.3)$$

The baseline age group and time period around which estimates of trend are centred, and the size of the time intervals considered — i.e. the position and scale parameters x_0, Δx, t_0 and Δt — are chosen in such a way that the expressions in brackets (the arguments of the polynomials) are the integers ...-2, -1, 0, 1, 2, ..., or else have values close to these integers if the periods of observation are irregular (for example, the values might be $x_0 = 50$, $\Delta x = 5$, $t_0 = 1970$, $\Delta t = 5$).

2. The age-cohort model

In this class of model, the age-specific incidence for subjects born in year u is considered to

Table 3.1: Matrix of rates by age and calendar period, showing extent of extrapolation from observed data required to estimate cumulative risk for age range 30-74 years for five-year birth cohorts 1910-1940 (rates for 1910 and 1940 cohorts shown in bold type): melanoma of the skin, females, mortality, England and Wales

| | | | | | Calendar period | | | | | | | | | | | |
| | | | | | 1955-59 | 1960-64 | 1965-69 | 1970-74 | 1975-79 | 1980-84 | 1985-88 | | | | | |
Age	Group	1	2	3	4	5	6	7	8	9	10	11	12	13	14	15
30-34	1	$r_{1,1}$	$r_{1,2}$	$r_{1,3}$	0.77	0.70	0.79	**0.70**	1.10	1.17	1.00					
35-39	2		$r_{2,2}$	$r_{2,3}$	0.99	1.05	1.36	1.29	**1.33**	1.51	1.34					
40-44	3			$r_{3,3}$	1.10	1.51	1.48	1.69	1.75	**1.60**	2.03					
45-49	4				**1.15**	1.38	1.94	2.24	2.13	2.42	**2.58**					
50-54	5				1.31	**1.48**	1.87	2.53	2.88	3.01	3.11	$r_{5,11}$				
55-59	6				1.22	1.34	**1.68**	2.59	2.70	3.20	3.21	$r_{6,11}$	$r_{6,12}$			
60-64	7				1.31	1.38	1.75	**2.63**	3.47	3.81	3.90	$r_{7,11}$	$r_{7,12}$	$r_{7,13}$		
65-69	8				1.85	2.09	2.13	2.45	**3.13**	4.08	5.00	$r_{8,11}$	$r_{8,12}$	$r_{8,13}$	$r_{8,14}$	
70-74	9				2.53	2.45	2.76	3.06	3.60	**4.28**	5.80	$r_{9,11}$	$r_{9,12}$	$r_{9,13}$	$r_{9,14}$	$r_{9,15}$
Birth cohort (central year)											1910	.1915	1920	1925	1930	1935

1940

be proportional to the age-specific incidence of those born in a baseline year u_0, and the expectation of k_{xu}, the number of events in a given age group, x, for a particular birth cohort, u, is defined by equations 3.4 and 3.5:

$$E\left(k_{xu}\right) = \lambda_{xu}\, m_{xu} \qquad (3.4)$$

$$Log\, \lambda_{xu} = a\left(\frac{x - x_0}{\Delta x}\right) + c\left(\frac{u - u_0}{\Delta u}\right) \qquad (3.5)$$

where a and c are polynomials of degree l and n, respectively. In other words, the age-incidence curves for *successive birth cohorts* are considered to be parallel on a logarithmic scale.

The usual approach to fitting this class of model is to consider that the number of events (cases or deaths) and the person-years observed in a given cell of the Lexis diagram (see Figure 3.1) belong to the birth cohort for which the central year of birth is determined by the centre of the age-period cell. The data collected by cancer registries, however, are in age and period intervals which are not always regularly-spaced square cells, i.e. they are not always in quinary age-groups in the age range 30-74 years or for successive calendar quinquennia. The usual approach was therefore inapplicable to many of the data sets analysed here. In order to maintain a standard analytic approach for all the data sets, it was necessary to adapt the usual procedure by subdividing each age-time cell into sub-units defined by successive five-year intervals of year of birth. This approach amounts to subdividing each cell of the age-time matrix into seg-

ments defined by successive birth cohorts; each segment is then indexed by the age and time point defining its centre of gravity (x_i, t_i). This is illustrated in Figure 3.1 for the cohorts born in 1920 and 1925 and observed during the period 1968-71. The number of cases k_{xt} observed in such a rectangle has the following expectation (expression 3.6):

$$E\left(k_{xt}\right) = \lambda_{x_1 u_1} m_{x_1 u_1} + \lambda_{x_2 u_2} m_{x_2 u_2} + \lambda_{x_3 u_3} m_{x_3 u_3} \quad (3.6)$$

where x_i and $u_i = t_i - x_i$ are defined by the centres of gravity x_i and t_i of the corresponding age-period-cohort intervals, weighted by the person-years density, and where the age-cohort-specific incidence or mortality rates, λ_{xu}, are defined by the model under consideration. Thus the maximum likelihood method for generalised linear models with Poisson error applies without modification. The person-years density is estimated over the age-period range of interest using an algorithm by Schifflers *et al.*[258] The number of person-years m_{xu} accumulated in each interval is calculated as the integral of this density over the corresponding range of age and period (see below).

3. *The age-period-cohort model*

In this class of model, the expectation of k_{xt} depends on age, calendar period and year of birth. The same principles as before are used, but now the age-specific incidence for the cohort born in year u is written (expression 3.7):

$$Log\, \lambda_{xu} = a\left(\frac{x - x_0}{\Delta x}\right) + p\left(\frac{t - t_0}{\Delta t}\right) + c\left(\frac{u - u_0}{\Delta u}\right) (3.7)$$

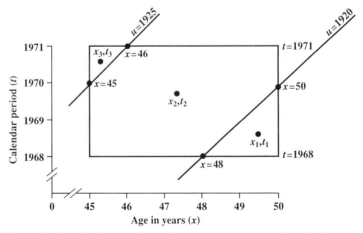

Figure 3.1 Subdivision of a Lexis diagram age-period cell by birth cohort.

where a, p and c are polynomials of degree l, m and n, respectively. In other words, the age-incidence curves for successive birth cohorts are no longer parallel: the relative risk of a given cohort is modified at each age by a factor which depends only on the period of observation. In order to ensure identifiability of all parameters in these models, there is no term of degree zero in the polynomials p and c, and no linear term in the polynomial c. The model may be rewritten (expression 3.8):

$$Log\ \lambda_{xt} = \alpha_0 + \alpha_1 \left(\frac{x - x_0}{\Delta x} \right) + a_2(x)$$

$$+ \beta_1 \left(\frac{t - t_0}{\Delta t} \right) + p_2(t) + c_2(t - x) \quad (3.8)$$

where the polynomials a_2, p_2 and c_2 contain only terms of degree two or greater in age, period and cohort, respectively.

Alternatively, the model may be written as a function of age and year of birth in the following way (expression 3.9):

$$Log\ \lambda_{xu} = \alpha_0 + \left(\alpha_1 + \beta_1 \frac{\Delta x}{\Delta t} \right) \left(\frac{x - x_0}{\Delta x} \right) + a_2(x)$$

$$+ \gamma_1 \left(\frac{u - u_0}{\Delta u} \right) + c_2(u) + p_2(u + x) \quad (3.9)$$

The expression:

$$e^\delta - 1 \quad (3.10)$$

where

$$\delta = \frac{\beta_1}{\Delta t} = \frac{\gamma_1}{\Delta u} \quad (3.11)$$

then provides the percentage increase in the rate per year in the neighbourhood of period t_0 or year of birth u_0. The parameter delta, called the 'drift', is the sum of the linear components of increase in the logarithm of the rate due to period and cohort effects combined[55,56]; it is identifiable, and may be estimated at the same time as the coefficients of the polynomials a_2, p_2 and c_2. For data sets best fitted by a model including only linear terms for period or cohort, and thus for which the incidence or mortality rate is chan-

ging at a constant rate over time, the 'drift' is the same as the slope of the line plotted in a graph of the logarithm of the incidence or mortality rate against time. For data sets best fitted by a model including non-linear terms for period or cohort, the change in the rate is varying over time, but it can be considered to have several components of change: linear, quadratic, etc. For such models, 'drift' is the linear component of the overall rate of change in the incidence or mortality rate with time. In many cases, the 'drift' is by far the largest component of the rate of change.

It should be noted, however, that in this polynomial version of the age-period-cohort model the value of the drift is strongly influenced by the degree of the polynomials included in the final model. The degree of each polynomial is determined by statistical criteria (see below). It would be inappropriate for the value of the linear drift to be dependent on statistical fluctuations in the data. For these reasons, the drift parameter has not been used to characterise the recent linear trend; instead, an overall linear trend has been preferred, calculated over the last three consecutive periods for which data were available, providing that 1985 or later years were included.

Estimation of person-years

In most data sets reported in *Cancer Incidence in Five Continents*, the 'person-years at risk' — the denominators of the age-specific rates — were calculated from the size of the population estimated in five-year age groups for the central year of the period of observation. It is widely accepted that the product of these numbers by the length of the period of observation is a reasonable approximation of the person-years at risk in a given age group. As explained for age-cohort models above, however, this approximation could not be used systematically here, because some data sets were available for irregular periods of time (1-7 years), and because the population estimates (census, projection or interpolation) used to calculate incidence rates for *Cancer Incidence in Five Continents* were not always in the centre of the period of observation in which the cases were registered, and estimates of the person-years accumulated by all birth cohorts which might have contributed cases of cancer were required.

If the size of the population in each single-year age group were precisely known from two censuses taken on dates t_0 and t_1, then, in the absence of migration, the person-years accumulated between the two censuses by the number of persons (s_0) who were aged x_0 at the first census would simply be:

$$\left(\frac{s_0 + s_1}{2}\right) \cdot (t_1 - t_0) \qquad (3.12)$$

where s_1 is the number of persons in the same birth cohort at the time of the second census, when the survivors have reached the age x_1, i.e. $x_0 + (t_1 - t_0)$. More generally, the number of person-years is the integral of the population density over the corresponding parallelogram of age and time[258]. When each rectangular domain of the Lexis diagram in which the cancer observations are made is decomposed into similar parallelograms and triangles of age and time (Figure 3.2), the person-years accumulated by the relevant cohorts in any age-time domain can be estimated, and thus the quantities m_{xu} in expression 3.6, required at the start of the algorithm for likelihood maximisation, can be obtained.

Example

In order to carry out this estimation in practice, the size of the various registry populations by five-year age group, and the date of the census or estimate from which these population figures were obtained, were abstracted from the six volumes of *Cancer Incidence in Five Continents*. The required density was then obtained by spline interpolation of the cumulative number of persons in the population between 0 and 90 years of age[258].

As an example, the estimation of person-years for male Filipinos in Hawaii between 1960 (volume II) and 1970 (volume III) is presented. Figure 3.3 shows the distribution of the population as recorded at the two censuses, and the corresponding interpolated population densities by single year of age. It is of interest to note the very irregular population structure and the shift of the peak age group with time. The incidence rates for the period 1960-64 for male Filipinos in Hawaii, as published in volume II, were calculated from the numbers of cases observed during 1960-64 and the census population of 1960 multiplied by five, a method which would give a correct (unbiased) estimate only if the population structure were stationary. It can be seen from the subsequent census that this was not in fact the case (Figure 3.3), and that interpolation of the population by cohort will produce more accurate denominators for calculating the age-specific rates. Table 3.2 gives the figures calculated by this method compared with the denominator actually used in volume II.

Another example is given by the estimation of the population of Cali (Colombia) for 1979 (submitted with the data for 1977-81 and used in volume V), which had been calculated by a cross-sectional extrapolation. Using the method described above, the 1979 population figures given in volume V were simply ignored, and the person-years were estimated by interpolation between the populations given in volumes IV and VI, which were virtually the same as the population of the 1973 and 1985 censuses, and thus much less prone to error. Table 3.2 gives the person-years as publi-

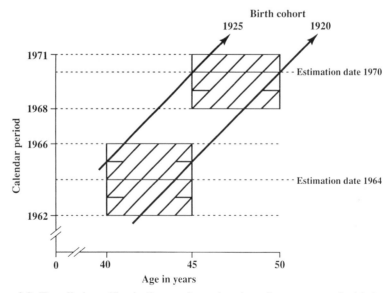

Figure 3.2 Tessellation of Lexis diagram for estimation of person-years by birth cohort

shed in volumes V and VI, compared with those obtained by interpolation along the birth cohort, which were used for the analyses in this book.

In most cases, however, the difference between the person-years provided by the successive volumes of *Cancer Incidence in Five Continents* and those calculated by this method in each age-period cell of the Lexis diagram was no more than 5%. This is important, because the recent linear trends presented in the bar chart diagrams were calculated using the denominators provided by the *Cancer Incidence in Five Continents* database, whereas the truncated rate graphs were calculated using the method of cohort interpolation of the population (see Chapter 4). In modelling the logarithm of the age-specific rates, as described earlier in this chapter, the logarithm of the person-years in each age-period interval was used as the offset, and such a difference in population numbers is equivalent to a maximum difference in the offset of ±0.05. It was unusual for such small discrepancies to create inconsistencies between the trend in the truncated rate and the recent linear trend. In the rare situations where this did occur, there were differences between the population estimations obtained from the two methods, and in these circumstances greater weight should be given in the interpretation to the trend in the truncated rate. Even so, the recent linear trends are calculated directly from the population denominators as published.

A further advantage of this approach to calculating the denominator, which was used even for data that were available in regular five-year age-period cells, such as most mortality data, is that the person-years denominators are estimated for birth cohorts defined by a single year of birth. Data for five-year birth cohorts are therefore available, calculated on the diagonal of the Lexis diagram, in contrast to the usual overlapping 10-year birth cohorts calculated for, say, individuals aged 50-54 in 1970-74, who were born between 1915 and 1924.

Choice of the best model

It is clear from the previous discussion that age-period and age-cohort models are sub-classes of the age-period-cohort model. Without *a priori* information on which type of model is appropriate for a given data set, all models have to be considered as belonging to the age-period-cohort class[94,95]. An age-period model will therefore be a model in which any non-linear cohort effect is not significant, and an age-cohort model will be one in which any non-linear period effect is not significant: linear cohort or period effects cannot be excluded. A model in which neither age-period nor age-cohort effects are significant will be called an age-drift model. These various models will be denoted $A_lP_mC_n$, A_lP_m, A_lC_n, and A_lD respectively. When a significant time trend exists, the model will be chosen from one of these four classes, using a strategy described below. When no significant time trend exists, the model will

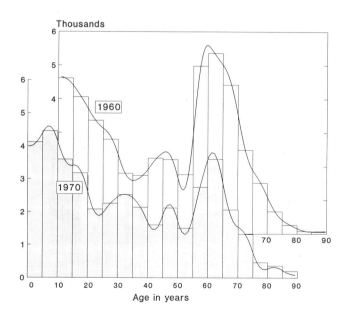

Figure 3.3 Interpolation of population age-structure in thousands for Filipino males in Hawaii for 1960 and 1970

Table 3.2 Population denominators (thousands of person-years): longitudinal interpolation vs. cross-sectional estimates used in *Cancer Incidence in Five Continents*

(a) Hawaii (USA), Filipino males, volumes II and III

Age	From longitudinal interpolation		From 1960 and 1970 censuses, multiplied by five	
	1960-64	1968-72	1960-64	1968-72
30-34	9.81	13.58	11.2	12.6
35-39	11.11	11.37	11.0	10.7
40-44	8.78	9.43	8.7	8.0
45-49	14.99	11.05	24.9	10.6
50-54	24.58	8.41	26.8	7.5
55-59	22.65	13.81	22.1	13.7
60-64	14.99	18.70	12.4	18.0
65-69	8.42	12.06	7.5	10.3
70-74	4.42	6.52	3.3	6.6

(b) Cali (Colombia), males, volumes V and VI

Age	From longitudinal interpolation		From cross-sectional extrapolation	
	1977-81	1982-86	1977-81	1982-86
30-34	189.5	245.0	167.3	238.1
35-39	153.4	203.4	140.7	197.2
40-44	123.9	161.5	126.1	155.3
45-49	106.9	127.9	96.0	123.7
50-54	85.2	110.2	80.3	108.6
55-59	67.3	87.7	57.2	84.0
60-64	48.7	67.4	47.7	65.2
65-69	36.0	46.6	29.5	43.8
70-74	24.1	32.5	22.0	31.5

(c) Cali (Colombia), females, volumes V and VI

Age	From longitudinal interpolation		From cross-sectional extrapolation	
	1977-81	1982-86	1977-81	1982-86
30-34	223.9	280.8	192.5	272.0
35-39	169.9	234.0	174.2	229.8
40-44	142.7	175.5	143.1	165.2
45-49	124.5	143.0	114.4	141.4
50-54	98.8	127.6	91.5	125.6
55-59	78.3	100.1	66.5	95.7
60-64	58.0	78.4	56.2	76.5
65-69	43.8	57.4	35.6	54.4
70-74	29.8	40.9	27.9	39.5

simply be an age model, A_l. It must be emphasised that whatever the final choice of model, only the *sum* of the linear period and cohort effects is estimable, in addition to any non-linear period and cohort effects[55,56,131].

The strategy adopted to identify the model which best describes a given data set was driven by several considerations.

First, it was considered essential that the same analytic strategy and model selection procedures should be applied to all the data sets, and that these should be explicit, objective and reproducible. For incidence alone, there were almost 2900 data sets to be examined (48 sex-site combinations for 60 populations), and a further 1500 or so mortality data sets. For each data set, it was necessary to fit and compare a number of statistical models. The potential number of models to be examined was considered too great for manual evaluation and comparison. An algorithm was therefore developed to provide automatically the optimal description of each data set in turn, by fitting a series of models in a defined sequence, applying standard tests to detect the best model, and providing both an audit trail of the models fitted and a standard set of statistical and graphical representations of the data, including the trend in the age-standardised (truncated) rate over time, the trend in the cumulative risk in successive birth cohorts, and the recent linear trend.

Second, a compromise was required between precision and simplicity. As explained earlier, the polynomials were required to be of the lowest degree compatible with an acceptable description of the data; as a consequence, it was decided to use a forward regression algorithm in which terms of higher degree were added to the model as long as they significantly improved the fit.

Third, no *a priori* information being available as to the appropriateness of a particular class of model, the decision as to whether a period and/or a cohort effect existed for each data set was made on statistical criteria.

Algorithm for selection of best model

Under these principles, the following algorithm was developed to select the best fitting model for each data set:

(i) Determine the degree l of the polynomial describing the marginal age-incidence curve, A_l, by adding terms of increasing degree in age as long as the corresponding coefficients are significant. In order to obtain the best possible description, the procedure stops when at least two successive coefficients are non-significant. In other words, l is defined as the integer for

which $\alpha_0, \alpha_1, \alpha_2, \ldots a_l$ are significantly different from zero, whereas neither α_{l+1} nor α_{l+2} are significant.

(ii) Evaluate the age-drift model A_lD by adding to the best age model a term for constant linear change in the logarithm of the rate with time.

(iii) Determine the degree m of the polynomial describing the crude period effect, A_lP_m, by a forward procedure starting from the A_lP_2 model and adding non-linear terms in t from degree 3 to degree m, m being defined as the first integer for which β_{m+1} and β_{m+2} are not significantly different from zero.

(iv) Determine the degree n of the polynomial describing the crude cohort effect, A_lC_n, by a forward procedure starting from the A_lC_2 model and adding non-linear terms in u from degree 3 to degree n, n being defined as the first integer for which γ_{n+1} and γ_{n+2} are not significantly different from zero.

(v) The model $A_lP_mC_n$ is then fitted to the data and considered as the age-period-cohort model of minimum complexity to use as the starting point in the search for the best-fitting model overall.

(vi) The best-fitting model is then determined in the following way:
compare the models $A_lP_mC_n$ and A_lC_n, and decide that there is no (non-linear) period effect if the improvement in deviance with the period term is not significant;
compare the models $A_lP_mC_n$ and A_lP_m, and decide that there is no (non-linear) cohort effect if the improvement in deviance with the cohort term is not significant.

When both terms are significant, the best-fitting model is the age-period-cohort model, $A_lP_mC_n$. When either the period effect or the cohort effect is significant, but not both, the best-fitting model is either an age-period model (A_lP_m) or an age-cohort model (A_lC_n), respectively. When neither is significant, age-drift and age models are compared $(A_lD$ and $A_l)$; if the improvement in deviance is significant, the best-fitting model is an age-drift model (A_lD), otherwise it is an age model (A_l).

Statistical significance

When evaluating the addition of successive terms in age, period or cohort to each model in the forward regression approach described above, an additional term was considered significant if the deviance of the model was reduced by 4 or more:

this amounts to a slightly conservative test (the critical value of a chi square on 1 degree of freedom for a probability of 5% being 3.84), and was adopted in order to avoid adding new terms if they were only of borderline statistical significance.

When evaluating the significance of period, cohort or drift (see step (vi) above), a model was considered significantly better than another model if the reduction in deviance was significant at the 5% level on the basis of a chi square distribution with the relevant degrees of freedom.

Goodness of fit

An evaluation of the goodness of fit of the best model obtained so far was then made from its deviance, D, which is a chi square with v degrees of freedom when the model fits adequately. The deviance was transformed in the usual way to obtain a standard Normal deviate, V, which was used to assess the goodness of fit:

$$V = \sqrt{(2D)} - \sqrt{(2v-1)} \qquad (3.13)$$

The goodness of fit was considered acceptable if V was less than 1.0. If the fit was satisfactory, the search stopped there. If not, a saturated age-period-cohort model — for our purposes, a model in which the degrees of the polynomials are the maximum compatible with the data, subject to a maximum of 9 — was then fitted to the data. This model was used as the basis for finding the best overall model, as follows.

If the saturated model itself fitted adequately, i.e. if the value of V was less than 1.0, the saturated model was retained for further testing. If not, the saturated model was evaluated on the basis of an F-statistic, comparing the improvement in deviance it provided over the best model so far with the residual deviance (this is equivalent to considering the log of the rate as a Normal variate which is modelled with a weighted least squares approach). If the saturated model did not improve the deviance, the best model identified so far was considered as the best model overall. If the saturated model did improve the deviance, the period and cohort effects were then tested in the same way as before (see step (vi) above), in order to make the final choice of the best model from within the saturated model. This was done in order to avoid retaining period or cohort effects the significance of which would have been overstated when tested against a poorly-fitting unsaturated model using the Poisson distribution.

Cohort cumulative risks

The presentation of cumulative risks by birth cohort is a departure from usual practice, and merits explanation. Cumulative risks are usually calculated in cross-sectional fashion, by using a set of age-specific rates observed over a short period of time for an age range such as 0-64 or 0-74 years, and they are often used to represent the 'lifetime' risk of developing the malignancy in question over that age span — or of dying from it in the absence of other causes of death. The rates conventionally used are the most recent available, in effect, the current rates. The cumulative risk is an accurate summary of the current force of morbidity, and it is in fact equivalent to a directly standardised risk with a uniform standard population[68]. The interpretation of a cumulative risk (0-64 years), so calculated, of 10 per 1000 for colon cancer is that, for a hypothetical person to whom the age-specific rates observed today were to apply over that person's lifetime, there would be a 1% chance of developing cancer of the colon before his or her 65th birthday. This would be a satisfactory estimate of the lifetime risk of a person in the corresponding population only if the age-specific rates are not changing with time. From this point of view, use of the conventional, cross-sectionally derived estimate of cumulative risk to examine *trends* in cancer risk may be misleading, for the same reasons which apply to the examination of trends using age-standardised rates.

Use of cumulative risks for successive birth cohorts carries the advantage that, for any given birth cohort (e.g. persons born in the period 1925-29), the observed age-specific rates used to estimate the cumulative risk are those actually experienced by persons in that birth cohort, and thus represent that part of the true lifetime risk of interest which has actually been observed longitudinally, with the passage of time. The difficulty is the requirement to use statistical models to estimate those components of the cumulative risk for each birth cohort which have *not* been observed: the rates up to age 74 years for those who have not yet reached that age, and the rates at age 30-44 years or so for those who are now around 70 years old, since the data do not go back far enough (Table 3.1). Clearly, estimation of cumulative risks for the oldest and the youngest birth cohorts requires progressively greater dependence on values derived by extrapolation from the chosen model than for the central cohorts, born around 1920-30, and for whom data are available for much of the age range 30-74 years. The adequacy of this extrapolation depends on the extent to which the age effect (i.e. the shape of the age-incidence or age-mortality curve determined by the model) is appropriate for describing the risk in each successive birth cohort. This is strictly the case only if an age-cohort model reflects the biological truth, and this is more likely to be so when the best fitting model is an age-cohort model.

Use of the cohort cumulative risk as a summary statistic for presenting cancer trends does not necessarily imply that an age-cohort model fits the data best. In fact, however, where an age-cohort (including age-drift) model was not the best model overall, the difference in the adequacy of fit between the best-fitting age-cohort model and the best model overall was often minor. The loss of precision in using the best age-cohort model to derive estimates of trend in the cumulative risk was outweighed by two advantages. It provided a consistent approach to the estimation of trends in cohort cumulative risk for all data sets. It also avoided over-fitting, since cohort effects adjusted for period were not reliable enough to be used in a systematic fashion. In any case, the lack of identifiability of the linear period and cohort effects[130] makes it almost illusory to adjust cohort effects for calendar period, since in many cases most of the observed trend is accounted for by the linear component. The best-fitting age-cohort model was therefore used to obtain a set of estimates of the underlying age-specific rates for each calendar period and age group in the required range, and these were then used to calculate the cumulative risk by birth cohort.

There is a further advantage to using the cohort-specific cumulative risk, however, since, like a directly age-standardised rate, it provides a measure of the *absolute* risk over a defined age span (generally 30-74 years in this book). By contrast, the standardised cohort mortality ratio, like the conventional SMR, only provides an estimate of the risk relative to some arbitrary standard, such as the first cohort or the marginal population. The use of such a standard for these analyses was considered inappropriate. The cohort cumulative risk enables direct comparison between the absolute levels of risk in successive cohorts in a given population, or between different populations at the same period.

Finally, use of the cohort cumulative risk offered the most succinct method of presenting trends for many populations in a single graphic, since the curve for each population summarises the information which would be presented as a family of age-incidence curves for successive birth cohorts in classical age-cohort analyses. This allows direct visual comparison between populations in the same geographical region. Tables are used to provide statistical summaries of the data as a further aid to interpretation.

Recent linear trend

The recent linear trend may be considered as the average of the percentage linear change in the age-specific rates over the age range 30-74 years, weighted by their precision. As explained above, it is a parameter obtained by fitting a linear function of calendar time to the age-specific data by Poisson regression. The recent linear trend is expressed as a percentage change per five-year period both for all ages and for three broad age groups within this range.

A quinquennial measure of trend is preferred to the more conventional annual percentage rate of change, despite the fact that annual rates of change may seem more intuitive. First, data were available only for five-year age groups and, for incidence data, generally for five-year calendar periods: presentation of annual rates of change would suggest greater precision in the methodology than is actually warranted. Second, cancer incidence and mortality rates do not in general change very rapidly over short periods of time, and a quinquennial rate of change estimated over a 15-year period seemed a more suitable summary measure for quantifying trends than an annual rate of change. The quinquennial trend is slightly greater than five times the corresponding annual rate of change, which is compounded in successive years. For small rates of change, however, the difference is small: 10% per five-year period is equivalent to 1.9%, i.e. $(1.10^{1/5} - 1)$% per year rather than 2% per year. If the best model is an age-drift model, implying that a linear increase in the rates fits the data best, the quinquennial trend can also be used as a first approximation of the likely rate of change in the truncated rate over the 5-10 years following the period for which data are available.

The relative disposition of the age-specific trend bars provides a rough guide to the underlying pattern of change. Thus, for example, the overall rate of decline of 2.4% every five years in lung cancer incidence among males in Scotland is made up of a small rate of decline in the elderly (0.6% per five years), a moderate rate of decline in the middle-aged (3.7%) and a rapid rate of decline in younger males (16.2% per five years, 3 standard errors). The bar charts have been drawn from the figures cited here, although the figures are not shown in the tables. These patterns imply a small recent decline in lung cancer incidence among males in Scotland which is likely to accelerate with time as the population ages, since the decline is most marked in the young. This is clearly seen in the graph of cumulative risk, showing a decline in risk for males born after about 1925. Reference to the incidence table shows that this trend is based on large annual numbers of cases of lung cancer: an estimated 2369 cases in 1985.

Similarly, the large recent increase in lung cancer in Scottish females (26.2% per five years) is composed of a decline (10.3%) in younger women, an increase (13.9%) in middle-aged women and a very rapid rate of increase (46.2% per five years) in elderly women. These patterns, which are also based on large numbers (an estimated 1076 cases in 1985) suggest that the apparently inexorable increase in lung cancer incidence among Scottish females is likely to decelerate soon. This is borne out by examination of the graphs, which show a recent slight deceleration in the steep increase of the truncated rate between 1965 and 1985, and a clear plateau in the cumulative risk (30-74 years) for women born around 1930, with a subsequent small decline. The cumulative risk plateau obviously carries a measure of extrapolation from the data under the best-fitting model, suggesting that the peak in the (cross-sectional) truncated rates (30-74 years) is likely to be seen in about the year 2004, when the women born around 1930 attain the age of 75.

The trends in incidence of myeloma among black females in New Orleans (USA) exemplify some of the limitations of the modelling approach using polynomial functions, especially when the data are relatively sparse, contain considerable variation and do not cover the complete period of interest. Only three data sets were available for this population, covering the period 1974-87, and the number of cases in the central period was substantially smaller than in the first and last periods, around 1975 and 1985. This is shown in the V-shaped curve of truncated rates, for which the best model was a parabola, or quadratic in period

(A_1P_2). Backward extrapolation of this curve for the (longer than usual) period of five years required to reach the reference year of 1970 led to the 'estimate' of 99 cases a year around 1970, which is italicised in the table to alert the reader to the caution necessary when interpreting this figure. Comparison of the truncated rate for 1970 with the other data in the table shows clearly the extent to which it is an outlier. The trends for melanoma among males in Cluj (Romania) provide a further example of this pattern.

Another example of the difficulty in interpreting sparse data is provided by the trend in the incidence of cervical cancer among non-Jews in Israel, which is based on an average of only three cases a year. The recent linear trend is estimated as a non-significant 21.2% increase every five years over the last 15 years, but the overall trend in the truncated rate shows a steady and significant decline over the entire 27-year period of observation. This leads to an apparent contradiction. A true recent increase would imply curvature in the period effect, but this curvature is not significant, and it is therefore not retained in the best model, which is an age-cohort model. By contrast, the increase among younger females, seen in the histogram, is captured by the modelling process as a significant cohort effect, which can also be seen as a clear increase in lifetime (30-74 years) risk for women born since 1930 in the graph of cumulative risk.

These examples may assist the reader with simultaneous interpretation of the three components of statistical analysis used in this book, and they serve as a reminder that satisfactory interpretation of time trends can rarely be achieved from analysis of a single function of calendar time.

Chapter 4

PRESENTATION OF RESULTS

Results are presented in separate chapters for each of 25 malignant neoplasms in adults. A separate chapter covers leukaemia and all malignancies combined in children (0-14 years). The age range is 30-74 years for adults, except for cancer of the testis (15-64 years) and Hodgkin's disease (15-74 years): these exceptions to the usual age range apply throughout the description in this chapter.

Geographical regions

For each cancer, results are presented for six regions of the world: Europe (excluding the member states of the European Community), Europe (European Community), Asia, Oceania (including Australia and New Zealand), the Americas (except USA) and Americas (USA). These regional groupings were identified partly on the basis of geography, but also for clarity in the graphs and histograms. Results for Europe were sufficiently diverse to warrant presentation of incidence and mortality data from many countries, too numerous to be presented clearly on a single graph, and Europe was therefore divided into two regions: the south and west, represented by member states of the European Community (EC), and the Nordic and central and eastern countries. There is considerable regional variation in cancer incidence in the USA, and a selection of the many population-based cancer registries was made in an effort to represent this variation: results for these registries are shown separately from those for the rest of the Americas. Mortality data for the Americas are presented together. Similar considerations applied for Asia and Oceania, for which incidence data are presented separately, and mortality data together. The arrangement of results by data type and geographical region is thus as follows:

Europe (except EC), incidence
Europe (EC), incidence
Europe (except EC), mortality
Europe (EC), mortality
Asia, incidence
Oceania, incidence
Asia and Oceania, mortality
Americas (except USA), incidence
Americas (USA), incidence
Americas, mortality

Presentation of results

For each region, results are presented as a set of tables, graphs and histograms, first for incidence, then for mortality, by sex.

Tables are given of the numbers of cases or deaths in the age range 30-74 years among males and females in each of two reference years, together with the truncated incidence or mortality rates and the cumulative risks for the same age range. On the facing page, the evolution of the truncated rates over calendar time and of the cohort cumulative risks in successive birth cohorts is represented graphically. The overall (30-74 years) recent linear trend in the rate is given as the last column of each table, in the form of the percentage change per five-year period. Bar charts of the recent linear trends in incidence and mortality are given on subsequent pages, showing the trend separately for each of the three age groups 30-44, 45-64 and 65-74 years. For cancers of the testis, the age groups are 15-29, 30-44 and 45-64 years; for Hodgkin's disease, 15-44, 45-64 and 65-74 years.

Tables

The tables of incidence and mortality statistics and the corresponding graphs are on facing pages (same page for single-sex chapters). Populations and countries are listed in alphabetical order.

The *best model* is described in terms of the degree of the polynomial fitted in age (A), period (P) and cohort (C), such as A2C2 or A1P3. A model such as A2D implies that there is only linear change (drift) with time in the age-incidence or age-mortality curves, i.e. that there is no significant departure from linearity of the trend.

The *goodness of fit* statistic for the best model is a likelihood ratio chi square, transformed into a standard normal deviate (see Chapter 3).

The world-standardised truncated *rate* per 100 000 per year and the number of *cases* or *deaths* per year are estimated from the best model, for the age range 30-74 years and for the single years cited in the table, i.e. 1970 and 1985 for incidence and 1965 and 1985 for mortality. These are the central years of the first and last data sets available for most registries and countries, although for some registries it was necessary to extrapolate the data to the reference year, using the best-fitting model. The *cumulative risk* per 1000 for the age range 30-74 years is estimated from the best age-cohort model for birth cohorts with the central birth year cited in the tables, usually 1915 and 1940 for cancer incidence, and 1900 and 1940 for cancer mortality. These birth years were chosen to represent two successive generations for which adequately precise estimates of risk could be made.

The *recent linear trend* is an estimate of the underlying rate of change in incidence or mortality rates over the last 15 years or so of available data, usually up to 1987 for incidence and up to the last year available for mortality, usually 1987 or 1988 (see Chapter 3). It is only calculated if three data points are available in this period, and is thus not presented for Hamburg (FRG), São Paulo (Brazil) or Cuba, or for Chinese in the San Francisco Bay Area (USA): in each case, incidence data were not available for part of this period. For some countries, mortality data for certain cancers were not available for part of this period, and recent linear trends are not presented.

An *asterisk* (*) is used to indicate that there were too few cases or deaths for reliable estimation of the parameter in question, while a *dash* ('-') is used to indicate that a parameter could not be calculated because of missing or incomplete data for one or more of the age groups or time periods required. An asterisk is also used if no satisfactory model could be fitted to the data at all, when all the parameters are represented by two points (..) in the tables, as unavailable. *Italics* are used in the tables to indicate that the figures are considered less reliable than those in ordinary typeface. Thus where the truncated rates estimated from the chosen model for the reference years cited in the table required extrapolation beyond the midpoints of the first and last data sets, the rates are shown in italics. If the mean annual number of cases or deaths estimated from the model was less than 0.5, this is represented by an italicised zero; it implies that the associated rate is based on an estimated 2 cases or less per five-year period. Estimates of cumulative risk in excess of 20% (200 per 1000) and those based on only two age-period data points are also italicised, to alert the reader. Recent linear trends which are not significantly different from zero at the 5% level are also shown in italics.

Graphs

All graphs are semi-log plots, with a logarithmic scale chosen to reflect the multiplicative nature of the models. The scale was also chosen to show the full range of rates for each geographical region to best effect in the available space. The values on the vertical axis are therefore dependent on the data and the results of model fitting, instead of being arbitrarily fixed to the observed range of rates in one region. Visual comparisons of trends in the absolute levels of risk between populations in different geographical regions, or between the sexes within the same region, should therefore take account of any difference in the vertical scales used. As far as possible, the trends for registries or countries in each part of a given region are plotted in the same colour, but with a different trace pattern. In Asia and the USA, the same approach was used for the various ethnic or racial groups.

Truncated rates

The graphics on the left of each page show trends in the truncated rate per 100 000, derived from the best-fitting model and standardised[270] to the 'world' population for the age range 30-74 years. In contrast to the corresponding tables, the graphs are plotted only for the period for which data are available, i.e. without extrapolation.

Cumulative risks

The graphics on the right of each page show trends in the cumulative risk per 1000, derived from the best-fitting age-cohort model for the age range 30-74 years, for persons born between 1910 and 1940 for cancer incidence, and for those born between 1900 and 1940 for cancer mortality. The last year of birth plotted for testicular cancer and Hodgkin's disease is 1950.

Bar charts

These charts show the recent linear trends in incidence and mortality over the last 15 years or so of available data, by sex and broad age band. The trends are shown as rates of change per five-year period, not as absolute increases or decreases in the underlying rate. Thus a small percentage increase in a large underlying rate may imply a larger absolute increase in the rate than a large percentage increase in a small rate. The bar charts are intended to enable *rates of change* in cancer incidence or mortality to be compared between populations: the truncated rates themselves and the associated numbers of cases or deaths are shown in the tables.

The estimates of recent trend in each bar chart are ranked by the overall recent trend for ages 30-74 years in males. For convenience, trends for males and females in a given population are presented alongside one another. The trends for females are thus not necessarily shown in rank order. For each cancer, the same scale is used for incidence in both sexes and for all geographical regions, in order to facilitate visual comparisons: the same applies for the mortality charts. The recent trend in each population is shown for all ages (30-74 years) as a solid bar: this is the same as the value tabulated under 'recent trend' in the corresponding table. The constituent age-specific trends are also shown with successive bars for younger (30-44 years), middle-aged (45-64 years) and elderly (60-74 years) persons, respectively. Populations for which recent trends could not be calculated are not shown on the histograms.

The age-specific trends plotted in the bar charts should be interpreted in conjunction with the graphs showing the evolution of the truncated rate and the cumulative risk. When the best model is an age-period model, the recent linear trend is a good summary of the change in the truncated rate over the last 15 years of available data; this is particularly so when the best model is an age-drift model based on a large number of events. When an age-cohort model has been selected, the relative disposition of the age-specific trend bars provides a rough guide to the underlying pattern of changes, and should help in interpreting the graph of the change in cumulative risk with year of birth. Finally, when an age model has been selected, there is no significant overall trend in risk in the data set as a whole, and the recent linear trends are not statistically significant[1]. Nevertheless, where the lack of significance is due to small numbers of events, the disposition of the age-specific trends still enables the consistency of trend with other populations to be assessed from the bar chart.

Extreme values of recent linear trend are truncated, in order to avoid compressing the more reliable trend values in the bar charts. The value of the trend is shown at the end of each truncated bar.

The age-specific values for the recent linear trend are not shown in the tables. The percentages and their standard errors are available in a companion volume[60].

---

[1] On rare occasions, there are inconsistencies, due to the fact that the denominators for the modelling procedure and the recent linear trend are not calculated in the same way (see Chapter 3).

Chapter 5

LIP (MALES)

Cancer of the lip is uncommon in males and very rare in females, with less than one case per year in most populations covered by cancer registries. Consequently, time trends in lip cancer are reported only for males. The lower lip is involved much more frequently than the upper lip. Cancer of the lip accounts for a substantial though declining proportion of oral cancers in males. In Denmark, for example, the estimated proportion of lip cancers among all cancers of the buccal cavity and pharynx in the age range 30-74 years fell from 53% to 28% between 1970 and 1985, but only from 13% to 9% in South Thames (UK). Since the relative frequencies of lip, mouth, and pharynx cancer are changing over time, it is important to examine trends in the occurrence of these cancers separately.

High incidence rates for lip cancer are observed in Newfoundland (Canada) and in Australia, whereas the risk is uniformly low in Asia and among blacks in the USA. This cancer is clearly linked to outdoor occupations, implying heavy exposure to ultra-violet radiation, and some studies suggest that pipe smoking is a risk factor. The geographical distribution and time trends are difficult to interpret because of misclassification, which varies between registries and is changing over time. Lip cancer may be confused with cancer of the skin of the lip, or with cancer of the anterior part of the mouth. The frequency of lip cancer is decreasing everywhere, with some notable exceptions. It is likely that improvement in histological verification and the consequent reduction of misclassification explains part of the observed changes. Survival from cancer of the lip is good, however, and mortality from lip cancer is generally extremely low, rendering mortality data of limited value for studying trends in the risk of this cancer.

Europe

The incidence of lip cancer is decreasing everywhere in Europe, except in Navarra and Zaragoza (Spain), where it is significantly increasing, and in Bas-Rhin and Doubs (France), where the number of cases is too small to permit any firm conclusion to be drawn. The rate of decline in eastern European populations is slower, and it is not significant in Hungary. The changes generally seem to be related to calendar period, consistent with an improvement in classification being responsible for part of the decreasing trend. As a consequence, the cumulative risk graphs are not always relevant for interpreting the trends. The abrupt change in Navarra and the high incidence now observed in both Navarra and Zaragoza (Spain) suggest differences in the coding rules adopted by these registries.

The truncated mortality rate is 0.5 per 100 000 or less in most countries, but higher in eastern Europe: the rate exceeds 1.0 in Hungary and Poland. Despite the small numbers, lip cancer mortality is decreasing significantly in most European countries. The most recent mortality data for Poland are from 1971, and no conclusion can be drawn about recent trends. The recent linear trends are mostly negative. The positive trends in Scotland and Czechoslovakia are not significant, and there is no overall change in mortality. In Austria and Sweden, the overall trend is significantly downward, and the positive recent linear trends are not significant (see Chapter 3).

Asia and Oceania

Except in Bombay (India), where the truncated incidence rate is similar to the lowest rate in Europe, cancer of the lip is almost unknown in Asia; the significant downward trends in Shanghai (China) and in Hong Kong may be due to improved classification.

Incidence is remarkably high in South Australia, and it has increased substantially during the period for which data are available. Incidence is more than three times higher than in New South Wales (Australia), where it is similar to the rate among non-Maoris in New Zealand. The estimated rate in South Australia in 1985 is even greater than in Newfoundland (Canada). Mortality has decreased slightly in Australia but not in New Zealand; mortality is low, and similar to the level in the European Community.

Americas

In Canada, the incidence rate has decreased in the five populations studied. Incidence is still remarkably high in Newfoundland, where the

continued page 63

LIP (ICD-9 140)

EUROPE (non-EC), INCIDENCE

MALES	Best model	Goodness of fit	1970 Rate	1970 Cases	1985 Rate	1985 Cases	Cumulative risk 1915	Cumulative risk 1940	Recent trend
FINLAND	A2P2C3	-0.94	11.2	114	8.5	101	6.7	1.5	-6.5
HUNGARY									
County Vas	A2	1.30	13.8	11	13.8	10	8.4	8.4	*2.8*
Szabolcs-Szatmar	A8P4C9	-0.88	22.8	29	13.9	18	8.7	6.2	*0.8*
ISRAEL									
All Jews	A1P3	-0.83	7.7	35	6.7	40	3.6	5.6	-9.2
Non-Jews	A1D	0.38	5.5	1	2.9	1	2.7	0.9	*-15.1*
NORWAY	A2P4C3	1.22	7.1	77	5.3	63	4.0	2.8	-12.1
POLAND									
Warsaw City	A1	0.27	3.7	10	3.7	14	2.4	2.4	*-9.5*
ROMANIA									
Cluj	A2D	0.33	*36.0*	*56*	12.6	22	17.3	3.0	-29.5
SWEDEN	A2C2	-0.91	5.2	127	3.9	106	3.1	1.4	-12.4
SWITZERLAND									
Geneva	A2	-0.34	2.2	1	2.2	2	1.1	1.1	*-16.0*
YUGOSLAVIA									
Slovenia	A2P2	0.10	9.9	36	4.8	21	4.3	2.3	-28.6

* : not enough cases for reliable estimation
– : incomplete or missing data
Best model: polynomial of the given degree in age (A), period (P) or cohort (C), or linear drift (D) model.
Goodness of fit: the normalised likelihood ratio chi-square for the best model (see Method).
Rate: world-standardised truncated rate per 100 000 per year (30-74 years) and number of **cases** are both estimated from the best-fitting model for the single years cited.
Cumulative risk per 1000 (30-74 years) is estimated from the best-fitting *age-cohort* model for cohorts of central birth year cited.
Recent trend: estimated mean percentage change per five-year period in the age-specific rates (30-74 years) over the period 1973-1987.
Italics denote recent trends not significant at 5 per cent level, or other figures which should be interpreted with caution (see Method).

MALES

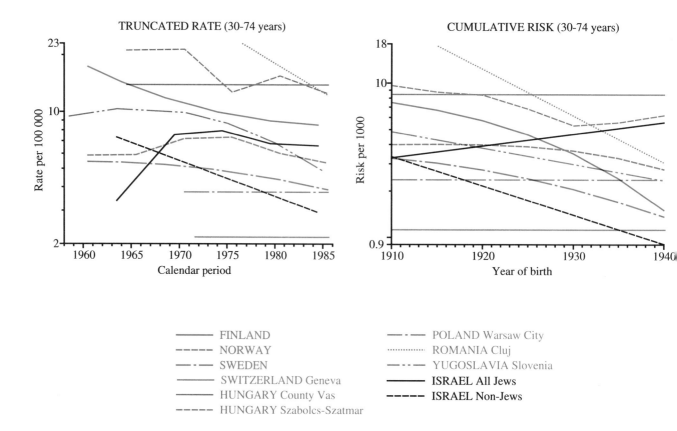

TRUNCATED RATE (30-74 years) — Rate per 100 000 — Calendar period

CUMULATIVE RISK (30-74 years) — Risk per 1000 — Year of birth

FINLAND
NORWAY
SWEDEN
SWITZERLAND Geneva
HUNGARY County Vas
HUNGARY Szabolcs-Szatmar
POLAND Warsaw City
ROMANIA Cluj
YUGOSLAVIA Slovenia
ISRAEL All Jews
ISRAEL Non-Jews

LIP (ICD-9 140)

EUROPE (non-EC), INCIDENCE
Percentage change per five-year period, 1973-1987

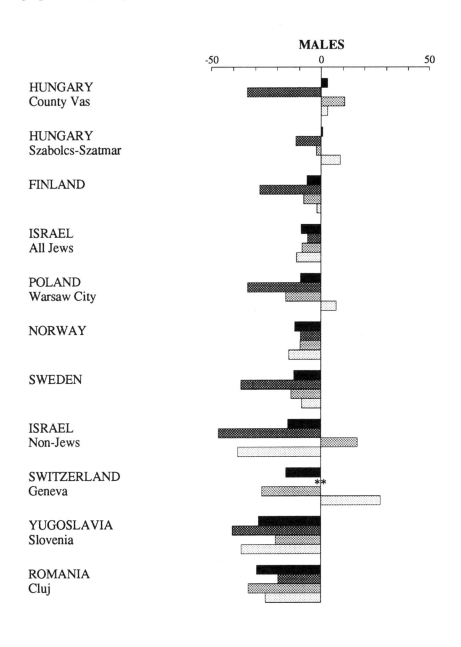

MALES

HUNGARY
County Vas

HUNGARY
Szabolcs-Szatmar

FINLAND

ISRAEL
All Jews

POLAND
Warsaw City

NORWAY

SWEDEN

ISRAEL
Non-Jews

SWITZERLAND
Geneva

YUGOSLAVIA
Slovenia

ROMANIA
Cluj

30-74
30-44
45-64
65-74

LIP (ICD-9 140)

EUROPE (EC), INCIDENCE

MALES	Best model	Goodness of fit	1970 Rate	1970 Cases	1985 Rate	1985 Cases	Cumulative risk 1915	Cumulative risk 1940	Recent trend
DENMARK	A2P6C4	-1.84	8.2	106	5.2	73	4.6	2.2	-19.4
FRANCE									
Bas-Rhin	A1	-1.15	*0.9*	*2*	0.9	1	0.6	0.6	*13.4*
Doubs	*	..	..	..	..	..	..	..	..
GERMANY (FRG)									
Hamburg	A2D	1.82	1.6	8	*0.4*	*1*	0.8	*0.1*	–
Saarland	A1	-0.38	2.3	6	2.3	6	1.4	1.4	*11.8*
GERMANY (GDR)	A4P4C6	-0.87	7.1	315	2.9	107	3.0	0.7	-27.5
ITALY									
Varese	A8C7	0.11	*	*	4.1	7	3.6	0.7	*-23.1*
SPAIN									
Navarra	A2P2	0.41	*0.0*	*0*	14.1	19	6.5	*238.0*	111.0
Zaragoza	A5P2C3	-0.15	16.7	31	21.9	51	8.1	10.6	38.4
UK									
Birmingham	A8P5	0.51	2.0	26	0.4	5	0.8	0.1	-55.0
Scotland	A2P3	1.17	4.5	61	3.2	44	2.6	1.2	-17.7
South Thames	A2P3	-0.68	1.3	33	0.8	15	0.7	0.3	-29.1

* : not enough cases for reliable estimation
– : incomplete or missing data
Best model: polynomial of the given degree in age (A), period (P) or cohort (C), or linear drift (D) model.
Goodness of fit: the normalised likelihood ratio chi-square for the best model (see Method).
Rate: world-standardised truncated rate per 100 000 per year (30-74 years) and number of **cases** are both estimated from the best-fitting model for the single years cited.
Cumulative risk per 1000 (30-74 years) is estimated from the best-fitting *age-cohort* model for cohorts of central birth year cited.
Recent trend: estimated mean percentage change per five-year period in the age-specific rates (30-74 years) over the period 1973-1987.
Italics denote recent trends not significant at 5 per cent level, or other figures which should be interpreted with caution (see Method).

MALES

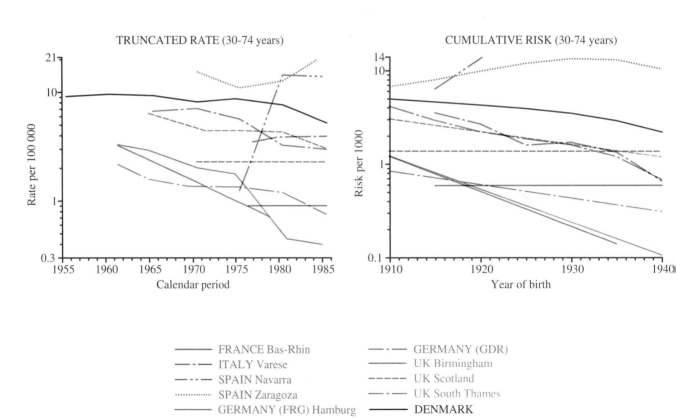

LIP (ICD-9 140)

EUROPE (EC), INCIDENCE
Percentage change per five-year period, 1973-1987

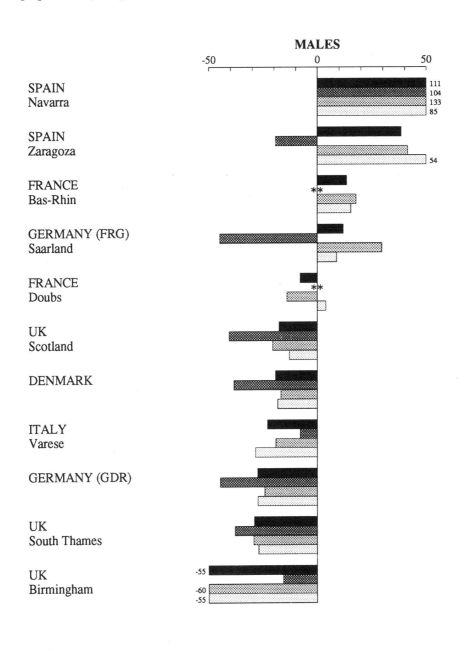

LIP (ICD-9 140)

EUROPE (non-EC), MORTALITY

MALES	Best model	Goodness of fit	1965 Rate	1965 Deaths	1985 Rate	1985 Deaths	Cumulative risk 1900	Cumulative risk 1940	Recent trend
AUSTRIA	A1D	0.47	0.3	5	0.1	2	0.2	0.1	*13.2*
CZECHOSLOVAKIA	A3	0.32	0.5	19	0.5	20	0.4	0.4	*8.6*
FINLAND	A1D	-0.30	0.8	7	0.2	2	0.6	0.0	*-21.0*
HUNGARY	A3D	0.14	*1.7*	42	1.1	31	*1.1*	0.5	*-9.5*
NORWAY	A1	-1.37	0.3	3	0.3	3	0.2	0.2	*0.4*
POLAND	A8D	-1.17	1.4	79	*2.4*	*181*	1.0	*3.0*	–
ROMANIA	–	–	–	–	–	–	–	–	–
SWEDEN	A1D	-0.26	0.1	3	0.1	2	0.1	0.0	*27.4*
SWITZERLAND	A3P2	-1.11	0.3	4	0.1	2	0.2	0.1	-39.3
YUGOSLAVIA	A2P2	0.93	0.5	17	0.6	31	0.4	0.6	*-3.6*

* : not enough deaths for reliable estimation
– : incomplete or missing data
Best model: polynomial of the given degree in age (A), period (P) or cohort (C), or linear drift (D) model.
Goodness of fit: the normalised likelihood ratio chi-square for the best model (see Method).
Rate: world-standardised truncated rate per 100 000 per year (30-74 years) and number of **deaths** are both estimated from the best-fitting model for the single years cited.
Cumulative risk per 1000 (30-74 years) is estimated from the best-fitting *age-cohort* model for cohorts of central birth year cited.
Recent trend: estimated mean percentage change per five-year period in the age-specific rates (30-74 years) over the period 1975-1988.
Italics denote recent trends not significant at 5 per cent level, or other figures which should be interpreted with caution (see Method).

MALES

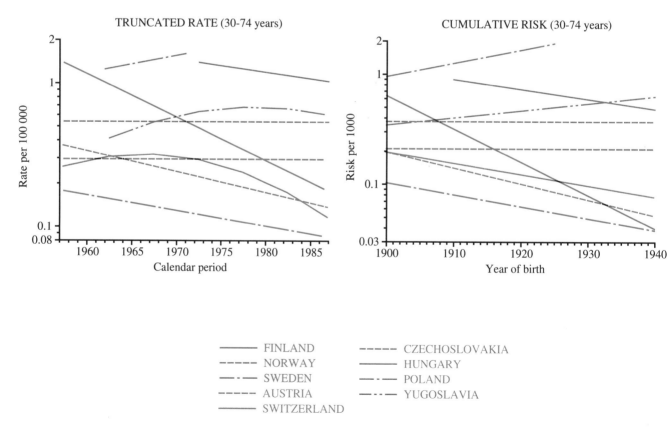

48

LIP (ICD-9 140)

EUROPE (non-EC), MORTALITY
Percentage change per five-year period, 1975-1988

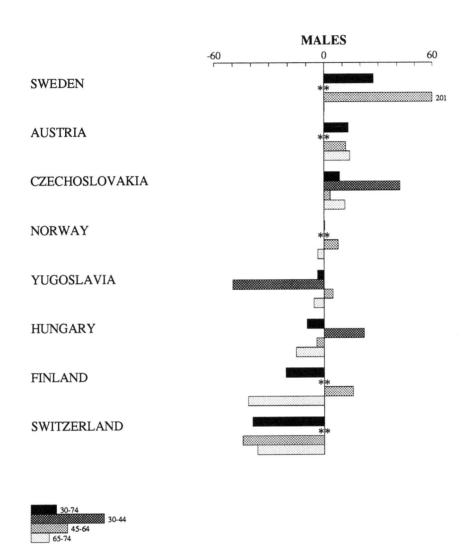

LIP (ICD-9 140)

EUROPE (EC), MORTALITY

MALES	Best model	Goodness of fit	1965 Rate	1965 Deaths	1985 Rate	1985 Deaths	Cumulative risk 1900	Cumulative risk 1940	Recent trend
BELGIUM	A1D	-0.60	0.4	9	0.2	4	0.3	0.1	*-15.7*
DENMARK	A1C2	0.97	0.3	4	0.2	3	0.2	0.0	*-15.4*
FRANCE	A2P2	0.00	0.4	55	0.2	26	0.3	0.1	-30.9
GERMANY (FRG)	A2P2	-1.46	0.3	42	0.1	21	0.2	0.1	-22.3
GREECE	A1	0.65	*0.3*	*4*	0.3	7	*0.2*	0.2	-28.6
IRELAND	A3D	-0.84	1.3	10	0.5	4	0.9	0.1	*-5.1*
ITALY	A2P6	1.17	0.8	97	0.5	77	0.5	0.1	*-5.2*
NETHERLANDS	A1D	1.31	0.2	6	0.1	3	0.1	0.0	-42.1
PORTUGAL	–	–	–	–	–	–	–	–	
SPAIN	A2D	1.10	0.7	45	0.4	36	0.4	0.1	-15.8
UK ENGLAND & WALES	A2C3	-1.16	0.2	25	0.1	13	0.1	0.0	-25.5
UK SCOTLAND	A1	-1.84	0.1	1	0.1	2	0.1	0.1	*23.4*

* : not enough deaths for reliable estimation
– : incomplete or missing data
Best model: polynomial of the given degree in age (A), period (P) or cohort (C), or linear drift (D) model.
Goodness of fit: the normalised likelihood ratio chi-square for the best model (see Method).
Rate: world-standardised truncated rate per 100 000 per year (30-74 years) and number of **deaths** are both estimated from the best-fitting model for the single years cited.
Cumulative risk per 1000 (30-74 years) is estimated from the best-fitting *age-cohort* model for cohorts of central birth year cited.
Recent trend: estimated mean percentage change per five-year period in the age-specific rates (30-74 years) over the period 1975-1988.
Italics denote recent trends not significant at 5 per cent level, or other figures which should be interpreted with caution (see Method).

MALES

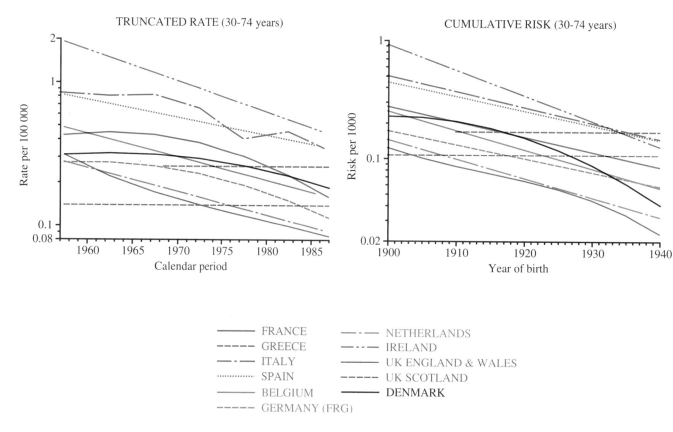

TRUNCATED RATE (30-74 years) — Rate per 100 000 — Calendar period

CUMULATIVE RISK (30-74 years) — Risk per 1000 — Year of birth

FRANCE   NETHERLANDS
GREECE   IRELAND
ITALY   UK ENGLAND & WALES
SPAIN   UK SCOTLAND
BELGIUM   DENMARK
GERMANY (FRG)

LIP (ICD-9 140)

EUROPE (EC), MORTALITY
Percentage change per five-year period, 1975-1988

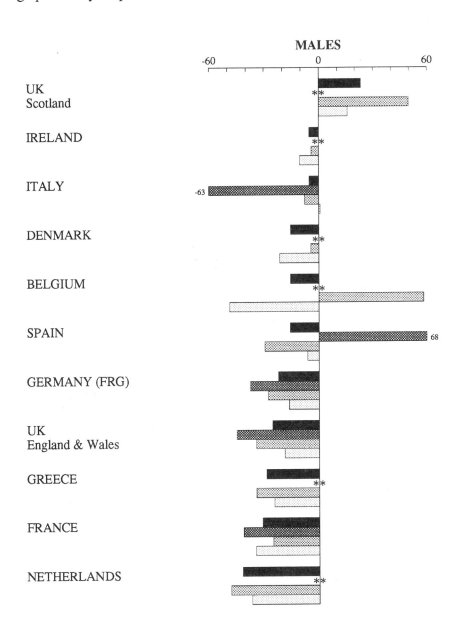

LIP (ICD-9 140)

ASIA, INCIDENCE

MALES	Best model	Goodness of fit	1970 Rate	Cases	1985 Rate	Cases	Cumulative risk 1915	1940	Recent trend
CHINA									
Shanghai	A1D	0.52	*1.4*	*12*	0.2	2	0.6	0.0	-51.7
HONG KONG	A2D	-0.73	*1.2*	*5*	0.3	2	0.5	0.0	-41.5
INDIA									
Bombay	A3	1.10	0.6	4	0.6	7	0.3	0.3	*28.3*
JAPAN									
Miyagi	A2	-1.15	*0.3*	*0*	0.3	1	0.2	0.2	*-8.1*
Nagasaki	A0	-1.43	*0.3*	*0*	*0.3*	*0*	0.1	0.1	*
Osaka	A1	-0.18	0.1	1	0.1	2	0.1	0.1	*-15.1*
SINGAPORE									
Chinese	A1	-1.57	*0.2*	*0*	*0.2*	*0*	0.1	0.1	*37.2*
Indian	–	–	–	–	–	–	–	–	–
Malay	*	..	..	..	..	..	..	..	..

* : not enough cases for reliable estimation
– : incomplete or missing data
Best model: polynomial of the given degree in age (A), period (P) or cohort (C), or linear drift (D) model.
Goodness of fit: the normalised likelihood ratio chi-square for the best model (see Method).
Rate: world-standardised truncated rate per 100 000 per year (30-74 years) and number of **cases** are both estimated from the best-fitting model for the single years cited.
Cumulative risk per 1000 (30-74 years) is estimated from the best-fitting *age-cohort* model for cohorts of central birth year cited.
Recent trend: estimated mean percentage change per five-year period in the age-specific rates (30-74 years) over the period 1973-1987.
Italics denote recent trends not significant at 5 per cent level, or other figures which should be interpreted with caution (see Method).

MALES

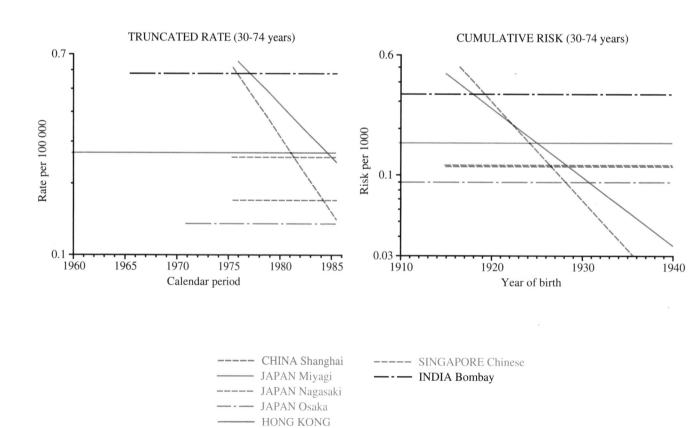

TRUNCATED RATE (30-74 years)   CUMULATIVE RISK (30-74 years)

----- CHINA Shanghai   ----- SINGAPORE Chinese
——— JAPAN Miyagi   —·— INDIA Bombay
----- JAPAN Nagasaki
—·— JAPAN Osaka
——— HONG KONG

LIP (ICD-9 140)

ASIA, INCIDENCE
Percentage change per five-year period, 1973-1987

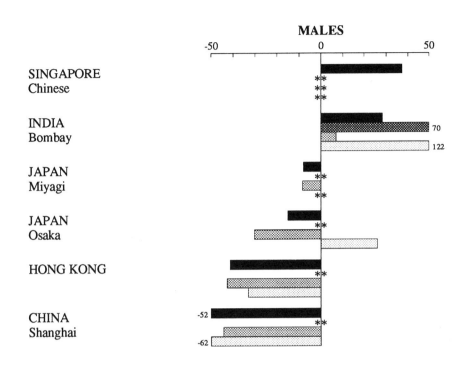

MALES

SINGAPORE
Chinese

INDIA
Bombay

JAPAN
Miyagi

JAPAN
Osaka

HONG KONG

CHINA
Shanghai

30-74
30-44
45-64
65-74

LIP (ICD-9 140)

OCEANIA, INCIDENCE

MALES	Best model	Goodness of fit	1970 Rate	1970 Cases	1985 Rate	1985 Cases	Cumulative risk 1915	Cumulative risk 1940	Recent trend
AUSTRALIA									
New South Wales	A2D	0.29	*10.8*	*111*	8.0	105	5.5	3.4	-9.4
South	A2D	0.69	*9.8*	*21*	25.7	87	8.9	43.7	38.9
HAWAII									
Caucasian	A8	0.54	5.7	2	5.7	3	2.6	2.6	*21.8*
Chinese	–	–	–	–	–	–	–	–	–
Filipino	–	–	–	–	–	–	–	–	–
Hawaiian	–	–	–	–	–	–	–	–	–
Japanese	*	..	..	..	..	..	..	..	..
NEW ZEALAND									
Maori	*	..	..	..	..	..	..	..	..
Non-Maori	A3P4	-0.28	5.6	31	8.5	58	3.2	5.1	33.4

* : not enough cases for reliable estimation
– : incomplete or missing data
Best model: polynomial of the given degree in age (A), period (P) or cohort (C), or linear drift (D) model.
Goodness of fit: the normalised likelihood ratio chi-square for the best model (see Method).
Rate: world-standardised truncated rate per 100 000 per year (30-74 years) and number of **cases** are both estimated from the best-fitting model for the single years cited.
Cumulative risk per 1000 (30-74 years) is estimated from the best-fitting *age-cohort* model for cohorts of central birth year cited.
Recent trend: estimated mean percentage change per five-year period in the age-specific rates (30-74 years) over the period 1973-1987.
Italics denote recent trends not significant at 5 per cent level, or other figures which should be interpreted with caution (see Method).

MALES

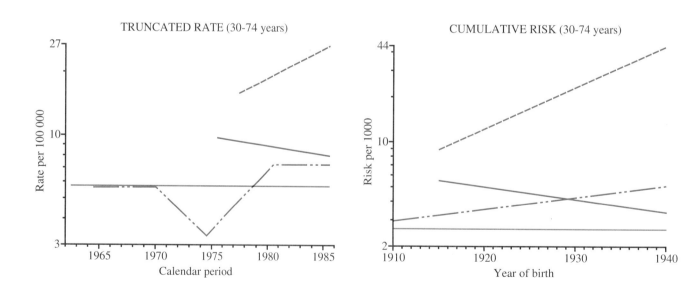

AUSTRALIA New South Wales
AUSTRALIA South
NEW ZEALAND Non-Maori
HAWAII Caucasian

54

LIP (ICD-9 140)

OCEANIA, INCIDENCE
Percentage change per five-year period, 1973-1987

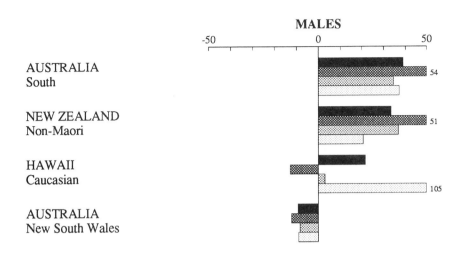

LIP (ICD-9 140)

ASIA and OCEANIA, MORTALITY

MALES	Best model	Goodness of fit	1965 Rate	Deaths	1985 Rate	Deaths	Cumulative risk 1900	1940	Recent trend
AUSTRALIA	A2D	-0.25	0.3	8	0.2	8	0.2	0.1	*-6.1*
HONG KONG	*	..	..	..	..	..	..	..	..
JAPAN	A3D	-0.42	0.0	6	0.0	5	0.0	0.0	*0.9*
MAURITIUS	A0	-1.50	*0.2*	*0*	*0.2*	*0*	*0.1*	0.1	*
NEW ZEALAND	A1	0.32	0.3	1	0.3	2	0.2	0.2	*8.4*
SINGAPORE	*	..	..	..	..	..	..	..	..

* : not enough deaths for reliable estimation
− : incomplete or missing data
Best model: polynomial of the given degree in age (A), period (P) or cohort (C), or linear drift (D) model.
Goodness of fit: the normalised likelihood ratio chi-square for the best model (see Method).
Rate: world-standardised truncated rate per 100 000 per year (30-74 years) and number of **deaths** are both estimated from the best-fitting model for the single years cited.
Cumulative risk per 1000 (30-74 years) is estimated from the best-fitting *age-cohort* model for cohorts of central birth year cited.
Recent trend: estimated mean percentage change per five-year period in the age-specific rates (30-74 years) over the period 1975-1988.
Italics denote recent trends not significant at 5 per cent level, or other figures which should be interpreted with caution (see Method).

MALES

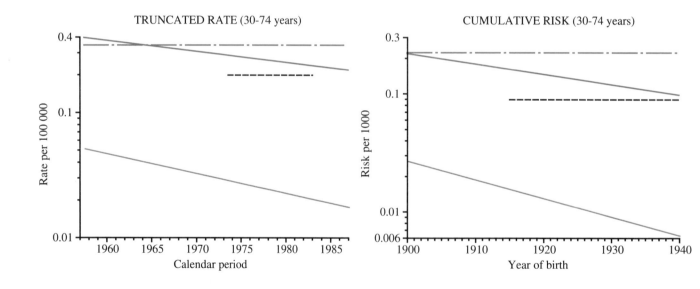

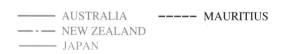

56

LIP (ICD-9 140)

ASIA and OCEANIA, MORTALITY
Percentage change per five-year period, 1975-1988

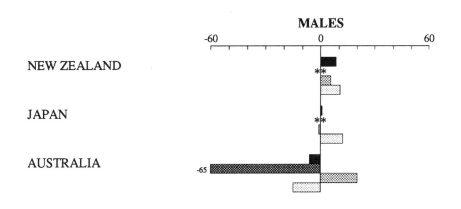

LIP (ICD-9 140)

AMERICAS (except USA), INCIDENCE

MALES	Best model	Goodness of fit	1970 Rate	1970 Cases	1985 Rate	1985 Cases	Cumulative risk 1915	Cumulative risk 1940	Recent trend
BRAZIL									
Sao Paulo	A2	-0.74	7.5	60	*7.5*	72	3.3	*3.3*	–
CANADA									
Alberta	A2C2	0.35	23.8	73	12.7	56	12.6	3.0	-16.4
British Columbia	A4P3C2	1.21	6.9	32	4.4	31	6.0	1.0	-35.4
Maritime Provinces	A2P2	0.36	22.1	70	9.3	33	9.0	2.3	-18.4
Newfoundland	A2P2	-0.15	51.4	44	20.7	23	20.8	10.9	-33.1
Quebec	A3P3C2	-0.15	9.3	100	4.7	67	5.0	1.0	-27.5
COLOMBIA									
Cali	A1P3	0.04	*1.4*	*0*	*0.4*	*0*	1.0	0.2	-41.6
CUBA	A2P2	-0.09	5.1	76	4.6	93	2.7	*2.5*	–
PUERTO RICO	A1D	1.70	2.8	12	1.4	9	1.3	0.4	-27.2

* : not enough cases for reliable estimation
– : incomplete or missing data
Best model: polynomial of the given degree in age (A), period (P) or cohort (C), or linear drift (D) model.
Goodness of fit: the normalised likelihood ratio chi-square for the best model (see Method).
Rate: world-standardised truncated rate per 100 000 per year (30-74 years) and number of **cases** are both estimated from the best-fitting model for the single years cited.
Cumulative risk per 1000 (30-74 years) is estimated from the best-fitting *age-cohort* model for cohorts of central birth year cited.
Recent trend: estimated mean percentage change per five-year period in the age-specific rates (30-74 years) over the period 1973-1987.
Italics denote recent trends not significant at 5 per cent level, or other figures which should be interpreted with caution (see Method).

MALES

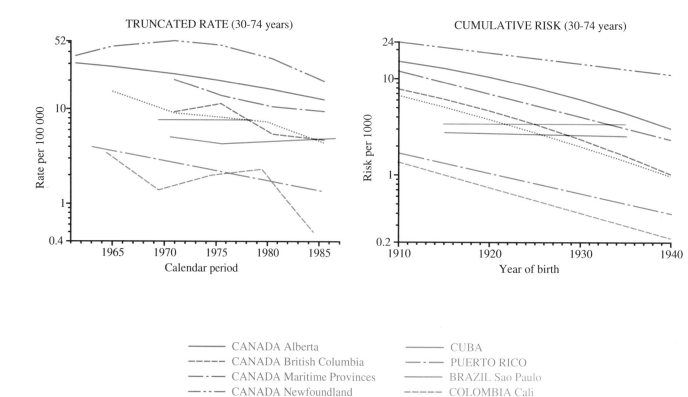

TRUNCATED RATE (30-74 years)

CUMULATIVE RISK (30-74 years)

———— CANADA Alberta
------ CANADA British Columbia
—·— CANADA Maritime Provinces
—··— CANADA Newfoundland
·········· CANADA Quebec
———— CUBA
—·— PUERTO RICO
———— BRAZIL Sao Paulo
------ COLOMBIA Cali

LIP (ICD-9 140)

AMERICAS (except USA), INCIDENCE
Percentage change per five-year period, 1973-1987

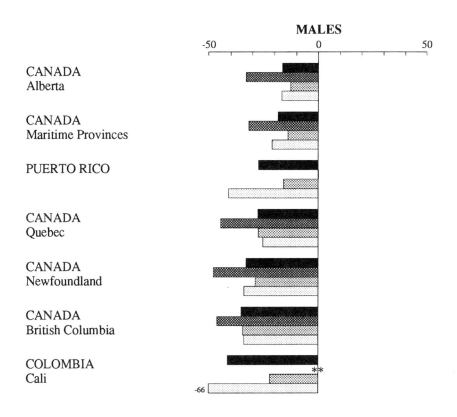

LIP (ICD-9 140)

AMERICAS (USA), INCIDENCE

MALES	Best model	Goodness of fit	1970 Rate	1970 Cases	1985 Rate	1985 Cases	Cumulative risk 1915	Cumulative risk 1940	Recent trend
USA									
Bay Area, Black	*	..	..	..	..	..	..	..	..
Bay Area, Chinese	–	–	–	–	–	–	–	–	–
Bay Area, White	A2C2	1.88	7.7	45	3.3	20	4.1	0.7	-28.6
Connecticut	A1P2	0.49	3.9	25	1.2	9	1.6	0.4	-34.8
Detroit, Black	A0	-1.16	0.2	0	0.2	0	0.1	0.1	*
Detroit, White	A2P3	0.75	2.0	15	2.0	14	1.5	1.0	-17.2
Iowa	A2D	0.44	9.9	66	8.3	57	5.5	4.1	-2.7
New Orleans, Black	A1D	-2.16	26.0	13	0.0	0	996.1	0.1	*
New Orleans, White	A2	-0.29	4.6	6	4.6	7	2.4	2.4	-19.5
Seattle	A2P2	2.02	32.0	153	3.3	21	3.8	0.7	-28.8

* : not enough cases for reliable estimation
– : incomplete or missing data
Best model: polynomial of the given degree in age (A), period (P) or cohort (C), or linear drift (D) model.
Goodness of fit: the normalised likelihood ratio chi-square for the best model (see Method).
Rate: world-standardised truncated rate per 100 000 per year (30-74 years) and number of **cases** are both estimated from the best-fitting model for the single years cited.
Cumulative risk per 1000 (30-74 years) is estimated from the best-fitting *age-cohort* model for cohorts of central birth year cited.
Recent trend: estimated mean percentage change per five-year period in the age-specific rates (30-74 years) over the period 1973-1987.
Italics denote recent trends not significant at 5 per cent level, or other figures which should be interpreted with caution (see Method).

MALES

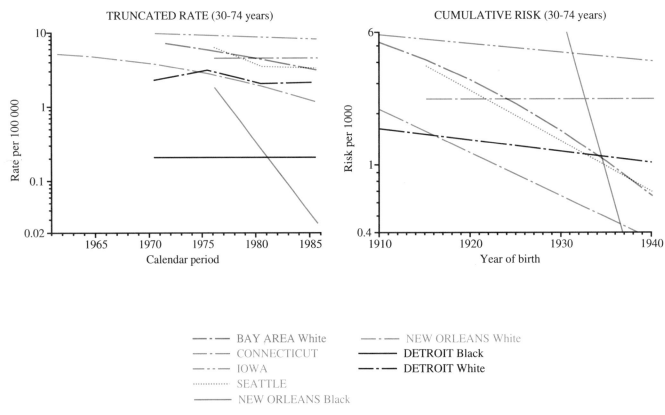

TRUNCATED RATE (30-74 years)

CUMULATIVE RISK (30-74 years)

—·— BAY AREA White   —·— NEW ORLEANS White
—·— CONNECTICUT   —— DETROIT Black
—··— IOWA   —··— DETROIT White
············ SEATTLE
—— NEW ORLEANS Black

60

LIP (ICD-9 140)

AMERICAS (USA), INCIDENCE
Percentage change per five-year period, 1973-1987

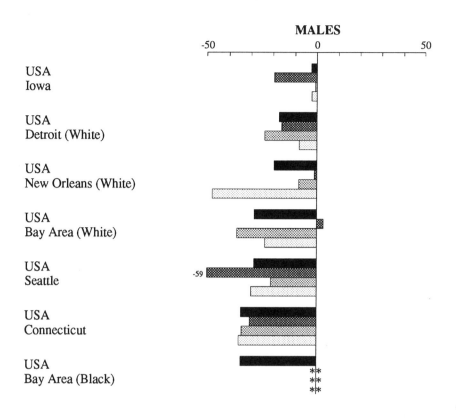

LIP (ICD-9 140)

AMERICAS, MORTALITY

MALES	Best model	Goodness of fit	1965		1985		Cumulative risk		Recent trend
			Rate	Deaths	Rate	Deaths	1900	1940	
CANADA	A5D	1.42	0.5	18	0.2	9	0.3	0.0	-42.5
CHILE	A1	0.27	0.2	2	*0.2*	*3*	0.1	*0.1*	–
COSTA RICA	–	–	–	–	–	–	–	–	–
PANAMA	–	–	–	–	–	–	–	–	–
PUERTO RICO	–	–	–	–	–	–	–	–	–
URUGUAY	–	–	–	–	–	–	–	–	–
USA	A2P6	0.31	0.2	80	0.1	53	0.2	0.0	-28.7
VENEZUELA	A2D	-1.04	0.2	1	*0.1*	*1*	0.2	*0.0*	–

* : not enough deaths for reliable estimation
− : incomplete or missing data
Best model: polynomial of the given degree in age (A), period (P) or cohort (C), or linear drift (D) model.
Goodness of fit: the normalised likelihood ratio chi-square for the best model (see Method).
Rate: world-standardised truncated rate per 100 000 per year (30-74 years) and number of **deaths** are both estimated from the best-fitting model for the single years cited.
Cumulative risk per 1000 (30-74 years) is estimated from the best-fitting *age-cohort* model for cohorts of central birth year cited.
Recent trend: estimated mean percentage change per five-year period in the age-specific rates (30-74 years) over the period 1975-1988.
Italics denote recent trends not significant at 5 per cent level, or other figures which should be interpreted with caution (see Method).

MALES

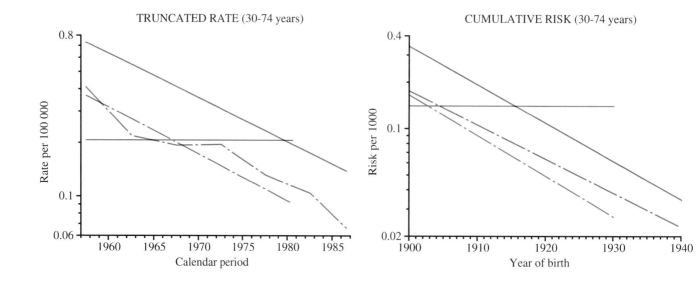

LIP (ICD-9 140)

AMERICAS, MORTALITY
Percentage change per five-year period, 1975-1988

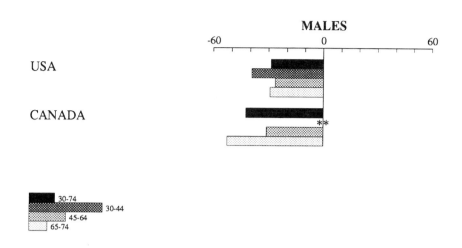

from page 43

rate of 20.8 per 100 000 is of the same order of magnitude as in South Australia and Spain. The rate has also decreased in Puerto Rico and Cali (Colombia) where it was already low (less than 3 per 100 000 in 1970); incidence did not change substantially in Cuba, nor in São Paulo (Brazil), where it remains moderately high on a world scale (5-10 per 100 000).

In the USA, incidence has decreased regularly on a period basis in Connecticut, and on a cohort basis among Bay Area whites. The decrease is more modest elsewhere, especially in the higher-risk region of Iowa, where the rate is still more than 8 per 100 000 per year. The rate among blacks is very low (less than 0.5 per 100 000); the large negative slope observed for blacks in New Orleans is the effect of small numbers: no case was observed in the age range 30-74 years in the period 1983-87.

Mortality from cancer of the lip of has decreased substantially in the USA, Canada, and Venezuela over the period of study. The truncated rate

was already lower in Chile than in Venezuela in 1957, and this may be partly responsible for the absence of a significant trend in Chile.

Comment

Few other reports on trends in lip cancer are available. There was a marked decline in squamous cell carcinoma (but not basal cell carcinoma) of the lip in males in south-east Netherlands during the period 1975-88. Little change was seen among females[57]. The decline in lip cancer mortality in the Federal Republic of Germany between 1952 and 1986 has also been noted[209], together with an increase in mortality from other cancers in the oral cavity. In Connecticut (USA), age-adjusted incidence of lip cancer in males fell five-fold during the period 1935-85, but did not change for females[52], and the overall male-to-female ratio fell from 15.0 to 6.0.

Chapter 6

TONGUE

Cancer of the tongue represents about 20% of cancers of the buccal cavity. The cumulative risk (30-74 years) is of the order of 1% in high-risk countries and less than one in a thousand in low-risk countries. The highest risks occur in Indian populations and among males in France and Switzerland. The sex ratio is of the order of 3 in India, 8 in Geneva (Switzerland) and 13 in Bas-Rhin (France). The main risk factors are tobacco (especially pipe) smoking, tobacco and betel chewing, and alcohol. Overall survival from cancer of the tongue is still mediocre (relative survival at five years is usually less than 50%), but it could be much higher if tumours were diagnosed at an early stage. It has been suggested that secondary prevention (screening) for cancer of the tongue should be evaluated.

Europe

There is no doubt that the frequency of cancer of the tongue is increasing in Europe, but it is difficult to estimate the rate of change with precision, since the number of cases recorded each year is small in most registry populations, especially for females.

For males, the recent linear trends are systematically positive, except in Doubs (France) and Varese (Italy). The small upward trend in Finland is not significant, although the estimate is based on more than 15 cases per year. The trends are often best described by an age-cohort model, or by an exponential increase (age-drift model). The most impressive rates of increase are seen in Germany, Scotland and Denmark, where recent linear trends have been 30% or more every five years for males and 10% or more for females. Sizeable increases are also observed in other Scandinavian countries, and in Slovenia. In Birmingham and South Thames (UK), the period effects are similar, but in Birmingham the risk has started to decrease again for cohorts born after 1930. In Geneva (Switzerland), where the risk among males is high (1.8%), the rate of increase is rapid (22% every five years), but the population is small, and the trend is based on relatively small numbers of cases each year. Similarly, in eastern countries of Europe other than Slovenia, the rates of increase are high or even very high, but they are based on small numbers of cases, and the age-specific trends are unstable.

In females, the trends are difficult to evaluate because of the lack of precision, except in Denmark, the German Democratic Republic and in South Thames (UK), where the population at risk is large (over 1.5 million), the risk is high, and there has been a rapid change. There are large and continuing increases in Denmark and the GDR among successive birth cohorts, while there is a marked period effect in South Thames, with a small recent decline. The rapid trends in Spain are unstable.

Because the mortality data are based on larger numbers of events, and are statistically more precise, the pattern of trends reveals more international contrast, especially for females. The risk of dying from cancer of the tongue is increasing in most European countries: the trends for male cohorts born after 1930 are strongly positive in Belgium, Germany, Spain, Denmark and eastern European countries, and moderately so in Switzerland, Italy, the Netherlands, the UK, and Sweden, but negative in Norway, France and Ireland. However, there are often strong period effects in the best models, and the predictions which can be made from even the best age-cohort models may not be reliable.

Among females, the pattern of mortality may be summarised by a decrease in Sweden, Finland, and Scotland; a moderate increase or little change in England and Wales and the south of Europe, and an increase in eastern European countries. The data also show that in France, where tongue cancer risk has been the highest in Europe, the increase in mortality among females has stopped, or may even have reversed for those born after 1930.

Asia and Oceania

The risk of tongue cancer in Bombay (India) is much higher than in other Asian populations, and is similar to the higher levels seen in Europe, although the underlying causes are more related to tobacco and betel chewing than to alcohol, the chief cause in Europe. There has been a notable decrease in risk among both males and females in Bombay in successive birth cohorts, and the lifetime risk for males in the 1940 birth cohort is now less than 5%, less than half the risk for the 1915 birth cohort. Recent linear trends suggest a conti-

continued page 86

TONGUE (ICD-9 141)

EUROPE (non-EC), INCIDENCE

MALES	Best model	Goodness of fit	1970 Rate	1970 Cases	1985 Rate	1985 Cases	Cumulative risk 1915	Cumulative risk 1940	Recent trend
FINLAND	A2	-0.60	1.6	16	1.6	19	0.9	0.9	*12.0*
HUNGARY									
County Vas	A8C9	0.33	1.3	1	8.7	5	2.7	99.9	200.5
Szabolcs-Szatmar	A2D	0.86	1.9	2	7.7	10	2.1	22.4	66.1
ISRAEL									
All Jews	A1D	0.28	0.9	4	1.6	9	0.8	2.0	*11.2*
Non-Jews	A1	-1.10	*1.0*	*0*	*1.0*	*0*	0.6	0.6	*42.6*
NORWAY	A2C5	-0.34	1.7	17	2.6	29	1.1	2.4	18.8
POLAND									
Warsaw City	A2D	-0.07	2.2	6	3.9	15	1.6	3.9	*16.8*
ROMANIA									
Cluj	A1D	-0.01	*0.5*	*0*	2.0	3	0.7	6.4	*52.5*
SWEDEN	A2D	-0.91	1.3	31	2.1	51	1.0	2.1	14.2
SWITZERLAND									
Geneva	A8C8	0.23	6.0	4	10.3	9	2.8	18.7	*21.9*
YUGOSLAVIA									
Slovenia	A2D	-0.11	4.6	16	9.5	41	3.5	11.5	18.5

FEMALES	Best model	Goodness of fit	1970 Rate	1970 Cases	1985 Rate	1985 Cases	Cumulative risk 1915	Cumulative risk 1940	Recent trend
FINLAND	A1	0.89	1.0	12	1.0	14	0.6	0.6	*-10.7*
HUNGARY									
County Vas	*	..	..	..	..	..	..	..	..
Szabolcs-Szatmar	*	..	..	..	..	..	..	..	..
ISRAEL									
All Jews	A1	0.52	0.8	3	0.8	4	0.5	0.5	*3.8*
Non-Jews	A0C2	-1.99	*3.3*	*0*	*0.2*	*0*	19.3	0.1	*
NORWAY	A1C2	0.26	0.7	8	1.0	12	0.5	1.2	25.3
POLAND									
Warsaw City	A1	-1.17	0.6	2	0.6	3	0.4	0.4	*15.6*
ROMANIA									
Cluj	A2C2	-2.54	*7.0*	*13*	0.6	1	0.5	3.6	*-7.5*
SWEDEN	A8P5C9	0.47	0.6	16	0.9	23	0.4	0.7	*2.4*
SWITZERLAND									
Geneva	A2	0.03	1.5	1	1.5	1	0.8	0.8	*-17.9*
YUGOSLAVIA									
Slovenia	A1D	0.37	0.4	2	0.7	3	0.3	0.7	68.7

* : not enough cases for reliable estimation
– : incomplete or missing data
Best model: polynomial of the given degree in age (A), period (P) or cohort (C), or linear drift (D) model.
Goodness of fit: the normalised likelihood ratio chi-square for the best model (see Method).
Rate: world-standardised truncated rate per 100 000 per year (30-74 years) and number of **cases** are both estimated from the best-fitting model for the single years cited.
Cumulative risk per 1000 (30-74 years) is estimated from the best-fitting *age-cohort* model for cohorts of central birth year cited.
Recent trend: estimated mean percentage change per five-year period in the age-specific rates (30-74 years) over the period 1973-1987.
Italics denote recent trends not significant at 5 per cent level, or other figures which should be interpreted with caution (see Method).

TONGUE (ICD-9 141)

EUROPE (non-EC), INCIDENCE

MALES

TRUNCATED RATE (30-74 years)

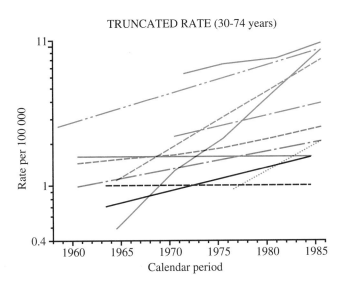

CUMULATIVE RISK (30-74 years)

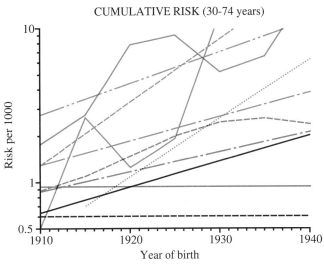

FEMALES

TRUNCATED RATE (30-74 years)

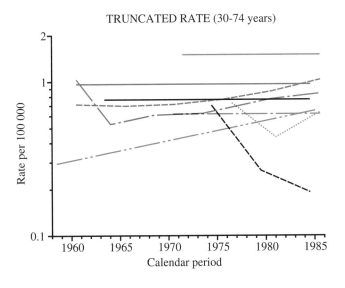

CUMULATIVE RISK (30-74 years)

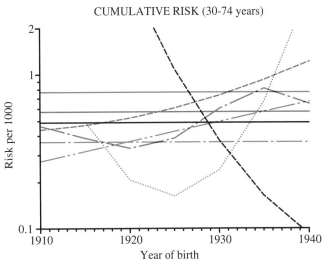

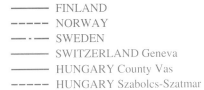

—— FINLAND	—·—· POLAND Warsaw City
----- NORWAY	········· ROMANIA Cluj
—··—·· SWEDEN	—···—··· YUGOSLAVIA Slovenia
—— SWITZERLAND Geneva	—— ISRAEL All Jews
—— HUNGARY County Vas	----- ISRAEL Non-Jews
----- HUNGARY Szabolcs-Szatmar	

TONGUE (ICD-9 141)

EUROPE (EC), INCIDENCE

MALES	Best model	Goodness of fit	1970 Rate	1970 Cases	1985 Rate	1985 Cases	Cumulative risk 1915	Cumulative risk 1940	Recent trend
DENMARK	A2P2C4	2.11	0.9	12	2.2	29	0.7	3.1	41.2
FRANCE									
Bas-Rhin	A3D	-0.95	*11.4*	*23*	22.2	45	7.4	22.2	25.1
Doubs	A3C2	-0.11	*36.3*	*21*	15.5	16	10.0	10.0	*-6.7*
GERMANY (FRG)									
Hamburg	A1D	-0.55	2.0	10	*3.1*	*12*	1.4	*3.0*	–
Saarland	A3C2	1.22	4.1	11	9.4	26	2.7	14.1	40.6
GERMANY (GDR)	A4C3	0.63	1.0	42	3.1	118	0.8	7.7	51.5
ITALY									
Varese	A2	1.01	*6.5*	*10*	6.5	13	3.5	3.5	*-8.1*
SPAIN									
Navarra	A2	0.63	*4.7*	*5*	4.7	6	2.4	2.4	*13.6*
Zaragoza	A2P2C2	1.17	4.6	8	8.0	17	1.8	11.7	60.2
UK									
Birmingham	A2P2C5	0.11	1.7	22	2.1	30	1.0	0.9	19.0
Scotland	A2C3	1.06	1.5	19	2.7	35	1.0	4.9	36.5
South Thames	A2P2C3	-1.00	1.4	35	1.9	34	0.9	1.3	17.1

FEMALES	Best model	Goodness of fit	1970 Rate	1970 Cases	1985 Rate	1985 Cases	Cumulative risk 1915	Cumulative risk 1940	Recent trend
DENMARK	A2C3	0.81	0.6	8	1.0	15	0.4	1.3	30.6
FRANCE									
Bas-Rhin	A1	0.16	*1.6*	*4*	1.6	3	0.8	0.8	*11.6*
Doubs	A2C3	-2.23	*7.5*	*7*	1.4	1	7.0	0.2	*-8.8*
GERMANY (FRG)									
Hamburg	A1	0.16	0.8	5	*0.8*	*3*	0.4	*0.4*	–
Saarland	A2	0.25	1.1	3	1.1	3	0.6	0.6	*22.3*
GERMANY (GDR)	A2D	-0.81	0.4	25	0.6	30	0.3	0.5	16.5
ITALY									
Varese	A1	0.08	*0.7*	*1*	0.7	1	0.4	0.4	*32.4*
SPAIN									
Navarra	A0	0.09	*0.5*	*0*	*0.5*	*0*	0.2	0.2	*-28.1*
Zaragoza	A1D	-0.66	*0.3*	*0*	1.2	3	0.6	7.2	*51.3*
UK									
Birmingham	A2	0.11	0.8	12	0.8	13	0.5	0.5	*-0.1*
Scotland	A3	-0.35	1.0	17	1.0	17	0.6	0.6	*10.1*
South Thames	A2P3	0.06	0.8	23	0.9	18	0.5	0.6	*-6.7*

* : not enough cases for reliable estimation
– : incomplete or missing data
Best model: polynomial of the given degree in age (A), period (P) or cohort (C), or linear drift (D) model.
Goodness of fit: the normalised likelihood ratio chi-square for the best model (see Method).
Rate: world-standardised truncated rate per 100 000 per year (30-74 years) and number of **cases** are both estimated from the best-fitting model for the single years cited.
Cumulative risk per 1000 (30-74 years) is estimated from the best-fitting *age-cohort* model for cohorts of central birth year cited.
Recent trend: estimated mean percentage change per five-year period in the age-specific rates (30-74 years) over the period 1973-1987.
Italics denote recent trends not significant at 5 per cent level, or other figures which should be interpreted with caution (see Method).

TONGUE (ICD-9 141)

EUROPE (EC), INCIDENCE

MALES

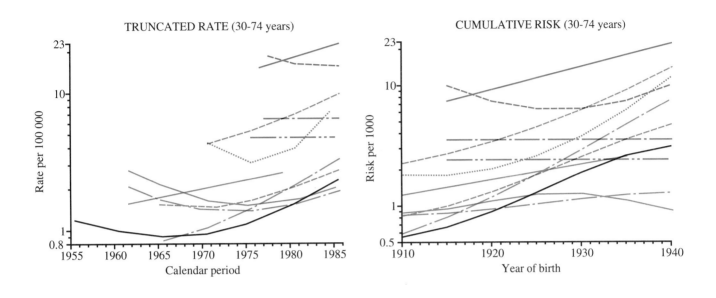

TRUNCATED RATE (30-74 years) — Rate per 100 000 / Calendar period

CUMULATIVE RISK (30-74 years) — Risk per 1000 / Year of birth

FEMALES

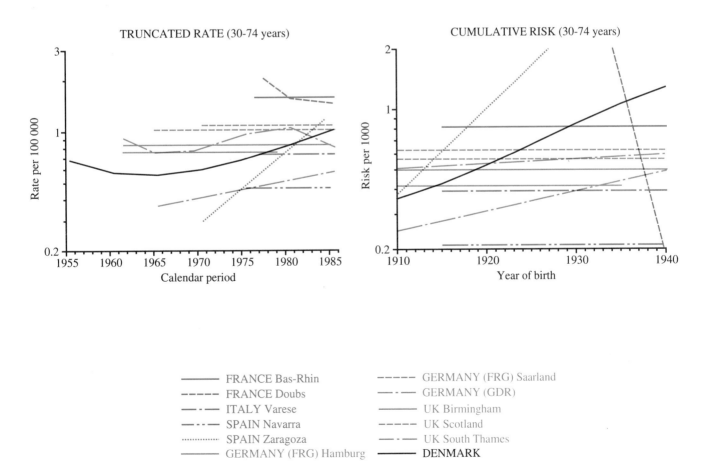

TRUNCATED RATE (30-74 years) — Rate per 100 000 / Calendar period

CUMULATIVE RISK (30-74 years) — Risk per 1000 / Year of birth

——— FRANCE Bas-Rhin	– – – GERMANY (FRG) Saarland
– – – FRANCE Doubs	–·–·– GERMANY (GDR)
–·–·– ITALY Varese	——— UK Birmingham
–··–··– SPAIN Navarra	– – – UK Scotland
············ SPAIN Zaragoza	–·–·– UK South Thames
——— GERMANY (FRG) Hamburg	——— DENMARK

TONGUE (ICD-9 141)

EUROPE (non-EC), INCIDENCE
Percentage change per five-year period, 1973-1987

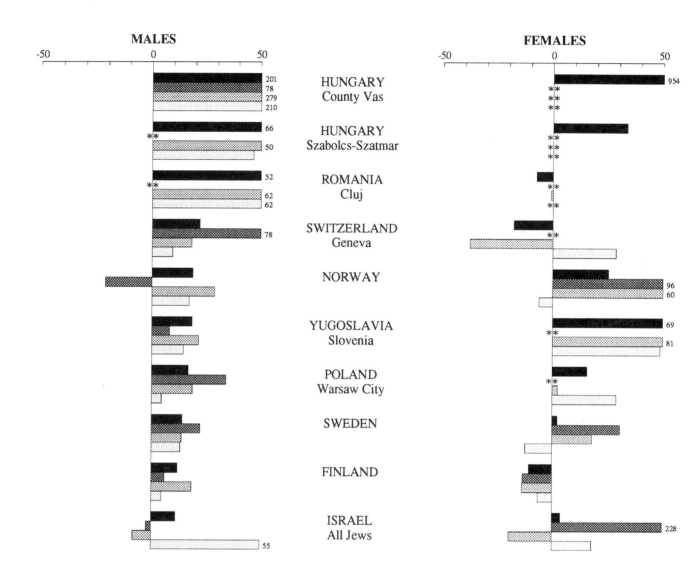

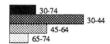

TONGUE (ICD-9 141)

EUROPE (EC), INCIDENCE
Percentage change per five-year period, 1973-1987

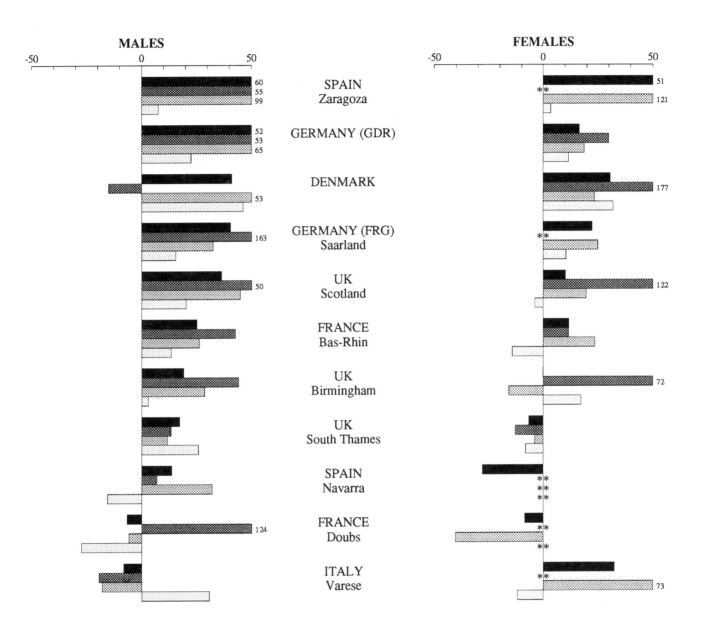

TONGUE (ICD-9 141)

EUROPE (non-EC), MORTALITY

MALES	Best model	Goodness of fit	1965 Rate	1965 Deaths	1985 Rate	1985 Deaths	Cumulative risk 1900	Cumulative risk 1940	Recent trend
AUSTRIA	A4P4C6	1.31	1.4	27	3.6	64	1.1	6.9	9.3
CZECHOSLOVAKIA	A3P5C2	0.34	0.8	28	3.7	130	0.5	14.2	44.4
FINLAND	A2C2	-0.75	0.8	7	0.9	10	0.5	0.7	*10.4*
HUNGARY	A3C2	3.11	*1.9*	*50*	7.8	208	*1.1*	26.1	55.3
NORWAY	A8C9	0.49	0.9	9	1.0	12	0.5	0.2	*4.5*
POLAND	A2D	-0.17	0.6	37	*1.5*	*120*	0.3	*2.2*	–
ROMANIA	*	..	..	..	..	..	..	..	..
SWEDEN	A2D	-1.51	0.6	13	1.0	24	0.4	1.0	*4.4*
SWITZERLAND	A8P6C9	-0.53	1.2	16	2.9	48	1.0	4.1	*-5.1*
YUGOSLAVIA	A3P4C2	1.85	1.0	35	3.5	179	0.6	7.6	26.9

FEMALES	Best model	Goodness of fit	1965 Rate	1965 Deaths	1985 Rate	1985 Deaths	Cumulative risk 1900	Cumulative risk 1940	Recent trend
AUSTRIA	A4C2	0.15	0.2	6	0.4	10	0.1	0.7	31.3
CZECHOSLOVAKIA	A1P4	2.38	0.1	5	0.3	15	0.1	0.3	*12.9*
FINLAND	A2D	-0.89	0.5	6	0.3	5	0.3	0.1	*-24.4*
HUNGARY	A8C8	-0.37	*0.1*	*3*	0.6	18	*0.0*	1.7	34.5
NORWAY	A1	0.81	0.3	4	0.3	4	0.2	0.2	*16.7*
POLAND	A2	0.02	0.1	9	*0.1*	*12*	0.1	*0.1*	–
ROMANIA	*	..	..	..	..	..	..	..	..
SWEDEN	A1D	1.52	0.4	9	0.2	7	0.2	0.1	*3.0*
SWITZERLAND	A1C3	0.69	0.3	4	0.4	8	0.1	0.3	*-0.2*
YUGOSLAVIA	A2D	1.05	0.1	5	0.4	22	0.1	0.7	38.7

* : not enough deaths for reliable estimation
– : incomplete or missing data
Best model: polynomial of the given degree in age (A), period (P) or cohort (C), or linear drift (D) model.
Goodness of fit: the normalised likelihood ratio chi-square for the best model (see Method).
Rate: world-standardised truncated rate per 100 000 per year (30-74 years) and number of **deaths** are both estimated from the best-fitting model for the single years cited.
Cumulative risk per 1000 (30-74 years) is estimated from the best-fitting *age-cohort* model for cohorts of central birth year cited.
Recent trend: estimated mean percentage change per five-year period in the age-specific rates (30-74 years) over the period 1975-1988.
Italics denote recent trends not significant at 5 per cent level, or other figures which should be interpreted with caution (see Method).

TONGUE (ICD-9 141)

EUROPE (non-EC), MORTALITY

MALES

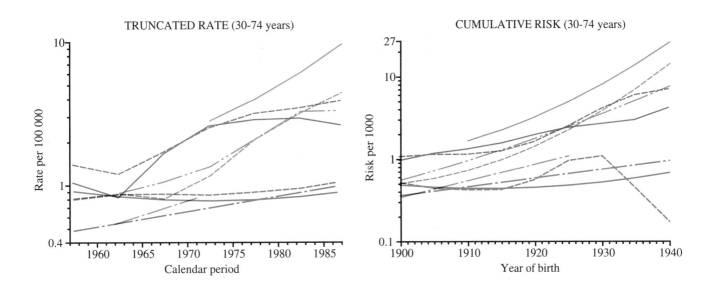

FEMALES

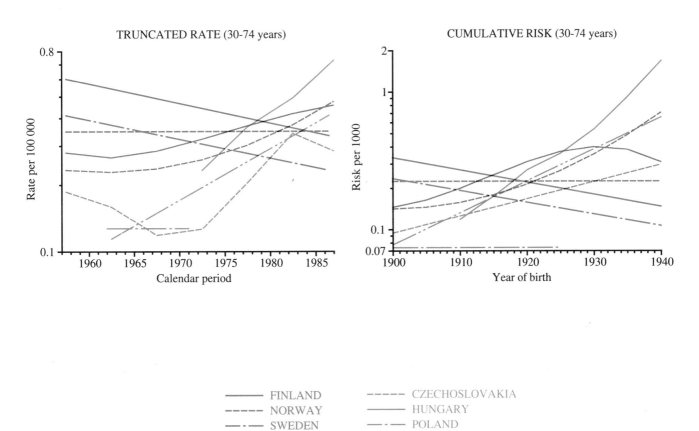

—— FINLAND	----- CZECHOSLOVAKIA	
----- NORWAY	—— HUNGARY	
—·— SWEDEN	—·— POLAND	
---- AUSTRIA	—··— YUGOSLAVIA	
—— SWITZERLAND		

TONGUE (ICD-9 141)

EUROPE (EC), MORTALITY

MALES	Best model	Goodness of fit	1965 Rate	1965 Deaths	1985 Rate	1985 Deaths	Cumulative risk 1900	Cumulative risk 1940	Recent trend
BELGIUM	A8C9	0.89	0.9	24	2.1	53	0.6	5.8	46.3
DENMARK	A8P6C9	0.25	0.4	5	1.5	20	0.3	2.1	28.5
FRANCE	A4P3C8	6.81	5.8	701	7.1	959	3.5	5.1	-8.2
GERMANY (FRG)	A4P4C4	2.70	0.8	118	2.7	428	0.5	7.1	29.0
GREECE	A2	0.74	*0.6*	*11*	0.6	16	*0.4*	0.4	*0.8*
IRELAND	A1C4	0.99	1.9	13	1.6	12	1.1	0.9	*6.8*
ITALY	A6P2C4	1.72	2.4	294	2.5	389	1.5	2.6	*2.1*
NETHERLANDS	A2C2	-2.27	0.7	18	0.7	26	0.4	0.8	23.8
PORTUGAL	*	..	..	..	..	..	..	..	..
SPAIN	A8P6C9	0.54	1.7	116	3.2	296	1.0	5.4	14.3
UK ENGLAND & WALES	A2C3	3.49	1.1	147	1.2	162	0.7	1.2	10.7
UK SCOTLAND	A8C9	-0.07	1.1	13	1.2	15	0.8	1.6	38.0

FEMALES	Best model	Goodness of fit	1965 Rate	1965 Deaths	1985 Rate	1985 Deaths	Cumulative risk 1900	Cumulative risk 1940	Recent trend
BELGIUM	A8D	0.12	0.2	6	0.3	10	0.1	0.3	*31.4*
DENMARK	A1C2	0.32	0.3	4	0.4	6	0.2	0.4	*12.1*
FRANCE	A3P3C7	1.53	0.4	52	0.6	94	0.2	0.4	*2.9*
GERMANY (FRG)	A3C4	1.47	0.2	41	0.4	78	0.1	0.5	20.7
GREECE	A1	-0.52	*0.2*	*4*	0.2	5	*0.1*	0.1	*-21.8*
IRELAND	A2	1.06	0.6	4	0.6	4	0.3	0.3	*-3.5*
ITALY	A2D	0.10	0.3	43	0.4	65	0.2	0.3	10.8
NETHERLANDS	A1C4	-1.30	0.3	11	0.3	11	0.2	0.3	*15.6*
PORTUGAL	*	..	..	..	..	..	..	..	..
SPAIN	A8P6C9	0.71	0.4	30	0.3	31	0.2	0.3	*-9.8*
UK ENGLAND & WALES	A2P3C2	0.38	0.4	70	0.5	79	0.3	0.3	*1.8*
UK SCOTLAND	A2D	0.71	0.6	10	0.4	7	0.4	0.2	*0.2*

* : not enough deaths for reliable estimation
− : incomplete or missing data
Best model: polynomial of the given degree in age (A), period (P) or cohort (C), or linear drift (D) model.
Goodness of fit: the normalised likelihood ratio chi-square for the best model (see Method).
Rate: world-standardised truncated rate per 100 000 per year (30-74 years) and number of **deaths** are both estimated from the best-fitting model for the single years cited.
Cumulative risk per 1000 (30-74 years) is estimated from the best-fitting *age-cohort* model for cohorts of central birth year cited.
Recent trend: estimated mean percentage change per five-year period in the age-specific rates (30-74 years) over the period 1975-1988.
Italics denote recent trends not significant at 5 per cent level, or other figures which should be interpreted with caution (see Method).

TONGUE (ICD-9 141)

EUROPE (EC), MORTALITY

MALES

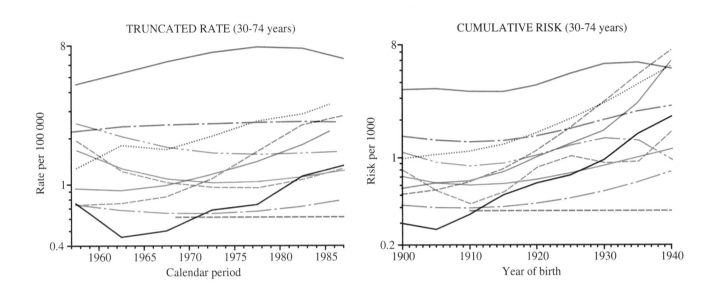

FEMALES

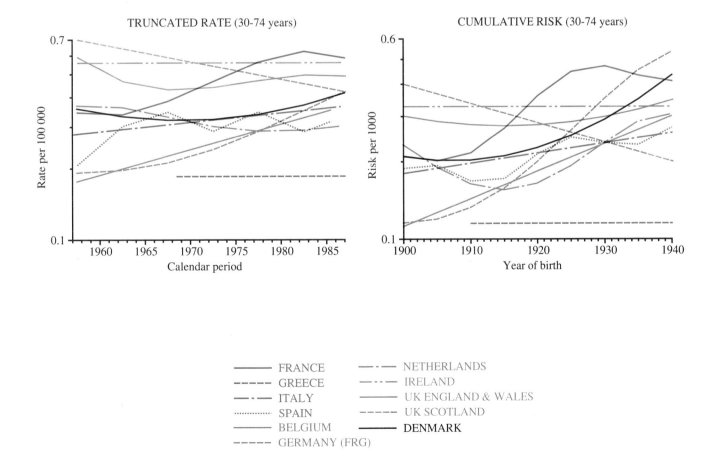

—————— FRANCE	—— · —— NETHERLANDS
– – – – GREECE	—— ·· —— IRELAND
— · — · ITALY	—————— UK ENGLAND & WALES
·············· SPAIN	– – – – UK SCOTLAND
—————— BELGIUM	—————— DENMARK
– – – – GERMANY (FRG)	

TONGUE (ICD-9 141)

EUROPE (non-EC), MORTALITY
Percentage change per five-year period, 1975-1988

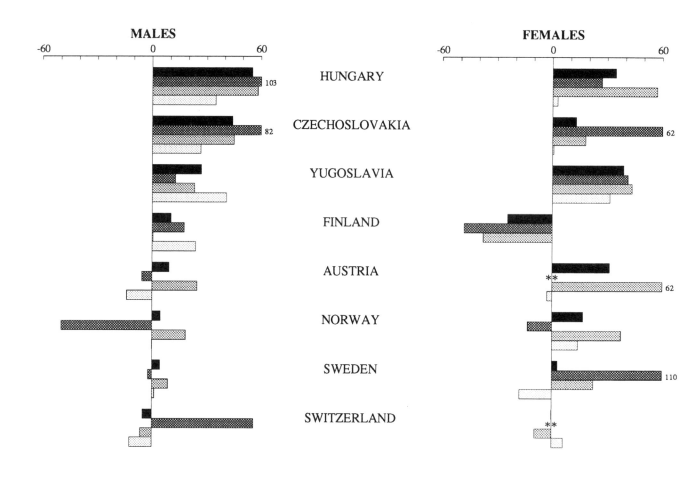

TONGUE (ICD-9 141)

EUROPE (EC), MORTALITY
Percentage change per five-year period, 1975-1988

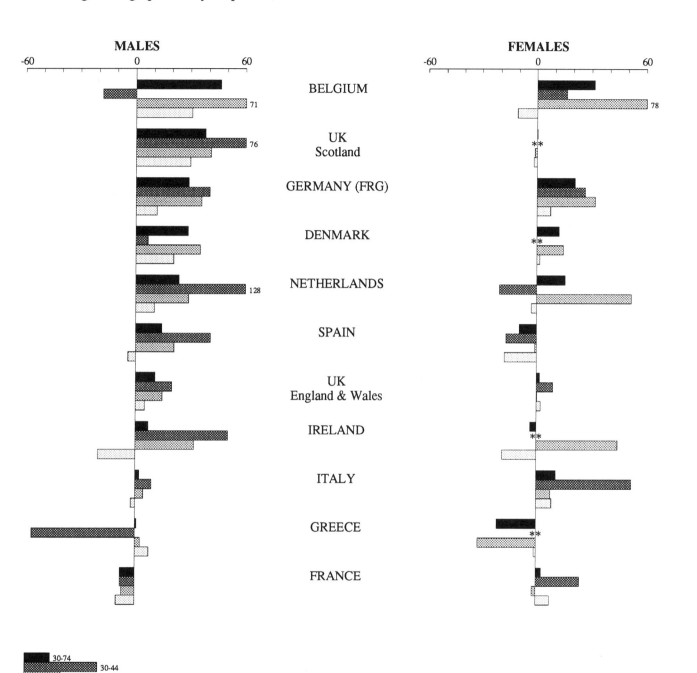

TONGUE (ICD-9 141)

ASIA, INCIDENCE

MALES	Best model	Goodness of fit	1970 Rate	1970 Cases	1985 Rate	1985 Cases	Cumulative risk 1915	Cumulative risk 1940	Recent trend
CHINA									
Shanghai	A1	-1.23	*1.0*	*10*	1.0	17	0.6	0.6	*0.0*
HONG KONG	A2	0.55	*5.0*	*29*	5.0	58	2.8	2.8	*4.8*
INDIA									
Bombay	A8P4C9	0.55	24.3	193	14.9	182	11.3	4.7	-12.0
JAPAN									
Miyagi	A1D	0.36	1.6	5	3.0	16	1.5	4.0	41.9
Nagasaki	A1	0.22	*3.7*	*3*	3.7	4	2.0	2.0	*7.0*
Osaka	A2C2	0.54	2.5	30	2.6	52	1.2	2.3	14.1
SINGAPORE									
Chinese	A2	-0.64	3.3	6	3.3	10	1.9	1.9	*-7.5*
Indian	A1	1.08	10.5	2	10.5	4	7.0	7.0	*0.1*
Malay	A3	-1.30	*2.6*	*0*	2.6	1	1.8	1.8	*-27.8*

FEMALES	Best model	Goodness of fit	1970 Rate	1970 Cases	1985 Rate	1985 Cases	Cumulative risk 1915	Cumulative risk 1940	Recent trend
CHINA									
Shanghai	A1C2	1.28	*1.1*	*14*	0.9	15	0.6	0.3	*-11.2*
HONG KONG	A3	2.35	*2.3*	*13*	2.3	24	1.2	1.2	*7.9*
INDIA									
Bombay	A2C2	1.57	7.0	36	5.4	49	3.9	1.9	-16.8
JAPAN									
Miyagi	A1C2	1.84	0.9	3	0.9	5	0.4	0.6	*13.8*
Nagasaki	A1C5	-0.25	*1.6*	*1*	0.9	1	1.9	0.2	*-10.6*
Osaka	A2C2	0.84	1.0	14	1.2	26	0.5	1.0	*14.3*
SINGAPORE									
Chinese	A1D	-0.12	1.2	2	0.9	3	0.6	0.4	*7.5*
Indian	*	..	..	..	..	..	..	..	..
Malay	*	..	..	..	..	..	..	..	..

* : not enough cases for reliable estimation
– : incomplete or missing data
Best model: polynomial of the given degree in age (A), period (P) or cohort (C), or linear drift (D) model.
Goodness of fit: the normalised likelihood ratio chi-square for the best model (see Method).
Rate: world-standardised truncated rate per 100 000 per year (30-74 years) and number of **cases** are both estimated from the best-fitting model for the single years cited.
Cumulative risk per 1000 (30-74 years) is estimated from the best-fitting *age-cohort* model for cohorts of central birth year cited.
Recent trend: estimated mean percentage change per five-year period in the age-specific rates (30-74 years) over the period 1973-1987.
Italics denote recent trends not significant at 5 per cent level, or other figures which should be interpreted with caution (see Method).

TONGUE (ICD-9 141)

ASIA, INCIDENCE

MALES

TRUNCATED RATE (30-74 years)

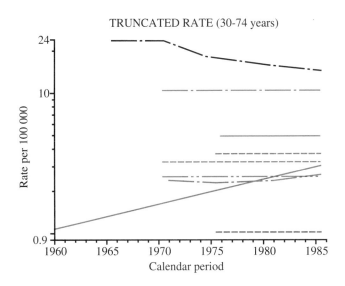

CUMULATIVE RISK (30-74 years)

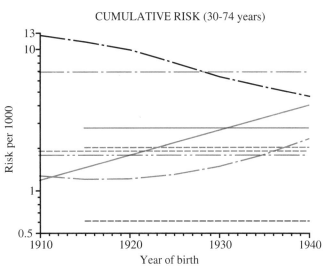

FEMALES

TRUNCATED RATE (30-74 years)

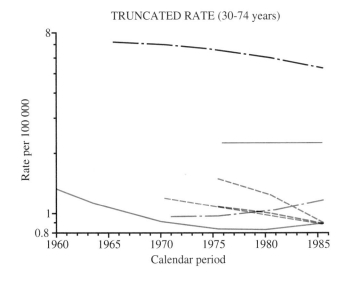

CUMULATIVE RISK (30-74 years)

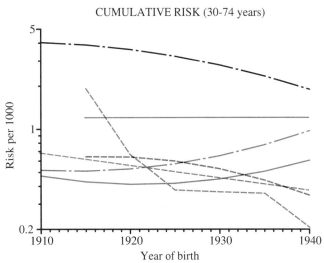

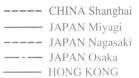

----- CHINA Shanghai
——— JAPAN Miyagi
----- JAPAN Nagasaki
—·—· JAPAN Osaka
——— HONG KONG

----- SINGAPORE Chinese
—·—· SINGAPORE Indian
—··—·· SINGAPORE Malay
—··—·· INDIA Bombay

TONGUE (ICD-9 141)

OCEANIA, INCIDENCE

MALES	Best model	Goodness of fit	1970 Rate	1970 Cases	1985 Rate	1985 Cases	Cumulative risk 1915	Cumulative risk 1940	Recent trend
AUSTRALIA									
New South Wales	A2D	0.05	*3.2*	*33*	4.8	62	2.2	4.4	14.4
South	A2	-0.25	*3.9*	*7*	3.9	13	2.3	2.3	*-14.3*
HAWAII									
Caucasian	A4P4	0.15	8.5	3	11.1	6	4.8	4.6	41.8
Chinese	A0	-0.51	3.6	*0*	*3.6*	*0*	1.6	1.6	20.5
Filipino	A1	-1.62	*2.7*	*0*	2.7	1	1.9	1.9	*19.1*
Hawaiian	A2	-1.00	*5.8*	*0*	5.8	1	3.1	3.1	*-10.5*
Japanese	A1	-0.02	3.7	1	3.7	3	2.1	2.1	*16.2*
NEW ZEALAND									
Maori	A1	-0.70	*2.0*	*0*	*2.0*	*0*	1.2	1.2	*25.3*
Non-Maori	A2	2.50	2.7	15	2.7	18	1.5	1.5	*8.9*

FEMALES	Best model	Goodness of fit	1970 Rate	1970 Cases	1985 Rate	1985 Cases	Cumulative risk 1915	Cumulative risk 1940	Recent trend
AUSTRALIA									
New South Wales	A2	0.52	*1.6*	*19*	1.6	22	0.9	0.9	*12.2*
South	A2	-0.06	*1.7*	*3*	1.7	5	0.9	0.9	*13.5*
HAWAII									
Caucasian	A2	-1.85	3.7	1	3.7	2	2.1	2.1	*0.9*
Chinese	A1	-2.20	2.0	*0*	*2.0*	*0*	1.3	1.3	*
Filipino	*	..	..	..	..	..	..	..	..
Hawaiian	A1	-1.19	*2.9*	*0*	2.9	*0*	1.9	1.9	*-34.0*
Japanese	A1	-0.14	*1.5*	*0*	1.5	1	0.9	0.9	*6.2*
NEW ZEALAND									
Maori	A0	-1.46	*1.0*	*0*	*1.0*	*0*	0.4	0.4	*-31.7*
Non-Maori	A2C2	0.14	1.0	6	1.5	10	0.6	1.7	*4.2*

* : not enough cases for reliable estimation
– : incomplete or missing data
Best model: polynomial of the given degree in age (A), period (P) or cohort (C), or linear drift (D) model.
Goodness of fit: the normalised likelihood ratio chi-square for the best model (see Method).
Rate: world-standardised truncated rate per 100 000 per year (30-74 years) and number of **cases** are both estimated from the best-fitting model for the single years cited.
Cumulative risk per 1000 (30-74 years) is estimated from the best-fitting *age-cohort* model for cohorts of central birth year cited.
Recent trend: estimated mean percentage change per five-year period in the age-specific rates (30-74 years) over the period 1973-1987.
Italics denote recent trends not significant at 5 per cent level, or other figures which should be interpreted with caution (see Method).

TONGUE (ICD-9 141)

OCEANIA, INCIDENCE

MALES

TRUNCATED RATE (30-74 years)

CUMULATIVE RISK (30-74 years)

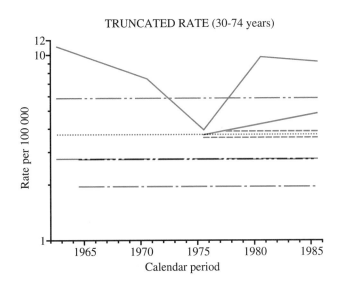

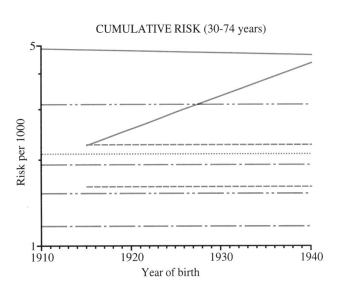

FEMALES

TRUNCATED RATE (30-74 years)

CUMULATIVE RISK (30-74 years)

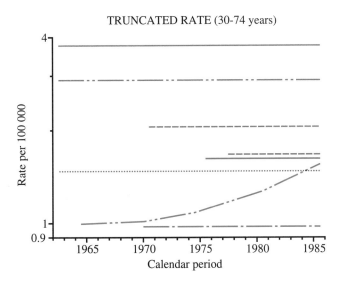

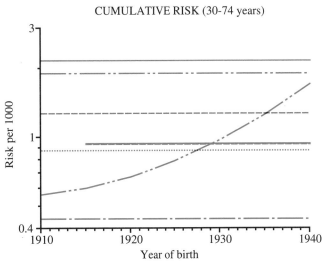

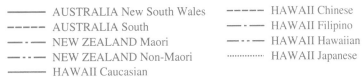

—— AUSTRALIA New South Wales	----- HAWAII Chinese
---- AUSTRALIA South	-·-·- HAWAII Filipino
-·-·- NEW ZEALAND Maori	-··-··- HAWAII Hawaiian
-··-··- NEW ZEALAND Non-Maori	············· HAWAII Japanese
—— HAWAII Caucasian	

TONGUE (ICD-9 141)

ASIA, INCIDENCE
Percentage change per five-year period, 1973-1987

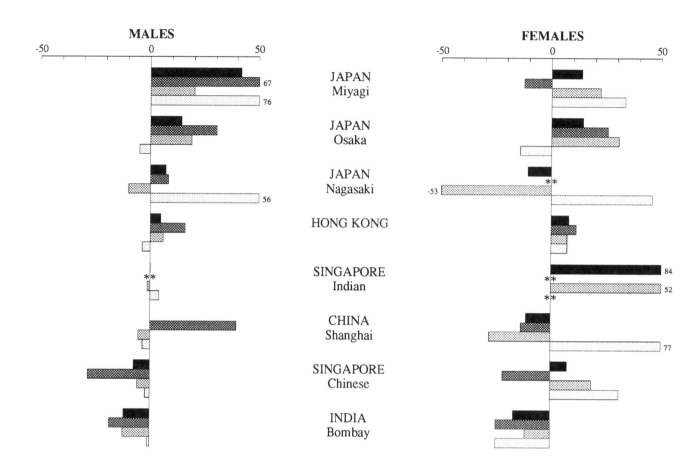

TONGUE (ICD-9 141)

OCEANIA, INCIDENCE
Percentage change per five-year period, 1973-1987

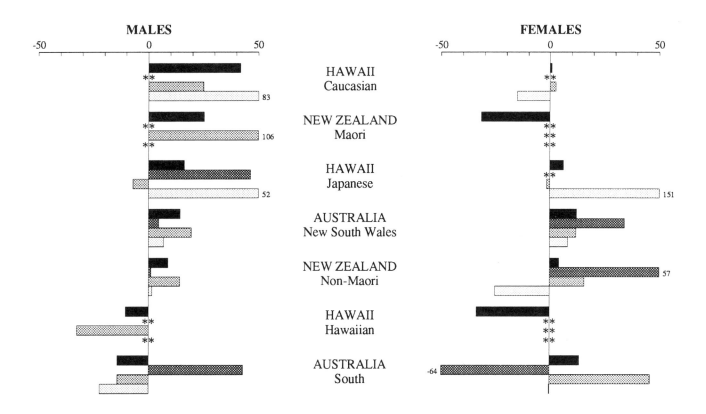

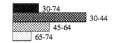

TONGUE (ICD-9 141)

ASIA and OCEANIA, MORTALITY

MALES	Best model	Goodness of fit	1965 Rate	1965 Deaths	1985 Rate	1985 Deaths	Cumulative risk 1900	Cumulative risk 1940	Recent trend
AUSTRALIA	A2C5	0.77	1.6	38	2.4	88	0.9	1.6	15.9
HONG KONG	A2C2	0.88	*1.4*	7	2.0	19	*0.7*	1.0	*-11.8*
JAPAN	A8P6C9	0.21	1.1	194	1.0	303	0.7	0.7	-5.3
MAURITIUS	A1	1.23	*1.4*	*1*	1.4	1	*0.8*	0.8	*73.8*
NEW ZEALAND	A4	1.52	1.4	7	1.4	10	0.9	0.9	*-4.7*
SINGAPORE	A1	0.83	2.2	3	2.2	5	*1.2*	1.2	–

FEMALES	Best model	Goodness of fit	1965 Rate	1965 Deaths	1985 Rate	1985 Deaths	Cumulative risk 1900	Cumulative risk 1940	Recent trend
AUSTRALIA	A2D	0.36	0.5	13	0.7	26	0.3	0.5	*14.4*
HONG KONG	A2	-0.69	*0.7*	*3*	0.7	6	*0.4*	0.4	-19.8
JAPAN	A1P2	-0.19	0.5	100	0.3	119	0.3	0.2	-19.3
MAURITIUS	*	..	..	..	..	..	..	..	..
NEW ZEALAND	A2	-0.17	0.5	3	0.5	4	0.3	0.3	*4.5*
SINGAPORE	A1	-0.43	*0.5*	*0*	0.5	1	*0.2*	0.2	–

* : not enough deaths for reliable estimation
– : incomplete or missing data
Best model: polynomial of the given degree in age (A), period (P) or cohort (C), or linear drift (D) model.
Goodness of fit: the normalised likelihood ratio chi-square for the best model (see Method).
Rate: world-standardised truncated rate per 100 000 per year (30-74 years) and number of **deaths** are both estimated from the best-fitting model for the single years cited.
Cumulative risk per 1000 (30-74 years) is estimated from the best-fitting *age-cohort* model for cohorts of central birth year cited.
Recent trend: estimated mean percentage change per five-year period in the age-specific rates (30-74 years) over the period 1975-1988.
Italics denote recent trends not significant at 5 per cent level, or other figures which should be interpreted with caution (see Method).

TONGUE (ICD-9 141)

ASIA and OCEANIA, MORTALITY

MALES

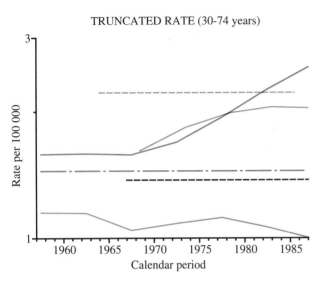

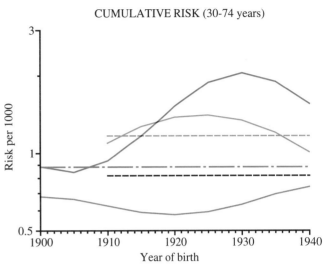

FEMALES

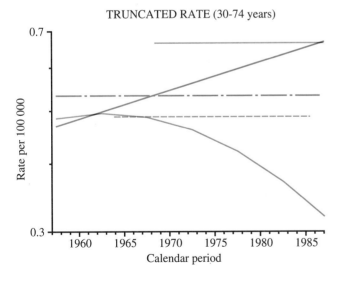

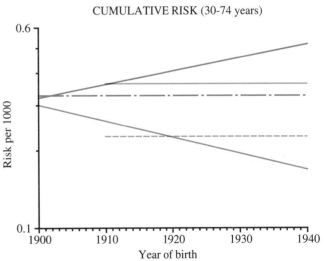

—— AUSTRALIA	—— HONG KONG
—·— NEW ZEALAND	----- SINGAPORE
—— JAPAN	==== MAURITIUS

TONGUE (ICD-9 141)

ASIA and OCEANIA, MORTALITY
Percentage change per five-year period, 1975-1988

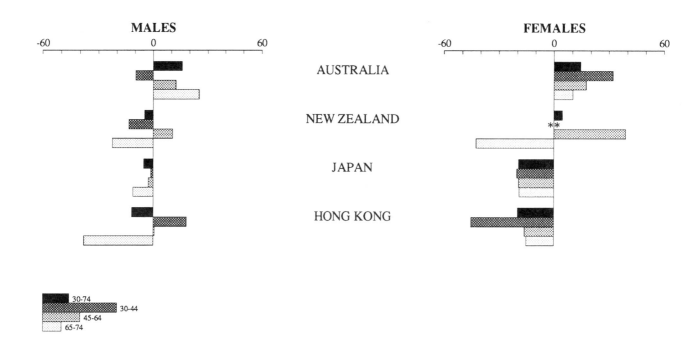

from page 65

nuing decline of 12% and 17% every five years among males and females respectively. By contrast, in Japan, where risks have been very low, there have been substantial recent rates of increase in successive birth cohorts in both sexes, particularly among males. The trends are well fitted by age-cohort models, except for males in Bombay, where a period effect is needed to describe a change in the early 1970s. A significant overall decrease in risk has occurred among Chinese females in Shanghai (China) and in Singapore, due mainly to a decrease in young females.

The mortality data in Japan are consistent with the increased incidence in young male generations, but there has been a small overall decrease in recent periods. Mortality among Japanese females has fallen significantly in successive calendar periods; these period effects may well be explained by an improvement in survival in Japan. There has been a significant increase in mortality among males in Hong Kong since 1968, although the rate of increase has flattened sharply and the recent linear trend of 10% every five years is not significant: this trend is not consistent with the incidence data, which show no significant change.

Incidence data show a significant increase of risk among males in New South Wales (Australia) at a rate of 14% every five years, and a significant increase among successive birth cohorts of non-Maori women in New Zealand. The sharp dip in incidence among male Caucasians in Hawaii is statistically significant, and it gives rise to a spurious recent trend. It is based on relatively small numbers, and it is likely that the risk of cancer of the tongue has remained almost constant at 5 per 1000 over the period examined, and that tongue cancer may have been under-registered in the period 1973-77. Tongue cancer risk in the other populations has not changed.

The mortality data for Australia show a large increase in risk, which is consistent with the incidence data for New South Wales. There is a significant reduction in risk for males born after 1930. The increase in incidence among non-Maori females in New Zealand is not reflected in mortality data, but the numbers of deaths are small.

Americas

Tongue cancer risk has been high in Puerto Rico, Cuba and Cali (Colombia), but there has been a major decline in risk in all these populations, although the decrease is not significant for females in Cali. In contrast, the risk of cancer of the tongue among males in Canada has been low, but it is increasing rapidly in all the provinces studied except Newfoundland, where there are still only 2 or 3 cases a year. The risk has changed little among females in Canada.

The risk of cancer of the tongue among males has increased in several of the US populations which have been studied. The rates of increase are larger among blacks in the San Francisco Bay Area and whites in Detroit, and in Iowa. The interpretation of the trends in Seattle and among blacks in Detroit is unclear, given the large period effects. Tongue cancer risk is also increasing among females, except for small declines in successive birth cohorts among Bay Area whites and in Seattle. The trend in New Orleans is unstable.

Mortality data for tongue cancer in the Americas are sparse, but there is a marked increase in mortality in successive birth cohorts among males in Canada, with a significant recent rate of increase of 9% every five years, and this probably reflects the trends in incidence. There is a plateau in mortality among Canadian females, and the large recent increase among younger females is not significant. Mortality has declined substantially in both sexes in Venezuela. Mortality has increased among males in Chile, but the cohort

effect suggests this may have stopped for males born after 1930.

Comment

In the UK, where long-term mortality data of sufficient quality are available, a decrease in mortality from cancer of the tongue has been observed for successive generations born up to 1910[213]. The risk has increased in cohorts born after 1910 in Scotland[172], however. In France, mortality (35-64 years) increased by around 2.4% per year in both sexes in the 30 years to 1985, although the recent decline in tongue cancer mortality among males and the plateau in females were noted; three-quarters of tongue cancer deaths are attributed to tobacco, alcohol or both[128].

A shift to younger age at presentation was noted among males with tongue cancer in a New York (USA) hospital in 1984[265]. Mortality data from the USA confirmed a two-fold increase among males aged 10-29 years between the 1950s and 1980-82, not seen for other sites in the oral cavity nor for older males, and increasing use of oral snuff was implicated[72]. Tongue cancer incidence in nine SEER registry areas in the USA increased three-fold among 30-39 year-old males between 1973 and 1984[67], also attributed to increasing use of smokeless tobacco products among young males.

TONGUE (ICD-9 141)

AMERICAS (except USA), INCIDENCE

MALES	Best model	Goodness of fit	1970		1985		Cumulative risk		Recent trend
			Rate	Cases	Rate	Cases	1915	1940	
BRAZIL									
Sao Paulo	A2D	-0.46	10.2	72	*16.4*	*138*	5.4	*11.9*	–
CANADA									
Alberta	A2D	0.70	2.2	6	3.4	14	1.7	3.5	28.5
British Columbia	A2D	0.06	3.0	14	4.2	28	2.0	3.4	*12.1*
Maritime Provinces	A2D	1.04	1.6	5	3.9	13	1.5	6.1	32.4
Newfoundland	A1	-0.28	2.6	2	2.6	3	1.6	1.6	*1.4*
Quebec	A3C2	1.08	4.5	48	5.6	80	2.8	5.6	14.5
COLOMBIA									
Cali	A2D	-0.44	3.8	2	2.0	2	1.7	0.6	*-27.4*
CUBA	A8C7	0.40	7.6	113	4.1	82	3.3	*2.1*	–
PUERTO RICO	A3D	1.34	13.5	61	10.1	67	7.0	4.3	-11.4

FEMALES	Best model	Goodness of fit	1970		1985		Cumulative risk		Recent trend
			Rate	Cases	Rate	Cases	1915	1940	
BRAZIL									
Sao Paulo	A1	0.59	1.6	11	*1.6*	*15*	0.8	*0.8*	–
CANADA									
Alberta	A2	1.16	1.1	3	1.1	5	0.7	0.7	*3.1*
British Columbia	A2	1.14	2.0	9	2.0	15	1.1	1.1	*7.9*
Maritime Provinces	A2	-0.74	1.0	3	1.0	3	0.6	0.6	*19.5*
Newfoundland	A1	-0.65	*0.8*	*0*	0.8	1	0.5	0.5	*26.7*
Quebec	A2	0.82	1.2	14	1.2	20	0.7	0.7	16.6
COLOMBIA									
Cali	A2	-0.18	1.5	1	1.5	2	0.9	0.9	*-18.2*
CUBA	A2P2	-0.32	2.1	26	1.5	29	1.0	*0.6*	–
PUERTO RICO	A2D	0.58	3.1	14	2.0	15	1.5	0.8	-17.6

* : not enough cases for reliable estimation
– : incomplete or missing data
Best model: polynomial of the given degree in age (A), period (P) or cohort (C), or linear drift (D) model.
Goodness of fit: the normalised likelihood ratio chi-square for the best model (see Method).
Rate: world-standardised truncated rate per 100 000 per year (30-74 years) and number of **cases** are both estimated from the best-fitting model for the single years cited.
Cumulative risk per 1000 (30-74 years) is estimated from the best-fitting *age-cohort* model for cohorts of central birth year cited.
Recent trend: estimated mean percentage change per five-year period in the age-specific rates (30-74 years) over the period 1973-1987.
Italics denote recent trends not significant at 5 per cent level, or other figures which should be interpreted with caution (see Method).

TONGUE (ICD-9 141)

AMERICAS (except USA), INCIDENCE

MALES

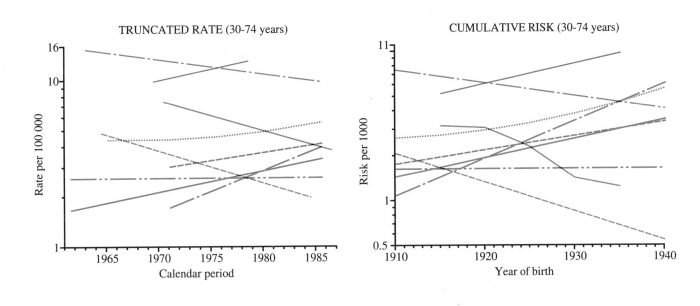

TRUNCATED RATE (30-74 years)

CUMULATIVE RISK (30-74 years)

FEMALES

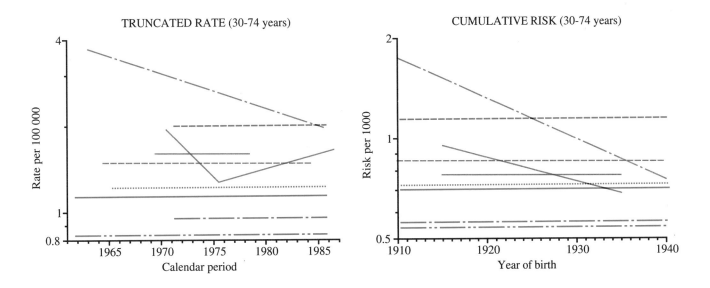

TRUNCATED RATE (30-74 years)

CUMULATIVE RISK (30-74 years)

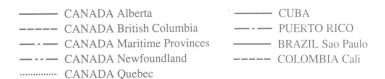

——— CANADA Alberta
– – – CANADA British Columbia
–·–· CANADA Maritime Provinces
–··–·· CANADA Newfoundland
·········· CANADA Quebec

——— CUBA
–·–· PUERTO RICO
——— BRAZIL Sao Paulo
– – – COLOMBIA Cali

TONGUE (ICD-9 141)

AMERICAS (USA), INCIDENCE

MALES	Best model	Goodness of fit	1970 Rate	Cases	1985 Rate	Cases	Cumulative risk 1915	1940	Recent trend
USA									
Bay Area, Black	A2D	-0.59	4.4	2	9.2	7	3.2	10.8	29.8
Bay Area, Chinese	A1	-0.35	2.8	0	2.8	1	1.6	1.6	–
Bay Area, White	A3	0.81	6.3	37	6.3	39	3.7	3.7	4.3
Connecticut	A2	1.47	6.6	43	6.6	51	3.8	3.8	-1.4
Detroit, Black	A3P3	-0.87	8.1	11	8.7	14	4.0	5.6	7.7
Detroit, White	A2D	1.07	5.0	37	6.6	46	3.3	5.2	14.2
Iowa	A2D	-1.05	2.8	18	3.9	26	2.0	3.5	14.4
New Orleans, Black	A2	-1.14	8.0	4	8.0	4	4.0	4.0	-3.9
New Orleans, White	A3C2	-0.05	8.8	12	7.8	11	3.4	10.6	7.3
Seattle	A2P2	-0.25	15.5	73	5.6	36	2.7	5.6	16.6

FEMALES	Best model	Goodness of fit	1970 Rate	Cases	1985 Rate	Cases	Cumulative risk 1915	1940	Recent trend
USA									
Bay Area, Black	A8C8	0.71	2.3	1	2.1	2	0.3	0.0	28.3
Bay Area, Chinese	*	..	..	..	..	..	..	..	..
Bay Area, White	A2C2	1.06	3.2	21	3.5	24	2.2	1.4	4.9
Connecticut	A2D	0.18	1.8	13	2.4	21	1.2	1.9	3.3
Detroit, Black	A2	-0.67	2.8	4	2.8	5	1.4	1.4	13.0
Detroit, White	A2P3	-0.14	1.8	15	2.5	20	1.2	2.2	10.8
Iowa	A3D	-1.30	1.1	8	1.9	14	0.9	2.0	20.5
New Orleans, Black	A1	-0.36	1.6	1	1.6	1	0.9	0.9	-42.9
New Orleans, White	A8C7	-0.67	*	*	2.0	3	0.9	0.5	-2.3
Seattle	A2C3	0.35	2.7	12	2.6	19	2.0	0.8	-3.8

* : not enough cases for reliable estimation
– : incomplete or missing data
Best model: polynomial of the given degree in age (A), period (P) or cohort (C), or linear drift (D) model.
Goodness of fit: the normalised likelihood ratio chi-square for the best model (see Method).
Rate: world-standardised truncated rate per 100 000 per year (30-74 years) and number of **cases** are both estimated from the best-fitting model for the single years cited.
Cumulative risk per 1000 (30-74 years) is estimated from the best-fitting *age-cohort* model for cohorts of central birth year cited.
Recent trend: estimated mean percentage change per five-year period in the age-specific rates (30-74 years) over the period 1973-1987.
Italics denote recent trends not significant at 5 per cent level, or other figures which should be interpreted with caution (see Method).

TONGUE (ICD-9 141)

AMERICAS (USA), INCIDENCE

MALES

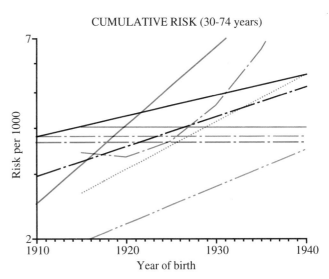

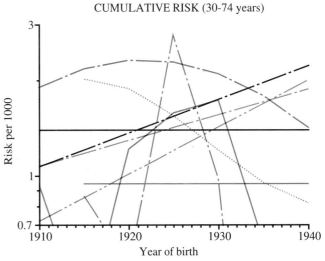

FEMALES

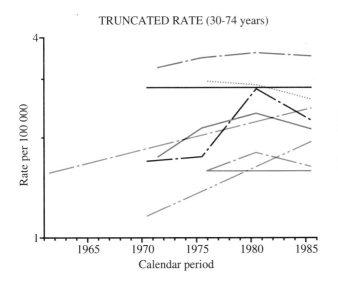

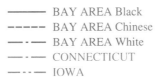

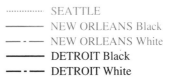

TONGUE (ICD-9 141)

AMERICAS (except USA), INCIDENCE
Percentage change per five-year period, 1973-1987

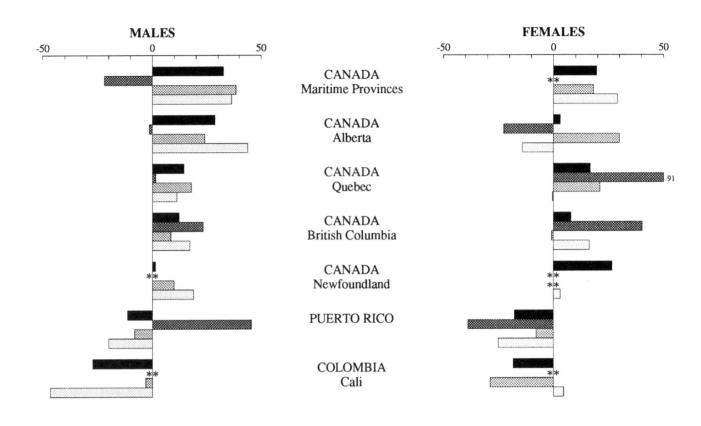

TONGUE (ICD-9 141)

AMERICAS (USA), INCIDENCE
Percentage change per five-year period, 1973-1987

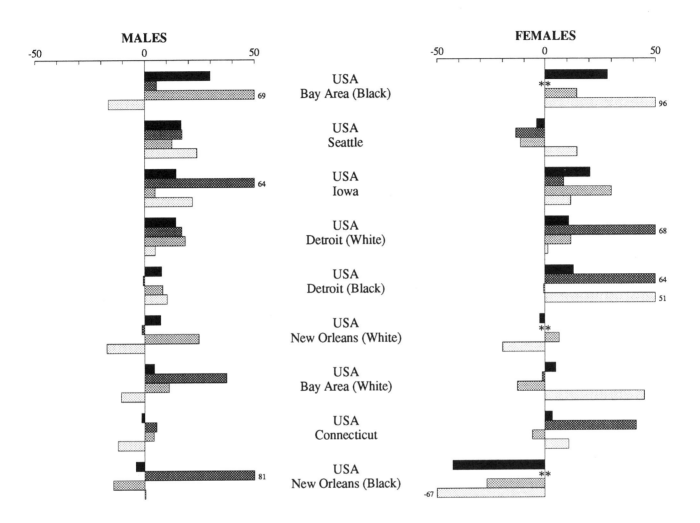

TONGUE (ICD-9 141)

AMERICAS, MORTALITY

MALES	Best model	Goodness of fit	1965 Rate	1965 Deaths	1985 Rate	1985 Deaths	Cumulative risk 1900	Cumulative risk 1940	Recent trend
CANADA	A3C2	1.23	1.6	60	2.1	119	1.0	2.2	8.6
CHILE	A2C3	1.45	1.0	12	*1.2*	*21*	0.5	*0.3*	–
COSTA RICA	*	..	..	..	..	..	..	..	..
PANAMA	*	..	..	..	..	..	..	..	..
PUERTO RICO	*	..	..	..	..	..	..	..	..
URUGUAY	*	..	..	..	..	..	..	..	..
USA	A5P2C7	0.80	2.3	956	1.8	1007	1.3	1.2	-7.8
VENEZUELA	A4D	-1.35	1.8	15	*0.9*	*13*	1.2	*0.3*	–

FEMALES	Best model	Goodness of fit	1965 Rate	1965 Deaths	1985 Rate	1985 Deaths	Cumulative risk 1900	Cumulative risk 1940	Recent trend
CANADA	A4P2	2.19	0.5	18	0.5	34	0.3	0.4	*0.1*
CHILE	A1	0.45	0.2	2	*0.2*	*4*	0.1	*0.1*	–
COSTA RICA	*	..	..	..	..	..	..	..	..
PANAMA	*	..	..	..	..	..	..	..	..
PUERTO RICO	*	..	..	..	..	..	..	..	..
URUGUAY	*	..	..	..	..	..	..	..	..
USA	A4P2C8	0.16	0.6	282	0.6	422	0.3	0.3	-4.7
VENEZUELA	A2D	1.11	1.2	10	*0.5*	*8*	0.9	*0.1*	–

* : not enough deaths for reliable estimation
– : incomplete or missing data
Best model: polynomial of the given degree in age (A), period (P) or cohort (C), or linear drift (D) model.
Goodness of fit: the normalised likelihood ratio chi-square for the best model (see Method).
Rate: world-standardised truncated rate per 100 000 per year (30-74 years) and number of **deaths** are both estimated from the best-fitting model for the single years cited.
Cumulative risk per 1000 (30-74 years) is estimated from the best-fitting *age-cohort* model for cohorts of central birth year cited.
Recent trend: estimated mean percentage change per five-year period in the age-specific rates (30-74 years) over the period 1975-1988.
Italics denote recent trends not significant at 5 per cent level, or other figures which should be interpreted with caution (see Method).

TONGUE (ICD-9 141)

AMERICAS, MORTALITY

MALES

TRUNCATED RATE (30-74 years)

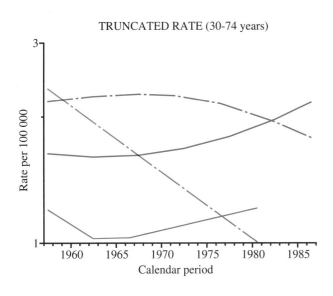

CUMULATIVE RISK (30-74 years)

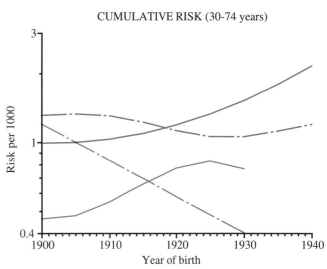

FEMALES

TRUNCATED RATE (30-74 years)

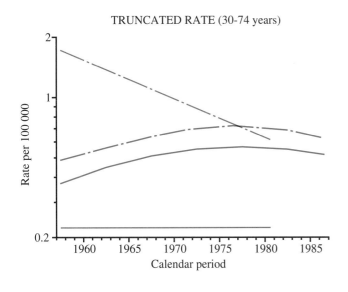

CUMULATIVE RISK (30-74 years)

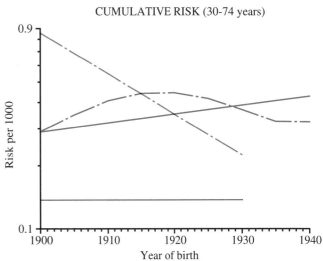

———— CANADA
—·—·— USA
———— CHILE
—··—··— VENEZUELA

TONGUE (ICD-9 141)

AMERICAS, MORTALITY
Percentage change per five-year period, 1975-1988

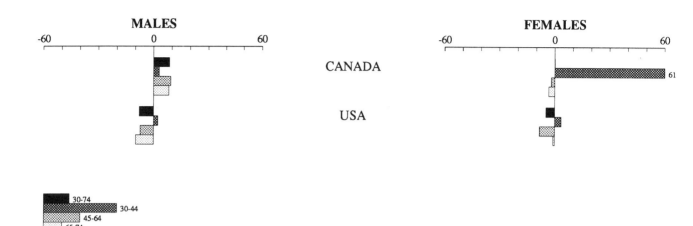

Chapter 7

MOUTH

Cancers of the mouth include those assigned to the gums, the floor of the mouth, the mucosa of the cheek, the hard and soft palate and the uvula (ICD-9 143-145). Cancers of the mouth and tongue combined may comprise up to 50% of all cancers in parts of India, where they are associated with chewing betel quid and tobacco[208]. In Europe and North America, both alcohol and tobacco are implicated. Cancer of the mouth usually represents 20-25% of all cancers of the oral cavity and pharynx (ICD-9 140-149), but in low-risk countries, this proportion may be lower (e.g. 10% in Finland). Survival at five years is only about 50%, but is much higher if the disease is diagnosed early. There are good indications for screening in high-risk populations, but except in India and Sri Lanka, no mass screening programmes have been seriously considered or evaluated.

In most countries, cancer of the mouth is uncommon in males, and rare in females: the cumulative risk (30-74 years) for the 1915 birth cohort is generally less than 1% and 0.2%, respectively. The chief exceptions are France, where the risk is higher in males (1.2% in Bas-Rhin) but low in females (0.1%), and various Indian populations, where the risk for the 1915 cohort is high among both males and females, e.g. 0.7% and 0.6%, respectively, in Bombay (India). The potential for prevention of cancer of the mouth is high (60-90%). If the risk for males in Bas-Rhin (France) could be reduced to that of males in Finland by suitable preventive strategies, for example, up to 94% of cancers of the mouth in Bas-Rhin would be preventable. A similar figure is obtained for females when comparing the risk among whites in the USA with that observed in Navarra (Spain). Comparison of the risk for Indians in India with that of Indian migrants in Fiji suggests that the potential for prevention in India is of the same order of magnitude, and could be achieved largely by the elimination of betel quid and tobacco chewing.

Europe

In many populations and countries in Europe, both incidence and mortality have increased in males. This increase is usually more striking on a cohort basis. The increase in incidence is especially impressive in Germany, Spain (especially Navarra), the Nordic countries (except Finland), Scotland, Slovenia, and Hungary. By contrast, the risk of cancer of the mouth among males has not changed substantially in Italian, French or English populations.

The general upward trend is confirmed by the mortality data, which show a dramatic increase in the risk of death from cancers of the mouth among males in most countries in Europe. Finland and Greece, however, remain at very low risk, and in Finland there is even a slight overall decrease in mortality, despite a small increase in incidence. The rate of increase in mortality in France and Italy, where the rates have been very high, is slower than in most other European countries, and there is evidence of a downturn in France. Mortality has increased substantially for successive birth cohorts in England and Wales, but especially in Scotland, Germany, Spain and Denmark, where the cumulative risk (30-74 years) for the 1940 birth cohort is now around 6 per 1000.

Trends in incidence are less uniform among females, mainly due to small numbers of cases. The upward trends among females in Scotland, Germany and Denmark are especially marked, however, at up to 30% or more every five years. The rate of increase is also significant in Finland (22%). Mortality data confirm the general increase in risk from cancer of the mouth among females in Europe, except in Ireland and Greece.

Asia and Oceania

In Asia, the most dramatic trend is the rapid increase in incidence in Japan for both males and females. Cancer of the mouth was extremely uncommon in Japan in 1970 (rates of 1 per 100 000 or less), but incidence has more than doubled in 15 years in Miyagi and Osaka, and is still rising at 30% or more every five years. The increases affect all age groups similarly, and age-period models fit well. In Bombay (India), and in the Indian population of Singapore, where incidence remains extremely high (10-15 per 100 000), there is some evidence of a decrease in successive birth cohorts, particularly among females. The populations of Indians and Malays in Singapore are small, however, and the trends

97

continued page 118

MOUTH (ICD-9 143-145)

EUROPE (non-EC), INCIDENCE

MALES	Best model	Goodness of fit	1970 Rate	1970 Cases	1985 Rate	1985 Cases	Cumulative risk 1915	Cumulative risk 1940	Recent trend
FINLAND	A2C2	1.11	1.4	13	1.6	18	0.7	1.4	*14.5*
HUNGARY									
County Vas	A3D	-1.34	1.5	1	4.1	3	1.9	10.4	*25.6*
Szabolcs-Szatmar	A1P2C4	0.29	1.5	2	4.2	5	1.0	7.6	99.6
ISRAEL									
All Jews	A2	0.85	1.7	8	1.7	10	1.0	1.0	-19.8
Non-Jews	A1D	0.05	*2.1*	*0*	*1.8*	*0*	1.2	0.9	*-16.6*
NORWAY	A2C2	0.74	2.1	23	3.4	38	1.4	5.0	28.1
POLAND									
Warsaw City	A3D	-0.75	2.6	7	4.2	16	1.8	4.1	*7.5*
ROMANIA									
Cluj	A2	-0.53	*1.6*	*2*	1.6	3	0.9	0.9	*-3.7*
SWEDEN	A2D	0.31	2.1	51	3.1	78	1.6	3.0	17.3
SWITZERLAND									
Geneva	A3P2	0.45	4.0	3	10.7	10	5.9	8.7	*-6.1*
YUGOSLAVIA									
Slovenia	A2C3	0.48	5.2	18	12.1	53	4.1	14.7	34.8

FEMALES	Best model	Goodness of fit	1970 Rate	1970 Cases	1985 Rate	1985 Cases	Cumulative risk 1915	Cumulative risk 1940	Recent trend
FINLAND	A1P2	0.66	0.8	10	1.2	18	0.6	0.6	22.2
HUNGARY									
County Vas	A1	-0.08	*1.0*	*0*	*1.0*	*0*	0.5	0.5	*21.3*
Szabolcs-Szatmar	A1	-1.27	*0.4*	*0*	*0.4*	*0*	0.2	0.2	*64.7*
ISRAEL									
All Jews	A1	1.66	1.0	4	1.0	6	0.6	0.6	*11.0*
Non-Jews	A0	-0.84	*0.7*	*0*	*0.7*	*0*	0.3	0.3	*-3.6*
NORWAY	A8D	0.81	1.0	12	1.3	17	0.8	1.2	*12.9*
POLAND									
Warsaw City	A2C3	-0.07	0.9	3	1.2	6	0.6	0.5	*10.6*
ROMANIA									
Cluj	A1	0.59	*0.7*	*1*	0.7	1	0.4	0.4	*38.8*
SWEDEN	A4D	1.81	1.1	27	1.2	33	0.7	0.9	*1.3*
SWITZERLAND									
Geneva	A1P2	0.15	*0.7*	*0*	2.1	2	1.3	1.5	*-14.9*
YUGOSLAVIA									
Slovenia	A1P4	0.74	0.4	1	1.1	5	0.4	0.6	*37.9*

* : not enough cases for reliable estimation
– : incomplete or missing data
Best model: polynomial of the given degree in age (A), period (P) or cohort (C), or linear drift (D) model.
Goodness of fit: the normalised likelihood ratio chi-square for the best model (see Method).
Rate: world-standardised truncated rate per 100 000 per year (30-74 years) and number of **cases** are both estimated from the best-fitting model for the single years cited.
Cumulative risk per 1000 (30-74 years) is estimated from the best-fitting *age-cohort* model for cohorts of central birth year cited.
Recent trend: estimated mean percentage change per five-year period in the age-specific rates (30-74 years) over the period 1973-1987.
Italics denote recent trends not significant at 5 per cent level, or other figures which should be interpreted with caution (see Method).

MOUTH (ICD-9 143-145)

EUROPE (non-EC), INCIDENCE

MALES

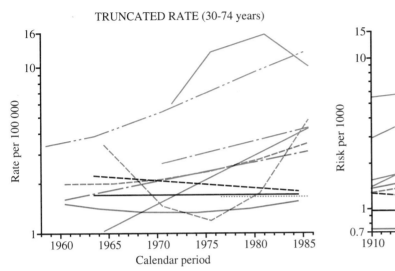

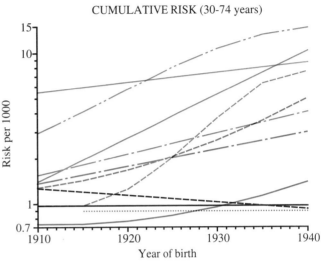

FEMALES

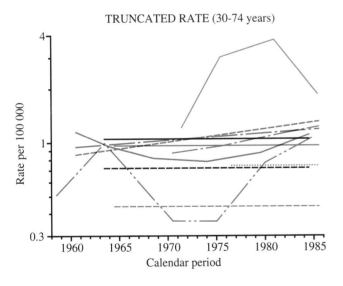

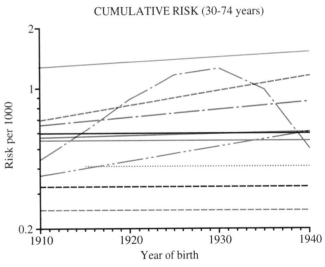

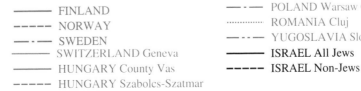

—————— FINLAND	— · — POLAND Warsaw City
- - - - - NORWAY	············ ROMANIA Cluj
— · — · SWEDEN	— ·· — YUGOSLAVIA Slovenia
—————— SWITZERLAND Geneva	—————— ISRAEL All Jews
—————— HUNGARY County Vas	- - - - - ISRAEL Non-Jews
- - - - - HUNGARY Szabolcs-Szatmar	

EUROPE (EC), INCIDENCE

MALES	Best model	Goodness of fit	1970 Rate	1970 Cases	1985 Rate	1985 Cases	Cumulative risk 1915	Cumulative risk 1940	Recent trend
DENMARK	A2C2	1.17	1.9	24	4.1	56	1.6	8.0	37.0
FRANCE									
Bas-Rhin	A3P2	0.92	6.7	13	31.5	64	11.9	20.8	12.8
Doubs	A2P2	0.08	0.0	0	14.5	15	8.5	5.5	-8.0
GERMANY (FRG)									
Hamburg	A2D	-0.16	2.4	11	5.4	22	1.7	6.7	–
Saarland	A4C2	1.26	3.4	9	10.3	28	2.4	28.2	49.7
GERMANY (GDR)	A4C4	1.85	1.1	48	3.4	131	0.9	9.9	42.7
ITALY									
Varese	A8C7	-1.01	*	*	5.8	12	2.9	10.8	-12.3
SPAIN									
Navarra	A2D	0.94	2.2	2	9.8	13	2.4	28.4	65.7
Zaragoza	A2P2	1.20	1.7	3	2.6	6	1.8	3.7	-3.6
UK									
Birmingham	A2	0.39	2.5	34	2.5	37	1.6	1.6	-1.5
Scotland	A2C3	0.19	2.2	30	4.7	63	1.9	11.9	29.7
South Thames	A2C3	0.56	1.9	46	2.0	36	1.1	1.3	5.8

FEMALES	Best model	Goodness of fit	1970 Rate	1970 Cases	1985 Rate	1985 Cases	Cumulative risk 1915	Cumulative risk 1940	Recent trend
DENMARK	A2C2	2.06	1.0	14	2.2	34	1.0	4.6	33.7
FRANCE									
Bas-Rhin	A2	0.70	2.0	4	2.0	4	1.0	1.0	15.7
Doubs	A1	0.45	1.3	1	1.3	1	0.7	0.7	109.1
GERMANY (FRG)									
Hamburg	A2	0.17	0.8	5	0.8	4	0.4	0.4	–
Saarland	A1D	1.07	0.6	2	1.2	4	0.5	1.5	30.1
GERMANY (GDR)	A2D	1.31	0.4	23	0.7	34	0.3	0.7	18.6
ITALY									
Varese	A1	0.09	1.1	1	1.1	2	0.6	0.6	57.8
SPAIN									
Navarra	A1	-0.32	0.5	0	0.5	0	0.3	0.3	6.8
Zaragoza	*	..	..	..	..	..	..	..	..
UK									
Birmingham	A2D	-1.30	1.0	14	1.1	17	0.6	0.7	9.9
Scotland	A2P2	0.18	1.2	19	2.0	31	0.9	1.5	32.3
South Thames	A2	-0.43	1.1	32	1.1	23	0.6	0.6	-3.6

* : not enough cases for reliable estimation
– : incomplete or missing data
Best model: polynomial of the given degree in age (A), period (P) or cohort (C), or linear drift (D) model.
Goodness of fit: the normalised likelihood ratio chi-square for the best model (see Method).
Rate: world-standardised truncated rate per 100 000 per year (30-74 years) and number of **cases** are both estimated from the best-fitting model for the single years cited.
Cumulative risk per 1000 (30-74 years) is estimated from the best-fitting *age-cohort* model for cohorts of central birth year cited.
Recent trend: estimated mean percentage change per five-year period in the age-specific rates (30-74 years) over the period 1973-1987.
Italics denote recent trends not significant at 5 per cent level, or other figures which should be interpreted with caution (see Method).

MOUTH (ICD-9 143-145)

EUROPE (EC), INCIDENCE

MALES

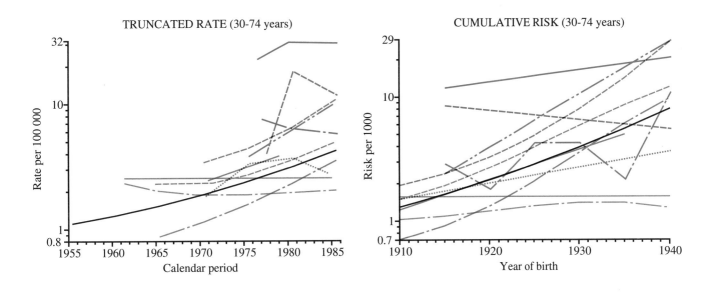

FEMALES

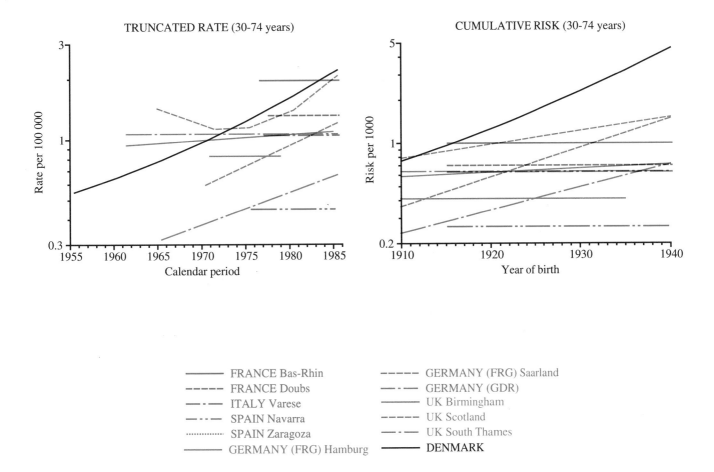

—— FRANCE Bas-Rhin	------ GERMANY (FRG) Saarland
- - - FRANCE Doubs	—·—· GERMANY (GDR)
—·—· ITALY Varese	—— UK Birmingham
—··—·· SPAIN Navarra	------ UK Scotland
············ SPAIN Zaragoza	—·—· UK South Thames
—— GERMANY (FRG) Hamburg	—— DENMARK

MOUTH (ICD-9 143-145)

EUROPE (non-EC), INCIDENCE

Percentage change per five-year period, 1973-1987

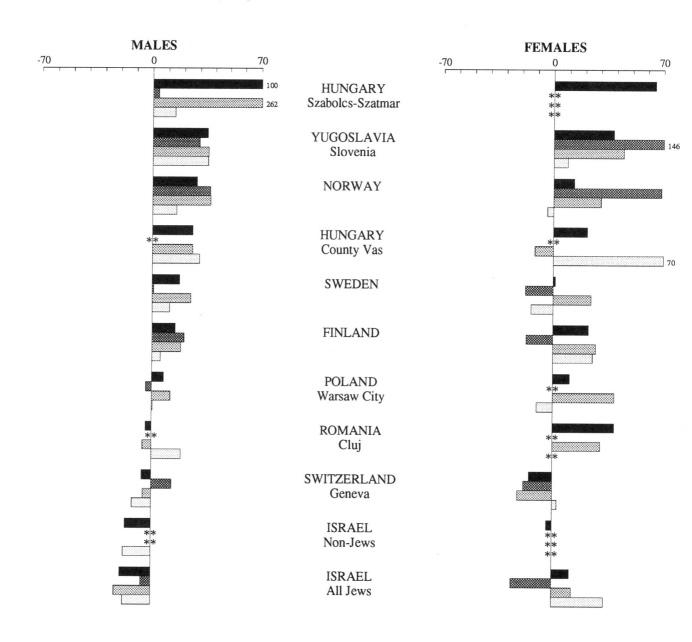

MOUTH (ICD-9 143-145)

EUROPE (EC), INCIDENCE
Percentage change per five-year period, 1973-1987

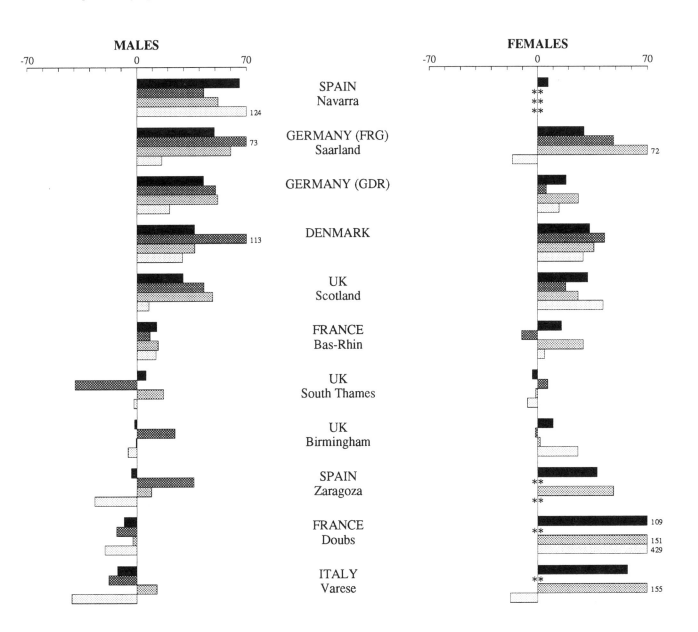

MALES

FEMALES

-70   0   70

SPAIN
Navarra

124

GERMANY (FRG)
Saarland

73

72

GERMANY (GDR)

DENMARK

113

UK
Scotland

FRANCE
Bas-Rhin

UK
South Thames

UK
Birmingham

SPAIN
Zaragoza

FRANCE
Doubs

109
151
429

ITALY
Varese

155

30-74
30-44
45-64
65-74

103

MOUTH (ICD-9 143-145)

EUROPE (non-EC), MORTALITY

MALES	Best model	Goodness of fit	1965 Rate	1965 Deaths	1985 Rate	1985 Deaths	Cumulative risk 1900	Cumulative risk 1940	Recent trend
AUSTRIA	A3D	-0.58	*0.7*	*13*	2.1	38	*0.3*	2.8	29.0
CZECHOSLOVAKIA	A3P3C4	2.29	1.9	67	2.6	92	1.1	3.9	35.3
FINLAND	A1D	0.49	0.7	6	0.7	7	0.4	0.4	*20.1*
HUNGARY	A3C2	-0.70	*0.4*	*11*	2.7	73	*0.3*	20.2	75.0
NORWAY	A2C2	1.06	1.2	12	1.3	15	0.8	1.2	26.6
POLAND	A2D	-0.35	1.0	59	*2.4*	*183*	0.6	*3.2*	–
ROMANIA	–	–	–	–	–	–	–	–	–
SWEDEN	A2D	-1.63	0.6	13	1.1	29	0.4	1.3	18.4
SWITZERLAND	A2C4	2.47	1.3	19	2.5	42	0.8	3.5	13.7
YUGOSLAVIA	A3P3C4	0.12	0.6	23	1.6	79	0.3	2.4	48.5

FEMALES	Best model	Goodness of fit	1965 Rate	1965 Deaths	1985 Rate	1985 Deaths	Cumulative risk 1900	Cumulative risk 1940	Recent trend
AUSTRIA	A2	1.31	*0.1*	*3*	0.1	3	*0.1*	0.1	*25.5*
CZECHOSLOVAKIA	A8P6	0.03	0.4	16	0.3	12	0.3	0.1	*10.5*
FINLAND	A1P2	-0.74	0.4	4	0.4	6	0.3	0.2	*27.0*
HUNGARY	A1D	1.09	*0.1*	*2*	0.4	12	*0.0*	1.0	49.7
NORWAY	A1	1.14	0.5	5	0.5	6	0.3	0.3	46.5
POLAND	A1C2	0.98	0.4	28	*0.3*	*30*	0.2	*0.1*	–
ROMANIA	–	–	–	–	–	–	–	–	–
SWEDEN	A2	0.34	0.4	9	0.4	10	0.2	0.2	*1.4*
SWITZERLAND	A4D	0.40	0.2	3	0.4	7	0.1	0.4	*9.7*
YUGOSLAVIA	A1	0.90	0.2	7	0.2	10	0.1	0.1	*8.0*

* : not enough deaths for reliable estimation
− : incomplete or missing data
Best model: polynomial of the given degree in age (A), period (P) or cohort (C), or linear drift (D) model.
Goodness of fit: the normalised likelihood ratio chi-square for the best model (see Method).
Rate: world-standardised truncated rate per 100 000 per year (30-74 years) and number of **deaths** are both estimated from the best-fitting model for the single years cited.
Cumulative risk per 1000 (30-74 years) is estimated from the best-fitting *age-cohort* model for cohorts of central birth year cited.
Recent trend: estimated mean percentage change per five-year period in the age-specific rates (30-74 years) over the period 1975-1988.
Italics denote recent trends not significant at 5 per cent level, or other figures which should be interpreted with caution (see Method).

MOUTH (ICD-9 143-145)

EUROPE (non-EC), MORTALITY

MALES

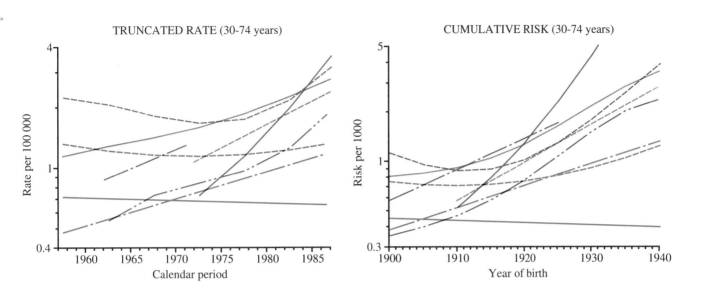

TRUNCATED RATE (30-74 years)

CUMULATIVE RISK (30-74 years)

FEMALES

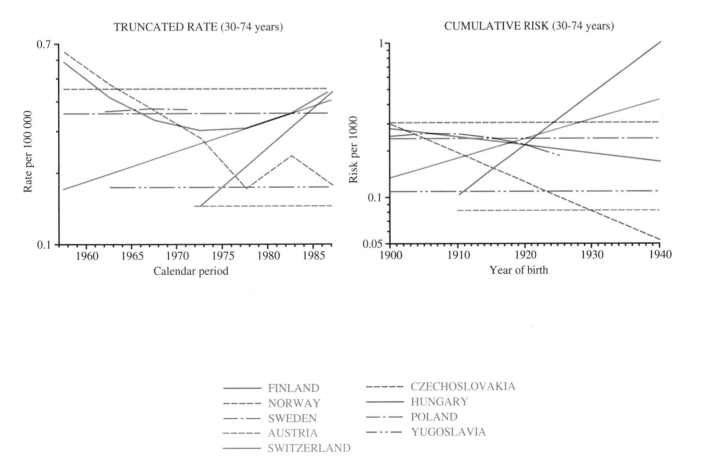

TRUNCATED RATE (30-74 years)

CUMULATIVE RISK (30-74 years)

——— FINLAND   ------ CZECHOSLOVAKIA
------ NORWAY   ——— HUNGARY
–·–· SWEDEN   –··– POLAND
------ AUSTRIA   –···– YUGOSLAVIA
——— SWITZERLAND

MOUTH (ICD-9 143-145)

EUROPE (EC), MORTALITY

MALES	Best model	Goodness of fit	1965 Rate	1965 Deaths	1985 Rate	1985 Deaths	Cumulative risk 1900	Cumulative risk 1940	Recent trend
BELGIUM	A3C2	-0.46	0.8	20	1.7	44	0.5	2.9	30.3
DENMARK	A4P3	0.14	0.5	6	1.9	27	0.4	3.5	43.2
FRANCE	A4P3C8	2.40	2.0	242	4.4	593	1.1	4.6	4.3
GERMANY (FRG)	A3P2	0.75	*1.6*	*223*	2.6	411	*0.2*	5.8	51.4
GREECE	A2	0.17	*0.4*	*8*	*0.4*	*12*	*0.3*	0.3	*4.1*
IRELAND	A3C2	-0.41	1.2	8	1.5	11	0.7	2.5	*19.3*
ITALY	A3P3C4	4.83	2.3	284	3.4	517	1.5	4.6	7.7
NETHERLANDS	A2C3	0.04	0.4	10	0.9	30	0.2	1.3	22.9
PORTUGAL	–	–	–	–	–	–	–	–	–
SPAIN	A5P4C4	-0.25	0.7	50	2.0	183	0.5	6.4	23.0
UK ENGLAND & WALES	A3P4C3	0.84	0.9	115	1.3	184	0.5	1.8	13.3
UK SCOTLAND	A2C2	0.08	1.0	13	1.7	22	0.7	6.6	25.3

FEMALES	Best model	Goodness of fit	1965 Rate	1965 Deaths	1985 Rate	1985 Deaths	Cumulative risk 1900	Cumulative risk 1940	Recent trend
BELGIUM	A8C9	1.17	0.2	4	0.3	9	0.1	0.2	*20.5*
DENMARK	A1C6	0.96	0.3	4	0.7	12	0.2	2.3	*13.5*
FRANCE	A2P4C3	0.99	0.1	21	0.5	69	0.1	0.6	19.1
GERMANY (FRG)	A3D	1.06	*0.1*	*18*	0.3	68	*0.0*	0.6	38.0
GREECE	A1	0.74	*0.1*	*2*	*0.1*	*3*	*0.1*	0.1	*-7.8*
IRELAND	A2D	-0.84	0.4	3	0.3	2	0.3	0.1	*18.8*
ITALY	A2C3	0.49	0.3	42	0.4	69	0.2	0.3	17.1
NETHERLANDS	A2P2	0.44	0.1	3	0.3	13	0.1	0.3	57.0
PORTUGAL	–	–	–	–	–	–	–	–	–
SPAIN	A1P4	-0.25	0.2	13	0.2	20	0.1	0.2	*-1.7*
UK ENGLAND & WALES	A2P2	-0.77	0.3	54	0.5	76	0.2	0.3	12.9
UK SCOTLAND	A2	0.77	0.5	8	0.5	8	0.3	0.3	38.9

* : not enough deaths for reliable estimation
– : incomplete or missing data
Best model: polynomial of the given degree in age (A), period (P) or cohort (C), or linear drift (D) model.
Goodness of fit: the normalised likelihood ratio chi-square for the best model (see Method).
Rate: world-standardised truncated rate per 100 000 per year (30-74 years) and number of **deaths** are both estimated from the best-fitting model for the single years cited.
Cumulative risk per 1000 (30-74 years) is estimated from the best-fitting *age-cohort* model for cohorts of central birth year cited.
Recent trend: estimated mean percentage change per five-year period in the age-specific rates (30-74 years) over the period 1975-1988.
Italics denote recent trends not significant at 5 per cent level, or other figures which should be interpreted with caution (see Method).

MOUTH (ICD-9 143-145)

EUROPE (EC), MORTALITY

MALES

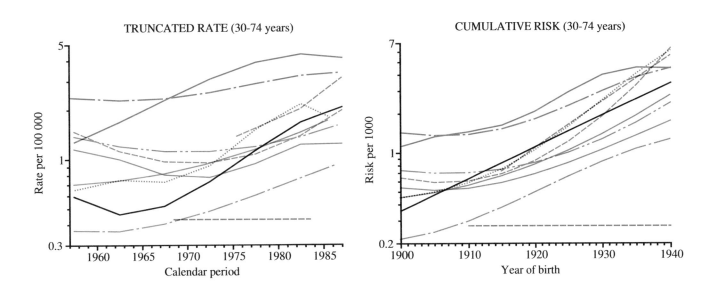

TRUNCATED RATE (30-74 years)

CUMULATIVE RISK (30-74 years)

FEMALES

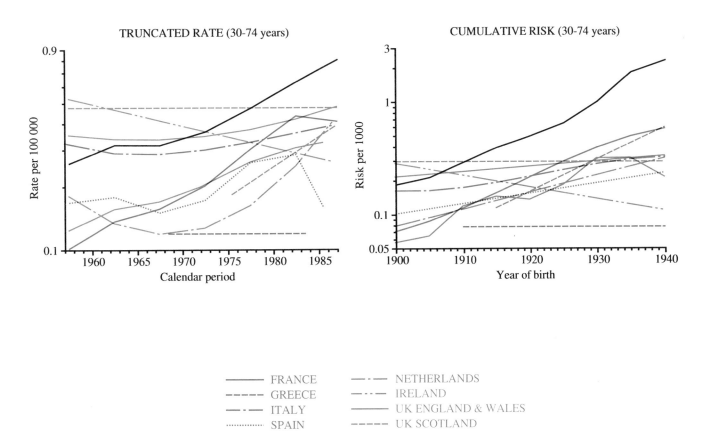

TRUNCATED RATE (30-74 years)

CUMULATIVE RISK (30-74 years)

FRANCE   NETHERLANDS
GREECE   IRELAND
ITALY   UK ENGLAND & WALES
SPAIN   UK SCOTLAND
BELGIUM   **DENMARK**
GERMANY (FRG)

MOUTH (ICD-9 143-145)

EUROPE (non-EC), MORTALITY
Percentage change per five-year period, 1975-1988

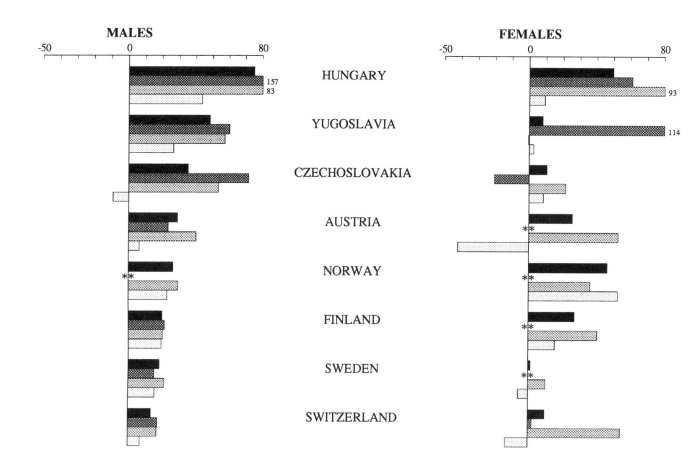

MOUTH (ICD-9 143-145)

EUROPE (EC), MORTALITY
Percentage change per five-year period, 1975-1988

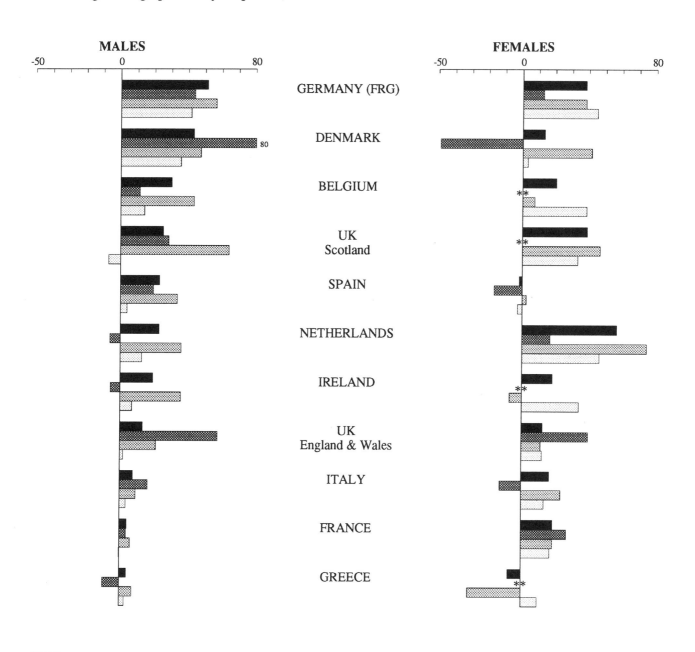

ASIA, INCIDENCE

MALES	Best model	Goodness of fit	1970 Rate	Cases	1985 Rate	Cases	Cumulative risk 1915	1940	Recent trend
CHINA									
Shanghai	A8C7	-0.50	*2.6*	27	1.4	24	1.3	0.4	-19.5
HONG KONG	A8C7	-0.24	*5.6*	*37*	4.0	46	2.3	1.6	-9.8
INDIA									
Bombay	A2P2C2	2.42	12.8	109	12.1	157	7.1	5.3	*1.1*
JAPAN									
Miyagi	A2P2	-0.19	0.8	2	1.7	8	0.8	1.4	53.9
Nagasaki	A1	-0.12	*2.8*	*2*	2.8	2	1.9	1.9	*10.7*
Osaka	A2P3	1.07	1.3	15	2.8	52	1.5	5.5	30.3
SINGAPORE									
Chinese	A2D	0.93	3.3	6	3.6	10	2.1	2.4	*10.2*
Indian	A2C7	0.57	8.5	2	9.7	4	5.3	0.0	*7.3*
Malay	A1D	-1.29	5.3	1	*0.4*	*0*	3.2	0.0	*-52.9*

FEMALES	Best model	Goodness of fit	1970 Rate	Cases	1985 Rate	Cases	Cumulative risk 1915	1940	Recent trend
CHINA									
Shanghai	A1	0.85	*1.3*	*15*	1.3	22	0.7	0.7	*-6.8*
HONG KONG	A1	1.39	*1.7*	*9*	1.7	19	1.0	1.0	*1.5*
INDIA									
Bombay	A3C2	0.07	11.8	64	9.1	88	6.3	3.4	-12.3
JAPAN									
Miyagi	A3P2	0.16	0.5	1	0.7	4	0.3	0.3	74.3
Nagasaki	A1D	0.34	*0.8*	*0*	1.0	1	0.6	0.8	*4.0*
Osaka	A2P3	1.72	0.3	3	0.8	17	0.5	1.6	23.7
SINGAPORE									
Chinese	A1	0.25	1.1	2	1.1	3	0.7	0.7	*-21.9*
Indian	A1	0.83	*15.2*	*0*	15.2	2	10.4	10.4	*-4.8*
Malay	A1C2	-1.68	2.3	*0*	*2.1*	*0*	2.9	0.0	*17.1*

* : not enough cases for reliable estimation
− : incomplete or missing data
Best model: polynomial of the given degree in age (A), period (P) or cohort (C), or linear drift (D) model.
Goodness of fit: the normalised likelihood ratio chi-square for the best model (see Method).
Rate: world-standardised truncated rate per 100 000 per year (30-74 years) and number of **cases** are both estimated from the best-fitting model for the single years cited.
Cumulative risk per 1000 (30-74 years) is estimated from the best-fitting *age-cohort* model for cohorts of central birth year cited.
Recent trend: estimated mean percentage change per five-year period in the age-specific rates (30-74 years) over the period 1973-1987.
Italics denote recent trends not significant at 5 per cent level, or other figures which should be interpreted with caution (see Method).

MOUTH (ICD-9 143-145)

ASIA, INCIDENCE

MALES

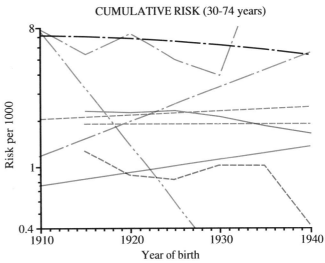

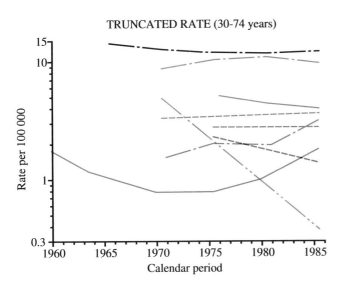

FEMALES

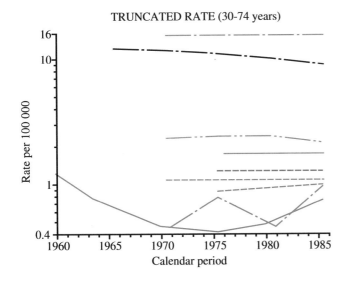

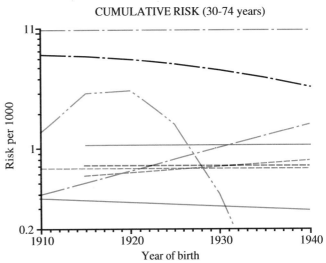

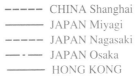

– – – – CHINA Shanghai	– – – – SINGAPORE Chinese
——— JAPAN Miyagi	—·—·— SINGAPORE Indian
– – – – JAPAN Nagasaki	——··— SINGAPORE Malay
—·—·— JAPAN Osaka	—··—·· **INDIA Bombay**
——— HONG KONG	

MOUTH (ICD-9 143-145)

OCEANIA, INCIDENCE

MALES	Best model	Goodness of fit	1970 Rate	1970 Cases	1985 Rate	1985 Cases	Cumulative risk 1915	Cumulative risk 1940	Recent trend
AUSTRALIA									
New South Wales	A2C5	1.56	*3.7*	*37*	6.2	81	2.6	5.0	15.8
South	A2	0.20	*4.2*	*9*	4.2	14	2.4	2.4	*30.1*
HAWAII									
Caucasian	A2	-0.28	11.0	3	11.0	6	6.7	6.7	*2.8*
Chinese	–	–	–	–	–	–	–	–	–
Filipino	A1	-0.09	5.3	1	5.3	2	3.4	3.4	*-28.9*
Hawaiian	A2D	-0.45	*6.6*	*0*	7.5	1	4.0	4.9	*-7.1*
Japanese	A1	0.70	2.7	1	2.7	2	1.8	1.8	*27.5*
NEW ZEALAND									
Maori	A1	-1.64	*3.0*	*0*	*3.0*	*0*	2.0	2.0	*-15.7*
Non-Maori	A2	1.01	3.0	17	3.0	20	1.8	1.8	*-2.5*

FEMALES	Best model	Goodness of fit	1970 Rate	1970 Cases	1985 Rate	1985 Cases	Cumulative risk 1915	Cumulative risk 1940	Recent trend
AUSTRALIA									
New South Wales	A2D	-0.54	*1.5*	*17*	2.3	31	1.1	2.1	14.4
South	A1D	-0.37	*0.3*	*0*	1.6	6	0.7	12.5	84.1
HAWAII									
Caucasian	A2	-0.40	6.6	2	6.6	3	3.7	3.7	*-19.7*
Chinese	*	..	..	..	..	..	..	..	..
Filipino	A1	-2.03	*4.3*	*0*	4.3	1	3.1	3.1	*-32.6*
Hawaiian	A1	-0.77	*3.0*	*0*	*3.0*	*0*	1.9	1.9	-53.8
Japanese	A1	-1.79	*1.0*	*0*	1.0	1	0.7	0.7	*13.6*
NEW ZEALAND									
Maori	*	..	..	..	..	..	..	..	..
Non-Maori	A2D	1.16	1.2	7	1.9	14	0.9	2.1	*5.3*

* : not enough cases for reliable estimation
– : incomplete or missing data
Best model: polynomial of the given degree in age (A), period (P) or cohort (C), or linear drift (D) model.
Goodness of fit: the normalised likelihood ratio chi-square for the best model (see Method).
Rate: world-standardised truncated rate per 100 000 per year (30-74 years) and number of **cases** are both estimated from the best-fitting model for the single years cited.
Cumulative risk per 1000 (30-74 years) is estimated from the best-fitting *age-cohort* model for cohorts of central birth year cited.
Recent trend: estimated mean percentage change per five-year period in the age-specific rates (30-74 years) over the period 1973-1987.
Italics denote recent trends not significant at 5 per cent level, or other figures which should be interpreted with caution (see Method).

MOUTH (ICD-9 143-145)

OCEANIA, INCIDENCE

MALES

TRUNCATED RATE (30-74 years)

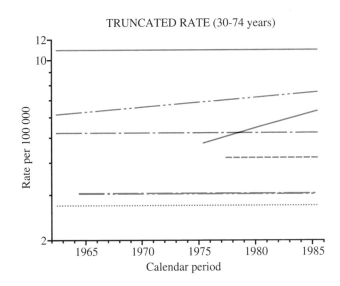

CUMULATIVE RISK (30-74 years)

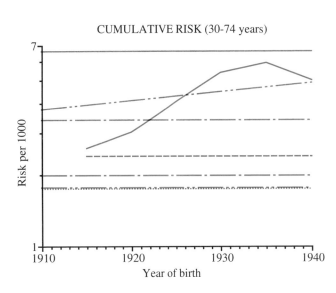

FEMALES

TRUNCATED RATE (30-74 years)

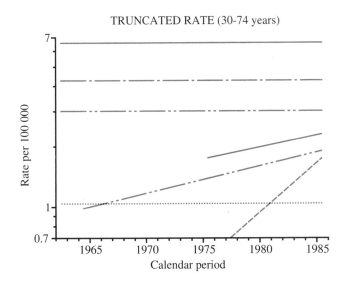

CUMULATIVE RISK (30-74 years)

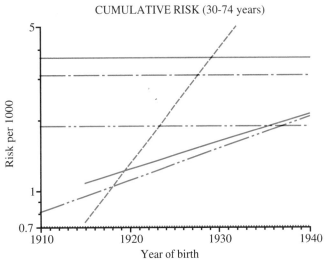

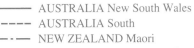

AUSTRALIA New South Wales
AUSTRALIA South
NEW ZEALAND Maori
NEW ZEALAND Non-Maori
HAWAII Caucasian

HAWAII Filipino
HAWAII Hawaiian
HAWAII Japanese

MOUTH (ICD-9 143-145)

ASIA, INCIDENCE
Percentage change per five-year period, 1973-1987

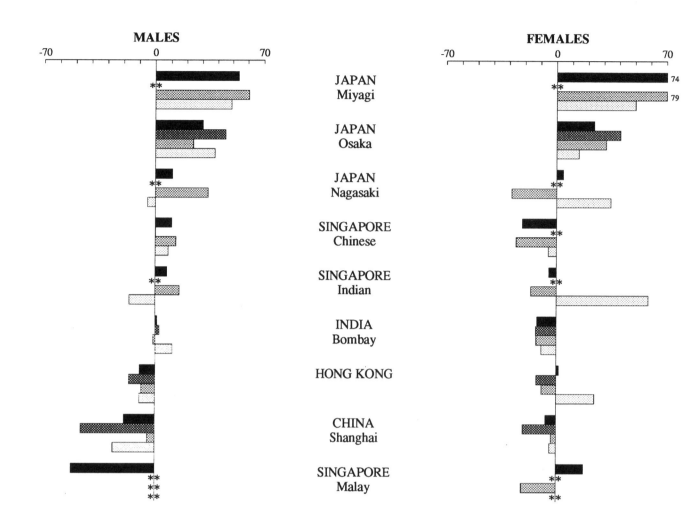

MOUTH (ICD-9 143-145)

OCEANIA, INCIDENCE
Percentage change per five-year period, 1973-1987

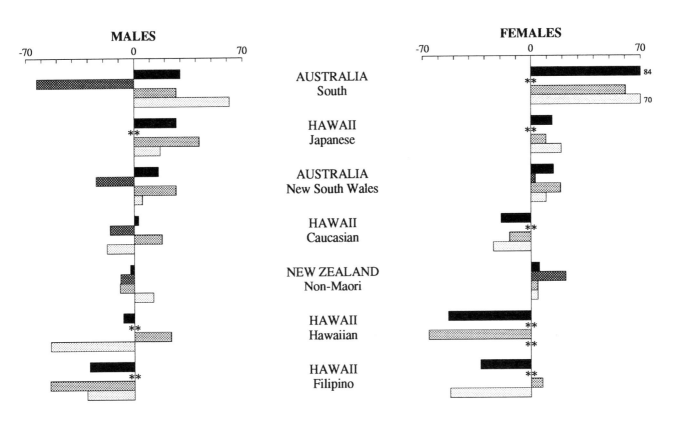

MALES | | FEMALES

-70   0   70   -70   0   70

AUSTRALIA
South

HAWAII
Japanese

AUSTRALIA
New South Wales

HAWAII
Caucasian

NEW ZEALAND
Non-Maori

HAWAII
Hawaiian

HAWAII
Filipino

- 30-74
- 30-44
- 45-64
- 65-74

MOUTH (ICD-9 143-145)

ASIA and OCEANIA, MORTALITY

MALES	Best model	Goodness of fit	1965 Rate	1965 Deaths	1985 Rate	1985 Deaths	Cumulative risk 1900	Cumulative risk 1940	Recent trend
AUSTRALIA	A4P2C3	1.34	1.2	29	1.7	63	0.7	1.3	*0.3*
HONG KONG	A2C3	0.38	*2.4*	*7*	1.5	13	*1.3*	0.5	*-7.9*
JAPAN	A2D	0.10	0.4	75	0.7	213	0.3	0.8	9.8
MAURITIUS	A2	-0.84	*0.8*	*0*	0.8	1	*0.4*	0.4	*-14.0*
NEW ZEALAND	A2D	1.01	1.2	6	1.6	11	0.8	1.3	*-12.6*
SINGAPORE	A1D	-1.00	1.0	1	1.3	3	*0.5*	0.8	–

FEMALES	Best model	Goodness of fit	1965 Rate	1965 Deaths	1985 Rate	1985 Deaths	Cumulative risk 1900	Cumulative risk 1940	Recent trend
AUSTRALIA	A2D	1.68	0.4	10	0.6	23	0.3	0.5	*3.0*
HONG KONG	A1C2	0.39	*0.5*	*2*	0.6	4	*0.3*	0.2	*24.5*
JAPAN	A2P3	-1.61	0.2	30	0.2	76	0.1	0.2	*2.5*
MAURITIUS	A1	-1.47	*0.4*	*0*	*0.4*	*0*	*0.3*	0.3	*18.3*
NEW ZEALAND	A1	-0.33	0.5	2	0.5	4	0.3	0.3	*-8.9*
SINGAPORE	A1C2	-0.11	*0.6*	*1*	0.7	1	*0.2*	0.1	–

* : not enough deaths for reliable estimation
− : incomplete or missing data
Best model: polynomial of the given degree in age (A), period (P) or cohort (C), or linear drift (D) model.
Goodness of fit: the normalised likelihood ratio chi-square for the best model (see Method).
Rate: world-standardised truncated rate per 100 000 per year (30-74 years) and number of **deaths** are both estimated from the best-fitting model for the single years cited.
Cumulative risk per 1000 (30-74 years) is estimated from the best-fitting *age-cohort* model for cohorts of central birth year cited.
Recent trend: estimated mean percentage change per five-year period in the age-specific rates (30-74 years) over the period 1975-1988.
Italics denote recent trends not significant at 5 per cent level, or other figures which should be interpreted with caution (see Method).

MOUTH (ICD-9 143-145)

ASIA and OCEANIA, MORTALITY

MALES

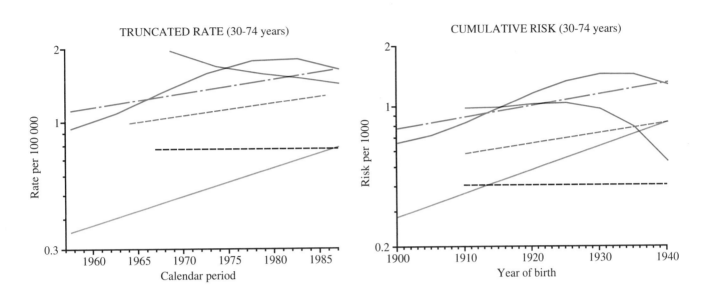

FEMALES

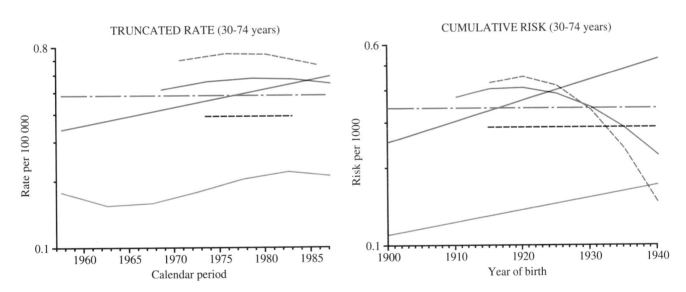

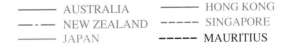

AUSTRALIA   HONG KONG
NEW ZEALAND   SINGAPORE
JAPAN   MAURITIUS

MOUTH (ICD-9 143-145)

ASIA and OCEANIA, MORTALITY
Percentage change per five-year period, 1975-1988

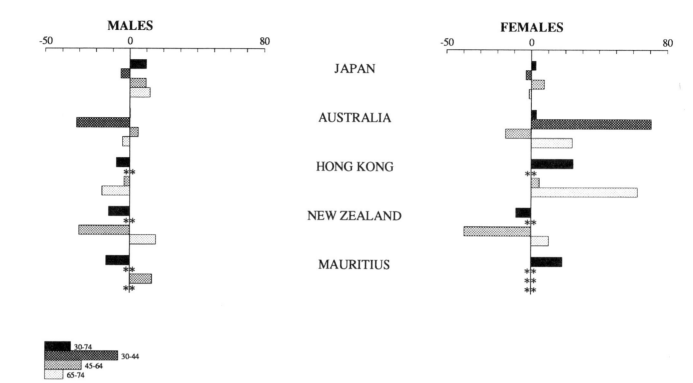

from page 97

are unstable: the risk estimate for the 1940 birth cohort in these populations is very imprecise.

The available data for Oceania show a positive trend in incidence for both males and females in Australia and for the non-Maori population in New Zealand. The mortality trend for these two countries is significant for males, but not for females in New Zealand, where few deaths have occurred each year. The age-specific rates for young adult males have started to fall in both New South Wales and South Australia. This decline is reflected in the trend of cumulative risk of cancer of the mouth in New South Wales for the most recent birth cohorts, and in the lower risk of mortality in Australia as a whole for the same cohorts.

Americas

In Central and South America, incidence is decreasing in Puerto Rico and in Cuba, but not in São Paulo (Brazil). Male populations in Brazil have the highest risks in the world for cancer of the mouth, after those in France and India[202,221]. Assessment of the most recent trends in Brazil is

difficult, however, because of the lack of incidence data spanning a long period, and the total absence of mortality data for cancer of the mouth.

In North America, there is a steep increase in cumulative risk among males in the Maritime Provinces (Canada), but a tendency for the risk to level off in Quebec. Overall, the risk of cancer of the mouth is increasing in successive birth cohorts in Canada, and this is reflected by the trend in mortality. The cumulative risk of death in Canada has more than doubled for both males and females between the 1900 and 1940 birth cohorts, and now exceeds the risk in the USA. The risk of cancer of the mouth has increased substantially in Detroit (USA) in both sexes, and in both blacks and whites. There have been only limited changes in incidence for males elsewhere in the USA. In contrast, incidence among females has decreased in the San Francisco Bay Area (whites), in Seattle and in New Orleans (blacks), but has increased substantially in Iowa and Connecticut. The trends among females are statistically unstable. The mortality data for the USA were incomplete (no data between 1967 and 1980); they suggest, however, a slight decrease in the most recent period.

118

Comment

It is especially important that the patterns of mouth cancer risk in Europe be further studied, because recent trends in young adults, particularly males, are very large, approaching 100% (doubling every five years) in some countries. Recent data suggest that the lifetime risk (30-74 years) of developing cancer in one of these oral sites will exceed 1% for males born around 1940 in several European countries, where previously this cancer was up to an order of magnitude less frequent. The increase in alcohol consumption among males in countries where the risk was low 20 years ago may be partly responsible for the increasing trends in cancers of the mouth, especially in Germany and Denmark, where all alcohol-related cancers are becoming more frequent. Trends in alcohol consumption seem unlikely to explain all the trends in cancer of the mouth, however, especially among females.

Age-standardised incidence of cancer of the mouth among males in Bombay (India) was stable between 1964 and 1982 (while that of the tongue declined steadily)[136], and there was little evidence of change in successive birth cohorts when these were examined over comparable 15-year age spans. In contrast, although the best model selected here for the data from Bombay was complex and did not fit well, inclusion of all the data to derive the projected lifetime risk for the 1940 birth cohort enables the significant reduction in risk relative to the 1915 cohort to be identified. The high risks for mouth cancer in São Paulo (Brazil) and Bombay (India) have been compared[120]: the male-to-female ratio of incidence rates is notably higher in São Paulo (3.64) than in Bombay (1.30), a difference attributed to the predomi-

nance of alcohol as the risk factor in Brazil. Betel (pan) chewing is common among females in India[208]. Oral cancers (including those of lip and tongue) ranked first among males seen in seven hospital centres in Pakistan during 1973-74, with 13.8% of non-metastatic tumours: the decline to second rank (8.6%) in six of the centres by 1977-80 was attributed to a switch in life-style, from chewing betel to smoking tobacco[176]: it can be calculated that the absolute number of cases of oral cancer in males seen each year in these centres also declined, from about 780 to 650. The recent decline in mortality from cancers of the tongue and mouth in Australia among both males and females aged less than 45 has been noted previously[183], together with the increase in incidence among females at all ages in South Australia up to 1986: these trends were closely related to time-lagged trends in the consumption of tobacco and alcohol in each sex.

Birth cohort analysis of mouth cancer mortality trends in the USA up to 1984 for whites and non-whites has revealed a decline in age-specific rates among younger white females born since 1920, and among younger non-white females born since about 1930. There was a continuing increase in mortality for younger males (35-39 years) born as late as 1945. These trends were related to patterns of tobacco smoking and chewing and alcohol consumption by age, race and sex[74]. Improvements in diagnosis and treatment were considered unlikely to have contributed greatly to the observed trends[75,271].

It must unfortunately be concluded that prevention of cancer of the mouth, largely feasible on the basis of current knowledge, has not yet been effective; in Europe and Japan, the situation has actually deteriorated.

AMERICAS (except USA), INCIDENCE

MALES	Best model	Goodness of fit	1970		1985		Cumulative risk		Recent trend
			Rate	Cases	Rate	Cases	1915	1940	
BRAZIL									
Sao Paulo	A7C6	-1.80	12.1	88	*64.2*	*1622*	5.0	*4.5*	–
CANADA									
Alberta	A4	0.24	3.6	10	3.6	16	2.0	2.0	*-2.5*
British Columbia	A2D	0.34	3.8	17	5.8	40	2.8	5.5	12.8
Maritime Provinces	A2C4	0.34	4.3	13	6.0	20	2.1	6.3	22.7
Newfoundland	A3	-0.49	2.7	2	2.7	3	1.8	1.8	*36.4*
Quebec	A5P4C3	-0.95	6.3	68	7.1	102	3.7	4.7	*1.6*
COLOMBIA									
Cali	A2	-0.32	3.2	2	3.2	4	1.9	1.9	*-16.8*
CUBA	A2D	-0.43	6.8	101	3.8	78	3.2	*1.2*	–
PUERTO RICO	A3D	1.58	14.7	66	12.4	81	7.8	6.0	*0.6*

FEMALES	Best model	Goodness of fit	1970		1985		Cumulative risk		Recent trend
			Rate	Cases	Rate	Cases	1915	1940	
BRAZIL									
Sao Paulo	A2D	-0.96	1.9	15	*5.3*	*54*	1.3	*6.6*	–
CANADA									
Alberta	A2D	0.33	1.4	4	2.4	11	1.1	2.5	28.0
British Columbia	A2C2	-0.47	2.0	9	2.9	22	1.7	1.6	20.6
Maritime Provinces	A4	-0.73	1.8	5	1.8	6	1.0	1.0	*6.1*
Newfoundland	A1	-1.28	*0.8*	*0*	0.8	1	0.6	0.6	*43.5*
Quebec	A4D	0.55	1.4	16	2.0	33	1.0	1.8	*8.8*
COLOMBIA									
Cali	A1D	-0.93	3.1	2	1.8	2	1.5	0.7	*-26.8*
CUBA	A2	0.21	2.2	27	2.2	45	1.5	*1.5*	–
PUERTO RICO	A2D	-0.54	4.1	18	2.7	20	2.0	1.0	-17.2

* : not enough cases for reliable estimation
– : incomplete or missing data
Best model: polynomial of the given degree in age (A), period (P) or cohort (C), or linear drift (D) model.
Goodness of fit: the normalised likelihood ratio chi-square for the best model (see Method).
Rate: world-standardised truncated rate per 100 000 per year (30-74 years) and number of **cases** are both estimated from the best-fitting model for the single years cited.
Cumulative risk per 1000 (30-74 years) is estimated from the best-fitting *age-cohort* model for cohorts of central birth year cited. ·
Recent trend: estimated mean percentage change per five-year period in the age-specific rates (30-74 years) over the period 1973-1987.
Italics denote recent trends not significant at 5 per cent level, or other figures which should be interpreted with caution (see Method).

MOUTH (ICD-9 143-145)

AMERICAS (except USA), INCIDENCE

MALES

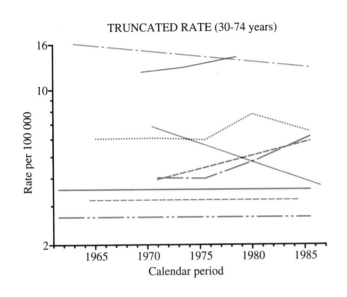

TRUNCATED RATE (30-74 years)

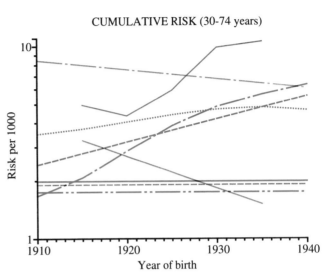

CUMULATIVE RISK (30-74 years)

FEMALES

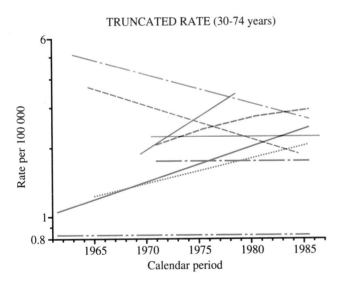

TRUNCATED RATE (30-74 years)

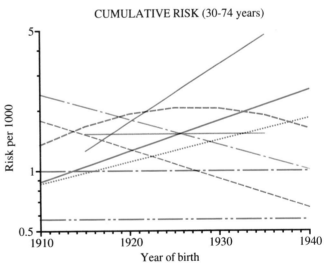

CUMULATIVE RISK (30-74 years)

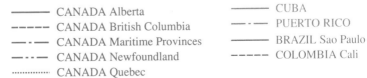

———— CANADA Alberta
– – – – CANADA British Columbia
– · – · – CANADA Maritime Provinces
– ·· – ·· CANADA Newfoundland
············ CANADA Quebec

———— CUBA
– · – · – PUERTO RICO
———— BRAZIL Sao Paulo
– – – – COLOMBIA Cali

AMERICAS (USA), INCIDENCE

MALES	Best model	Goodness of fit	1970 Rate	1970 Cases	1985 Rate	1985 Cases	Cumulative risk 1915	Cumulative risk 1940	Recent trend
USA									
Bay Area, Black	A2	0.22	11.9	6	11.9	9	6.2	6.2	*-4.1*
Bay Area, Chinese	A1D	-0.51	8.6	1	*1.2*	*0*	5.6	*0.2*	–
Bay Area, White	A2	-1.04	8.2	49	8.2	50	4.8	4.8	*-1.8*
Connecticut	A2P2	2.08	9.2	61	9.4	73	5.4	7.0	*-3.8*
Detroit, Black	A3P2	0.28	4.7	6	14.5	23	4.6	15.8	18.0
Detroit, White	A2P3	-1.96	7.5	56	9.2	65	4.3	7.4	16.5
Iowa	A3	1.42	5.7	37	5.7	37	3.2	3.2	*0.9*
New Orleans, Black	A2	1.19	*13.1*	*6*	13.1	7	7.5	7.5	*-5.5*
New Orleans, White	A2P2	-0.09	*43.8*	*63*	9.4	14	5.7	4.8	*-3.0*
Seattle	A2	0.95	*7.1*	*33*	7.1	46	4.2	4.2	*-1.5*

FEMALES	Best model	Goodness of fit	1970 Rate	1970 Cases	1985 Rate	1985 Cases	Cumulative risk 1915	Cumulative risk 1940	Recent trend
USA									
Bay Area, Black	A2P2	-0.35	*1.1*	*0*	3.3	3	1.8	2.7	*-18.0*
Bay Area, Chinese	A2D	-1.37	7.6	1	*0.1*	*0*	8.5	*0.0*	–
Bay Area, White	A2C2	0.36	4.9	33	5.1	35	3.2	2.0	*-1.0*
Connecticut	A2C2	1.22	2.9	22	4.0	36	2.1	2.5	7.8
Detroit, Black	A3C2	-1.25	3.4	5	4.9	9	1.6	5.3	*12.3*
Detroit, White	A2D	0.24	2.8	23	3.7	30	1.8	2.8	9.2
Iowa	A2D	0.36	1.6	12	2.9	22	1.3	3.5	36.8
New Orleans, Black	A1C3	-0.23	*32.9*	*27*	2.5	1	2.7	0.5	-38.3
New Orleans, White	A2	-0.93	*3.6*	*6*	3.6	6	2.0	2.0	*0.5*
Seattle	A3C3	0.57	*4.2*	*20*	4.0	30	3.3	1.1	*-4.0*

* : not enough cases for reliable estimation
– : incomplete or missing data
Best model: polynomial of the given degree in age (A), period (P) or cohort (C), or linear drift (D) model.
Goodness of fit: the normalised likelihood ratio chi-square for the best model (see Method).
Rate: world-standardised truncated rate per 100 000 per year (30-74 years) and number of **cases** are both estimated from the best-fitting model for the single years cited.
Cumulative risk per 1000 (30-74 years) is estimated from the best-fitting *age-cohort* model for cohorts of central birth year cited.
Recent trend: estimated mean percentage change per five-year period in the age-specific rates (30-74 years) over the period 1973-1987.
Italics denote recent trends not significant at 5 per cent level, or other figures which should be interpreted with caution (see Method).

MOUTH (ICD-9 143-145)

AMERICAS (USA), INCIDENCE

MALES

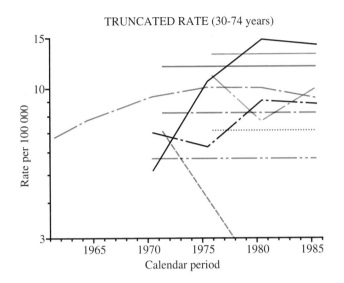

TRUNCATED RATE (30-74 years)

Rate per 100 000 · Calendar period

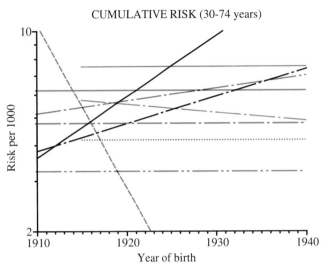

CUMULATIVE RISK (30-74 years)

Risk per 1000 · Year of birth

FEMALES

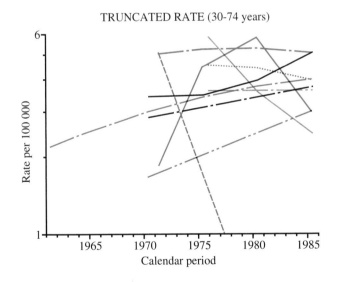

TRUNCATED RATE (30-74 years)

Rate per 100 000 · Calendar period

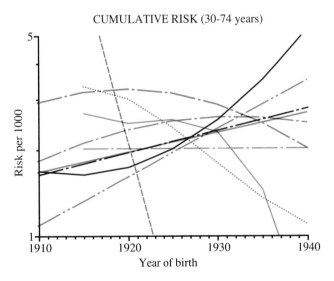

CUMULATIVE RISK (30-74 years)

Risk per 1000 · Year of birth

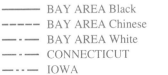

——— BAY AREA Black
– – – BAY AREA Chinese
–·–·– BAY AREA White
–··–··– CONNECTICUT
–···–···– IOWA

·········· SEATTLE
——— NEW ORLEANS Black
–·–·– NEW ORLEANS White
——— DETROIT Black
–··–··– DETROIT White

MOUTH (ICD-9 143-145)

AMERICAS (except USA), INCIDENCE
Percentage change per five-year period, 1973-1987

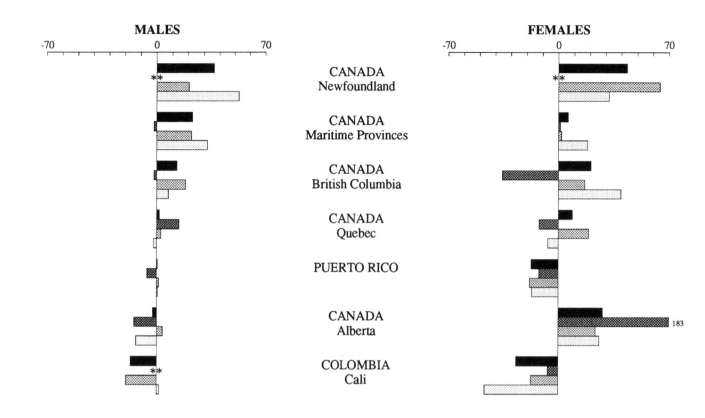

MALES

FEMALES

-70   0   70

-70   0   70

CANADA
Newfoundland

CANADA
Maritime Provinces

CANADA
British Columbia

CANADA
Quebec

PUERTO RICO

CANADA
Alberta

COLOMBIA
Cali

183

30-74
30-44
45-64
65-74

MOUTH (ICD-9 143-145)

AMERICAS (USA), INCIDENCE
Percentage change per five-year period, 1973-1987

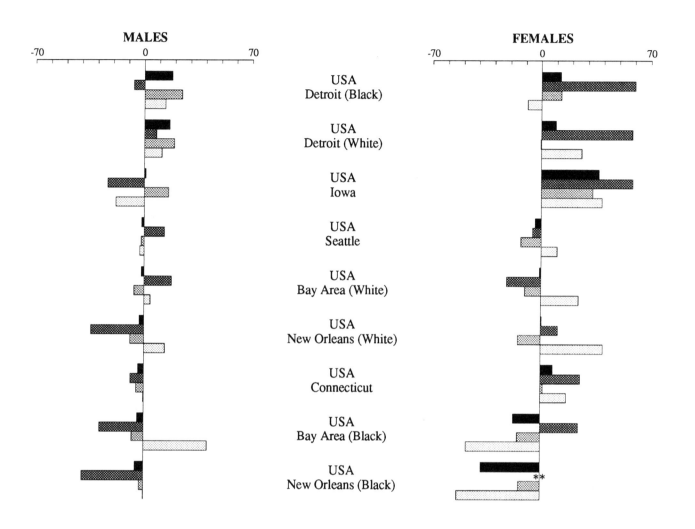

MOUTH (ICD-9 143-145)

AMERICAS, MORTALITY

MALES	Best model	Goodness of fit	1965 Rate	1965 Deaths	1985 Rate	1985 Deaths	Cumulative risk 1900	Cumulative risk 1940	Recent trend
CANADA	A4C5	1.10	1.3	50	1.8	104	0.8	1.7	_3.0_
CHILE	A2D	2.75	0.7	8	_1.6_	_30_	0.3	_1.9_	–
COSTA RICA	–	–	–	–	–	–	–	–	–
PANAMA	–	–	–	–	–	–	–	–	–
PUERTO RICO	–	–	–	–	–	–	–	–	–
URUGUAY	–	–	–	–	–	–	–	–	–
USA	–	–	–	–	–	–	–	–	–
VENEZUELA	A2	0.62	1.1	9	_1.1_	_17_	0.7	_0.7_	–

FEMALES	Best model	Goodness of fit	1965 Rate	1965 Deaths	1985 Rate	1985 Deaths	Cumulative risk 1900	Cumulative risk 1940	Recent trend
CANADA	A2C3	0.08	0.4	14	0.6	38	0.2	0.5	_7.6_
CHILE	*	..	..	..	..	..	..	..	..
COSTA RICA	–	–	–	–	–	–	–	–	–
PANAMA	–	–	–	–	–	–	–	–	–
PUERTO RICO	–	–	–	–	–	–	–	–	–
URUGUAY	–	–	–	–	–	–	–	–	–
USA	–	–	–	–	–	–	–	–	–
VENEZUELA	A2D	1.20	1.7	14	_0.9_	_14_	1.2	_0.3_	–

* : not enough deaths for reliable estimation
– : incomplete or missing data
Best model: polynomial of the given degree in age (A), period (P) or cohort (C), or linear drift (D) model.
Goodness of fit: the normalised likelihood ratio chi-square for the best model (see Method).
Rate: world-standardised truncated rate per 100 000 per year (30-74 years) and number of **deaths** are both estimated from the best-fitting model for the single years cited.
Cumulative risk per 1000 (30-74 years) is estimated from the best-fitting _age-cohort_ model for cohorts of central birth year cited.
Recent trend: estimated mean percentage change per five-year period in the age-specific rates (30-74 years) over the period 1975-1988.
Italics denote recent trends not significant at 5 per cent level, or other figures which should be interpreted with caution (see Method).

MOUTH (ICD-9 143-145)

AMERICAS, MORTALITY

MALES

TRUNCATED RATE (30-74 years)

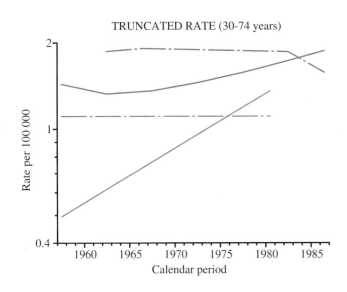

CUMULATIVE RISK (30-74 years)

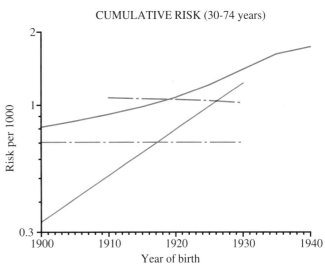

FEMALES

TRUNCATED RATE (30-74 years)

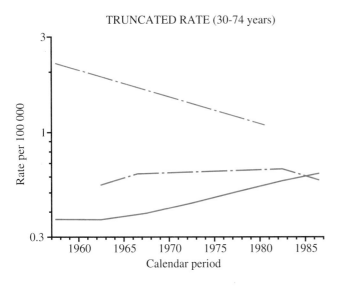

CUMULATIVE RISK (30-74 years)

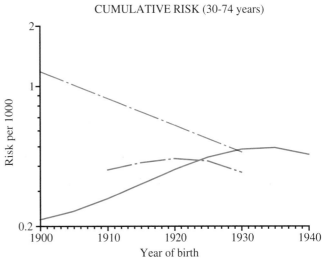

CANADA
USA
CHILE
VENEZUELA

MOUTH (ICD-9 143-145)

AMERICAS, MORTALITY
Percentage change per five-year period, 1975-1988

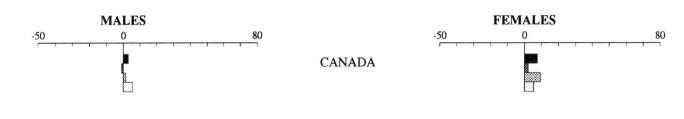

MALES   CANADA   FEMALES

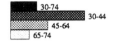

Chapter 8

PHARYNX

Cancers of the mouth and pharynx combined (ICD-9 140-149) ranked sixth in the world around 1980[219], with about 380 000 new cases a year, or 6% of all new cancers. Three-quarters of the cases arise in developing countries, where they rank third in frequency. Cancers of the pharynx (ICD-9 146-148) include those assigned to the oropharynx, tonsil and free border of the epiglottis (146), the nasopharynx (147) and the hypopharynx, including pyriform fossa or sinus (148). Cancers of these sites are usually treated together for epidemiological purposes, and this convention is followed here, even though there are several aetiological entities. Trends in cancer of the nasopharynx, in particular, would merit separate study in some countries, but suitable data were not available. Nasopharyngeal cancer is very common in several Chinese populations (especially in Hong Kong and southern China) and in other parts of south-east Asia, in particular the Philippines, Vietnam and Indonesia. High risks are also seen among Eskimos, and in North Africa and Sudan. Migrants from high-risk areas keep their risk differential for several generations. The male-to-female sex ratio is about three-fold. Survival from cancer of the pharynx is poor, and mortality is a reasonable indicator of trends in the risk where incidence data are unavailable.

It is often difficult to determine the precise anatomical origin of tumours in this region, and misclassification between the three-digit rubrics within the pharynx is more likely than in other parts of the body, particularly at death certification. Consequently, several countries until recently reported mortality only for a broader group of sites, including all sites in the mouth and pharynx (ICD-9 140-149) or, in the USA, this same group excluding salivary glands (ICD-9 142). In this chapter, therefore, in order to present the most complete set of mortality data available for this anatomical region, the mortality data examined for the Americas are those for the oral cavity and pharynx combined. It is important to note that these data are not directly comparable with incidence data for cancers of the pharynx in the Americas, nor with the mortality data for Europe, Asia and Oceania.

Cancers of the pharynx account for 15% to 50% of all cancers of the buccal cavity and pharynx combined, e.g. 17% in Finland and 53% in Bas-Rhin (France). Except in areas where the

risk of nasopharyngeal cancer is high, cancers of the pharynx comprise mainly those of the oropharynx and hypopharynx. For example, it can be calculated from volume VI of *Cancer Incidence in Five Continents*[221] that these two sites account for more than 80% of pharyngeal cancers in western European populations. High-risk regions for cancers of the oropharynx and hypopharynx are found in France, Switzerland and, to a lesser extent, Italy. Cancers of the pharynx are generally rare in females, except in some black American and Indian populations. In contrast to the situation for cancers of the mouth, however, the sex-ratio in Indian populations reflects the usual male predominance for epithelial tumours.

The risk factors for cancer of the oropharynx are similar to those for cancers of the tongue and mouth, including tobacco and alcohol, but these two factors do not entirely account for the observed geographical variation. Tobacco and alcohol consumption have multiplicative effects on cancer risk for both the hypopharynx and larynx[289]. Dietary and environmental factors, particularly consumption of salt fish and infection with Epstein-Barr virus, are implicated in the aetiology of nasopharyngeal carcinoma.

Europe

Trends in cancer of the pharynx are generally similar to those for cancer of the mouth.

Among males, there is a clear decrease of the cumulative risk in successive birth cohorts in Finland, and a plateau for males born in 1930 or later in Sweden. There are rapid upward trends in Slovenia, Hungary, Poland, Norway, Denmark, Germany and Spain (especially Navarra). Almost all models are age-cohort models, suggesting that trends in the cumulative risk are readily interpretable. Little change has occurred in France, Italy and Spain, countries where risk has been high. In England, the risk has remained low, despite a slight upward trend in Birmingham, which is now declining for cohorts born since 1930.

The mortality data for males are consistent with the incidence data, but are considerably less clear than for cancer of the mouth. The recent trend suggests that mortality from cancer of the pharynx is rising, especially among younger males, in most European countries except Finland, Sweden

129

continued page 150

EUROPE (non-EC), INCIDENCE

MALES	Best model	Goodness of fit	1970 Rate	1970 Cases	1985 Rate	1985 Cases	Cumulative risk 1915	Cumulative risk 1940	Recent trend
FINLAND	A2C2	0.35	3.1	31	2.5	29	1.8	0.9	-13.3
HUNGARY									
County Vas	A2D	-0.60	4.0	3	7.7	5	2.9	8.6	51.5
Szabolcs-Szatmar	A2D	1.89	2.8	3	9.1	12	2.5	17.9	23.8
ISRAEL									
All Jews	A2	0.63	3.0	14	3.0	18	1.6	1.6	17.1
Non-Jews	A1	1.52	2.9	1	2.9	1	1.6	1.6	*14.4*
NORWAY	A2C3	-0.72	2.6	28	4.1	45	1.8	5.4	17.5
POLAND									
Warsaw City	A2D	1.41	4.2	12	7.6	30	3.0	8.0	*6.9*
ROMANIA									
Cluj	A2	1.41	*6.9*	*10*	6.9	12	3.7	3.7	*5.7*
SWEDEN	A8C9	0.03	3.4	82	4.0	98	1.9	2.6	8.0
SWITZERLAND									
Geneva	A2	-0.68	22.3	17	22.3	20	12.2	12.2	*4.4*
YUGOSLAVIA									
Slovenia	A3P2C5	0.36	10.9	39	23.3	103	7.4	32.5	21.1

FEMALES	Best model	Goodness of fit	1970 Rate	1970 Cases	1985 Rate	1985 Cases	Cumulative risk 1915	Cumulative risk 1940	Recent trend
FINLAND	A2D	1.60	1.4	18	1.0	14	0.7	0.4	-19.3
HUNGARY									
County Vas	A1D	-0.72	*0.5*	*0*	2.2	1	0.7	7.3	*58.6*
Szabolcs-Szatmar	A2C2	0.20	*0.6*	*0*	1.6	2	0.3	2.5	*32.5*
ISRAEL									
All Jews	A1	0.67	1.2	5	1.2	8	0.6	0.6	*-3.9*
Non-Jews	A0	-0.68	*1.1*	*0*	1.1	1	0.5	0.5	*13.0*
NORWAY	A2C2	-1.82	0.9	11	1.3	14	0.5	1.4	*13.4*
POLAND									
Warsaw City	A2	2.25	1.4	5	1.4	7	0.8	0.8	*15.7*
ROMANIA									
Cluj	A2	-0.46	*2.0*	*3*	2.0	3	1.0	1.0	*15.7*
SWEDEN	A2C2	-2.31	1.4	37	1.2	30	0.7	0.6	*-5.1*
SWITZERLAND									
Geneva	A2	0.82	2.9	2	2.9	3	1.6	1.6	*-7.9*
YUGOSLAVIA									
Slovenia	A2C2	0.27	1.2	5	1.7	9	0.6	1.7	36.3

* : not enough cases for reliable estimation
− : incomplete or missing data
Best model: polynomial of the given degree in age (A), period (P) or cohort (C), or linear drift (D) model.
Goodness of fit: the normalised likelihood ratio chi-square for the best model (see Method).
Rate: world-standardised truncated rate per 100 000 per year (30-74 years) and number of **cases** are both estimated from the best-fitting model for the single years cited.
Cumulative risk per 1000 (30-74 years) is estimated from the best-fitting *age-cohort* model for cohorts of central birth year cited.
Recent trend: estimated mean percentage change per five-year period in the age-specific rates (30-74 years) over the period 1973-1987.
Italics denote recent trends not significant at 5 per cent level, or other figures which should be interpreted with caution (see Method).

PHARYNX (ICD-9 146-148)

EUROPE (non-EC), INCIDENCE

MALES

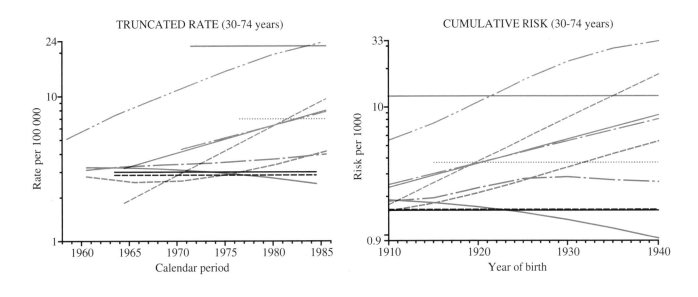

FEMALES

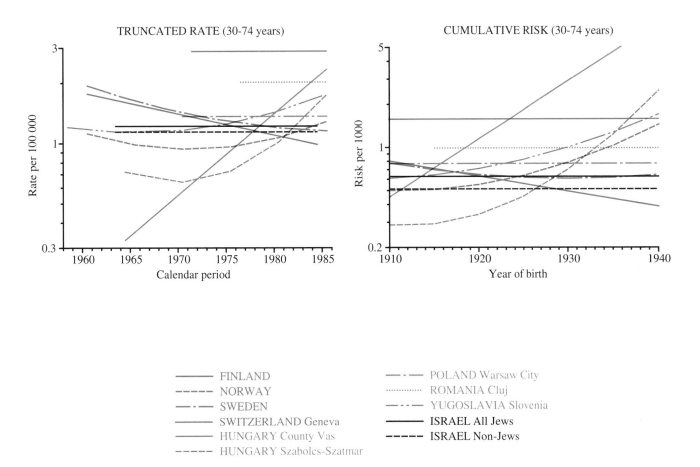

FINLAND
NORWAY
SWEDEN
SWITZERLAND Geneva
HUNGARY County Vas
HUNGARY Szabolcs-Szatmar

POLAND Warsaw City
ROMANIA Cluj
YUGOSLAVIA Slovenia
ISRAEL All Jews
ISRAEL Non-Jews

PHARYNX (ICD-9 146-148)

EUROPE (EC), INCIDENCE

MALES	Best model	Goodness of fit	1970 Rate	1970 Cases	1985 Rate	1985 Cases	Cumulative risk 1915	Cumulative risk 1940	Recent trend
DENMARK	A2C3	-0.52	2.2	28	5.6	75	2.0	10.1	33.7
FRANCE									
Bas-Rhin	A8C7	-1.07	*40.5*	*79*	62.9	129	24.7	39.6	16.4
Doubs	A3D	0.17	*27.6*	*22*	46.1	50	18.0	41.7	19.7
GERMANY (FRG)									
Hamburg	A1P2	2.50	3.0	15	*0.4*	*1*	3.3	*7.0*	–
Saarland	A3C2	0.00	6.5	18	11.7	32	3.0	17.5	43.1
GERMANY (GDR)	A3C4	1.03	2.2	94	5.3	204	1.5	13.5	45.3
ITALY									
Varese	A2	-0.49	*17.4*	*26*	17.4	35	10.0	10.0	*-1.0*
SPAIN									
Navarra	A2D	0.48	*2.2*	*2*	7.4	9	2.0	14.3	49.6
Zaragoza	A2P3	2.23	2.7	4	7.2	16	3.5	5.2	-26.5
UK									
Birmingham	A4C5	-0.34	3.8	50	3.9	57	2.0	2.2	11.9
Scotland	A2C2	-0.55	2.7	37	3.8	50	1.7	5.8	20.9
South Thames	A2C2	-1.69	3.6	90	3.0	56	1.9	1.8	*-2.9*

FEMALES	Best model	Goodness of fit	1970 Rate	1970 Cases	1985 Rate	1985 Cases	Cumulative risk 1915	Cumulative risk 1940	Recent trend
DENMARK	A2C3	0.86	0.9	12	1.9	27	0.7	2.4	25.4
FRANCE									
Bas-Rhin	A1	0.20	*2.0*	*5*	2.0	4	1.1	1.1	*0.3*
Doubs	A1C2	-0.33	*1.2*	*1*	1.6	1	0.6	0.8	*10.2*
GERMANY (FRG)									
Hamburg	A1	-0.88	1.2	8	*1.2*	*6*	0.7	*0.7*	–
Saarland	A2	1.11	1.6	5	1.6	5	0.8	0.8	*32.4*
GERMANY (GDR)	A2P3	-0.85	0.8	47	1.0	53	0.5	0.8	19.3
ITALY									
Varese	A2	0.01	*1.4*	*2*	1.4	3	0.7	0.7	*33.0*
SPAIN									
Navarra	A1	-0.32	*0.6*	*0*	*0.6*	*0*	0.3	0.3	*7.2*
Zaragoza	A1	0.22	0.9	1	0.9	2	0.5	0.5	*21.7*
UK									
Birmingham	A2C3	-0.29	2.2	31	1.6	24	1.1	0.6	-14.4
Scotland	A2C3	-0.42	1.8	29	1.5	24	1.0	0.6	*-9.6*
South Thames	A2P3	-0.72	2.1	61	1.3	27	0.9	0.5	-12.8

* : not enough cases for reliable estimation
– : incomplete or missing data
Best model: polynomial of the given degree in age (A), period (P) or cohort (C), or linear drift (D) model.
Goodness of fit: the normalised likelihood ratio chi-square for the best model (see Method).
Rate: world-standardised truncated rate per 100 000 per year (30-74 years) and number of **cases** are both estimated from the best-fitting model for the single years cited.
Cumulative risk per 1000 (30-74 years) is estimated from the best-fitting *age-cohort* model for cohorts of central birth year cited.
Recent trend: estimated mean percentage change per five-year period in the age-specific rates (30-74 years) over the period 1973-1987.
Italics denote recent trends not significant at 5 per cent level, or other figures which should be interpreted with caution (see Method).

PHARYNX (ICD-9 146-148)

EUROPE (EC), INCIDENCE

MALES

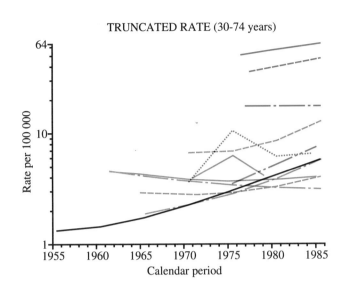

TRUNCATED RATE (30-74 years)

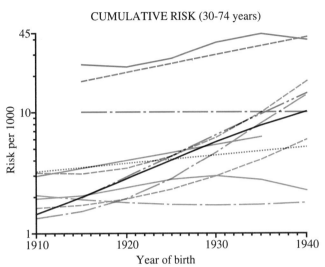

CUMULATIVE RISK (30-74 years)

FEMALES

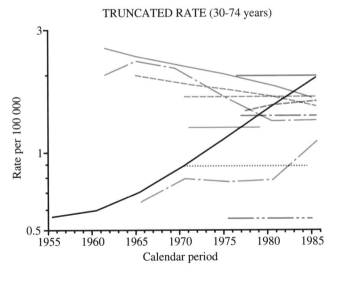

TRUNCATED RATE (30-74 years)

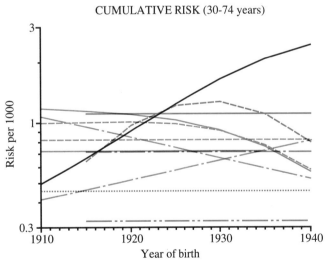

CUMULATIVE RISK (30-74 years)

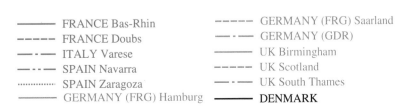

—— FRANCE Bas-Rhin	----- GERMANY (FRG) Saarland
----- FRANCE Doubs	—·—· GERMANY (GDR)
—·—· ITALY Varese	—— UK Birmingham
—··—·· SPAIN Navarra	----- UK Scotland
········ SPAIN Zaragoza	—·—· UK South Thames
—— GERMANY (FRG) Hamburg	—— DENMARK

PHARYNX (ICD-9 146-148)

EUROPE (non-EC), INCIDENCE
Percentage change per five-year period, 1973-1987

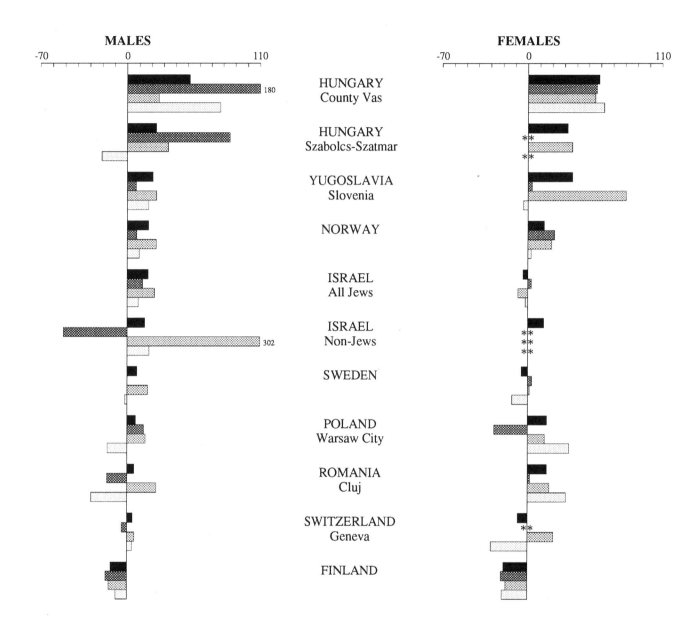

MALES

-70   0   110

FEMALES

-70   0   110

HUNGARY
County Vas

HUNGARY
Szabolcs-Szatmar

YUGOSLAVIA
Slovenia

NORWAY

ISRAEL
All Jews

ISRAEL
Non-Jews

SWEDEN

POLAND
Warsaw City

ROMANIA
Cluj

SWITZERLAND
Geneva

FINLAND

30-74
30-44
45-64
65-74

PHARYNX (ICD-9 146-148)

EUROPE (EC), INCIDENCE
Percentage change per five-year period, 1973-1987

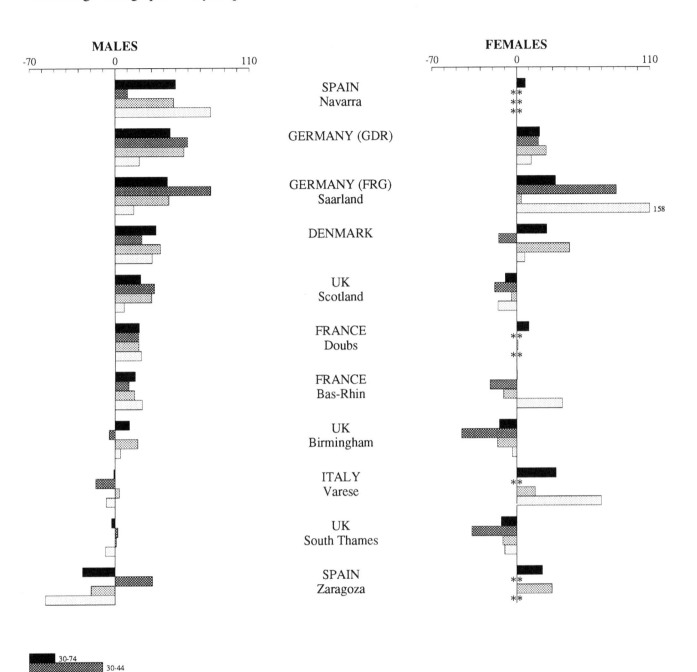

PHARYNX (ICD-9 146-148)

EUROPE (non-EC), MORTALITY

MALES	Best model	Goodness of fit	1965 Rate	Deaths	1985 Rate	Deaths	Cumulative risk 1900	1940	Recent trend
AUSTRIA	A3C3	1.09	*3.7*	*72*	4.3	76	*1.9*	5.2	24.1
CZECHOSLOVAKIA	A3P4C4	-1.39	1.8	62	6.1	214	1.0	15.7	58.9
FINLAND	A2	0.51	1.9	17	1.9	21	1.2	1.2	*-4.0*
HUNGARY	A3P3C2	-0.44	*71.4*	*1864*	9.5	253	*0.5*	59.0	84.1
NORWAY	A2C2	0.48	1.8	18	2.4	27	1.1	2.8	*9.1*
POLAND	A8P2C7	-1.34	2.4	144	*109.8*	*8661*	1.6	*2.3*	–
ROMANIA	–	–	–	–	–	–	–	–	–
SWEDEN	A2	-0.75	2.3	54	2.3	61	1.5	1.5	*2.0*
SWITZERLAND	A3P6C4	0.67	9.9	140	6.0	100	5.3	4.3	*6.0*
YUGOSLAVIA	A4P4C3	1.83	1.8	66	4.3	223	1.1	5.2	33.8

FEMALES	Best model	Goodness of fit	1965 Rate	Deaths	1985 Rate	Deaths	Cumulative risk 1900	1940	Recent trend
AUSTRIA	A2D	1.31	*0.4*	*10*	0.7	16	*0.2*	0.6	21.5
CZECHOSLOVAKIA	A3P6	-0.28	0.4	17	0.9	39	0.3	0.3	34.0
FINLAND	A2C3	0.61	0.8	10	0.6	9	0.5	0.1	*-18.4*
HUNGARY	A2D	2.14	*0.1*	*4*	0.8	26	*0.1*	2.4	51.9
NORWAY	A2D	0.30	0.9	10	0.4	5	0.6	0.1	*-4.9*
POLAND	A2	-0.31	0.7	51	*0.7*	*66*	0.4	*0.4*	–
ROMANIA	–	–	–	–	–	–	–	–	–
SWEDEN	A2D	1.63	1.3	32	0.5	15	0.9	0.2	-22.7
SWITZERLAND	A2P4C3	1.36	0.8	13	1.0	20	0.4	0.6	32.5
YUGOSLAVIA	A2P2	0.16	0.5	22	0.4	26	0.3	0.2	*6.3*

* : not enough deaths for reliable estimation
– : incomplete or missing data
Best model: polynomial of the given degree in age (A), period (P) or cohort (C), or linear drift (D) model.
Goodness of fit: the normalised likelihood ratio chi-square for the best model (see Method).
Rate: world-standardised truncated rate per 100 000 per year (30-74 years) and number of **deaths** are both estimated from the best-fitting model for the single years cited.
Cumulative risk per 1000 (30-74 years) is estimated from the best-fitting *age-cohort* model for cohorts of central birth year cited.
Recent trend: estimated mean percentage change per five-year period in the age-specific rates (30-74 years) over the period 1975-1988.
Italics denote recent trends not significant at 5 per cent level, or other figures which should be interpreted with caution (see Method).

136

PHARYNX (ICD-9 146-148)

EUROPE (non-EC), MORTALITY

MALES

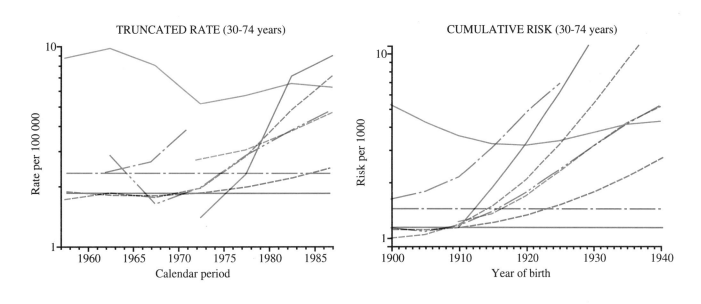

FEMALES

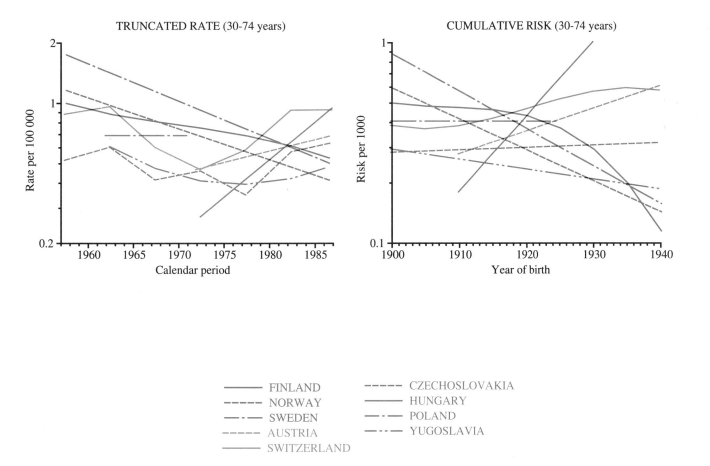

—— FINLAND	----- CZECHOSLOVAKIA
--- NORWAY	—— HUNGARY
—·— SWEDEN	—··— POLAND
----- AUSTRIA	—··— YUGOSLAVIA
—— SWITZERLAND	

PHARYNX (ICD-9 146-148)

EUROPE (EC), MORTALITY

MALES	Best model	Goodness of fit	1965 Rate	1965 Deaths	1985 Rate	1985 Deaths	Cumulative risk 1900	Cumulative risk 1940	Recent trend
BELGIUM	A2P4C2	0.29	1.9	49	1.8	47	1.1	1.2	27.4
DENMARK	A8P6	1.04	1.7	21	1.9	26	0.9	2.1	20.1
FRANCE	A3P6C9	8.84	10.9	1334	11.5	1549	5.4	10.7	6.2
GERMANY (FRG)	A3C3	3.58	*3.0*	*456*	4.6	732	*1.6*	6.8	30.5
GREECE	A2D	-0.39	*0.7*	*13*	1.1	29	*0.4*	0.9	*10.2*
IRELAND	A1P4C4	1.06	2.3	17	1.7	13	1.5	0.7	*14.2*
ITALY	A4P5C5	0.31	3.7	446	4.1	628	1.9	2.8	29.1
NETHERLANDS	A2C2	0.39	1.0	28	1.6	56	0.6	1.8	20.3
PORTUGAL	–	–	–	–	–	–	–	–	–
SPAIN	A3P6C4	-1.17	1.7	118	2.8	260	0.7	2.4	142.2
UK ENGLAND & WALES	A2C4	0.65	2.2	284	1.9	267	1.4	1.4	*0.6*
UK SCOTLAND	A8P6C9	0.69	2.5	32	2.1	28	1.3	1.7	16.5

FEMALES	Best model	Goodness of fit	1965 Rate	1965 Deaths	1985 Rate	1985 Deaths	Cumulative risk 1900	Cumulative risk 1940	Recent trend
BELGIUM	A2P4C2	0.13	0.4	12	0.5	14	0.2	0.4	*33.3*
DENMARK	A2C3	-2.47	0.6	8	0.8	11	0.3	0.5	*3.0*
FRANCE	A4C5	-0.46	0.5	74	0.9	130	0.3	0.9	23.0
GERMANY (FRG)	A3D	0.83	*0.3*	*66*	0.7	134	*0.2*	0.7	18.9
GREECE	A2	-1.89	*0.3*	*7*	0.3	9	*0.2*	0.2	*2.7*
IRELAND	A2P2	2.79	1.7	12	0.9	7	1.4	0.2	*2.2*
ITALY	A3P5C5	-0.54	0.7	95	0.6	98	0.3	0.2	26.0
NETHERLANDS	A2	1.26	0.4	12	0.4	16	0.2	0.2	*2.3*
PORTUGAL	–	–	–	–	–	–	–	–	–
SPAIN	A1P4	4.11	0.2	19	0.4	40	0.1	0.1	199.9
UK ENGLAND & WALES	A2C3	-0.37	1.5	233	0.9	143	1.0	0.3	-10.2
UK SCOTLAND	A2P4	-0.10	1.4	23	1.1	16	0.9	0.3	*4.0*

* : not enough deaths for reliable estimation
– : incomplete or missing data
Best model: polynomial of the given degree in age (A), period (P) or cohort (C), or linear drift (D) model.
Goodness of fit: the normalised likelihood ratio chi-square for the best model (see Method).
Rate: world-standardised truncated rate per 100 000 per year (30-74 years) and number of **deaths** are both estimated from the best-fitting model for the single years cited.
Cumulative risk per 1000 (30-74 years) is estimated from the best-fitting *age-cohort* model for cohorts of central birth year cited.
Recent trend: estimated mean percentage change per five-year period in the age-specific rates (30-74 years) over the period 1975-1988.
Italics denote recent trends not significant at 5 per cent level, or other figures which should be interpreted with caution (see Method).

PHARYNX (ICD-9 146-148)

EUROPE (EC), MORTALITY

MALES

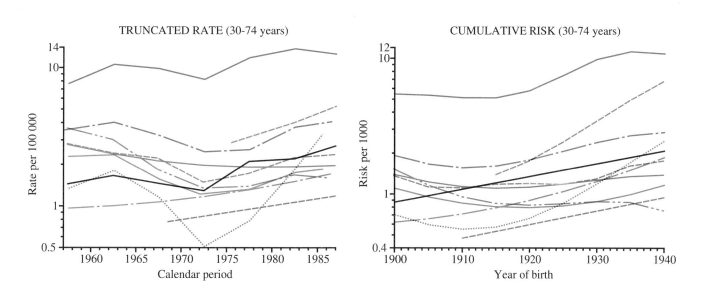

FEMALES

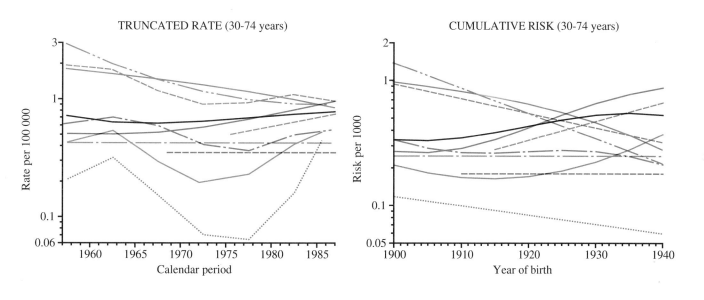

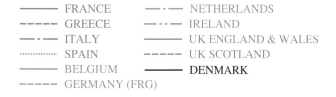

PHARYNX (ICD-9 146-148)

EUROPE (non-EC), MORTALITY
Percentage change per five-year period, 1975-1988

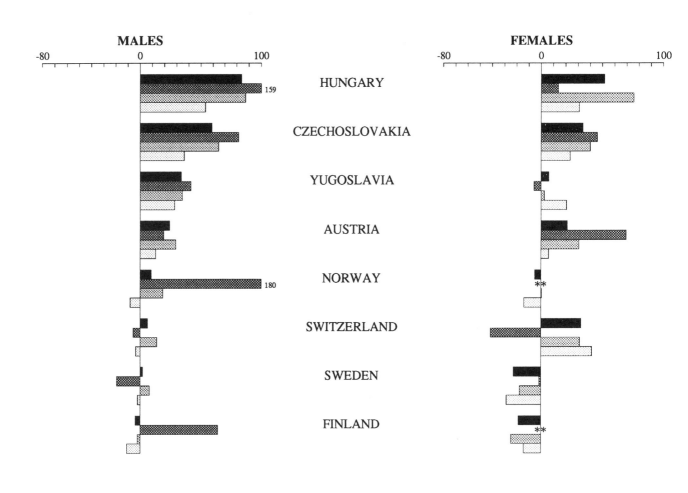

PHARYNX (ICD-9 146-148)

EUROPE (EC), MORTALITY
Percentage change per five-year period, 1975-1988

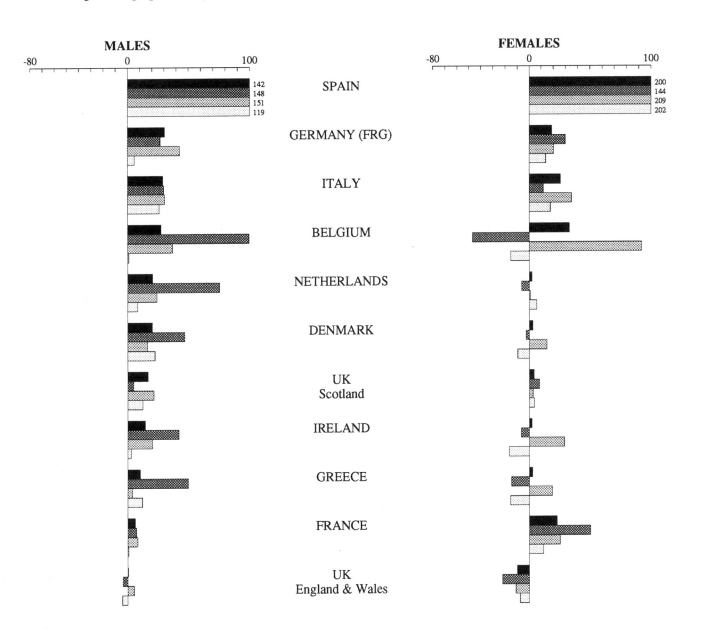

MALES

SPAIN	142 / 148 / 151 / 119
GERMANY (FRG)	
ITALY	
BELGIUM	
NETHERLANDS	
DENMARK	
UK Scotland	
IRELAND	
GREECE	
FRANCE	
UK England & Wales	

FEMALES

SPAIN	200 / 144 / 209 / 202

Legend:
- 30-74
- 30-44
- 45-64
- 65-74

ASIA, INCIDENCE

MALES	Best model	Goodness of fit	1970		1985		Cumulative risk		Recent trend
			Rate	Cases	Rate	Cases	1915	1940	
CHINA									
Shanghai	A2D	1.82	*14.9*	*175*	9.1	155	7.3	3.2	-15.3
HONG KONG	A3C2	-0.63	*68.6*	*520*	68.0	808	32.0	30.7	-4.2
INDIA									
Bombay	A2C4	3.33	28.8	225	24.1	290	15.8	9.5	-5.3
JAPAN									
Miyagi	A2D	1.85	1.5	5	3.0	16	1.4	4.3	46.5
Nagasaki	A1	0.49	*3.5*	*2*	3.5	3	2.1	2.1	*-1.9*
Osaka	A2D	-0.74	1.8	22	3.8	73	1.7	6.0	30.8
SINGAPORE									
Chinese	A3	-0.27	43.8	100	43.8	161	20.1	20.1	*-3.0*
Indian	A1	-1.06	9.4	2	9.4	3	5.8	5.8	*-15.2*
Malay	A2	-0.68	11.4	3	11.4	6	6.1	6.1	*-11.6*

FEMALES	Best model	Goodness of fit	1970		1985		Cumulative risk		Recent trend
			Rate	Cases	Rate	Cases	1915	1940	
CHINA									
Shanghai	A3D	2.22	*6.2*	*78*	4.3	73	3.1	1.7	-11.6
HONG KONG	A3D	1.17	*35.9*	*247*	25.0	273	17.5	9.6	-11.6
INDIA									
Bombay	A2D	0.70	7.8	41	5.9	58	3.8	2.4	-8.8
JAPAN									
Miyagi	A2D	1.34	0.5	1	0.9	5	0.3	0.9	*38.1*
Nagasaki	A0	-0.21	*0.6*	*0*	*0.6*	*0*	0.2	0.2	*10.7*
Osaka	A2C2	0.13	0.6	9	1.0	22	0.5	0.7	*12.7*
SINGAPORE									
Chinese	A2	0.02	16.3	40	16.3	64	7.4	7.4	*-0.7*
Indian	A1P2	-0.33	*1.0*	*0*	*1.9*	*0*	4.0	1.5	*-47.7*
Malay	A1	-0.44	3.6	1	3.6	1	1.9	1.9	*-4.5*

* : not enough cases for reliable estimation
− : incomplete or missing data
Best model: polynomial of the given degree in age (A), period (P) or cohort (C), or linear drift (D) model.
Goodness of fit: the normalised likelihood ratio chi-square for the best model (see Method).
Rate: world-standardised truncated rate per 100 000 per year (30-74 years) and number of **cases** are both estimated from the best-fitting model for the single years cited.
Cumulative risk per 1000 (30-74 years) is estimated from the best-fitting *age-cohort* model for cohorts of central birth year cited.
Recent trend: estimated mean percentage change per five-year period in the age-specific rates (30-74 years) over the period 1973-1987.
Italics denote recent trends not significant at 5 per cent level, or other figures which should be interpreted with caution (see Method).

PHARYNX (ICD-9 146-148)

ASIA, INCIDENCE

MALES

TRUNCATED RATE (30-74 years)

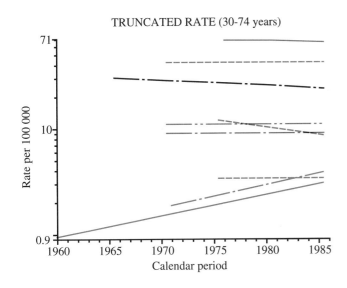

CUMULATIVE RISK (30-74 years)

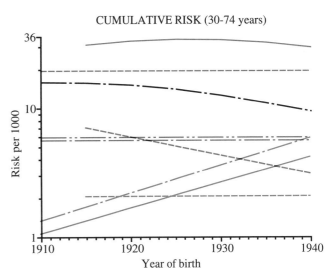

FEMALES

TRUNCATED RATE (30-74 years)

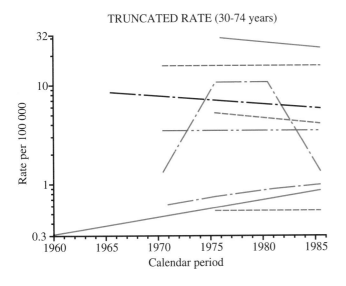

CUMULATIVE RISK (30-74 years)

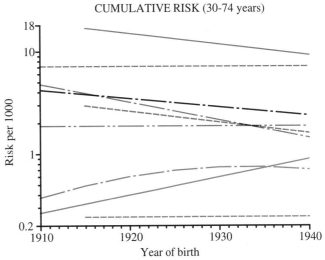

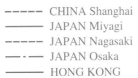

----- CHINA Shanghai
——— JAPAN Miyagi
----- JAPAN Nagasaki
—·— JAPAN Osaka
——— HONG KONG

----- SINGAPORE Chinese
—·— SINGAPORE Indian
—··— SINGAPORE Malay
—··— INDIA Bombay

OCEANIA, INCIDENCE

MALES	Best model	Goodness of fit	1970 Rate	Cases	1985 Rate	Cases	Cumulative risk 1915	1940	Recent trend
AUSTRALIA									
New South Wales	A4D	0.93	*5.0*	*51*	8.7	112	3.7	9.2	20.0
South	A2	-0.72	*6.2*	*13*	6.2	21	3.6	3.6	*5.0*
HAWAII									
Caucasian	A2	-0.54	12.0	4	12.0	7	7.2	7.2	*-9.8*
Chinese	A0	0.22	22.3	2	22.3	3	10.0	10.0	*28.3*
Filipino	A1	0.61	7.0	1	7.0	2	4.1	4.1	*18.1*
Hawaiian	A2D	-0.27	15.5	2	8.0	2	7.1	2.3	*-30.0*
Japanese	A2	-0.02	5.5	2	5.5	4	3.3	3.3	*-4.8*
NEW ZEALAND									
Maori	A2D	-1.80	*2.6*	*0*	7.8	2	2.6	15.9	*23.9*
Non-Maori	A2P4	2.72	3.0	16	5.9	40	2.6	7.4	14.0

FEMALES	Best model	Goodness of fit	1970 Rate	Cases	1985 Rate	Cases	Cumulative risk 1915	1940	Recent trend
AUSTRALIA									
New South Wales	A3D	-0.67	*1.1*	*12*	2.5	33	0.9	3.8	32.8
South	A1	-0.81	*1.5*	*2*	1.5	5	0.9	0.9	*1.5*
HAWAII									
Caucasian	A2	-0.24	6.5	2	6.5	3	3.7	3.7	*-14.0*
Chinese	A0	0.31	*8.5*	*0*	8.5	1	3.8	3.8	*12.9*
Filipino	A0C3	-0.78	*3.2*	*0*	3.8	1	1.3	3.6	*-8.2*
Hawaiian	A1	-1.80	*3.8*	*0*	3.8	1	2.6	2.6	*1.8*
Japanese	*	..	..	..	..	..	..	..	..
NEW ZEALAND									
Maori	A1	-0.47	*2.1*	*0*	*2.1*	*0*	1.2	1.2	*-15.6*
Non-Maori	A2C2	0.11	1.0	6	1.4	9	0.6	1.6	*15.9*

* : not enough cases for reliable estimation
− : incomplete or missing data
Best model: polynomial of the given degree in age (A), period (P) or cohort (C), or linear drift (D) model.
Goodness of fit: the normalised likelihood ratio chi-square for the best model (see Method).
Rate: world-standardised truncated rate per 100 000 per year (30-74 years) and number of **cases** are both estimated from the best-fitting model for the single years cited.
Cumulative risk per 1000 (30-74 years) is estimated from the best-fitting *age-cohort* model for cohorts of central birth year cited.
Recent trend: estimated mean percentage change per five-year period in the age-specific rates (30-74 years) over the period 1973-1987.
Italics denote recent trends not significant at 5 per cent level, or other figures which should be interpreted with caution (see Method).

PHARYNX (ICD-9 146-148)

OCEANIA, INCIDENCE

MALES

TRUNCATED RATE (30-74 years)

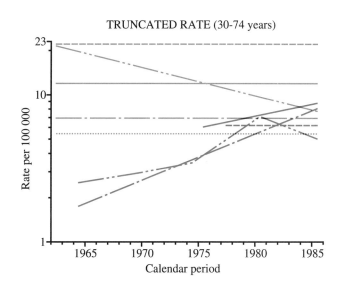

CUMULATIVE RISK (30-74 years)

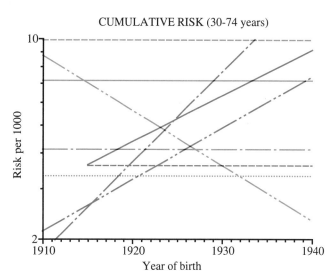

FEMALES

TRUNCATED RATE (30-74 years)

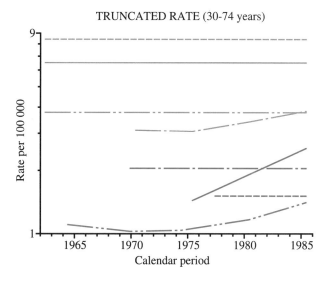

CUMULATIVE RISK (30-74 years)

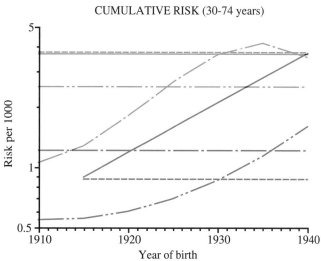

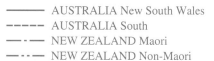

——————— AUSTRALIA New South Wales	— — — — HAWAII Chinese
— — — — AUSTRALIA South	—·—·—·— HAWAII Filipino
—·—·—·— NEW ZEALAND Maori	—··—··— HAWAII Hawaiian
—··—··— NEW ZEALAND Non-Maori	············ HAWAII Japanese
——————— HAWAII Caucasian	

PHARYNX (ICD-9 146-148)

ASIA, INCIDENCE
Percentage change per five-year period, 1973-1987

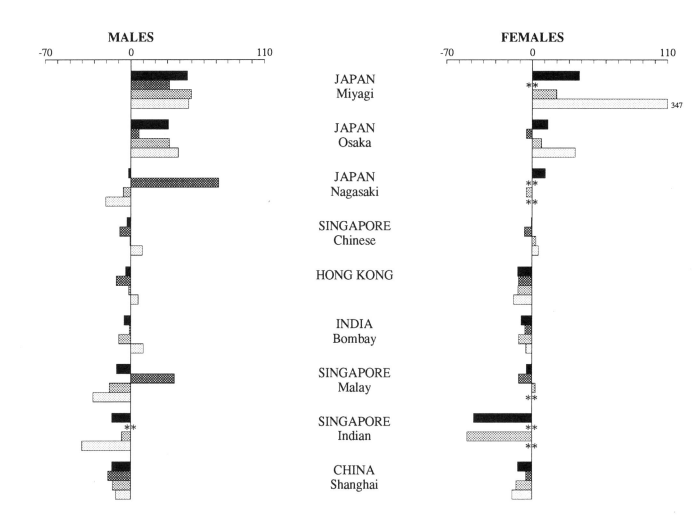

MALES

FEMALES

JAPAN
Miyagi

JAPAN
Osaka

JAPAN
Nagasaki

SINGAPORE
Chinese

HONG KONG

INDIA
Bombay

SINGAPORE
Malay

SINGAPORE
Indian

CHINA
Shanghai

30-74
30-44
45-64
65-74

PHARYNX (ICD-9 146-148)

OCEANIA, INCIDENCE
Percentage change per five-year period, 1973-1987

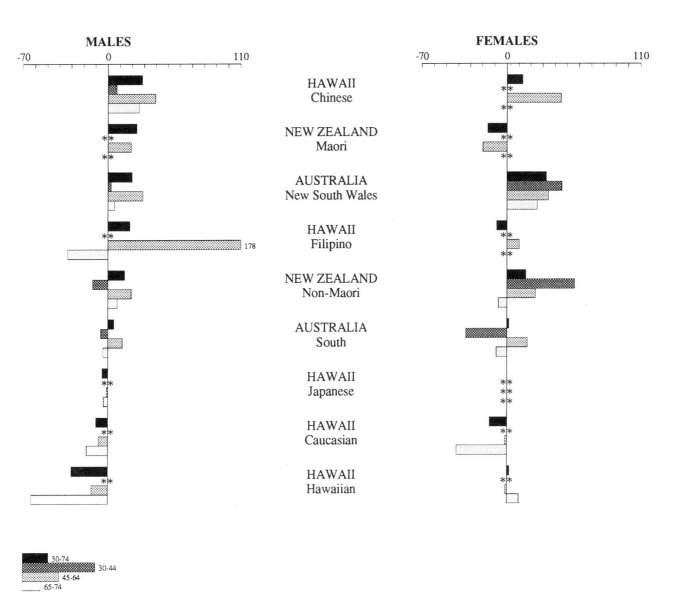

MALES   FEMALES

HAWAII
Chinese

NEW ZEALAND
Maori

AUSTRALIA
New South Wales

HAWAII
Filipino

NEW ZEALAND
Non-Maori

AUSTRALIA
South

HAWAII
Japanese

HAWAII
Caucasian

HAWAII
Hawaiian

30-74
30-44
45-64
65-74

PHARYNX (ICD-9 146-148)

ASIA and OCEANIA, MORTALITY

MALES	Best model	Goodness of fit	1965 Rate	Deaths	1985 Rate	Deaths	Cumulative risk 1900	1940	Recent trend
AUSTRALIA	A3C5	0.44	2.4	59	4.0	143	1.4	3.3	10.1
HONG KONG	A3P2C3	0.20	*33.7*	*197*	29.6	321	*18.0*	12.9	-13.5
JAPAN	A8P6C9	0.37	0.7	133	1.5	428	0.4	1.5	26.9
MAURITIUS	A2	1.23	*1.4*	*1*	1.4	1	*0.7*	0.7	*71.1*
NEW ZEALAND	A2C3	0.00	1.7	9	3.1	22	1.0	3.5	*12.8*
SINGAPORE	A7P4C8	-1.63	19.8	43	22.4	91	*13.1*	11.9	–

FEMALES	Best model	Goodness of fit	1965 Rate	Deaths	1985 Rate	Deaths	Cumulative risk 1900	1940	Recent trend
AUSTRALIA	A2D	-0.28	0.7	17	0.8	31	0.4	0.5	16.3
HONG KONG	A3C2	-0.08	*15.4*	*99*	9.0	88	*8.3*	3.2	-17.9
JAPAN	A2C4	1.76	0.3	64	0.3	120	0.2	0.2	*0.0*
MAURITIUS	A0	-0.97	*0.3*	*0*	*0.3*	*0*	*0.1*	0.1	*
NEW ZEALAND	A2	-0.02	0.7	4	0.7	5	0.4	0.4	*-1.3*
SINGAPORE	A2	-0.26	8.4	18	8.4	33	*3.6*	3.6	–

* : not enough deaths for reliable estimation
– : incomplete or missing data
Best model: polynomial of the given degree in age (A), period (P) or cohort (C), or linear drift (D) model.
Goodness of fit: the normalised likelihood ratio chi-square for the best model (see Method).
Rate: world-standardised truncated rate per 100 000 per year (30-74 years) and number of **deaths** are both estimated from the best-fitting model for the single years cited.
Cumulative risk per 1000 (30-74 years) is estimated from the best-fitting *age-cohort* model for cohorts of central birth year cited.
Recent trend: estimated mean percentage change per five-year period in the age-specific rates (30-74 years) over the period 1975-1988.
Italics denote recent trends not significant at 5 per cent level, or other figures which should be interpreted with caution (see Method).

PHARYNX (ICD-9 146-148)

ASIA and OCEANIA, MORTALITY

MALES

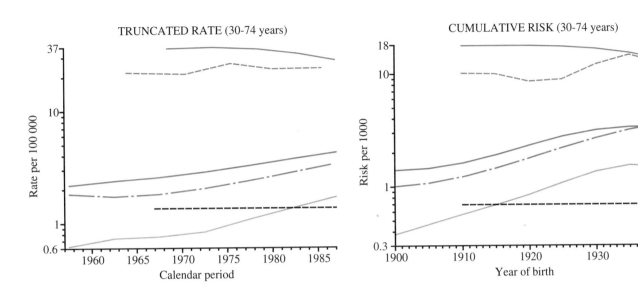

FEMALES

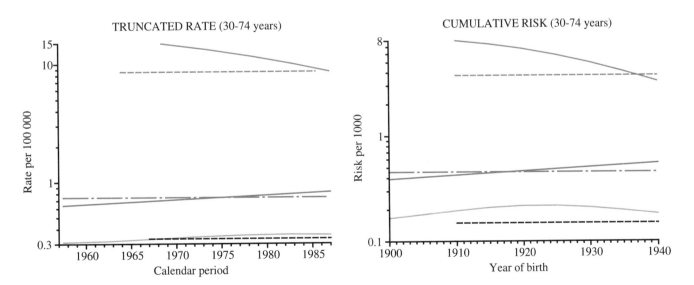

AUSTRALIA   HONG KONG
NEW ZEALAND   SINGAPORE
JAPAN   MAURITIUS

PHARYNX (ICD-9 146-148)

ASIA and OCEANIA, MORTALITY
Percentage change per five-year period, 1975-1988

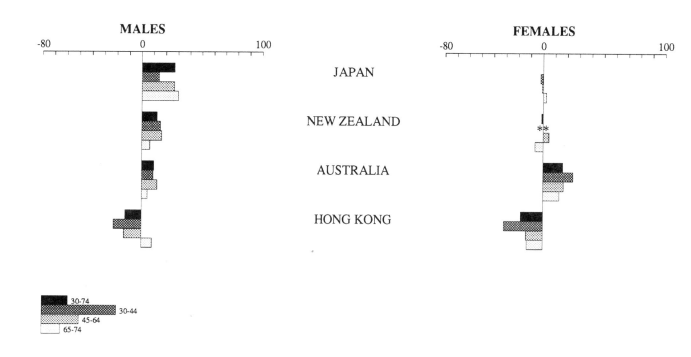

from page 129

and England and Wales. In Ireland, mortality among males fell steadily until the mid-1970s, and although the small recent increase in risk is not significant, it is also most marked in 30-44 year-old males, and the pattern is coherent with that in other western European countries. In France, the evolution of the risk by birth cohort has the characteristic double wave-shape seen for all alcohol-related cancers, and is similar to that observed for incidence, with a dip for males born around 1910, and a peak for those born around 1930.

Among females, incidence has increased significantly in Hungary, Slovenia, Denmark and Germany (GDR). In Norway, incidence has increased after reaching a nadir around 1970, and the age-specific rates are increasing most rapidly in younger females (30-44 years): this is very similar to the pattern for males in Norway. Incidence has decreased in Finland, Sweden and the UK. In Scotland, the small recent rate of decline in incidence among females (10% every five years) contrasts with the sharp increase seen for cancer of the mouth (32%). The mortality data are generally consistent with the incidence data, except for a significant decrease in mortality in Norway, which does not reflect the recent increase in inci-

dence in younger females. The mortality data reveal additional aspects of the trend patterns, including a recent increase in Switzerland that is not reflected by incidence in Geneva. There is also an increase in mortality in Belgium and in France, the latter increase not seen in the French incidence data, where the numbers of cases are small.

When all sites of the buccal cavity and pharynx (ICD-9 140-149) are grouped together, the increase in mortality from these cancers in females has been especially impressive in Denmark, France, Germany and Belgium, while mortality has been decreasing sharply in the UK (Figure 8.1). These remarkably divergent trends in risk are not easily explained.

Asia and Oceania

In examining trends for cancer of the pharynx in Asia, it is essential to note that cancers of the nasopharynx comprise more than 90% of the total in Chinese populations, 30% in Japanese, 28% in Singapore Indians, and only 7% in Bombay (India). The data from Singapore and Shanghai

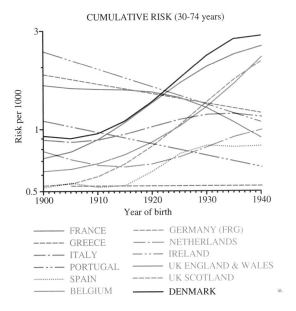

CUMULATIVE RISK (30-74 years)

FRANCE — — — — GERMANY (FRG)
— — — — GREECE — · — NETHERLANDS
— · — ITALY — · · — IRELAND
— · · — PORTUGAL ——— UK ENGLAND & WALES
············· SPAIN — — — — UK SCOTLAND
——— BELGIUM ——— DENMARK

Figure 8.1: Mortality from cancer of the buccal cavity and pharynx, females, Europe (EC).

(China), and from Hong Kong, especially for females, suggest a slight decrease in cancer of the nasopharynx. This trend is confirmed for Hong Kong by the mortality data. The more rapid decrease in females is seen both for incidence and for mortality. The observed trend in incidence and mortality from cancer of the pharynx in Japan suggests that cancers of the oropharynx and hypopharynx are increasing in frequency, much as for cancers of the mouth. These same cancers are decreasing slowly but steadily in Bombay (India) among both males and females, and among Indians in Singapore, although not significantly.

There has been a striking increase in the incidence of cancer of the pharynx among both males and females in New South Wales (Australia) and in New Zealand. The numbers of cases in Hawaii are small, but the data suggest a reduction of risk for Hawaiian males. The mortality data show an increasing trend in mortality from cancer of the pharynx for both males and females in Australia, and among males in New Zealand.

Americas

In Canada, the risk of cancer of the pharynx has increased for both males and females, although there is a deceleration among the younger birth cohorts in Quebec and British Columbia.

In Central and South America, the trends in incidence among males are diverse, with a large increase in São Paulo (Brazil) and a decrease in other populations, limited to more recent birth cohorts in Puerto Rico, where the risk in both sexes has been high for many years. The risk is also decreasing among females in Puerto Rico. There is no other significant change in incidence among females, although the recent linear trends in the age-specific rates are negative in Cali (Colombia).

Mortality from cancers of the mouth and pharynx combined in males reflects the incidence trends at these anatomical sites for Canada and Puerto Rico, and it provides additional information on trends in these cancers in Central and South America. There is a sharply increasing risk in Uruguay, where the risks for alcohol-related cancers are known to be high. Mortality is declining in Venezuela, but there has been little overall change in Panama or Chile. There is a recent period effect in Costa Rica. Among females, the mortality data for cancers of the mouth and pharynx combined show an overall increase in risk in Canada, and a decrease in Central and South America. The recent trend in women aged 30-44 years in Uruguay is significantly positive, however, as is the increase in the last period in Costa Rica.

In the USA, no significant change is seen among males, except in Detroit, where the risk has increased substantially, especially among blacks. Chinese in the San Francisco Bay Area have retained their high risk of cancer of the nasopharynx, but information was not available to assess recent trends. The other notable features are the large increase in risk among black females in Detroit, and the reduction of risk in younger cohorts of white females in the Bay Area, and in Seattle and Detroit, three populations for which age-cohort models fit the incidence data well. The same pattern is seen in Iowa, where a more complicated model is needed because of the very small risk estimated for the 1940 birth cohort (not shown on the graph).

The mortality data for cancers of the mouth and pharynx combined (ICD-9 140-141, 143-149) in the USA show a declining risk of death for both males and females. Among females, the decline in risk is more pronounced for younger cohorts, as suggested by the incidence data for several of the populations.

Comment

The results reported here are consistent with previous reports, although these do not always relate to the same anatomical groups. Most trends are attributed to trends in consumption of alcohol and tobacco, although other factors are involved in populations at high risk for nasopharyngeal carcinoma.

continued page 160

PHARYNX (ICD-9 146-148)

AMERICAS (except USA), INCIDENCE

MALES	Best model	Goodness of fit	1970 Rate	1970 Cases	1985 Rate	1985 Cases	Cumulative risk 1915	Cumulative risk 1940	Recent trend
BRAZIL									
Sao Paulo	A3D	1.33	8.8	64	*24.7*	*209*	5.5	*30.2*	–
CANADA									
Alberta	A5D	-0.53	3.3	10	5.6	25	2.4	5.7	*8.6*
British Columbia	A2P2C2	0.46	5.3	24	7.7	53	3.1	6.3	27.7
Maritime Provinces	A2D	-1.29	3.9	12	5.8	20	2.8	5.5	*11.9*
Newfoundland	A2	1.34	3.9	3	3.9	4	2.1	2.1	*-8.1*
Quebec	A3P4C6	2.04	7.9	86	9.4	136	4.2	6.3	7.1
COLOMBIA									
Cali	A2D	0.22	4.9	3	2.7	3	2.2	0.8	*-8.1*
CUBA	A4D	-0.15	8.4	124	5.8	117	4.3	*2.3*	–
PUERTO RICO	A8C9	0.93	17.7	80	16.4	108	9.7	5.5	*0.7*

FEMALES	Best model	Goodness of fit	1970 Rate	1970 Cases	1985 Rate	1985 Cases	Cumulative risk 1915	Cumulative risk 1940	Recent trend
BRAZIL									
Sao Paulo	A1	2.55	1.5	10	*1.5*	*14*	0.7	*0.7*	–
CANADA									
Alberta	A2D	0.18	1.3	3	2.0	9	0.8	1.7	*2.7*
British Columbia	A2C2	-0.21	1.5	6	2.7	19	1.1	2.1	27.9
Maritime Provinces	A2	1.05	1.4	4	1.4	5	0.8	0.8	33.4
Newfoundland	A2	-0.55	1.9	1	1.9	2	1.0	1.0	*3.7*
Quebec	A8P4C9	0.46	2.2	26	2.0	33	1.1	0.7	*3.4*
COLOMBIA									
Cali	A1	0.73	1.9	1	1.9	3	1.2	1.2	*-25.1*
CUBA	A1	0.88	1.8	22	1.8	36	1.1	*1.1*	–
PUERTO RICO	A2D	-0.04	3.5	15	2.0	15	1.6	0.6	*-6.0*

* : not enough cases for reliable estimation
– : incomplete or missing data
Best model: polynomial of the given degree in age (A), period (P) or cohort (C), or linear drift (D) model.
Goodness of fit: the normalised likelihood ratio chi-square for the best model (see Method).
Rate: world-standardised truncated rate per 100 000 per year (30-74 years) and number of **cases** are both estimated from the best-fitting model for the single years cited.
Cumulative risk per 1000 (30-74 years) is estimated from the best-fitting *age-cohort* model for cohorts of central birth year cited.
Recent trend: estimated mean percentage change per five-year period in the age-specific rates (30-74 years) over the period 1973-1987.
Italics denote recent trends not significant at 5 per cent level, or other figures which should be interpreted with caution (see Method).

PHARYNX (ICD-9 146-148)

AMERICAS (except USA), INCIDENCE

MALES

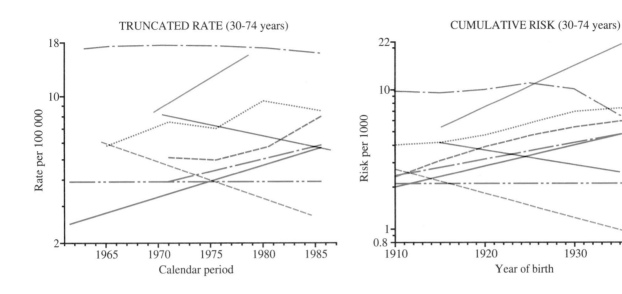

FEMALES

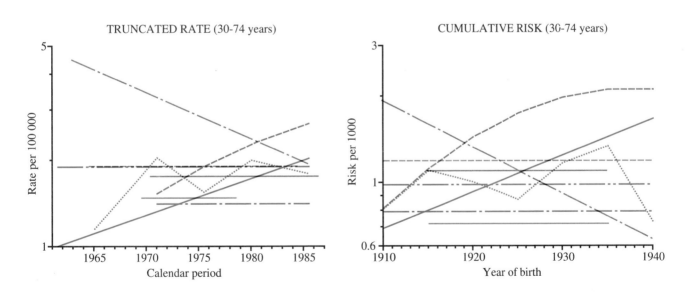

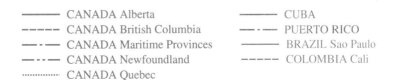

CANADA Alberta
CANADA British Columbia
CANADA Maritime Provinces
CANADA Newfoundland
CANADA Quebec
CUBA
PUERTO RICO
BRAZIL Sao Paulo
COLOMBIA Cali

AMERICAS (USA), INCIDENCE

MALES	Best model	Goodness of fit	1970		1985		Cumulative risk		Recent trend
			Rate	Cases	Rate	Cases	1915	1940	
USA									
Bay Area, Black	A2	-0.56	15.7	9	15.7	12	8.1	8.1	*9.7*
Bay Area, Chinese	A2	1.76	37.7	7	*37.7*	*18*	17.3	*17.3*	–
Bay Area, White	A2	0.52	9.6	57	9.6	59	5.8	5.8	*-3.7*
Connecticut	A4	-0.08	9.0	59	9.0	70	5.2	5.2	*2.9*
Detroit, Black	A2D	-0.63	7.1	10	19.7	33	5.9	32.0	38.2
Detroit, White	A2C3	0.98	7.5	55	9.5	67	4.4	8.9	19.2
Iowa	A3	0.42	6.4	42	6.4	43	3.7	3.7	*5.7*
New Orleans, Black	A2	0.96	*14.3*	*7*	14.3	8	7.4	7.4	*-19.1*
New Orleans, White	A2	1.28	*10.6*	*15*	10.6	16	6.2	6.2	*-5.4*
Seattle	A2	-0.83	*7.7*	*36*	7.7	50	4.5	4.5	*10.7*

FEMALES	Best model	Goodness of fit	1970		1985		Cumulative risk		Recent trend
			Rate	Cases	Rate	Cases	1915	1940	
USA									
Bay Area, Black	A2P2	-0.53	*0.9*	*0*	4.2	3	2.1	3.7	*-17.2*
Bay Area, Chinese	A0	0.76	14.7	2	*14.7*	*8*	6.6	*6.6*	–
Bay Area, White	A2C2	0.72	4.4	30	4.6	31	2.8	1.8	*-3.3*
Connecticut	A2C2	0.82	2.4	18	3.0	26	1.6	1.6	*8.6*
Detroit, Black	A2D	-0.68	2.3	3	5.2	10	1.4	5.2	29.6
Detroit, White	A2C2	0.45	2.1	17	2.5	20	1.4	1.1	*2.8*
Iowa	A8C8	0.67	1.5	11	1.5	12	0.9	0.1	*-3.8*
New Orleans, Black	A2	-0.25	*2.7*	*1*	2.7	2	1.3	1.3	*1.2*
New Orleans, White	A2	-1.21	*2.7*	*4*	2.7	5	1.5	1.5	*-22.8*
Seattle	A2C2	0.84	*3.2*	*15*	3.4	24	2.2	1.1	*0.4*

* : not enough cases for reliable estimation
– : incomplete or missing data
Best model: polynomial of the given degree in age (A), period (P) or cohort (C), or linear drift (D) model.
Goodness of fit: the normalised likelihood ratio chi-square for the best model (see Method).
Rate: world-standardised truncated rate per 100 000 per year (30-74 years) and number of **cases** are both estimated from the best-fitting model for the single years cited.
Cumulative risk per 1000 (30-74 years) is estimated from the best-fitting *age-cohort* model for cohorts of central birth year cited.
Recent trend: estimated mean percentage change per five-year period in the age-specific rates (30-74 years) over the period 1973-1987.
Italics denote recent trends not significant at 5 per cent level, or other figures which should be interpreted with caution (see Method).

PHARYNX (ICD-9 146-148)

AMERICAS (USA), INCIDENCE

MALES

TRUNCATED RATE (30-74 years)

CUMULATIVE RISK (30-74 years)

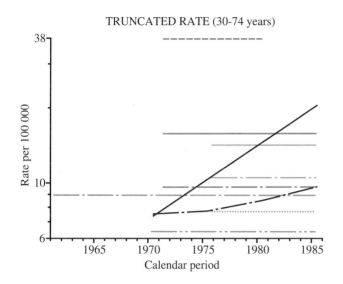

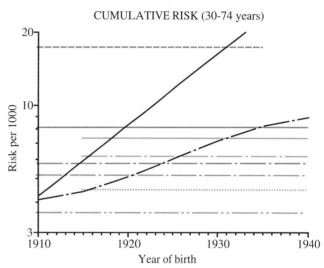

FEMALES

TRUNCATED RATE (30-74 years)

CUMULATIVE RISK (30-74 years)

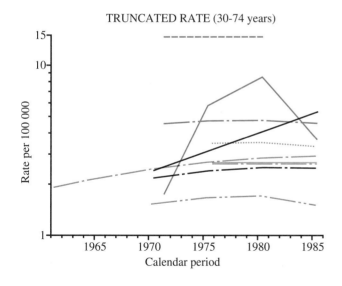

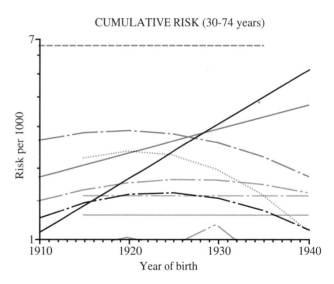

——— BAY AREA Black	·········· SEATTLE
– – – BAY AREA Chinese	——— NEW ORLEANS Black
–·–·– BAY AREA White	–·–·– NEW ORLEANS White
–··–··– CONNECTICUT	——— DETROIT Black
–···–···– IOWA	–··–··– DETROIT White

PHARYNX (ICD-9 146-148)

AMERICAS (except USA), INCIDENCE
Percentage change per five-year period, 1973-1987

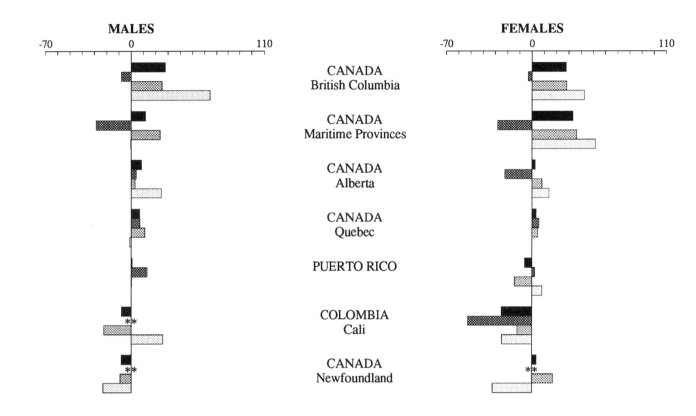

PHARYNX (ICD-9 146-148)

AMERICAS (USA), INCIDENCE
Percentage change per five-year period, 1973-1987

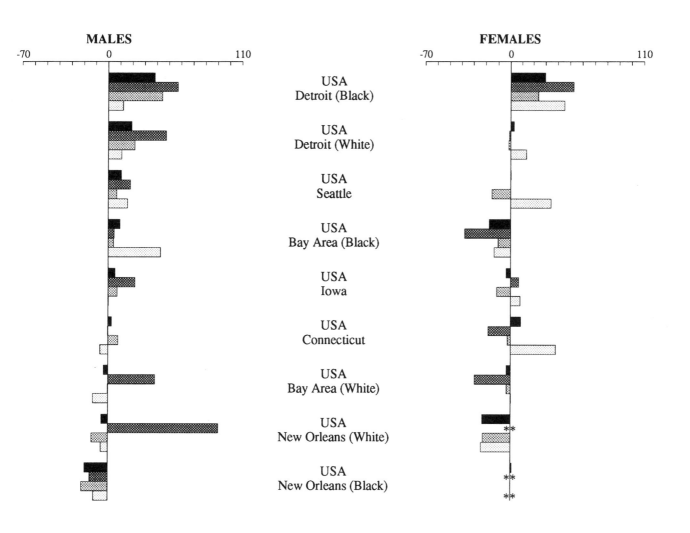

MALES		FEMALES

USA
Detroit (Black)

USA
Detroit (White)

USA
Seattle

USA
Bay Area (Black)

USA
Iowa

USA
Connecticut

USA
Bay Area (White)

USA
New Orleans (White)

USA
New Orleans (Black)

30-74
30-44
45-64
65-74

157

AMERICAS, MORTALITY

MALES	Best model	Goodness of fit	1965		1985		Cumulative risk		Recent trend
			Rate	Deaths	Rate	Deaths	1900	1940	
CANADA	A8P6C9	0.20	7.0	265	8.4	481	4.3	6.8	*3.8*
CHILE	A4P2C7	-0.24	4.2	49	4.9	86	2.1	2.5	*-4.9*
COSTA RICA	A8P4C9	-0.51	*4.3*	*6*	4.2	12	*2.7*	1.5	*11.9*
PANAMA	A4	0.50	4.7	6	4.7	13	3.1	3.1	–
PUERTO RICO	A2P3	1.83	*19.1*	*78*	18.5	93	*12.0*	9.0	*-1.7*
URUGUAY	A3D	-0.37	10.9	65	15.1	108	5.9	11.2	15.1
USA	A5P3C7	5.51	9.2	3908	8.1	4413	5.3	4.7	-9.5
VENEZUELA	A8P5	0.73	6.5	55	*5.1*	*82*	3.8	1.9	–

FEMALES	Best model	Goodness of fit	1965		1985		Cumulative risk		Recent trend
			Rate	Deaths	Rate	Deaths	1900	1940	
CANADA	A4C3	0.95	2.0	79	2.5	161	1.2	1.7	*3.0*
CHILE	A2D	0.48	1.5	18	1.0	20	0.9	0.4	*-3.5*
COSTA RICA	A1P2	0.93	*2.6*	*2*	1.6	3	*1.2*	0.7	*38.3*
PANAMA	A1P2	-0.07	3.2	4	3.0	8	2.6	1.2	–
PUERTO RICO	A2C2	0.85	*4.1*	*16*	2.7	13	*2.7*	0.7	-17.3
URUGUAY	A1P3	0.79	2.0	12	1.6	13	1.0	0.8	27.0
USA	A4P5C6	2.27	2.5	1169	2.7	1780	1.3	1.3	-5.9
VENEZUELA	A2D	2.29	5.1	43	*2.4*	*37*	3.5	0.8	–

* : not enough deaths for reliable estimation
– : incomplete or missing data
Best model: polynomial of the given degree in age (A), period (P) or cohort (C), or linear drift (D) model.
Goodness of fit: the normalised likelihood ratio chi-square for the best model (see Method).
Rate: world-standardised truncated rate per 100 000 per year (30-74 years) and number of **deaths** are both estimated from the best-fitting model for the single years cited.
Cumulative risk per 1000 (30-74 years) is estimated from the best-fitting *age-cohort* model for cohorts of central birth year cited.
Recent trend: estimated mean percentage change per five-year period in the age-specific rates (30-74 years) over the period 1975-1988.
Italics denote recent trends not significant at 5 per cent level, or other figures which should be interpreted with caution (see Method).

MOUTH AND PHARYNX (ICD-9 140-149)

AMERICAS, MORTALITY

MALES

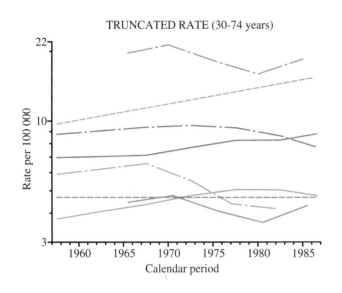

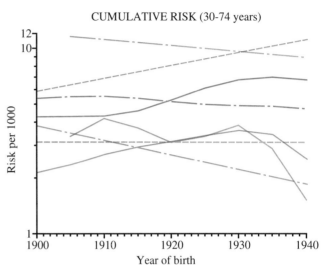

FEMALES

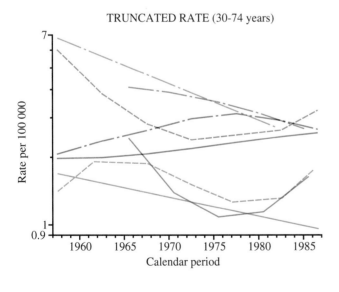

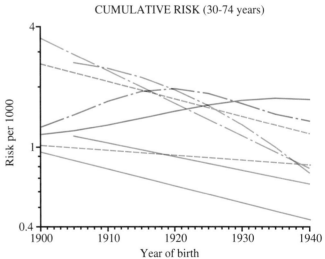

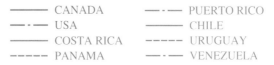

CANADA	PUERTO RICO
USA	CHILE
COSTA RICA	URUGUAY
PANAMA	VENEZUELA

MOUTH AND PHARYNX (ICD-9 140-149)

AMERICAS, MORTALITY
Percentage change per five-year period, 1975-1988

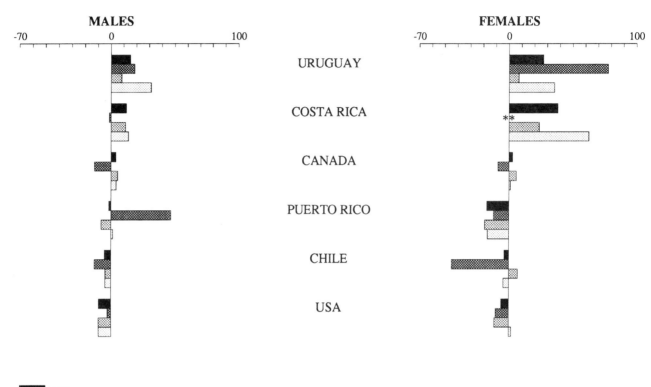

MALES | FEMALES

URUGUAY

COSTA RICA

CANADA

PUERTO RICO

CHILE

USA

30-74
30-44
45-64
65-74

from page 151

Cancer of the pharynx was reported[260] as the only cancer for which incidence among males in Doubs (France) increased in younger birth cohorts during 1979-86: exceptionally high relative risks are seen for heavy smokers who are also heavy drinkers. The very rapid increase in mortality from cancers of the pharynx in Czechoslovakia seen in the analyses reported here (59% every five years in males, 34% in females) is only partly reflected by the change in incidence of cancers of the mouth and pharynx combined in Slovakia (the eastern part of the former Czechoslovakia): there was a 24% increase between the two quinquennia ending in 1988 for males, but a 5% decline for females[237].

There was a small decline in the incidence of nasopharyngeal carcinoma (ICD-9 147) among Chinese males in Singapore in the 15-year period 1968-82 (average fall of 0.4% a year)[154], which corresponds to the small overall decline seen here for all cancers of the pharynx (ICD-9 146-148). In Bombay (India), the small overall decline in incidence of cancers of the pharynx appears to be composed of a small increase in cancers of the hypopharynx and a larger fall in cancers of the oropharynx[136]. There was a decline in the relative frequency of pharyngeal cancers in a Pakistan hospital series during the 1970s among males, but not among females[176]. The small increases in incidence of cancer of the pharynx in South Australia, particularly in females, and the corresponding increase in mortality, have been attributed to increases in tobacco and alcohol consumption[183].

Age-adjusted incidence of pharyngeal cancer in Ontario (Canada) fell by 2.9% among males, but increased by 4.3% among females, between the two quinquennia ending in 1988[182], similar to the recent trends observed here for Newfoundland. A peak in cohort mortality for cancers of the mouth and pharynx combined (ICD-9 141, 143-149) among females in the USA who were born around 1915-20 has been noted[77]: it is reflected in several of the incidence curves here. The peak was tentatively attributed to poor nutrition during the childbearing period in the 1930s and 1940s.

160

Chapter 9

OESOPHAGUS

Cancer of the oesophagus was estimated as the seventh most common cancer in the world in 1980, with some 310 000 new cases a year, or about 5% of all cancers[219]. Oesophageal cancer ranks fourth in the developing world (and second only to stomach cancer in China), but no higher than fifteenth in developed countries, where it ranks alongside cancers of the liver and larynx. Geographical variation in risk is particularly marked, with some sharply localised areas of very high incidence near the Caspian sea in Kazakhstan and Iran, in Brittany (France), and especially in China, which accounts for more than half of all the cases in the world each year[204]. There are also sharp differences in incidence between various racial and ethnic groups[263]. Alcohol[288] and tobacco consumption are major risk factors for oesophageal cancer in Europe and the Americas, but they do not explain the very high incidence in parts of China and Iran, where poor nutrition and ingestion of opium pyrolysates are involved[204]. Survival from oesophageal cancer is poor, typically 5-10% or less at five years.

Europe

The pattern of incidence and mortality in Europe is diverse. Finland stands out for several reasons: there has been a clear-cut decrease in incidence and mortality of about 10% every five years in both sexes. Incidence has fallen from around 10-12 per 100 000 in the 1960s to about half that level today, and mortality has dropped commensurately. The sex ratio is close to unity, and females in Finland have had the highest risk in Europe, although this is now falling quickly, and females in the 1940 cohort appear likely to have lifetime (30-74 years) risks of less than 1 per 1000, well within the European range. Incidence data for Finland are well fitted by age-cohort models, and there have been recent increases in risk among young males and females born since 1935, although these are not significant. The mortality data are well fitted by age-period models, showing a steady and significant decline of around 10% every five years, but while there is a deceleration in the rate of decline, the mortality trends do not at present reflect the recent upward trend in incidence among persons aged less than 45 years. In Denmark, there has been a sharp increase in incidence and mortality among males, and to a lesser extent among females. In Norway and Sweden, there has been a slight increase in incidence and mortality among males and, in Sweden, a slight decrease among females.

Incidence has increased sharply among males in Hungary to about 10 per 100 000 per year, whereas in Warsaw City (Poland), where incidence was already at this level in the 1960s, there has been little change. In Slovenia, where incidence among males was already among the highest in Europe in the 1970s (12 per 100 000), it has increased significantly, and is still rising at around 16% every five years. Mortality is increasing rapidly among males in Hungary, Poland and Czechoslovakia, and in the former Yugoslavia as a whole. These patterns suggest that if current trends continue, oesophageal cancer will kill 1-3% of males in the 1940 birth cohort in eastern European countries before their 75th birthday. Romania appears to be the exception, in that incidence and mortality are moderate by European standards, and are not increasing; mortality is declining significantly in females.

In western Europe, incidence is exceptionally high among males in Bas-Rhin and Doubs (France), with truncated rates up to 40 per 100 000. In Bas-Rhin, the trend in risk among successive birth cohorts has the characteristic pattern of other alcohol-related cancers, seen also for cancers of the tongue, mouth, pharynx and larynx. This is closely mirrored in the mortality trend for males in France as a whole: there is a dip in the cohort cumulative risk for males born around 1915-20, who were young during the second world war, followed by a peak for males born around 1935, then a further decline for later birth cohorts.

The most remarkable increase in the risk of oesophageal cancer in males has occurred among all three German populations: cumulative risks (30-74 years) quadrupled between the 1915 and 1940 birth cohorts, and are now similar to the risks observed in France. Recent data from Navarra (Spain) suggest almost as rapid a rate of increase in successive birth cohorts. In the UK, incidence is increasing in all three populations in males, though less rapidly in Birmingham than in Scotland or South Thames.

Incidence among females in the UK is the highest in Europe, alongside that in Finland, but in contrast to the declining trend in Finland, incidence is still increasing in all three UK populations at similar rates: these trends contrast with the declines in risk for other alcohol-related cancers of the buccal cavity and pharynx among females in the UK. The

continued page 182

OESOPHAGUS (ICD-9 150)

EUROPE (non-EC), INCIDENCE

MALES	Best model	Goodness of fit	1970 Rate	1970 Cases	1985 Rate	1985 Cases	Cumulative risk 1915	Cumulative risk 1940	Recent trend
FINLAND	A8C9	0.26	8.3	85	4.9	58	3.5	2.9	-9.0
HUNGARY									
County Vas	A3C2	-0.32	2.6	2	8.8	6	2.9	66.3	*30.3*
Szabolcs-Szatmar	A2P2	-0.46	2.0	2	11.3	15	3.7	58.3	118.0
ISRAEL									
All Jews	A2D	0.52	3.7	15	2.4	12	1.9	0.9	-19.4
Non-Jews	A1	0.80	*2.0*	*0*	2.0	1	1.1	1.1	*1.2*
NORWAY	A2C2	-0.05	4.9	55	5.1	62	3.1	5.0	*2.1*
POLAND									
Warsaw City	A3	-0.23	9.9	27	9.9	38	6.3	6.3	*-0.9*
ROMANIA									
Cluj	A2	1.40	*2.9*	*4*	2.9	5	1.8	1.8	*25.4*
SWEDEN	A4D	0.84	5.1	129	6.0	162	3.8	5.0	6.2
SWITZERLAND									
Geneva	A2C2	1.36	17.6	13	16.7	15	7.8	26.5	*2.5*
YUGOSLAVIA									
Slovenia	A3C4	0.72	11.8	44	15.8	68	7.2	20.6	16.2

FEMALES	Best model	Goodness of fit	1970 Rate	1970 Cases	1985 Rate	1985 Cases	Cumulative risk 1915	Cumulative risk 1940	Recent trend
FINLAND	A2C3	0.82	5.5	78	3.0	52	2.7	0.5	-14.8
HUNGARY									
County Vas	A1	-2.06	*0.4*	*0*	*0.4*	*0*	0.3	0.3	*
Szabolcs-Szatmar	A1D	-1.01	*0.2*	*0*	0.8	1	0.4	3.2	*109.1*
ISRAEL									
All Jews	A8C9	0.83	3.0	11	1.5	9	1.3	0.0	-16.7
Non-Jews	*	..	..	..	..	..	..	..	..
NORWAY	A3	-0.70	1.2	15	1.2	17	0.8	0.8	*6.6*
POLAND									
Warsaw City	A1D	-0.66	2.4	10	1.6	8	1.3	0.7	*-7.3*
ROMANIA									
Cluj	*	..	..	..	..	..	..	..	..
SWEDEN	A2D	1.15	1.6	46	1.3	41	1.0	0.7	*-6.2*
SWITZERLAND									
Geneva	A1	0.21	2.2	2	2.2	2	1.5	1.5	59.0
YUGOSLAVIA									
Slovenia	A2C3	-0.69	1.7	8	1.2	7	1.0	0.2	*-15.4*

* : not enough cases for reliable estimation
– : incomplete or missing data
Best model: polynomial of the given degree in age (A), period (P) or cohort (C), or linear drift (D) model.
Goodness of fit: the normalised likelihood ratio chi-square for the best model (see Method).
Rate: world-standardised truncated rate per 100 000 per year (30-74 years) and number of **cases** are both estimated from the best-fitting model for the single years cited.
Cumulative risk per 1000 (30-74 years) is estimated from the best-fitting *age-cohort* model for cohorts of central birth year cited.
Recent trend: estimated mean percentage change per five-year period in the age-specific rates (30-74 years) over the period 1973-1987.
Italics denote recent trends not significant at 5 per cent level, or other figures which should be interpreted with caution (see Method).

OESOPHAGUS (ICD-9 150)

EUROPE (non-EC), INCIDENCE

MALES

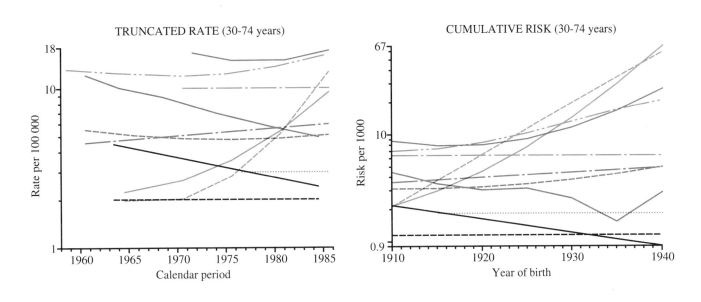

FEMALES

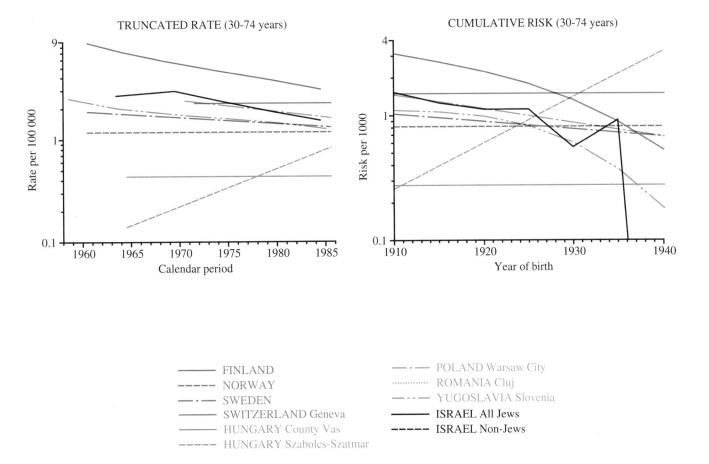

—————— FINLAND	—·—·— POLAND Warsaw City
— — — NORWAY	············· ROMANIA Cluj
—·—·— SWEDEN	—··—··— YUGOSLAVIA Slovenia
—————— SWITZERLAND Geneva	—————— ISRAEL All Jews
—————— HUNGARY County Vas	— — — ISRAEL Non-Jews
— — — HUNGARY Szabolcs-Szatmar	

OESOPHAGUS (ICD-9 150)

EUROPE (EC), INCIDENCE

MALES	Best model	Goodness of fit	1970 Rate	1970 Cases	1985 Rate	1985 Cases	Cumulative risk 1915	Cumulative risk 1940	Recent trend
DENMARK	A2P3C3	0.47	5.0	67	7.5	107	3.8	7.3	20.9
FRANCE									
Bas-Rhin	A8C7	-0.91	*36.1*	*77*	40.3	83	19.9	25.4	*7.7*
Doubs	A4	-0.57	*26.1*	*18*	26.1	28	15.6	15.6	*14.7*
GERMANY (FRG)									
Hamburg	A2P2C2	-0.02	5.3	29	*26.7*	*105*	4.6	*29.5*	–
Saarland	A8C8	-0.25	8.8	25	12.0	34	4.1	15.6	13.5
GERMANY (GDR)	A5C5	1.48	5.1	246	7.6	285	3.1	16.5	18.4
ITALY									
Varese	A3	-0.81	*14.1*	*18*	14.1	29	8.8	8.8	*5.9*
SPAIN									
Navarra	A2C2	0.51	*15.4*	*18*	14.6	19	6.4	21.7	*6.1*
Zaragoza	A3C4	1.23	7.7	14	10.2	23	4.2	11.3	*0.6*
UK									
Birmingham	A2D	0.75	8.8	119	10.1	153	6.4	8.1	*0.1*
Scotland	A4C2	0.68	10.3	140	16.0	224	9.3	15.5	12.6
South Thames	A2C3	0.31	7.9	203	11.5	222	6.5	13.3	14.9

FEMALES	Best model	Goodness of fit	1970 Rate	1970 Cases	1985 Rate	1985 Cases	Cumulative risk 1915	Cumulative risk 1940	Recent trend
DENMARK	A2C3	0.69	1.8	27	2.3	37	1.3	2.3	*10.2*
FRANCE									
Bas-Rhin	A3	-2.54	*1.9*	*5*	1.9	4	1.1	1.1	*3.9*
Doubs	A1C3	-2.12	*41.0*	*0*	2.1	2	0.6	10.8	*69.0*
GERMANY (FRG)									
Hamburg	A1	-0.25	1.4	11	*1.4*	*7*	0.9	*0.9*	–
Saarland	A2C2	1.99	1.5	6	1.3	4	0.7	2.0	*5.0*
GERMANY (GDR)	A2C2	0.18	0.9	70	1.0	57	0.6	1.3	*2.5*
ITALY									
Varese	A1	-0.88	*1.2*	*1*	1.2	3	0.9	0.9	*-15.1*
SPAIN									
Navarra	A1	0.46	*1.5*	*2*	1.5	2	1.0	1.0	*-29.3*
Zaragoza	A2D	0.20	1.7	4	0.6	1	0.6	0.1	-45.4
UK									
Birmingham	A8C9	-0.10	5.0	79	6.3	107	4.0	4.2	10.1
Scotland	A4C2	1.16	5.8	102	7.5	134	4.9	5.2	*5.3*
South Thames	A2D	2.27	4.1	136	5.2	123	3.2	4.7	7.6

* : not enough cases for reliable estimation
− : incomplete or missing data
Best model: polynomial of the given degree in age (A), period (P) or cohort (C), or linear drift (D) model.
Goodness of fit: the normalised likelihood ratio chi-square for the best model (see Method).
Rate: world-standardised truncated rate per 100 000 per year (30-74 years) and number of **cases** are both estimated from the best-fitting model for the single years cited.
Cumulative risk per 1000 (30-74 years) is estimated from the best-fitting *age-cohort* model for cohorts of central birth year cited.
Recent trend: estimated mean percentage change per five-year period in the age-specific rates (30-74 years) over the period 1973-1987.
Italics denote recent trends not significant at 5 per cent level, or other figures which should be interpreted with caution (see Method).

OESOPHAGUS (ICD-9 150)

EUROPE (EC), INCIDENCE

MALES

TRUNCATED RATE (30-74 years)

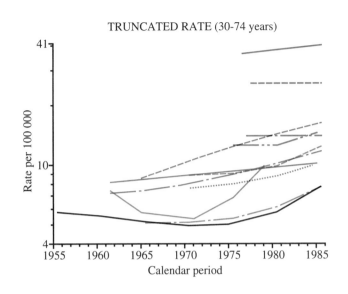

CUMULATIVE RISK (30-74 years)

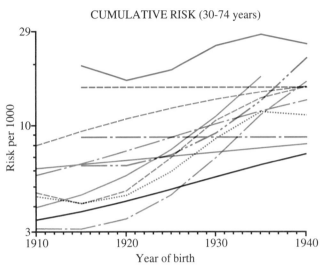

FEMALES

TRUNCATED RATE (30-74 years)

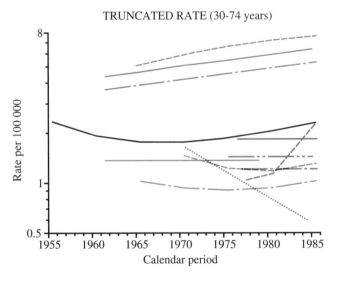

CUMULATIVE RISK (30-74 years)

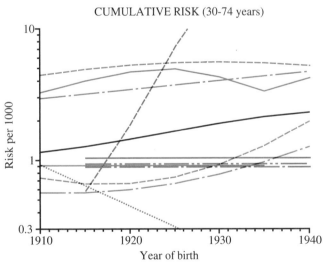

——— FRANCE Bas-Rhin	– – – GERMANY (FRG) Saarland
– – – FRANCE Doubs	–·–·– GERMANY (GDR)
–··–··– ITALY Varese	——— UK Birmingham
–···–···– SPAIN Navarra	– – – UK Scotland
·········· SPAIN Zaragoza	–·–·– UK South Thames
——— GERMANY (FRG) Hamburg	——— DENMARK

OESOPHAGUS (ICD-9 150)

EUROPE (non-EC), INCIDENCE
Percentage change per five-year period, 1973-1987

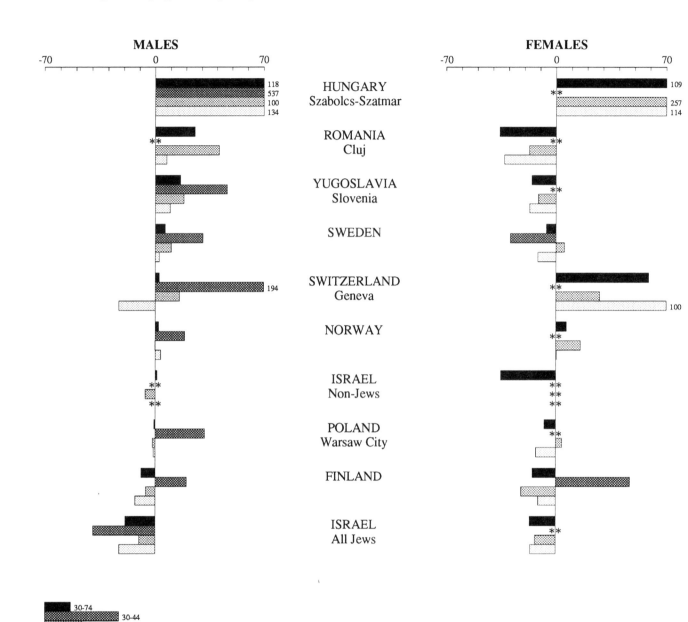

OESOPHAGUS (ICD-9 150)

EUROPE (EC), INCIDENCE
Percentage change per five-year period, 1973-1987

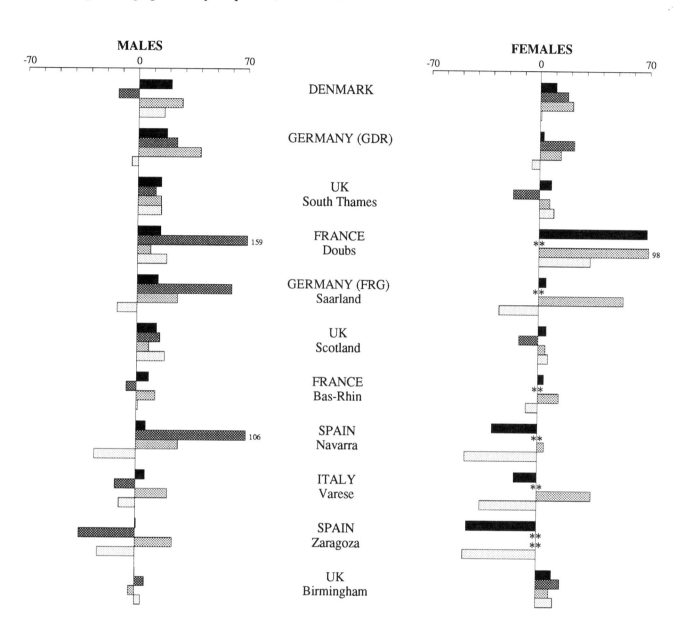

OESOPHAGUS (ICD-9 150)

EUROPE (non-EC), MORTALITY

MALES	Best model	Goodness of fit	1965		1985		Cumulative risk		Recent trend
			Rate	Deaths	Rate	Deaths	1900	1940	
AUSTRIA	A8P5C6	1.03	7.6	153	7.8	141	4.9	9.4	_1.4_
CZECHOSLOVAKIA	A3C4	1.62	4.5	157	7.4	266	2.9	18.6	25.6
FINLAND	A2P2	0.01	9.4	85	4.7	55	6.6	1.4	_-8.0_
HUNGARY	A3P4C4	0.84	4.6	119	12.0	324	2.9	32.3	44.3
NORWAY	A2C2	-0.06	4.6	49	4.5	56	3.1	4.0	_-6.2_
POLAND	A3P5C4	4.27	8.9	520	10.0	776	6.0	9.4	15.5
ROMANIA	A2C2	1.24	3.7	147	_3.4_	_182_	2.3	2.8	−
SWEDEN	A4D	-0.85	4.5	107	5.4	149	3.1	4.4	_2.2_
SWITZERLAND	A3C3	2.16	16.7	239	10.9	188	11.0	8.2	-11.1
YUGOSLAVIA	A3P4C4	1.94	4.3	155	8.2	410	2.8	12.1	12.6

FEMALES	Best model	Goodness of fit	1965		1985		Cumulative risk		Recent trend
			Rate	Deaths	Rate	Deaths	1900	1940	
AUSTRIA	A8C9	0.40	1.0	27	0.7	18	0.7	0.3	_-10.5_
CZECHOSLOVAKIA	A2D	1.77	0.9	37	0.6	30	0.6	0.3	_4.4_
FINLAND	A2P2	0.39	6.0	77	2.6	45	4.4	0.6	-11.3
HUNGARY	A3C2	-0.91	0.9	27	1.0	35	0.5	1.1	19.6
NORWAY	*	..	..	..	..	..	..	..	..
POLAND	A2P2	0.23	2.3	173	1.4	139	1.5	0.5	-7.9
ROMANIA	A2D	-0.52	1.2	57	_0.8_	_51_	0.8	0.4	−
SWEDEN	A2D	-1.17	1.6	41	1.0	32	1.1	0.5	_-4.5_
SWITZERLAND	A2P5	1.06	1.8	33	1.6	34	1.1	0.7	20.6
YUGOSLAVIA	A2D	-0.52	1.0	42	1.4	82	0.6	1.2	_7.7_

* : not enough deaths for reliable estimation
− : incomplete or missing data
Best model: polynomial of the given degree in age (A), period (P) or cohort (C), or linear drift (D) model.
Goodness of fit: the normalised likelihood ratio chi-square for the best model (see Method).
Rate: world-standardised truncated rate per 100 000 per year (30-74 years) and number of **deaths** are both estimated from the best-fitting model for the single years cited.
Cumulative risk per 1000 (30-74 years) is estimated from the best-fitting *age-cohort* model for cohorts of central birth year cited.
Recent trend: estimated mean percentage change per five-year period in the age-specific rates (30-74 years) over the period 1975-1988.
Italics denote recent trends not significant at 5 per cent level, or other figures which should be interpreted with caution (see Method).

OESOPHAGUS (ICD-9 150)

EUROPE (non-EC), MORTALITY

MALES

TRUNCATED RATE (30-74 years)

CUMULATIVE RISK (30-74 years)

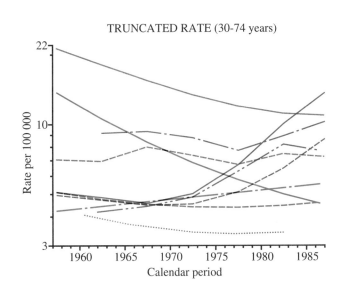
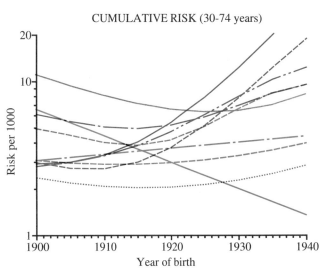

FEMALES

TRUNCATED RATE (30-74 years)

CUMULATIVE RISK (30-74 years)

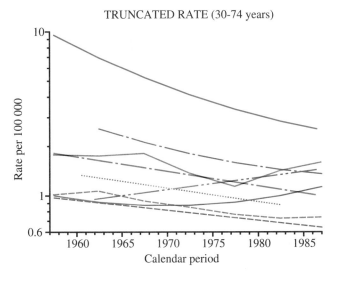
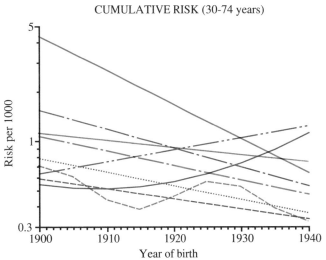

—— FINLAND	--- - CZECHOSLOVAKIA
--- NORWAY	—— HUNGARY
—·—· SWEDEN	—··— POLAND
----- AUSTRIA	······· ROMANIA
—— SWITZERLAND	—···— YUGOSLAVIA

OESOPHAGUS (ICD-9 150)

EUROPE (EC), MORTALITY

MALES	Best model	Goodness of fit	1965 Rate	Deaths	1985 Rate	Deaths	Cumulative risk 1900	1940	Recent trend
BELGIUM	A3C2	0.85	6.4	169	8.7	235	4.1	9.7	13.1
DENMARK	A2P3C3	-0.11	4.3	56	8.2	120	3.0	11.0	24.2
FRANCE	A6P4C8	12.20	27.7	3427	25.5	3490	17.5	17.5	-7.2
GERMANY (FRG)	A4P6C6	4.39	6.0	935	9.0	1432	4.0	20.0	20.5
GREECE	A2	1.89	3.3	62	3.3	92	2.2	2.2	-11.3
IRELAND	A2C4	-0.48	9.1	68	11.6	92	6.0	10.4	*4.3*
ITALY	A3P2C4	5.45	8.4	1020	9.0	1390	5.3	9.8	*1.1*
NETHERLANDS	A4P2C6	0.20	4.5	127	7.1	251	3.2	8.9	22.4
PORTUGAL	A2P3	1.09	10.8	197	11.0	278	6.3	7.8	*-0.8*
SPAIN	A3P5C6	1.28	7.3	501	10.4	990	4.7	15.9	*2.1*
UK ENGLAND & WALES	A2P4C5	1.71	7.6	983	11.9	1735	5.0	12.3	15.1
UK SCOTLAND	A2C3	-0.29	9.9	129	16.2	225	6.3	17.6	13.2

FEMALES	Best model	Goodness of fit	1965 Rate	Deaths	1985 Rate	Deaths	Cumulative risk 1900	1940	Recent trend
BELGIUM	A2C3	-2.22	1.4	46	1.6	52	0.9	1.2	*8.2*
DENMARK	A2P3C2	0.99	1.4	20	2.1	35	1.0	3.2	*12.3*
FRANCE	A8P6C9	0.04	1.6	264	1.8	297	1.1	1.6	*-0.2*
GERMANY (FRG)	A3P3C6	4.08	1.3	290	1.2	268	0.8	1.5	9.8
GREECE	A1C2	0.12	1.2	27	0.8	27	*0.8*	0.3	*-14.7*
IRELAND	A3C2	0.32	7.1	54	6.4	56	4.6	2.9	*-1.5*
ITALY	A2D	0.61	1.4	208	1.2	233	0.9	0.7	-7.4
NETHERLANDS	A3C2	-1.05	1.6	52	2.0	84	1.1	2.4	13.8
PORTUGAL	A2P2C4	1.10	3.5	82	2.1	68	2.4	1.0	-15.5
SPAIN	A2P3C4	0.52	1.9	157	1.0	118	1.2	0.5	-21.4
UK ENGLAND & WALES	A3C3	0.01	4.0	660	4.9	849	2.6	2.9	2.9
UK SCOTLAND	A3C3	0.90	5.3	91	6.7	120	3.4	3.5	7.0

* : not enough deaths for reliable estimation
– : incomplete or missing data
Best model: polynomial of the given degree in age (A), period (P) or cohort (C), or linear drift (D) model.
Goodness of fit: the normalised likelihood ratio chi-square for the best model (see Method).
Rate: world-standardised truncated rate per 100 000 per year (30-74 years) and number of **deaths** are both estimated from the best-fitting model for the single years cited.
Cumulative risk per 1000 (30-74 years) is estimated from the best-fitting *age-cohort* model for cohorts of central birth year cited.
Recent trend: estimated mean percentage change per five-year period in the age-specific rates (30-74 years) over the period 1975-1988.
Italics denote recent trends not significant at 5 per cent level, or other figures which should be interpreted with caution (see Method).

OESOPHAGUS (ICD-9 150)

EUROPE (EC), MORTALITY

MALES

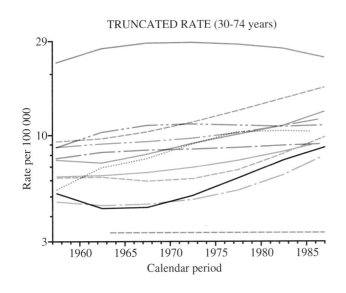

TRUNCATED RATE (30-74 years)

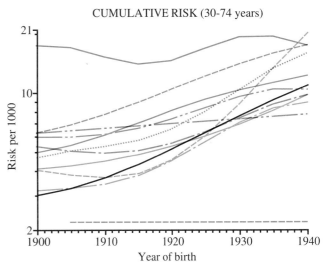

CUMULATIVE RISK (30-74 years)

FEMALES

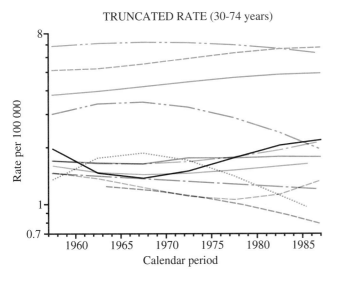

TRUNCATED RATE (30-74 years)

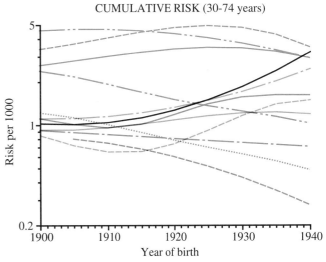

CUMULATIVE RISK (30-74 years)

—— FRANCE	- - - - GERMANY (FRG)
- - - GREECE	—·—· NETHERLANDS
—·—· ITALY	—··—·· IRELAND
—··—·· PORTUGAL	—— UK ENGLAND & WALES
········ SPAIN	- - - UK SCOTLAND
—— BELGIUM	—— DENMARK

OESOPHAGUS (ICD-9 150)

EUROPE (non-EC), MORTALITY
Percentage change per five-year period, 1975-1988

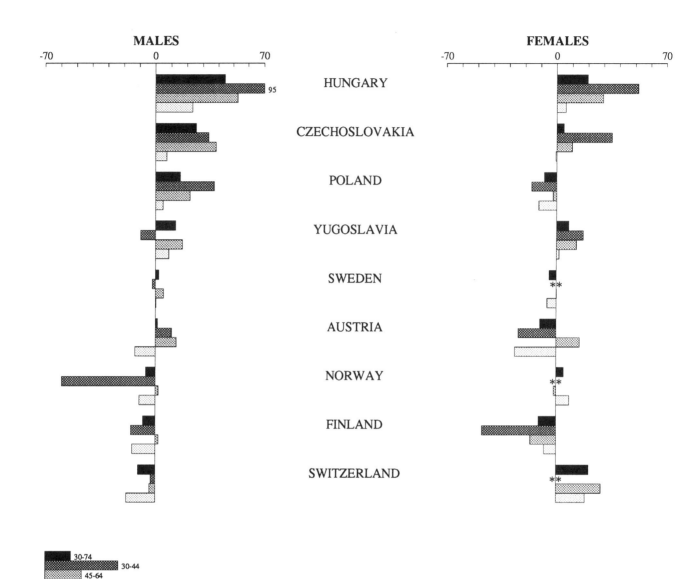

MALES

FEMALES

-70 0 70

-70 0 70

HUNGARY

CZECHOSLOVAKIA

POLAND

YUGOSLAVIA

SWEDEN

AUSTRIA

NORWAY

FINLAND

SWITZERLAND

30-74
30-44
45-64
65-74

OESOPHAGUS (ICD-9 150)

EUROPE (EC), MORTALITY
Percentage change per five-year period, 1975-1988

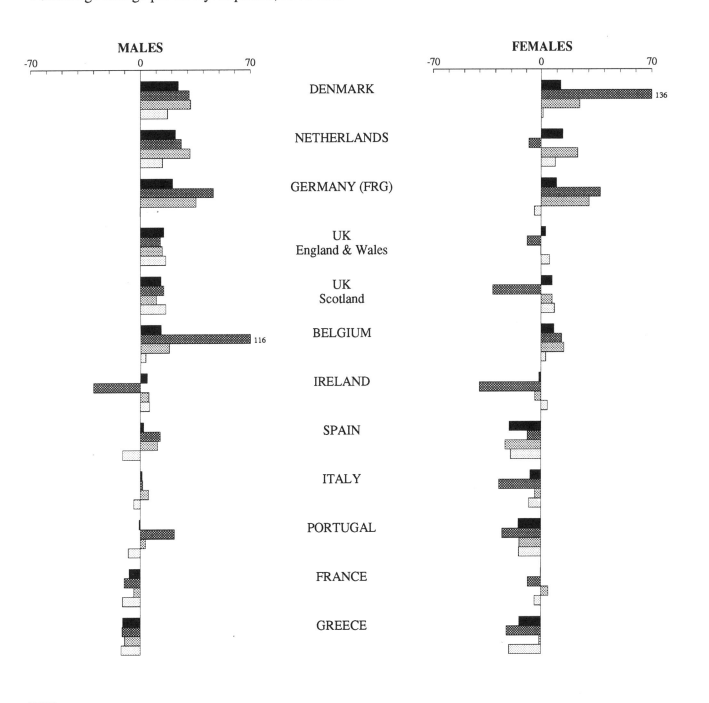

OESOPHAGUS (ICD-9 150)

ASIA, INCIDENCE

MALES	Best model	Goodness of fit	1970 Rate	1970 Cases	1985 Rate	1985 Cases	Cumulative risk 1915	Cumulative risk 1940	Recent trend
CHINA									
Shanghai	A2C6	1.75	*49.7*	*517*	26.3	454	28.5	2.2	-29.0
HONG KONG	A4C3	2.38	*36.1*	*192*	36.6	422	21.7	18.4	*-1.9*
INDIA									
Bombay	A2P3C3	-1.55	26.5	190	21.0	232	14.3	8.4	-9.6
JAPAN									
Miyagi	A3P2C4	0.30	24.4	81	27.1	142	15.6	26.6	7.2
Nagasaki	A2	-0.50	*14.6*	*11*	14.6	15	9.1	9.1	*2.7*
Osaka	A3C7	1.46	20.1	232	15.0	274	9.3	12.9	*-2.1*
SINGAPORE									
Chinese	A4C3	1.00	38.4	77	19.2	56	18.0	5.1	-22.4
Indian	A2	0.77	12.0	3	12.0	4	7.7	7.7	*-23.9*
Malay	*	..	..	..	..	..	..	..	..

FEMALES	Best model	Goodness of fit	1970 Rate	1970 Cases	1985 Rate	1985 Cases	Cumulative risk 1915	Cumulative risk 1940	Recent trend
CHINA									
Shanghai	A2P2C2	0.18	*6.9*	*77*	11.7	218	11.4	2.2	-21.4
HONG KONG	A2D	0.27	*13.4*	*72*	6.6	76	5.9	1.8	-22.2
INDIA									
Bombay	A3D	-0.31	21.4	105	16.9	158	11.0	7.5	-11.0
JAPAN									
Miyagi	A2P2	0.33	6.4	25	4.4	28	3.3	1.3	*-2.7*
Nagasaki	A2	0.17	*2.5*	*2*	2.5	3	1.6	1.6	*-28.9*
Osaka	A2P3	0.36	5.8	79	3.2	71	2.4	1.3	*-7.5*
SINGAPORE									
Chinese	A8P3C8	-0.02	11.1	25	3.2	10	4.3	0.1	-18.8
Indian	A1	-0.61	*10.4*	*0*	10.4	2	6.2	6.2	*-34.4*
Malay	A2D	-1.15	9.6	2	*1.2*	*0*	3.1	0.1	*-45.2*

* : not enough cases for reliable estimation
− : incomplete or missing data
Best model: polynomial of the given degree in age (A), period (P) or cohort (C), or linear drift (D) model.
Goodness of fit: the normalised likelihood ratio chi-square for the best model (see Method).
Rate: world-standardised truncated rate per 100 000 per year (30-74 years) and number of **cases** are both estimated from the best-fitting model for the single years cited.
Cumulative risk per 1000 (30-74 years) is estimated from the best-fitting *age-cohort* model for cohorts of central birth year cited.
Recent trend: estimated mean percentage change per five-year period in the age-specific rates (30-74 years) over the period 1973-1987.
Italics denote recent trends not significant at 5 per cent level, or other figures which should be interpreted with caution (see Method).

174

OESOPHAGUS (ICD-9 150)

ASIA, INCIDENCE

MALES

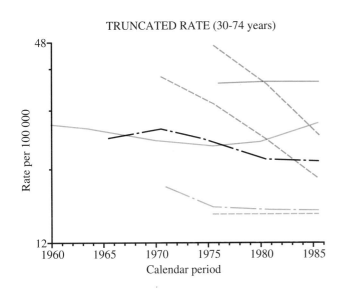

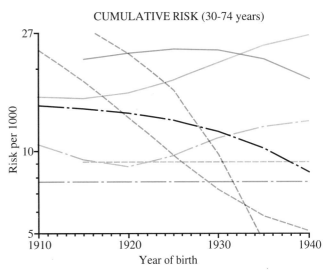

FEMALES

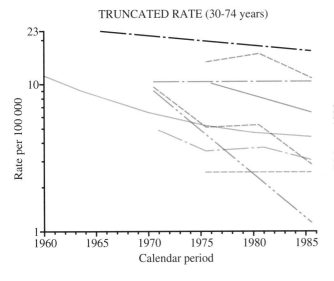

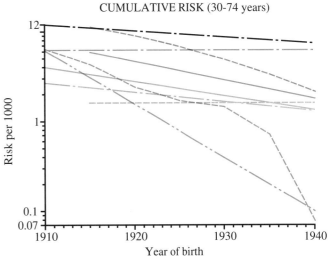

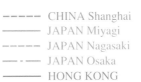

----- CHINA Shanghai
—— JAPAN Miyagi
----- JAPAN Nagasaki
—·— JAPAN Osaka
—— HONG KONG

----- SINGAPORE Chinese
—·— SINGAPORE Indian
—··— SINGAPORE Malay
—··— INDIA Bombay

OESOPHAGUS (ICD-9 150)

OCEANIA, INCIDENCE

MALES	Best model	Goodness of fit	1970 Rate	1970 Cases	1985 Rate	1985 Cases	Cumulative risk 1915	Cumulative risk 1940	Recent trend
AUSTRALIA									
New South Wales	A2P2	1.59	*12.9*	*132*	7.5	100	4.9	4.3	*-2.4*
South	A2	-0.33	*7.4*	*13*	7.4	26	4.6	4.6	*-0.4*
HAWAII									
Caucasian	A2	0.25	8.0	2	8.0	4	5.0	5.0	*24.1*
Chinese	A1D	-1.81	10.7	1	*3.4*	*0*	4.8	0.7	-57.9
Filipino	A1P2	-2.03	9.0	2	3.0	1	4.4	3.5	-50.4
Hawaiian	A2P2	1.40	27.2	3	16.1	3	13.5	9.8	-36.1
Japanese	A1D	-0.49	8.4	3	6.6	6	4.9	3.3	*0.2*
NEW ZEALAND									
Maori	A2	0.28	11.3	1	11.3	3	7.5	7.5	*10.2*
Non-Maori	A8P4	1.06	6.7	37	9.1	64	6.2	7.9	*-0.2*

FEMALES	Best model	Goodness of fit	1970 Rate	1970 Cases	1985 Rate	1985 Cases	Cumulative risk 1915	Cumulative risk 1940	Recent trend
AUSTRALIA									
New South Wales	A2P2C2	-0.62	*5.4*	*63*	3.9	60	2.7	1.6	10.8
South	A2	-1.03	*2.6*	*4*	2.6	10	1.7	1.7	*13.1*
HAWAII									
Caucasian	A2C2	-3.12	3.7	1	2.1	1	2.6	0.0	*-24.4*
Chinese	*	..	..	..	..	..	..	..	..
Filipino	A2C2	-2.07	*0.7*	*0*	4.7	1	1.2	0.0	*85.1*
Hawaiian	A1C2	-0.33	*3.3*	*0*	5.0	1	3.3	1.4	*-15.5*
Japanese	A2	-1.87	*0.6*	*0*	*0.6*	*0*	0.4	0.4	*0.9*
NEW ZEALAND									
Maori	A1C2	-1.01	*1.9*	*0*	*2.1*	*0*	2.2	0.1	*-29.4*
Non-Maori	A2	0.11	3.6	23	3.6	29	2.4	2.4	*3.9*

* : not enough cases for reliable estimation
– : incomplete or missing data
Best model: polynomial of the given degree in age (A), period (P) or cohort (C), or linear drift (D) model.
Goodness of fit: the normalised likelihood ratio chi-square for the best model (see Method).
Rate: world-standardised truncated rate per 100 000 per year (30-74 years) and number of **cases** are both estimated from the best-fitting model for the single years cited.
Cumulative risk per 1000 (30-74 years) is estimated from the best-fitting *age-cohort* model for cohorts of central birth year cited.
Recent trend: estimated mean percentage change per five-year period in the age-specific rates (30-74 years) over the period 1973-1987.
Italics denote recent trends not significant at 5 per cent level, or other figures which should be interpreted with caution (see Method).

OESOPHAGUS (ICD-9 150)

OCEANIA, INCIDENCE

MALES

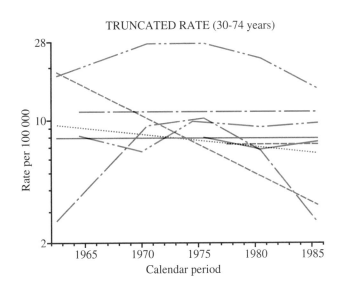

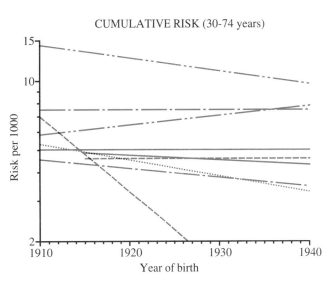

FEMALES

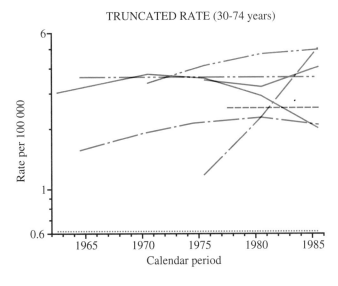

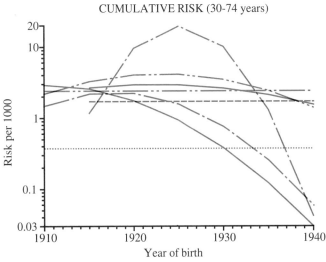

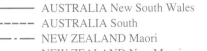

———— AUSTRALIA New South Wales	– – – – HAWAII Chinese
– – – – AUSTRALIA South	–·–·– HAWAII Filipino
–·–·– NEW ZEALAND Maori	–··–··– HAWAII Hawaiian
–··–··– NEW ZEALAND Non-Maori	············ HAWAII Japanese
———— HAWAII Caucasian	

OESOPHAGUS (ICD-9 150)

ASIA, INCIDENCE
Percentage change per five-year period, 1973-1987

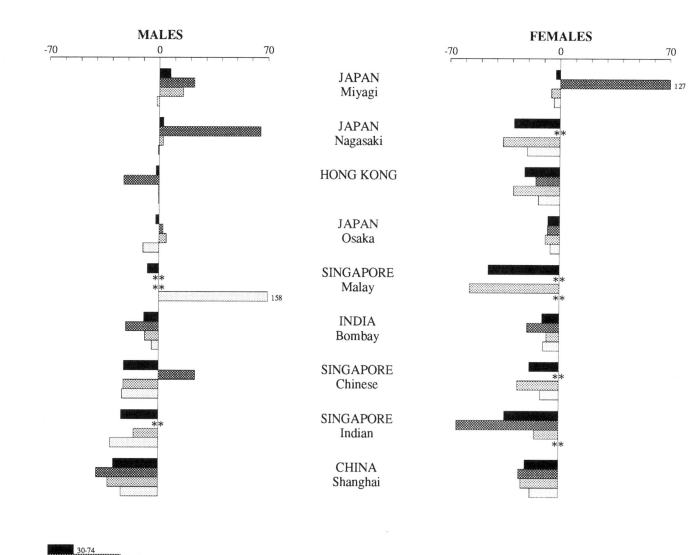

178

OESOPHAGUS (ICD-9 150)

OCEANIA, INCIDENCE
Percentage change per five-year period, 1973-1987

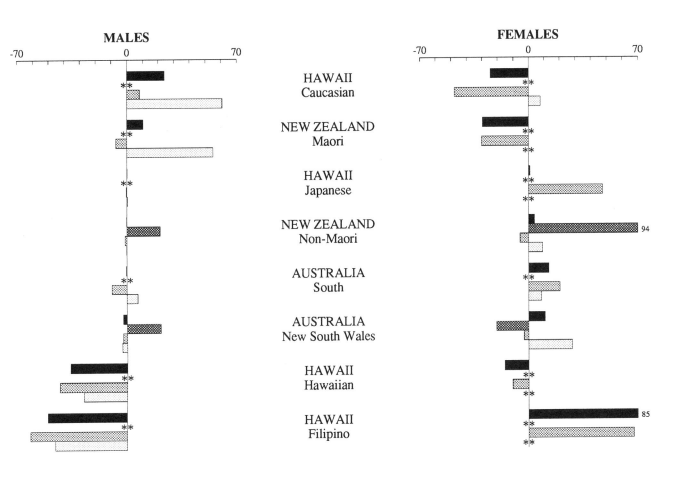

MALES

FEMALES

HAWAII
Caucasian

NEW ZEALAND
Maori

HAWAII
Japanese

NEW ZEALAND
Non-Maori

AUSTRALIA
South

AUSTRALIA
New South Wales

HAWAII
Hawaiian

HAWAII
Filipino

30-74
30-44
45-64
65-74

ASIA and OCEANIA, MORTALITY

MALES	Best model	Goodness of fit	1965		1985		Cumulative risk		Recent trend
			Rate	Deaths	Rate	Deaths	1900	1940	
AUSTRALIA	A2P2C6	0.03	6.0	142	8.1	298	3.9	5.8	*3.6*
HONG KONG	A3P3C4	0.84	21.7	85	23.1	221	*13.7*	11.2	-8.3
JAPAN	A8P6C8	7.52	13.6	2377	13.0	3741	9.7	9.3	*-0.9*
MAURITIUS	A4C2	0.64	6.0	5	6.1	6	*3.0*	1.2	*15.5*
NEW ZEALAND	A2D	-0.46	6.5	34	9.4	70	4.3	9.1	*4.5*
SINGAPORE	A2C3	1.01	*22.8*	*42*	11.6	27	*12.6*	2.7	–

FEMALES	Best model	Goodness of fit	1965		1985		Cumulative risk		Recent trend
			Rate	Deaths	Rate	Deaths	1900	1940	
AUSTRALIA	A3P2C5	2.19	2.2	60	2.8	118	1.4	1.6	*2.3*
HONG KONG	A2P2C2	0.42	5.2	25	3.6	29	*3.8*	1.2	-23.0
JAPAN	A2P6C5	3.68	3.8	755	1.9	682	2.8	0.4	-19.1
MAURITIUS	A2C2	0.36	1.8	1	2.8	3	*0.8*	1.2	*-3.1*
NEW ZEALAND	A3	-1.24	3.0	18	3.0	25	2.0	2.0	*-5.2*
SINGAPORE	A2P2	-0.95	*7.3*	*10*	2.5	6	*6.0*	0.7	–

* : not enough deaths for reliable estimation
− : incomplete or missing data
Best model: polynomial of the given degree in age (A), period (P) or cohort (C), or linear drift (D) model.
Goodness of fit: the normalised likelihood ratio chi-square for the best model (see Method).
Rate: world-standardised truncated rate per 100 000 per year (30-74 years) and number of **deaths** are both estimated from the best-fitting model for the single years cited.
Cumulative risk per 1000 (30-74 years) is estimated from the best-fitting *age-cohort* model for cohorts of central birth year cited.
Recent trend: estimated mean percentage change per five-year period in the age-specific rates (30-74 years) over the period 1975-1988.
Italics denote recent trends not significant at 5 per cent level, or other figures which should be interpreted with caution (see Method).

OESOPHAGUS (ICD-9 150)

ASIA and OCEANIA, MORTALITY

MALES

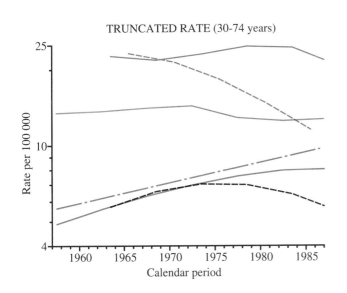

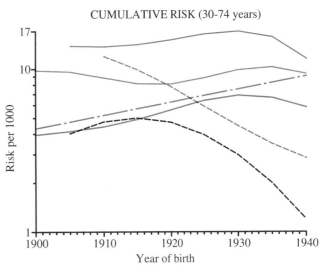

FEMALES

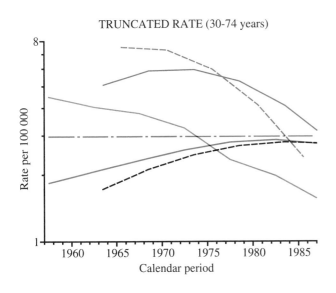

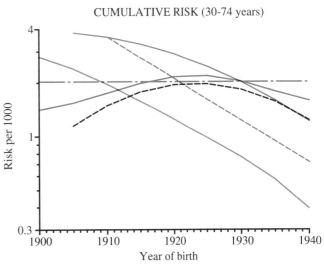

AUSTRALIA
NEW ZEALAND
JAPAN
HONG KONG
SINGAPORE
MAURITIUS

OESOPHAGUS (ICD-9 150)

ASIA and OCEANIA, MORTALITY
Percentage change per five-year period, 1975-1988

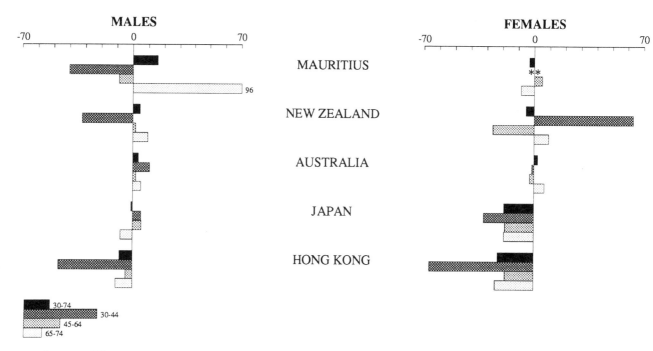

from page 161

risk among females in Saarland (FRG) and the GDR is also increasing in successive cohorts. Incidence among males in Geneva (Switzerland) is increasing slightly, although mortality among males in Switzerland as a whole is decreasing. Little change is seen in other western European countries, except for Doubs (France) and Zaragoza (Spain), where the estimates of trend are very imprecise.

Mortality trends for males in other European countries largely confirm the geographical patterns observed for oesophageal cancer incidence. They show a rapid increase in mortality in Belgium, Ireland and the Netherlands, for which incidence trends were not available. There is a small increase in mortality in successive cohorts in Italy, which is not seen in the incidence data from Varese. In Portugal, there is little change among males, but a decline in mortality among females, which is also seen in Spain and Greece.

Asia and Oceania

Oesophageal cancer incidence in Chinese populations in Shanghai (China), Singapore and to some extent in Hawaii has been higher than elsewhere in the region, but it is now falling steadily in both sexes at 20% or more every five years. In Hong Kong, the

rate of decline is also about 20% among females, but for males the decline is apparent only for recent birth cohorts. Mortality trends in Singapore and Hong Kong confirm these patterns.

Incidence in the Japanese prefectures of Miyagi and Osaka is increasing among males in successive cohorts born since 1920, but decreasing by calendar period among females. There is no significant trend in Nagasaki (Japan), but there are few cases. There is little change in mortality among males in Japan, but the birth cohort pattern closely resembles the inflection seen in France, albeit at about half the level of risk (1%). Among females in Japan, there has been a rapid decline of about 20% every five years, parallel with the declines among females in Hong Kong and Singapore.

There has been little change in incidence among males in Australia and New Zealand. There has been a slight but significant fall in risk among females in more recent birth cohorts in New South Wales (Australia). Other trends in Oceania are based on very small numbers of cases, and the cohort risk curves are uninterpretable (see Chapter 3). In Australia, mortality has increased in both sexes, but there is a slight decline in more recent birth cohorts in both sexes; the age-specific trends among non-Maori males in New Zealand suggest that the current steady rate of increase of about 5% every five years may also slow down during the 1990s.

182

Americas

In Central and South America, the estimated overall incidence of oesophageal cancer around 1980 was two to three times higher than in North America[219]. The data from Cali (Colombia) suggest an exception to this pattern, with incidence rates around 5 per 100 000 per year in both sexes, similar to the rates in North America, and little evidence of change in either sex. In São Paulo (Brazil), incidence is among the highest in the Americas in both sexes (around 35 and 10 per 100 000 in males and females, respectively), and was increasing steadily up to 1978, although more recent data were not available.

With the exception of Panama, mortality was also much higher in South America than in North America until recently, but there have been significant declines in both sexes in the countries of Central and South America for which mortality data were available. Estimated lifetime mortality risks from oesophageal cancer for recent birth cohorts in these countries are now similar to or less than those for Canada and the USA, around 5 per 1000 in males and 1 per 1000 in females. The exception is Uruguay, where mortality appears to be declining much more slowly, and the lifetime risk for recent birth cohorts is still around 13 and 2 per 1000 in males and females, respectively, twice as high as elsewhere in South America.

In Puerto Rico, where both incidence and mortality from oesophageal cancer were very high in the 1960s, there has been a rapid decline in both sexes since the 1970s, particularly in females: the recent rates of decline are about 13% and 37% every five years in males and females, respectively. This is best explained by a cohort effect.

Oesophageal cancer incidence among males is increasing in all five Canadian provinces or regions examined here, significantly so in British Columbia, Quebec and the Maritime Provinces. Mortality among Canadian males reflects these changes in incidence; it has been increasing by 10% every five years (19% in 30-44 year-olds). There has been little change in Canadian females, and rates remain low.

In the USA, blacks in Detroit now have among the highest incidence rates in the Americas in both sexes, along with other black populations in the San Francisco Bay Area and New Orleans. Although there is a three-fold difference between blacks and whites in the San Francisco Bay Area, there has been a parallel and accelerating increase in risk in both racial groups for successive cohorts born since 1925. A similar pattern, though less marked, can be seen for males in Connecticut, where the incidence was five-fold higher in blacks than in whites in both sexes in 1978-82[202], as elsewhere in the USA, and

although only about 10% of the Connecticut population is black, it is possible that the increase in Connecticut as a whole is partly due to rising incidence in the black population. Both in Connecticut and among blacks in Detroit, the recent increases are greatest among 30-44 year-olds. Estimated incidence among males in Seattle and Iowa was relatively low (around 8 per 100 000) in 1970, but it has been increasing steadily at over 10% every five years, and incidence rates are now at the level of other white populations in the USA. The racial differences in incidence are similar in females, but in contrast to the pattern seen for males, there has been a significant decline in incidence among females born since 1925 in several populations, both white and black.

Mortality in Canada and, to a lesser extent, the USA is rising in successive birth cohorts for males, but there are signs of a deceleration in the overall rate of increase in the USA, particularly among females, for whom cumulative risk appears to have peaked for the 1920-30 birth cohorts, and to have been declining since: this suggests an imminent decline in mortality in the mid-1990s, in parallel with the observed declines in incidence in the same birth cohorts. Cross-sectional mortality among females has already reached a plateau in the USA, and it is declining by 20% every five years among 30-44 year-old females in both countries.

Comment

Most previous reports on trends in oesophageal cancer in many countries are consistent with the trends reported here. These reports often implicate trends in alcohol and tobacco consumption, and improvements in less well defined nutritional deficiencies, as being likely to underlie the observed changes in risk; some analyses have incorporated data on trends in these risk factors, or surrogates for them.

In one analysis of trends in oesophageal cancer mortality in 17 European countries, percentage changes in the standardised mortality ratios (SMR) between 1956 and 1985 were correlated with the corresponding change in the SMR for lung cancer and liver cirrhosis, as surrogates for tobacco and alcohol consumption[53]. The trends in oesophageal cancer were considered paradoxical, in that the correlations between the percentage changes in the SMRs were weak. Correlations between percentage changes in the age-specific rates were also generally weak, and correlations of the change in SMR with lagged changes in alcohol consumption were not significant. There were significant inverse correlations between changes in oesophageal cancer and changes in the consumption of fresh fruit,

continued page 188

OESOPHAGUS (ICD-9 150)

AMERICAS (except USA), INCIDENCE

MALES	Best model	Goodness of fit	1970 Rate	1970 Cases	1985 Rate	1985 Cases	Cumulative risk 1915	Cumulative risk 1940	Recent trend
BRAZIL									
Sao Paulo	A3D	-0.82	21.9	138	*36.9*	*275*	12.8	*30.5*	–
CANADA									
Alberta	A2D	-0.41	4.2	12	6.3	28	3.6	7.1	*14.5*
British Columbia	A2D	-0.32	5.9	27	8.1	58	4.7	8.0	15.7
Maritime Provinces	A2D	0.59	4.4	14	7.6	27	4.1	10.2	22.9
Newfoundland	A1P3	1.00	10.6	9	6.9	8	4.8	3.4	*6.0*
Quebec	A2C3	1.13	6.0	64	8.1	117	4.6	8.0	9.6
COLOMBIA									
Cali	A2P2	-1.02	5.3	3	6.1	8	3.4	2.5	*15.4*
CUBA	A8C7	0.28	8.9	131	7.8	156	5.4	*3.3*	–
PUERTO RICO	A3C3	0.70	29.9	136	18.4	126	15.0	6.2	-12.7

FEMALES	Best model	Goodness of fit	1970 Rate	1970 Cases	1985 Rate	1985 Cases	Cumulative risk 1915	Cumulative risk 1940	Recent trend
BRAZIL									
Sao Paulo	A1D	-0.95	3.4	21	*12.7*	*111*	3.4	29.9	–
CANADA									
Alberta	A2	0.88	1.5	4	1.5	7	0.9	0.9	*-7.6*
British Columbia	A2D	-0.97	3.5	16	2.4	19	1.8	1.0	*-10.2*
Maritime Provinces	A2	-2.17	1.8	6	1.8	7	1.2	1.2	*12.4*
Newfoundland	A1D	-1.28	2.8	2	1.6	2	1.4	0.5	*-22.0*
Quebec	A2	-1.36	1.9	22	1.9	32	1.2	1.2	*4.9*
COLOMBIA									
Cali	A1	-1.83	2.7	1	2.7	4	1.8	1.8	*-4.9*
CUBA	A8C7	-0.90	3.7	47	2.6	52	1.9	*2.4*	–
PUERTO RICO	A3P2C2	2.72	11.1	50	3.9	31	4.9	0.5	-37.2

* : not enough cases for reliable estimation
– : incomplete or missing data
Best model: polynomial of the given degree in age (A), period (P) or cohort (C), or linear drift (D) model.
Goodness of fit: the normalised likelihood ratio chi-square for the best model (see Method).
Rate: world-standardised truncated rate per 100 000 per year (30-74 years) and number of **cases** are both estimated from the best-fitting model for the single years cited.
Cumulative risk per 1000 (30-74 years) is estimated from the best-fitting *age-cohort* model for cohorts of central birth year cited.
Recent trend: estimated mean percentage change per five-year period in the age-specific rates (30-74 years) over the period 1973-1987.
Italics denote recent trends not significant at 5 per cent level, or other figures which should be interpreted with caution (see Method).

OESOPHAGUS (ICD-9 150)

AMERICAS (except USA), INCIDENCE

MALES

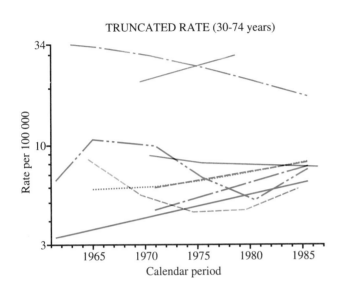

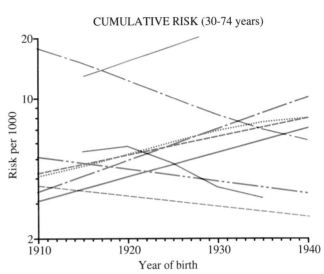

FEMALES

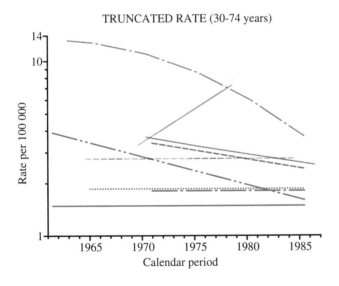

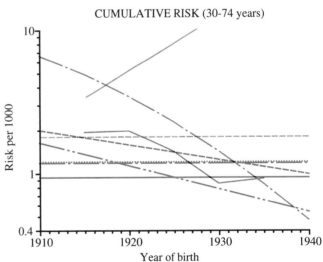

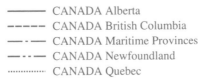

--- CANADA Alberta
- - - - CANADA British Columbia
-·-·- CANADA Maritime Provinces
-··-··- CANADA Newfoundland
············ CANADA Quebec

--- CUBA
-·-·- PUERTO RICO
--- BRAZIL Sao Paulo
- - - - COLOMBIA Cali

OESOPHAGUS (ICD-9 150)

AMERICAS (USA), INCIDENCE

MALES	Best model	Goodness of fit	1970 Rate	1970 Cases	1985 Rate	1985 Cases	Cumulative risk 1915	Cumulative risk 1940	Recent trend
USA									
Bay Area, Black	A4C2	-0.26	32.3	17	26.8	21	14.2	21.7	*7.6*
Bay Area, Chinese	A1	0.11	13.1	2	*13.1*	*6*	8.7	*8.7*	–
Bay Area, White	A2C3	-0.25	7.8	46	7.4	46	4.8	6.3	*0.0*
Connecticut	A3C2	-3.02	11.2	74	12.2	97	6.9	10.6	7.3
Detroit, Black	A8D	0.25	26.6	37	33.4	56	14.9	21.8	*6.3*
Detroit, White	A2	0.34	8.5	62	8.5	62	5.5	5.5	-6.8
Iowa	A2D	0.55	5.7	38	7.2	50	4.1	6.0	11.1
New Orleans, Black	A2	0.79	*29.6*	*15*	29.6	17	15.9	15.9	*-4.5*
New Orleans, White	A2	-0.05	*8.0*	*11*	8.0	12	4.9	4.9	*17.3*
Seattle	A2D	-0.86	*5.6*	*26*	8.9	59	4.8	10.4	17.1

FEMALES	Best model	Goodness of fit	1970 Rate	1970 Cases	1985 Rate	1985 Cases	Cumulative risk 1915	Cumulative risk 1940	Recent trend
USA									
Bay Area, Black	A3C2	-0.55	7.2	4	8.0	7	5.1	1.8	*0.3*
Bay Area, Chinese	A1C2	-0.70	*4.6*	*0*	*0.7*	*0*	7.0	*0.0*	–
Bay Area, White	A4C4	-0.82	4.0	29	3.4	26	2.7	0.8	-5.5
Connecticut	A3D	0.30	2.6	20	3.5	32	1.8	3.0	-5.4
Detroit, Black	A2C2	1.13	8.5	12	10.3	21	5.7	4.8	*1.1*
Detroit, White	A2D	0.10	2.3	19	2.4	21	1.5	1.6	-1.9
Iowa	A2	-1.11	1.6	12	1.6	12	1.0	1.0	*6.4*
New Orleans, Black	A2C2	-1.14	*5.1*	*3*	7.9	6	4.9	1.6	*14.0*
New Orleans, White	A2P2	-0.56	*0.0*	*0*	1.5	2	1.1	1.0	-0.9
Seattle	A2C2	0.37	*2.3*	*11*	2.5	19	1.9	0.4	*-1.0*

* : not enough cases for reliable estimation
– : incomplete or missing data
Best model: polynomial of the given degree in age (A), period (P) or cohort (C), or linear drift (D) model.
Goodness of fit: the normalised likelihood ratio chi-square for the best model (see Method).
Rate: world-standardised truncated rate per 100 000 per year (30-74 years) and number of **cases** are both estimated from the best-fitting model for the single years cited.
Cumulative risk per 1000 (30-74 years) is estimated from the best-fitting *age-cohort* model for cohorts of central birth year cited.
Recent trend: estimated mean percentage change per five-year period in the age-specific rates (30-74 years) over the period 1973-1987.
Italics denote recent trends not significant at 5 per cent level, or other figures which should be interpreted with caution (see Method).

OESOPHAGUS (ICD-9 150)

AMERICAS (USA), INCIDENCE

MALES

TRUNCATED RATE (30-74 years)

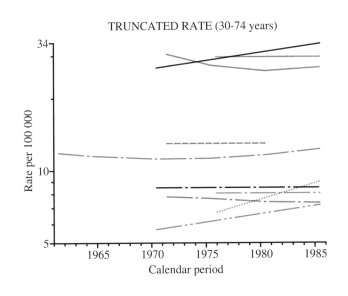

CUMULATIVE RISK (30-74 years)

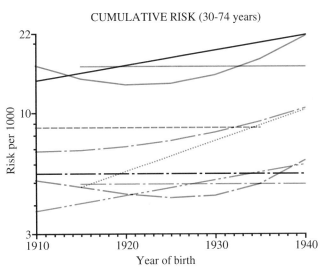

FEMALES

TRUNCATED RATE (30-74 years)

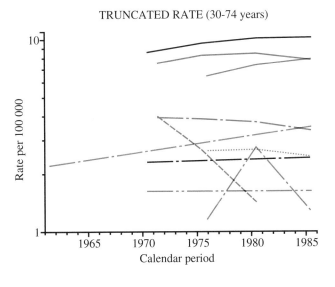

CUMULATIVE RISK (30-74 years)

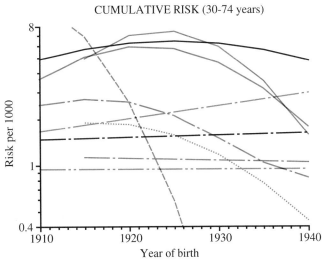

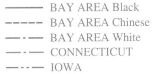

—— BAY AREA Black	·········· SEATTLE
– – – BAY AREA Chinese	—— NEW ORLEANS Black
–·–·– BAY AREA White	–··– NEW ORLEANS White
–·–·– CONNECTICUT	—— DETROIT Black
–··–··– IOWA	–··–··– DETROIT White

OESOPHAGUS (ICD-9 150)

AMERICAS (except USA), INCIDENCE
Percentage change per five-year period, 1973-1987

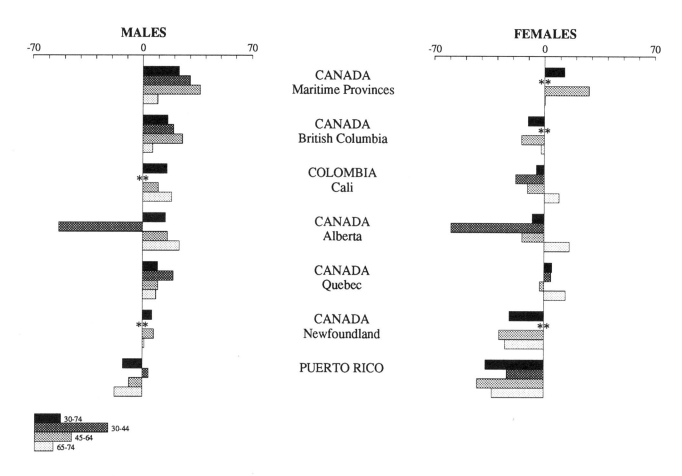

from page 183

which is protective[204]. The results were interpreted as suggesting that oesophageal cancer risk would have declined dramatically in Europe without the influence of alcohol and tobacco, since nutritional improvements appeared largely to have offset the adverse effect of these carcinogenic exposures. Increasing mortality in England and Wales up to 1980 has been attributed largely to alcohol, with an additional cohort effect due to tobacco in males; a small cohort decline in females was attributed to nutritional improvement[213]. Mortality increased by 4% per year among males in Northern Ireland (UK) during 1979-88[224]: the rate is similar to that in the rest of the UK, as is the pattern of increase seen for successive birth cohorts since 1910, with a 20% increase every five years since 1975 (data not shown). Studies in Birmingham (UK)[243] and in the SEER group of registries in the USA[29] have documented an increase in the incidence of adenocarcinoma of the middle and lower thirds of the oesophagus and of the adjacent gastric cardia, with no change in the incidence either of squamous cell carcinoma in these sites or of adenocarcinoma in the upper oesophagus or other parts of the stomach: the trends were not attributable to improved endoscopic diagnosis and localisation of tumours.

The rapid increase in mortality in Spain among males aged 40-79 in the period 1951-85 (5% per year) was closely correlated with consumption of cigarettes and alcohol, particularly spirits[51]. Among males in Vaud (Switzerland), incidence fell by 15% per five years in the decade 1979-88[164], similar to the rate of decline in national mortality, but the decline among females (12%) is not reflected in the mortality, which has recently been rising at 20% every five years, although it has fluctuated more than in other countries. Incidence trends reported for Slovakia[237] and for the whole of the former Czechoslovakia[80] reflect the trends seen here for mortality, with an increase of some 30% every five years among males and little change among females.

continued page 192

OESOPHAGUS (ICD-9 150)

AMERICAS (USA), INCIDENCE
Percentage change per five-year period, 1973-1987

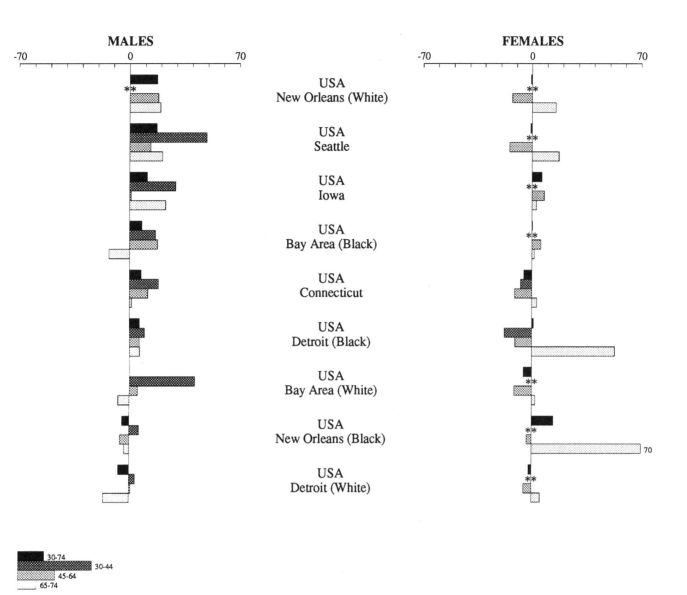

OESOPHAGUS (ICD-9 150)

AMERICAS, MORTALITY

MALES	Best model	Goodness of fit	1965 Rate	1965 Deaths	1985 Rate	1985 Deaths	Cumulative risk 1900	Cumulative risk 1940	Recent trend
CANADA	A3C3	0.43	5.5	209	7.7	446	3.6	7.5	10.0
CHILE	A3P2C2	1.88	18.5	208	13.5	233	12.2	4.7	-10.6
COSTA RICA	A6C3	1.00	*9.0*	*13*	5.1	15	*5.5*	0.8	*-14.2*
PANAMA	A4	1.20	3.5	4	3.5	10	2.3	2.3	–
PUERTO RICO	A3C2	-0.19	29.5	121	18.4	85	*18.9*	5.1	-17.3
URUGUAY	A3P3	0.54	27.4	162	22.0	162	17.5	13.1	-11.5
USA	A4C5	2.20	7.6	3236	9.0	4994	4.6	6.0	2.7
VENEZUELA	A2C2	-0.52	6.9	56	*4.9*	*70*	4.7	1.6	–

FEMALES	Best model	Goodness of fit	1965 Rate	1965 Deaths	1985 Rate	1985 Deaths	Cumulative risk 1900	Cumulative risk 1940	Recent trend
CANADA	A2C3	-0.47	1.9	73	1.9	125	1.2	0.8	*-1.6*
CHILE	A8P6C9	0.45	9.6	120	5.1	104	5.8	1.6	-13.7
COSTA RICA	A1D	1.64	*4.2*	*4*	2.2	4	*2.9*	0.8	*2.5*
PANAMA	A1	-0.25	1.5	2	1.5	4	1.1	1.1	–
PUERTO RICO	A2C2	1.33	11.3	45	3.6	17	*8.3*	0.4	-35.9
URUGUAY	A2C2	2.10	8.2	50	5.0	42	5.5	2.5	*-7.4*
USA	A4P3C4	0.42	1.8	864	2.3	1497	1.0	1.0	*0.8*
VENEZUELA	A2P2C3	0.41	4.8	41	*1.7*	*26*	3.3	0.7	–

* : not enough deaths for reliable estimation
– : incomplete or missing data
Best model: polynomial of the given degree in age (A), period (P) or cohort (C), or linear drift (D) model.
Goodness of fit: the normalised likelihood ratio chi-square for the best model (see Method).
Rate: world-standardised truncated rate per 100 000 per year (30-74 years) and number of **deaths** are both estimated from the best-fitting model for the single years cited.
Cumulative risk per 1000 (30-74 years) is estimated from the best-fitting *age-cohort* model for cohorts of central birth year cited.
Recent trend: estimated mean percentage change per five-year period in the age-specific rates (30-74 years) over the period 1975-1988.
Italics denote recent trends not significant at 5 per cent level, or other figures which should be interpreted with caution (see Method).

OESOPHAGUS (ICD-9 150)

AMERICAS, MORTALITY

MALES

TRUNCATED RATE (30-74 years)

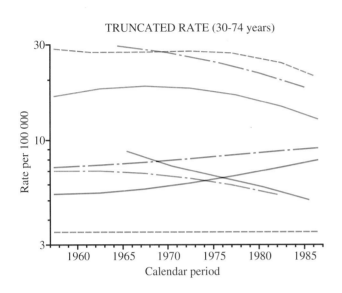

CUMULATIVE RISK (30-74 years)

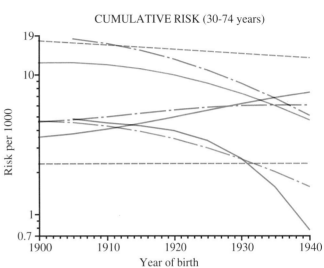

FEMALES

TRUNCATED RATE (30-74 years)

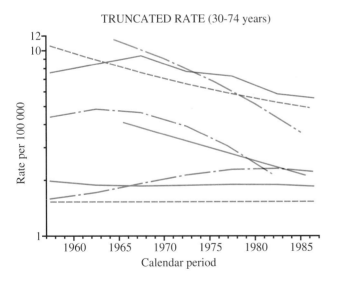

CUMULATIVE RISK (30-74 years)

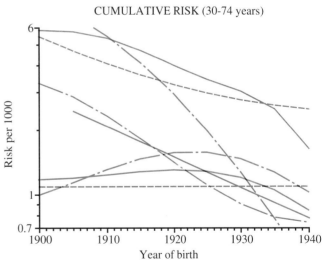

—— CANADA		—··— PUERTO RICO	
—·— USA		—— CHILE	
—— COSTA RICA		---- URUGUAY	
---- PANAMA		—··— VENEZUELA	

OESOPHAGUS (ICD-9 150)

AMERICAS, MORTALITY
Percentage change per five-year period, 1975-1988

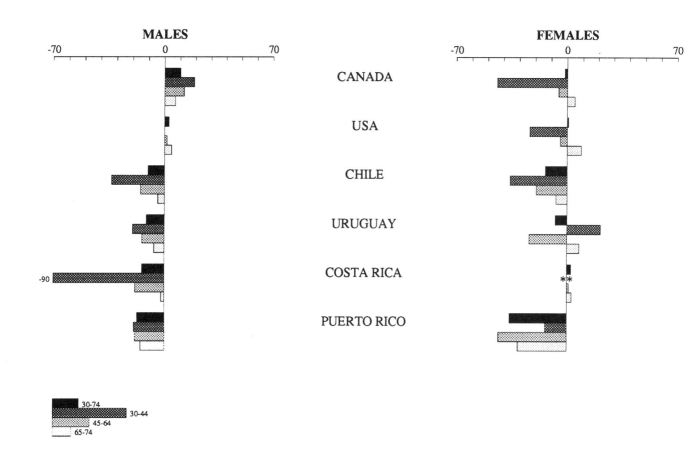

from page 188

In Henan province (China), where cancer of the oesophagus ranks first in both sexes, accounting for 42% and 39% of all cancer deaths in males and females, respectively, there was a slight fall during the period 1974-85 in the extremely high age-standardised rates, from 108 to 90 per 100 000 for males and from 62 to 48 for females[169]: this pattern may reflect improved nutrition, as in Shanghai. Small declines among males in successive birth cohorts have been reported previously from Singapore[154] and Bombay (India)[136]; the effect can be seen for males born around 1925 or later in the data reported here.

Incidence trends in Ontario (Canada) have been similar to those reported here for other Canadian provinces, with a 9% increase in males and an 8% fall in females between the two quinquennia ending in 1988[182]. In Kingston and St Andrew (Jamaica), a substantial fall in the incidence of oesophageal cancer has been reported in both sexes since the mid-

1960s, and attributed to improved nutrition[42].

A report on mortality in the USA during the decade 1970-80 identified increases in mortality of 56% and 19% among black males and females, respectively, and 8% and 7% among whites[17]. The different trends in incidence by race and sex in the USA reported here are reflected in more recent mortality trends by race. Analysis of US mortality data by race and sex for the period 1950-84[74] showed an increasing risk in successive cohorts among black males, for whom risk is already high, and a lesser increase or plateau for white males. There was a decline in risk among white females born after about 1920, and a later but more rapid decline among black females born after 1930. Among white females, the peak mortality for those born around 1915-20, who passed their childbearing years during the 1930s and 1940s, has been linked with poorer nutrition during this period[77].

192

Chapter 10

STOMACH

Cancer of the stomach is one of the most frequent cancers in the world, with an estimated 670 000 new cases per year world-wide around 1980[219]. The frequency of stomach cancer has been declining almost everywhere for a number of years, however[134], and it has almost certainly been replaced as the most frequent cancer in the world by cancer of the lung. Stomach cancer is about twice as common in males as in females. While the causes of stomach cancer and the reason for its decline are unclear, it is still a major public health problem, particularly in Japan, where it remains the most frequent cancer in both sexes, comprising 20-30% of all cancers, and the cumulative risk (30-74 years) for the 1915 birth cohort is around 10% for males and 5% for females. More than 90% of stomach cancers are adenocarcinomas, of which 'intestinal' and 'diffuse' categories have been described, with different distributions by age, sex and place, suggesting that adenocarcinoma of the stomach may comprise two or more distinct aetiological entities[134]. Longitudinal data to examine trends in these two sub-types of stomach cancer are not routinely available. Survival from stomach cancer is very poor, and has changed little in recent years, typically less than 10% of patients surviving five years from diagnosis. Trends in incidence in most countries are closely mirrored by trends in mortality.

Europe

Incidence and mortality from stomach cancer are lower in EC countries than elsewhere in Europe, but a decline has occurred in all parts of the continent. Truncated incidence rates generally fell by a third to a half in both sexes during the period 1970-85. Incidence is declining substantially in 22 of the 23 populations studied, recent trends ranging between 10% and 30% per five-year period for both sexes. The declines in EC countries are almost all in the narrower range of 10-20% per five-year period; Scotland and Birmingham (UK) show lesser rates of decline, particularly for males (3-4% every five years), although the decline in mortality in Scotland is similar to that seen in the rest of the European Community. In many populations the rate of decline in stomach cancer is greatest in older subjects and least (in some cases reversed) among younger subjects, providing some

evidence of an impending deceleration in the rate of decline in stomach cancer in Europe. This is reflected in the cumulative risk curves for successive birth cohorts. It is seen for incidence among females in Varese (Italy) and for both sexes in the German Democratic Republic, for example, and for mortality in Greece and several other countries. The deceleration of the rate of decline in risk affects countries spanning the entire range of stomach cancer risk in Europe. Even among the small population of non-Jews in Israel, for whom stomach cancer is uncommon, there has been an overall decline among males: the small recent increase is not significant. Among female non-Jews there has been no significant change, but there are very few cases.

Stomach cancer mortality in Yugoslavia and Greece is falling more slowly than in other European countries. Yugoslavia now has the same risk as in other east European countries, whereas 25 years ago there was a two-fold difference. Greece has now been replaced as the country with the lowest stomach cancer mortality in Europe by France and Denmark. Mortality in Spain only began to decline in the 1960s, later than in most other countries.

There are no suitable data to examine incidence trends in Portugal, where the risk is known to be very high[221], but in sharp contrast with other European countries, mortality was still increasing in both sexes until as late as 1970. The subsequent decline has been among the slowest in Europe, and the cohort risk curves show signs of further deceleration in the rate of decline in both sexes, reflected in the age-specific trends. Stomach cancer mortality in Portugal is now almost twice as high as elsewhere in the European Community, and is similar to that seen in Poland, Hungary, Czechoslovakia, Yugoslavia and Romania. These countries display a striking similarity in their levels of stomach cancer risk and the manner in which it is evolving; together with Portugal, which stands out as the exception in western Europe, they are becoming progressively more prominent as the areas of highest stomach cancer risk in Europe.

In most of the European countries for which data were examined, the rate of decline in mortality for females is slightly greater, by about 1-3% every five years, than that for males.

continued page 214

STOMACH (ICD-9 151)

EUROPE (non-EC), INCIDENCE

MALES	Best model	Goodness of fit	1970		1985		Cumulative risk		Recent trend
			Rate	Cases	Rate	Cases	1915	1940	
FINLAND	A3P2	2.62	60.8	620	34.2	407	27.9	9.5	-15.7
HUNGARY									
County Vas	A2D	0.20	77.4	63	57.9	44	41.0	25.5	*-7.6*
Szabolcs-Szatmar	A2P3C2	-0.41	60.7	81	54.3	76	39.5	17.3	*-4.4*
ISRAEL									
All Jews	A2C4	0.51	35.8	147	24.7	131	17.1	13.2	-12.1
Non-Jews	A2D	-0.22	19.4	6	11.4	5	9.2	3.8	*5.8*
NORWAY	A2D	2.30	42.9	480	26.8	332	21.0	9.7	-13.4
POLAND									
Warsaw City	A4D	0.10	61.9	172	38.9	148	30.3	14.1	-14.9
ROMANIA									
Cluj	A2C2	0.96	*142.2*	*224*	52.4	94	44.7	17.9	-24.7
SWEDEN	A2P2	-0.32	33.1	838	21.6	594	16.7	7.6	-12.6
SWITZERLAND									
Geneva	A1P3C3	0.34	22.3	17	19.3	17	18.3	5.1	-28.1
YUGOSLAVIA									
Slovenia	A8P5C9	0.84	76.1	287	47.2	202	36.6	17.3	-18.8

FEMALES	Best model	Goodness of fit	1970		1985		Cumulative risk		Recent trend
			Rate	Cases	Rate	Cases	1915	1940	
FINLAND	A8P5C9	0.17	29.1	405	17.7	283	13.7	7.0	-14.0
HUNGARY									
County Vas	A8D	0.60	30.2	27	18.3	15	13.8	6.0	*-8.3*
Szabolcs-Szatmar	A2C3	0.85	28.3	44	18.2	31	14.0	7.2	-14.2
ISRAEL									
All Jews	A2D	1.53	21.2	89	12.9	78	10.4	4.6	-17.3
Non-Jews	A1	1.71	7.4	2	7.4	4	4.8	4.8	*4.5*
NORWAY	A3C6	0.12	21.3	269	13.7	187	10.4	5.2	-11.1
POLAND									
Warsaw City	A1D	0.37	24.6	109	14.0	76	11.8	4.6	-18.8
ROMANIA									
Cluj	A1D	4.80	*77.3*	*146*	19.7	42	30.8	3.2	-35.9
SWEDEN	A4C2	0.57	16.9	461	10.8	316	8.1	4.5	-13.7
SWITZERLAND									
Geneva	A1D	1.52	17.4	18	7.4	8	7.5	1.8	-33.4
YUGOSLAVIA									
Slovenia	A2P2C4	-1.22	36.7	185	21.7	126	16.4	10.7	-16.9

* : not enough cases for reliable estimation
− : incomplete or missing data
Best model: polynomial of the given degree in age (A), period (P) or cohort (C), or linear drift (D) model.
Goodness of fit: the normalised likelihood ratio chi-square for the best model (see Method).
Rate: world-standardised truncated rate per 100 000 per year (30-74 years) and number of **cases** are both estimated from the best-fitting model for the single years cited.
Cumulative risk per 1000 (30-74 years) is estimated from the best-fitting *age-cohort* model for cohorts of central birth year cited.
Recent trend: estimated mean percentage change per five-year period in the age-specific rates (30-74 years) over the period 1973-1987.
Italics denote recent trends not significant at 5 per cent level, or other figures which should be interpreted with caution (see Method).

STOMACH (ICD-9 151)

EUROPE (non-EC), INCIDENCE

MALES

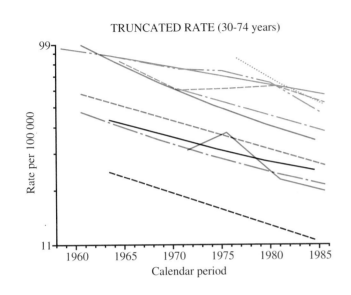

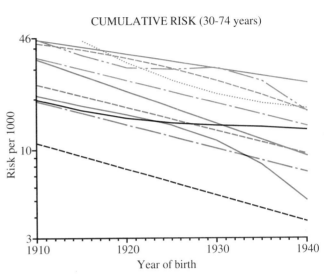

FEMALES

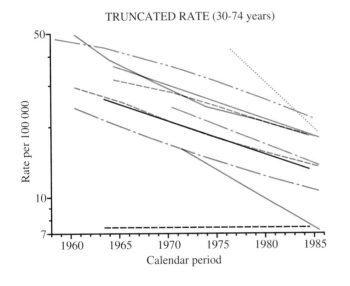

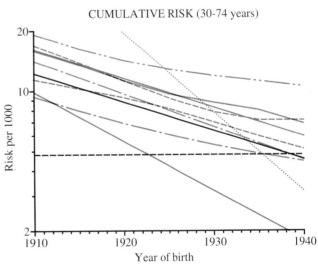

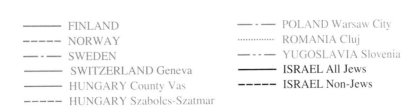

—— FINLAND	—·— POLAND Warsaw City
----- NORWAY	·········· ROMANIA Cluj
—·—·— SWEDEN	—··—··— YUGOSLAVIA Slovenia
—— SWITZERLAND Geneva	—— ISRAEL All Jews
—— HUNGARY County Vas	----- ISRAEL Non-Jews
----- HUNGARY Szabolcs-Szatmar	

STOMACH (ICD-9 151)

EUROPE (EC), INCIDENCE

MALES	Best model	Goodness of fit	1970 Rate	1970 Cases	1985 Rate	1985 Cases	Cumulative risk 1915	Cumulative risk 1940	Recent trend
DENMARK	A8P6C9	-0.11	33.7	464	22.3	329	15.1	8.1	-12.3
FRANCE									
Bas-Rhin	A2D	-1.19	*39.1*	*94*	26.1	52	19.8	10.1	-11.2
Doubs	A1	-0.22	*28.0*	*16*	28.0	30	18.1	18.1	*-10.4*
GERMANY (FRG)									
Hamburg	A2P4C4	0.68	51.6	288	*10.9*	*41*	25.0	*18.7*	–
Saarland	A2D	-0.01	56.7	164	36.9	103	28.2	13.9	-17.0
GERMANY (GDR)	A4P2C6	3.59	64.9	3083	41.2	1520	32.3	16.3	-15.0
ITALY									
Varese	A2D	-1.04	*90.9*	*99*	56.0	116	43.9	19.9	-15.0
SPAIN									
Navarra	A3D	0.10	*75.9*	*91*	48.4	67	37.3	17.7	-13.7
Zaragoza	A2P3	-0.42	56.9	107	38.8	93	26.7	9.3	-18.4
UK									
Birmingham	A2P4C3	4.09	44.5	603	38.9	593	26.6	14.1	*-2.7*
Scotland	A2C2	2.59	40.4	551	34.9	491	25.0	14.4	-4.0
South Thames	A2C4	-0.20	34.6	888	25.1	503	19.9	8.5	-12.3

FEMALES	Best model	Goodness of fit	1970 Rate	1970 Cases	1985 Rate	1985 Cases	Cumulative risk 1915	Cumulative risk 1940	Recent trend
DENMARK	A3C8	-0.25	15.4	242	9.4	154	6.4	3.3	-18.2
FRANCE									
Bas-Rhin	A1D	1.33	*16.9*	*56*	10.8	29	8.5	4.1	-13.1
Doubs	A8C7	-0.01	*12.3*	*12*	9.5	11	9.6	5.9	*-15.0*
GERMANY (FRG)									
Hamburg	A1C4	1.24	24.1	194	*16.6*	*93*	12.1	*6.2*	–
Saarland	A3P2	0.50	28.8	113	18.6	75	13.5	6.7	*-4.4*
GERMANY (GDR)	A4C3	2.79	30.1	2161	20.0	1149	14.8	8.8	-12.3
ITALY									
Varese	A1C2	0.79	*40.1*	*44*	23.2	62	17.1	10.8	-16.0
SPAIN									
Navarra	A1D	-0.47	*38.5*	*55*	18.3	29	17.3	5.1	-21.9
Zaragoza	A3D	1.10	30.3	69	12.4	36	12.1	2.8	-24.8
UK									
Birmingham	A2P2	0.44	18.5	300	13.8	239	10.0	5.2	-8.7
Scotland	A2C2	0.37	18.5	330	15.6	279	11.4	6.9	-5.6
South Thames	A2C4	0.56	13.7	459	9.3	226	7.2	3.8	-17.3

* : not enough cases for reliable estimation
– : incomplete or missing data
Best model: polynomial of the given degree in age (A), period (P) or cohort (C), or linear drift (D) model.
Goodness of fit: the normalised likelihood ratio chi-square for the best model (see Method).
Rate: world-standardised truncated rate per 100 000 per year (30-74 years) and number of **cases** are both estimated from the best-fitting model for the single years cited.
Cumulative risk per 1000 (30-74 years) is estimated from the best-fitting *age-cohort* model for cohorts of central birth year cited.
Recent trend: estimated mean percentage change per five-year period in the age-specific rates (30-74 years) over the period 1973-1987.
Italics denote recent trends not significant at 5 per cent level, or other figures which should be interpreted with caution (see Method).

196

STOMACH (ICD-9 151)

EUROPE (EC), INCIDENCE

MALES

TRUNCATED RATE (30-74 years)

CUMULATIVE RISK (30-74 years)

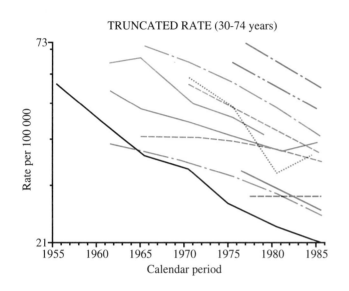
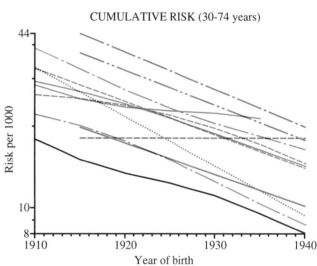

FEMALES

TRUNCATED RATE (30-74 years)

CUMULATIVE RISK (30-74 years)

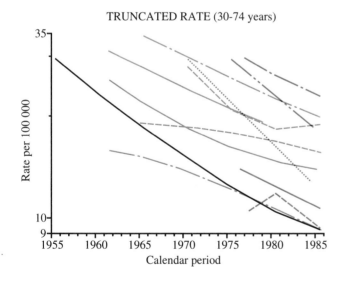
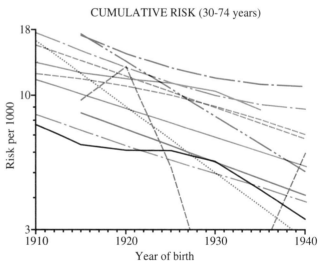

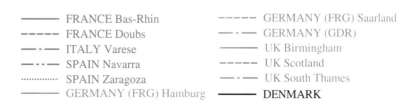

—— FRANCE Bas-Rhin	----- GERMANY (FRG) Saarland
- - - FRANCE Doubs	-·-·- GERMANY (GDR)
-·-·- ITALY Varese	—— UK Birmingham
-··-··- SPAIN Navarra	--- UK Scotland
·········· SPAIN Zaragoza	-·-·- UK South Thames
—— GERMANY (FRG) Hamburg	—— DENMARK

STOMACH (ICD-9 151)

EUROPE (non-EC), INCIDENCE
Percentage change per five-year period, 1973-1987

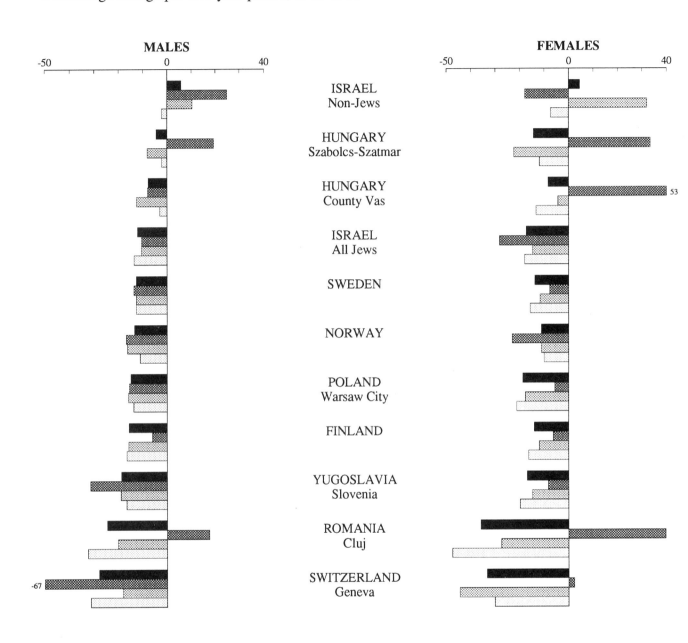

STOMACH (ICD-9 151)

EUROPE (EC), INCIDENCE
Percentage change per five-year period, 1973-1987

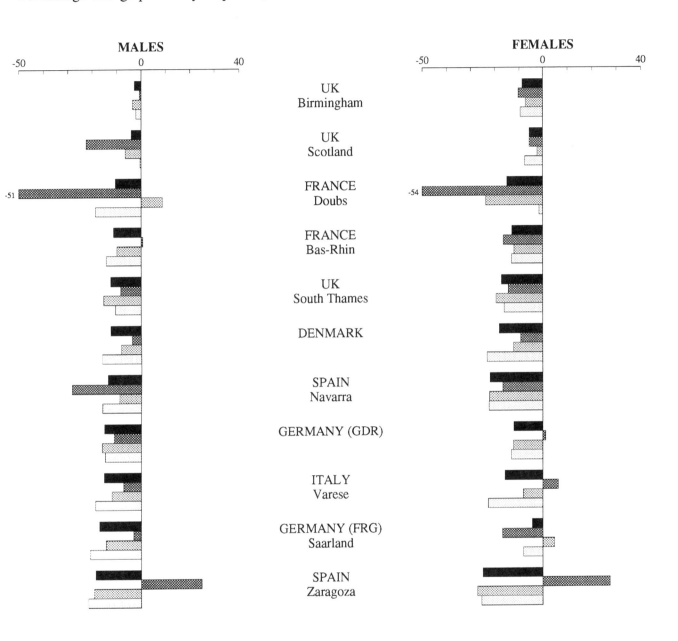

MALES

FEMALES

UK
Birmingham

UK
Scotland

FRANCE
Doubs

FRANCE
Bas-Rhin

UK
South Thames

DENMARK

SPAIN
Navarra

GERMANY (GDR)

ITALY
Varese

GERMANY (FRG)
Saarland

SPAIN
Zaragoza

30-74
30-44
45-64
65-74

STOMACH (ICD-9 151)

EUROPE (non-EC), MORTALITY

MALES	Best model	Goodness of fit	1965 Rate	1965 Deaths	1985 Rate	1985 Deaths	Cumulative risk 1900	Cumulative risk 1940	Recent trend
AUSTRIA	A2P2C3	2.23	72.0	1442	33.6	635	48.0	10.7	-19.9
CZECHOSLOVAKIA	A2P3C4	6.03	78.6	2764	38.3	1416	52.3	14.0	-17.3
FINLAND	A3C4	-0.04	71.3	649	25.5	302	49.9	7.2	-21.4
HUNGARY	A2P3C6	0.79	79.8	2081	46.4	1303	53.9	19.8	-16.0
NORWAY	A2C2	1.41	44.7	469	20.0	251	30.5	5.8	-17.3
POLAND	A8P5C9	5.87	85.7	5056	49.8	3828	54.4	20.0	-13.7
ROMANIA	A4P4C3	10.93	72.8	2923	*36.3*	*1907*	47.5	18.9	–
SWEDEN	A2D	0.72	35.3	833	16.0	447	24.1	5.0	-21.7
SWITZERLAND	A2P2C4	-1.36	43.9	629	17.5	311	30.0	5.9	-22.6
YUGOSLAVIA	A4P3C9	5.03	44.8	1604	35.9	1742	28.9	18.8	-10.7

FEMALES	Best model	Goodness of fit	1965 Rate	1965 Deaths	1985 Rate	1985 Deaths	Cumulative risk 1900	Cumulative risk 1940	Recent trend
AUSTRIA	A4P3C4	2.39	35.9	1024	14.9	403	23.7	6.0	-20.8
CZECHOSLOVAKIA	A8P5C4	3.20	38.1	1690	16.3	764	26.1	6.2	-17.5
FINLAND	A4P2C6	-0.60	33.3	420	13.7	220	22.8	4.5	-15.9
HUNGARY	A4P4C7	2.83	39.0	1268	17.9	649	27.4	7.6	-20.7
NORWAY	A3D	0.15	22.7	264	9.8	136	16.0	3.0	-15.5
POLAND	A8P4C4	2.78	39.5	3019	17.6	1779	26.9	5.9	-17.3
ROMANIA	A4P3C3	7.02	32.7	1590	*14.5*	*919*	24.1	6.1	–
SWEDEN	A3C2	-1.31	18.2	467	8.5	248	12.4	3.3	-18.0
SWITZERLAND	A4C6	0.85	20.9	383	7.3	155	15.4	2.8	-23.0
YUGOSLAVIA	A4P2C3	2.39	23.5	1015	15.8	953	15.8	7.5	-12.1

* : not enough deaths for reliable estimation
– : incomplete or missing data
Best model: polynomial of the given degree in age (A), period (P) or cohort (C), or linear drift (D) model.
Goodness of fit: the normalised likelihood ratio chi-square for the best model (see Method).
Rate: world-standardised truncated rate per 100 000 per year (30-74 years) and number of **deaths** are both estimated from the best-fitting model for the single years cited.
Cumulative risk per 1000 (30-74 years) is estimated from the best-fitting *age-cohort* model for cohorts of central birth year cited.
Recent trend: estimated mean percentage change per five-year period in the age-specific rates (30-74 years) over the period 1975-1988.
Italics denote recent trends not significant at 5 per cent level, or other figures which should be interpreted with caution (see Method).

STOMACH (ICD-9 151)

EUROPE (non-EC), MORTALITY

MALES

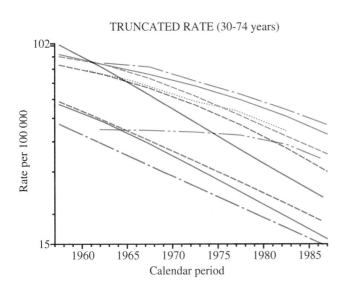

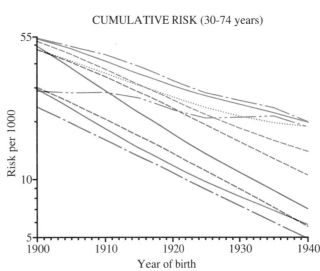

FEMALES

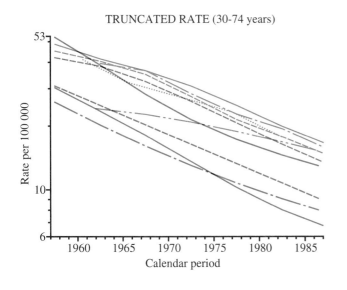

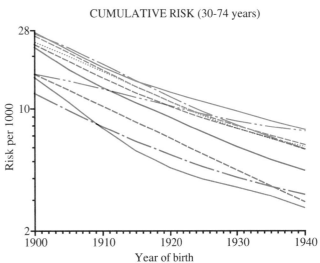

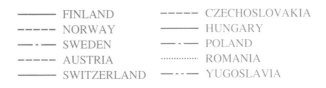

—————— FINLAND	------- CZECHOSLOVAKIA
--------- NORWAY	—————— HUNGARY
—·—·— SWEDEN	—·—·— POLAND
--------- AUSTRIA	·············· ROMANIA
—————— SWITZERLAND	—··—··— YUGOSLAVIA

STOMACH (ICD-9 151)

EUROPE (EC), MORTALITY

MALES	Best model	Goodness of fit	1965 Rate	1965 Deaths	1985 Rate	1985 Deaths	Cumulative risk 1900	Cumulative risk 1940	Recent trend
BELGIUM	A2P3C3	2.93	46.4	1241	20.8	571	31.2	6.4	-18.4
DENMARK	A3C4	-0.04	34.5	449	15.4	229	23.6	5.7	-16.4
FRANCE	A2P4C7	3.56	37.3	4619	16.9	2372	24.9	6.6	-18.2
GERMANY (FRG)	A3P6C4	11.36	62.5	9698	26.7	4252	41.4	9.6	-20.9
GREECE	A2C5	0.82	28.4	536	19.0	526	*18.9*	9.8	-13.4
IRELAND	A2C3	1.28	45.8	341	24.8	203	31.1	8.4	-18.1
ITALY	A3P5C9	14.13	62.7	7640	34.5	5446	40.4	14.4	-12.4
NETHERLANDS	A4C2	0.60	44.8	1267	23.6	847	30.3	7.7	-16.7
PORTUGAL	A2P2C4	-0.03	66.4	1205	48.3	1229	42.0	25.9	-14.5
SPAIN	A5P5C4	3.51	55.4	3827	27.3	2649	36.1	12.2	-22.3
UK ENGLAND & WALES	A2C7	1.93	43.5	5653	24.9	3725	29.4	7.8	-15.8
UK SCOTLAND	A3C3	-0.94	46.2	606	26.4	374	30.3	7.9	-14.4

FEMALES	Best model	Goodness of fit	1965 Rate	1965 Deaths	1985 Rate	1985 Deaths	Cumulative risk 1900	Cumulative risk 1940	Recent trend
BELGIUM	A2P4C5	2.10	22.7	748	8.2	271	15.9	2.9	-24.1
DENMARK	A1C6	0.20	17.1	253	7.4	125	11.9	2.6	-19.4
FRANCE	A8P2C3	0.65	16.0	2651	6.0	1016	11.3	2.0	-22.9
GERMANY (FRG)	A8P3C8	8.02	30.5	6726	13.2	2978	20.9	5.5	-19.0
GREECE	A2C5	2.19	17.1	377	9.5	303	*11.8*	4.3	-16.0
IRELAND	A4P3C3	0.33	27.3	215	10.0	89	19.8	3.6	-29.8
ITALY	A4P5C4	4.77	29.5	4470	14.4	2770	20.0	6.1	-15.0
NETHERLANDS	A8C4	-0.48	20.5	666	8.9	377	14.2	3.2	-18.2
PORTUGAL	A3P5C5	0.65	36.7	862	22.8	709	23.7	11.7	-15.1
SPAIN	A8P6C9	2.01	28.3	2416	11.4	1333	19.8	5.0	-27.9
UK ENGLAND & WALES	A2P2C2	0.74	19.1	3176	9.4	1665	13.1	2.9	-19.0
UK SCOTLAND	A2D	0.64	23.0	400	11.5	205	15.7	3.9	-14.8

* : not enough deaths for reliable estimation
– : incomplete or missing data
Best model: polynomial of the given degree in age (A), period (P) or cohort (C), or linear drift (D) model.
Goodness of fit: the normalised likelihood ratio chi-square for the best model (see Method).
Rate: world-standardised truncated rate per 100 000 per year (30-74 years) and number of **deaths** are both estimated from the best-fitting model for the single years cited.
Cumulative risk per 1000 (30-74 years) is estimated from the best-fitting *age-cohort* model for cohorts of central birth year cited.
Recent trend: estimated mean percentage change per five-year period in the age-specific rates (30-74 years) over the period 1975-1988.
Italics denote recent trends not significant at 5 per cent level, or other figures which should be interpreted with caution (see Method).

STOMACH (ICD-9 151)

EUROPE (EC), MORTALITY

MALES

TRUNCATED RATE (30-74 years)

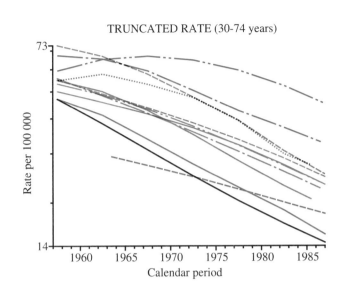

CUMULATIVE RISK (30-74 years)

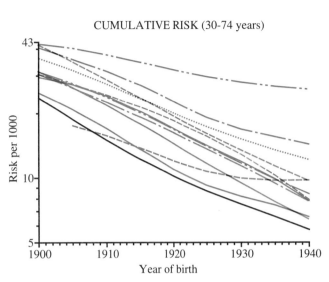

FEMALES

TRUNCATED RATE (30-74 years)

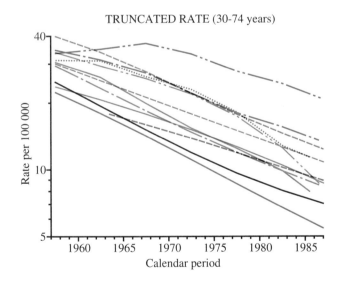

CUMULATIVE RISK (30-74 years)

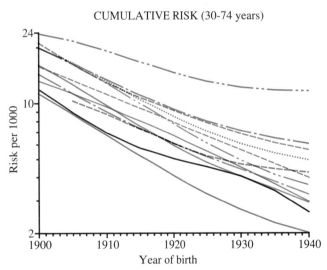

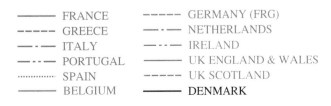

———— FRANCE	– – – – GERMANY (FRG)
– – – – GREECE	–·–·– NETHERLANDS
–·–·– ITALY	–··–··– IRELAND
–··–··– PORTUGAL	———— UK ENGLAND & WALES
·········· SPAIN	– – – – UK SCOTLAND
———— BELGIUM	———— DENMARK

STOMACH (ICD-9 151)

EUROPE (non-EC), MORTALITY
Percentage change per five-year period, 1975-1988

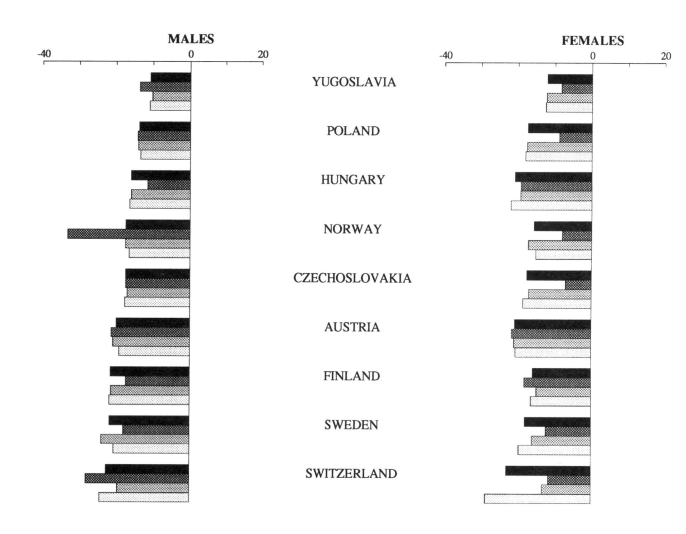

STOMACH (ICD-9 151)

EUROPE (EC), MORTALITY
Percentage change per five-year period, 1975-1988

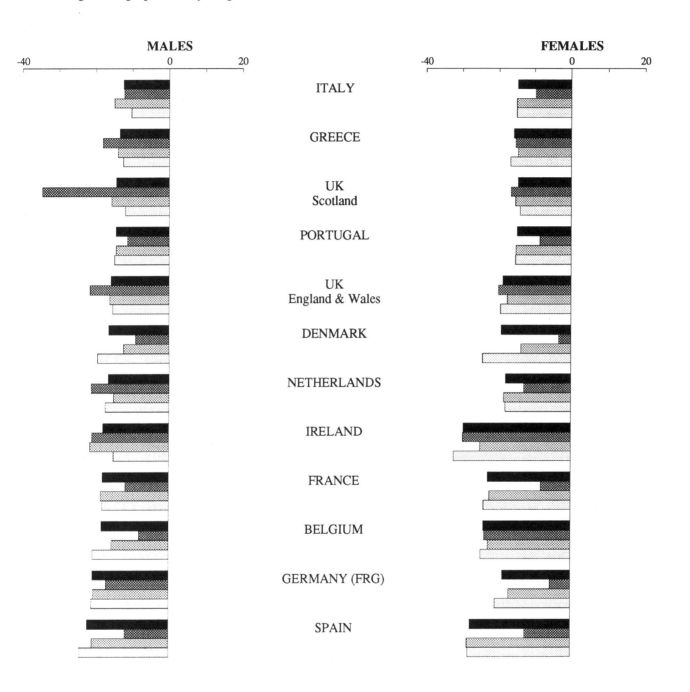

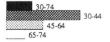

STOMACH (ICD-9 151)

ASIA, INCIDENCE

MALES	Best model	Goodness of fit	1970 Rate	1970 Cases	1985 Rate	1985 Cases	Cumulative risk 1915	Cumulative risk 1940	Recent trend
CHINA									
Shanghai	A5P2C3	1.00	*89.6*	*919*	97.5	1677	75.6	32.2	-11.5
HONG KONG	A8P2	0.80	*59.0*	*286*	39.0	448	23.3	25.1	*-0.6*
INDIA									
Bombay	A2D	3.20	16.4	116	13.1	151	8.8	6.0	-6.9
JAPAN									
Miyagi	A8P5	0.77	162.6	563	155.4	824	97.1	84.7	*-0.3*
Nagasaki	A2D	0.16	*225.1*	*182*	149.5	159	106.7	55.4	-12.7
Osaka	A2P2C2	1.31	172.0	2083	136.4	2560	85.4	74.3	-3.2
SINGAPORE									
Chinese	A2C2	2.07	89.2	182	62.0	184	50.1	17.3	-13.7
Indian	A1	0.29	35.0	8	35.0	13	23.1	23.1	*-10.0*
Malay	A1C2	1.29	19.4	6	12.5	5	12.4	2.1	*-20.8*

FEMALES	Best model	Goodness of fit	1970 Rate	1970 Cases	1985 Rate	1985 Cases	Cumulative risk 1915	Cumulative risk 1940	Recent trend
CHINA									
Shanghai	A5P2C6	1.48	*24.4*	*284*	42.3	769	30.1	16.6	-5.6
HONG KONG	A1P2	1.18	*28.5*	*155*	19.3	224	10.9	13.8	*4.1*
INDIA									
Bombay	A2D	1.28	10.2	48	8.7	77	5.6	4.3	*-4.5*
JAPAN									
Miyagi	A4P2	0.90	80.4	329	70.3	440	43.8	33.1	-5.5
Nagasaki	A1P2	-0.25	*225.0*	*232*	59.1	79	59.9	16.3	-23.2
Osaka	A8C8	0.67	84.9	1218	61.4	1397	41.7	27.5	-7.6
SINGAPORE									
Chinese	A2D	-0.20	35.6	80	27.3	96	19.1	12.4	*-6.3*
Indian	A1C2	1.23	33.0	2	17.5	2	20.1	2.8	*-22.6*
Malay	A4D	-0.13	20.5	5	10.3	4	9.2	3.0	*-10.3*

* : not enough cases for reliable estimation
– : incomplete or missing data
Best model: polynomial of the given degree in age (A), period (P) or cohort (C), or linear drift (D) model.
Goodness of fit: the normalised likelihood ratio chi-square for the best model (see Method).
Rate: world-standardised truncated rate per 100 000 per year (30-74 years) and number of **cases** are both estimated from the best-fitting model for the single years cited.
Cumulative risk per 1000 (30-74 years) is estimated from the best-fitting *age-cohort* model for cohorts of central birth year cited.
Recent trend: estimated mean percentage change per five-year period in the age-specific rates (30-74 years) over the period 1973-1987.
Italics denote recent trends not significant at 5 per cent level, or other figures which should be interpreted with caution (see Method).

STOMACH (ICD-9 151)

ASIA, INCIDENCE

MALES

TRUNCATED RATE (30-74 years)

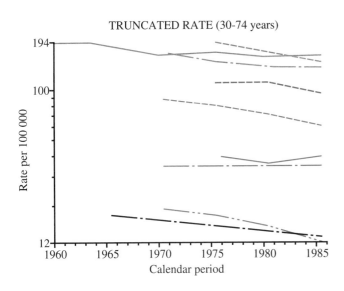

CUMULATIVE RISK (30-74 years)

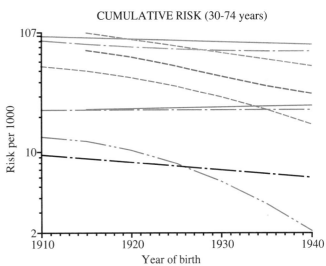

FEMALES

TRUNCATED RATE (30-74 years)

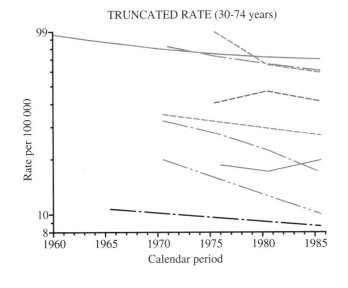

CUMULATIVE RISK (30-74 years)

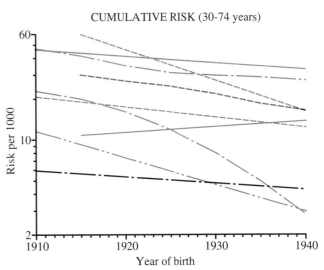

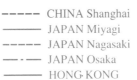

- CHINA Shanghai
- JAPAN Miyagi
- JAPAN Nagasaki
- JAPAN Osaka
- HONG-KONG
- SINGAPORE Chinese
- SINGAPORE Indian
- SINGAPORE Malay
- INDIA Bombay

STOMACH (ICD-9 151)

OCEANIA, INCIDENCE

MALES	Best model	Goodness of fit	1970 Rate	1970 Cases	1985 Rate	1985 Cases	Cumulative risk 1915	Cumulative risk 1940	Recent trend
AUSTRALIA									
New South Wales	A8C7	-1.17	*36.0*	*387*	20.6	277	13.2	10.5	-5.3
South	A2	-0.96	*22.9*	*37*	22.9	81	14.8	14.8	*-0.3*
HAWAII									
Caucasian	A2D	-0.31	27.4	8	17.7	10	13.7	6.6	*-13.1*
Chinese	A1	1.93	16.7	1	16.7	2	10.8	10.8	*18.9*
Filipino	A2	-0.95	12.4	3	12.4	4	7.6	7.6	*8.1*
Hawaiian	A1D	0.62	68.1	8	44.4	10	34.3	17.0	*-10.2*
Japanese	A1C3	0.55	60.2	28	37.1	33	31.2	9.7	-13.9
NEW ZEALAND									
Maori	A3D	0.83	68.9	13	50.3	15	35.5	21.2	-18.9
Non-Maori	A2D	0.34	28.1	158	21.1	151	15.4	9.6	-12.0

FEMALES	Best model	Goodness of fit	1970 Rate	1970 Cases	1985 Rate	1985 Cases	Cumulative risk 1915	Cumulative risk 1940	Recent trend
AUSTRALIA									
New South Wales	A1D	-0.07	*12.6*	*156*	8.4	122	6.4	3.3	-12.9
South	A1D	-0.57	*12.9*	*21*	7.1	28	6.1	2.3	*-16.6*
HAWAII									
Caucasian	A1D	0.12	11.7	4	6.4	4	5.6	2.0	*-14.8*
Chinese	A1D	0.58	17.5	1	9.7	1	8.5	3.2	*-8.2*
Filipino	A2	-0.35	*7.4*	*0*	7.4	2	4.2	4.2	*-7.6*
Hawaiian	A1D	-0.90	42.7	6	23.4	6	20.2	7.5	*-20.4*
Japanese	A1D	0.09	35.0	17	18.5	17	16.7	5.8	-16.8
NEW ZEALAND									
Maori	A1P3	-0.07	30.3	6	35.7	12	22.5	14.6	*-1.3*
Non-Maori	A1P3	0.23	10.7	67	8.4	67	6.3	3.2	-13.6

* : not enough cases for reliable estimation
– : incomplete or missing data
Best model: polynomial of the given degree in age (A), period (P) or cohort (C), or linear drift (D) model.
Goodness of fit: the normalised likelihood ratio chi-square for the best model (see Method).
Rate: world-standardised truncated rate per 100 000 per year (30-74 years) and number of **cases** are both estimated from the best-fitting model for the single years cited.
Cumulative risk per 1000 (30-74 years) is estimated from the best-fitting *age-cohort* model for cohorts of central birth year cited.
Recent trend: estimated mean percentage change per five-year period in the age-specific rates (30-74 years) over the period 1973-1987.
Italics denote recent trends not significant at 5 per cent level, or other figures which should be interpreted with caution (see Method).

STOMACH (ICD-9 151)

OCEANIA, INCIDENCE

MALES

TRUNCATED RATE (30-74 years)

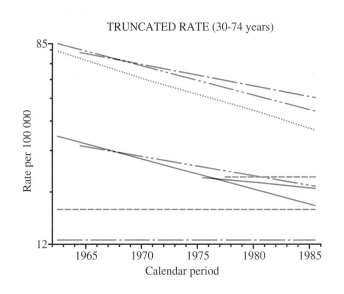

CUMULATIVE RISK (30-74 years)

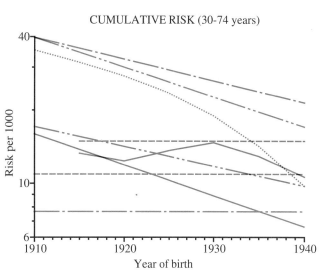

FEMALES

TRUNCATED RATE (30-74 years)

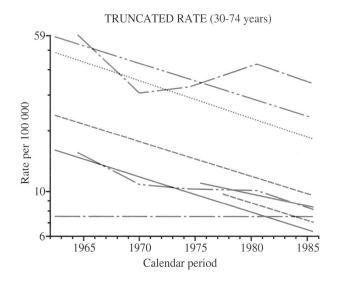

CUMULATIVE RISK (30-74 years)

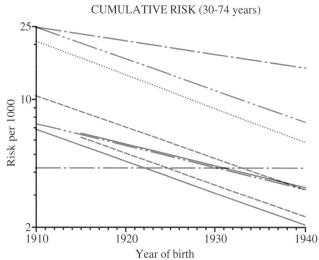

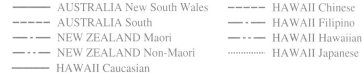

—— AUSTRALIA New South Wales	– – – HAWAII Chinese
– – – AUSTRALIA South	– · – HAWAII Filipino
– · – NEW ZEALAND Maori	– ·· – HAWAII Hawaiian
– ·· – NEW ZEALAND Non-Maori	·········· HAWAII Japanese
—— HAWAII Caucasian	

STOMACH (ICD-9 151)

ASIA, INCIDENCE
Percentage change per five-year period, 1973-1987

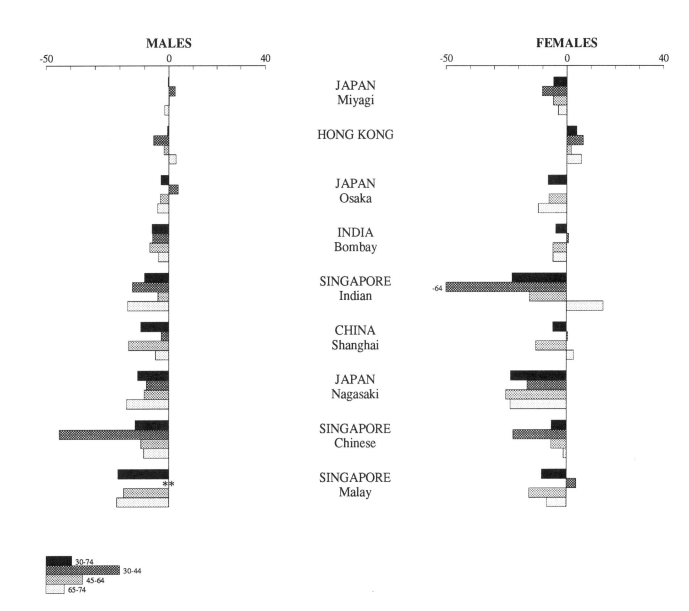

STOMACH (ICD-9 151)

OCEANIA, INCIDENCE
Percentage change per five-year period, 1973-1987

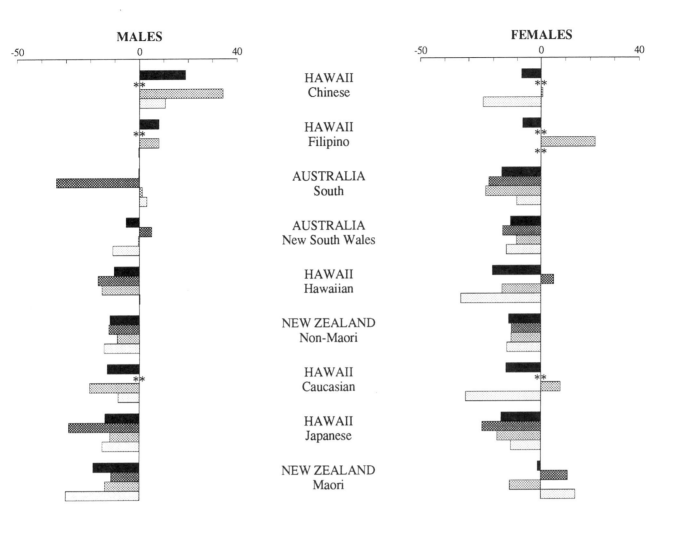

ASIA and OCEANIA, MORTALITY

MALES	Best model	Goodness of fit	1965 Rate	1965 Deaths	1985 Rate	1985 Deaths	Cumulative risk 1900	Cumulative risk 1940	Recent trend
AUSTRALIA	A8C9	1.04	28.2	676	14.7	550	18.8	4.9	-13.8
HONG KONG	A2C3	1.04	39.1	157	21.6	189	*26.4*	6.4	-20.5
JAPAN	A8P5C9	13.70	135.9	24089	72.1	20965	87.7	27.1	-17.3
MAURITIUS	A2C5	-0.03	31.0	24	29.1	30	*17.6*	13.3	-17.9
NEW ZEALAND	A2C3	-0.44	28.9	153	17.9	134	19.6	8.7	-13.5
SINGAPORE	A2C2	0.92	*61.2*	*116*	32.5	82	*34.2*	7.3	–

FEMALES	Best model	Goodness of fit	1965 Rate	1965 Deaths	1985 Rate	1985 Deaths	Cumulative risk 1900	Cumulative risk 1940	Recent trend
AUSTRALIA	A2P4C2	0.12	12.6	346	5.8	238	8.6	2.3	-18.7
HONG KONG	A2C2	-0.37	20.3	96	11.3	101	*13.6*	5.0	*-6.9*
JAPAN	A4P5C5	12.20	69.5	14028	33.6	11745	46.7	14.0	-21.5
MAURITIUS	A2	1.26	13.3	9	13.3	15	*8.4*	8.4	*1.1*
NEW ZEALAND	A2C2	-1.64	12.9	78	7.8	64	8.5	3.9	-13.1
SINGAPORE	A2C2	-0.61	*28.8*	*51*	16.1	45	*16.0*	4.5	–

* : not enough deaths for reliable estimation
– : incomplete or missing data
Best model: polynomial of the given degree in age (A), period (P) or cohort (C), or linear drift (D) model.
Goodness of fit: the normalised likelihood ratio chi-square for the best model (see Method).
Rate: world-standardised truncated rate per 100 000 per year (30-74 years) and number of **deaths** are both estimated from the best-fitting model for the single years cited.
Cumulative risk per 1000 (30-74 years) is estimated from the best-fitting *age-cohort* model for cohorts of central birth year cited.
Recent trend: estimated mean percentage change per five-year period in the age-specific rates (30-74 years) over the period 1975-1988.
Italics denote recent trends not significant at 5 per cent level, or other figures which should be interpreted with caution (see Method).

STOMACH (ICD-9 151)

ASIA and OCEANIA, MORTALITY

MALES

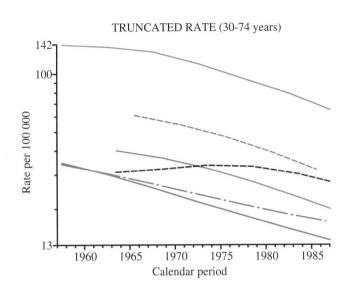

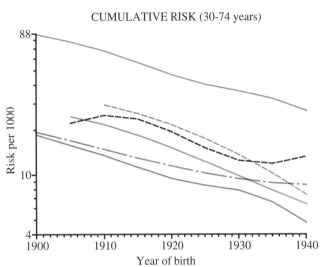

FEMALES

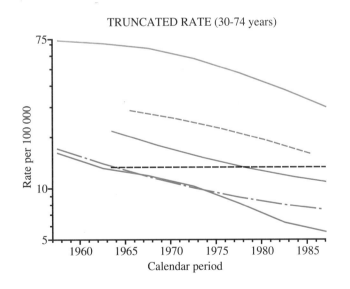

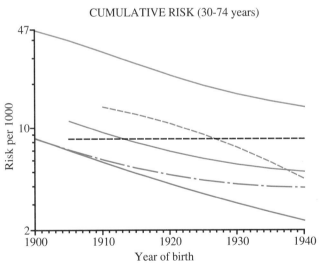

AUSTRALIA   HONG KONG
NEW ZEALAND   SINGAPORE
JAPAN   MAURITIUS

STOMACH (ICD-9 151)

ASIA and OCEANIA, MORTALITY
Percentage change per five-year period, 1975-1988

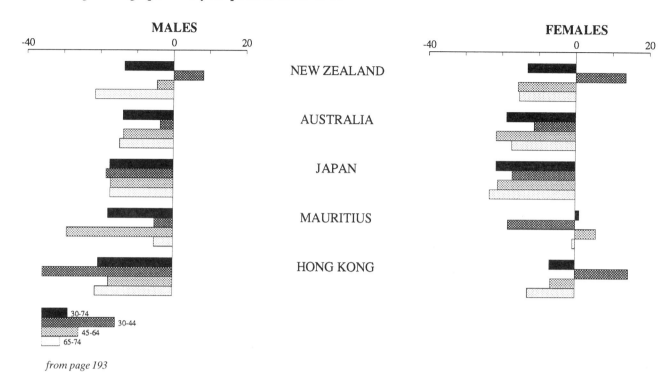

MALES

FEMALES

NEW ZEALAND

AUSTRALIA

JAPAN

MAURITIUS

HONG KONG

30-74
30-44
45-64
65-74

from page 193

Asia and Oceania

Japanese of both sexes have the highest recorded incidence of all the populations studied here, with truncated rates of around 140 per 100 000 in males and 60 in females, two to three times higher than the rates for lung cancer in the same populations. Incidence is declining in all the Asian populations with the exception of Hong Kong, where the slight recent increase is probably due to an artefact of registration (inclusion for 1983-87, only, of some 10% of cases diagnosed solely from a death certificate[221]); mortality in Hong Kong is declining at least as rapidly as elsewhere in Asia.

In Osaka and Miyagi (Japan), the rate of decline is small in females and negligible in males. Only in Nagasaki (Japan) do the recent trends approach the rates of decline seen in Europe, but this is consistent with the pattern of incidence in Nagasaki for many sites, and these data should be accorded less weight than the data from Osaka and Miyagi. Cumulative risks for the development of stomach cancer up to age 75 in the 1940 birth cohort in Japan are 6-8% in males and around 2% in females, the highest recorded anywhere, but even these risks are between a third and a half lower than the corresponding risks for the preceding generation, born around 1915 (8-10% in males, 4% in females). The rate of decline in mortality in Japan is similar to that seen elsewhere in

Asia and Europe, at around 20% every five years. The disparity between trends in incidence and mortality in Japan is striking.

In Bombay (India), stomach cancer is uncommon, with truncated rates around 10 per 100 000; Indians in Singapore have somewhat higher rates, but there has been a decline in incidence in both populations.

In New Zealand, the incidence of stomach cancer is more than twice as high in both sexes among Maoris than among non-Maoris, who comprise the great majority of the population, but the risks are declining at a similar rate in successive birth cohorts in both racial groups. Hawaiians and Japanese in Hawaii show closely similar risks and rates of decline to those of Maoris in New Zealand. The rate of decline in incidence among Japanese in Hawaii is notably quicker than in Japan, and the risk for the 1940 birth cohort in males is about 1%, a third of the level for the 1915 birth cohort.

Incidence rates among Australians, and in New Zealand non-Maoris, of similar racial stock, are up to 50% lower than in western European populations. The rates of decline are also slower. This is not easily reconciled with the mortality data, which show substantial rates of decline in Australia as a whole; although there may well be geographical variation in the incidence trends within Australia, suitable data are not available for other areas of the country, and New South Wales represents about a third of the national population. Mortality in Australia has been declining recently at around 14-19% per five-year period, much as in Japan and New Zealand. In New Zealand, however, age-specific rates of decline suggest that the overall decline will slow down further in the near future, particularly for females; the 14% increase among younger females (30-44 years) is not significant. This is reflected by the cumulative risk curve for successive birth cohorts, which shows signs of flattening of the downward slope. A similar deceleration is seen for females in Hong Kong.

Americas

Incidence and mortality from stomach cancer in the Americas are generally stable or declining. Most of the ten US populations analysed show declines in incidence, particularly for whites in the San Francisco Bay Area and in Connecticut, where about 90% of the population is white. Black males in New Orleans show a notable decrease, the cumulative risk falling from 2.5% to 0.7% between the birth cohorts of 1915 and 1940, but black females in New Orleans and blacks of both sexes in Detroit and the San Francisco Bay Area show no significant change in risk. In North America, mortality is slightly higher in Canada than in the USA, but it is falling at all ages and in both sexes at about 16% per five-year period in Canada and 11% in the USA. Truncated mortality rates around 1985 were about half those seen 20 years earlier. The rate of decline in mortality among males in the USA is decelerating slightly, as can be seen from the pattern of age-specific trends. These declines in mortality reflect the changes in incidence seen in four of the five Canadian provinces studied here, and in some but not all of the states in the USA. The declines in mortality in Canada and the USA are several percentage points quicker for both sexes than the declines in incidence in the 15 populations studied; this could represent more intense diagnostic activity, with wider access to endoscopy and biopsy of less aggressive lesions, or possibly some improvement in survival, or a combination of both factors.

In Central and South America, the rate of decline in incidence in Puerto Rico was around 16-18% every five years, also somewhat slower than the rate of decline in mortality (22%). Incidence in Cuba fell at a similar rate. The highest incidence recorded in South America was in Cali (Colombia), with truncated rates around 1970 of 80 and 40 per 100 000 in males and females, respectively, although it is likely that incidence in Chile was at least as high. The significant decline in incidence in Cali, similar in magnitude to that seen in North America, has been most marked in younger individuals. Although the latest available data for São Paulo (Brazil) were for 1978, the rates were as high as in Colombia, and the underlying trend appeared to be upward; this is the only apparent exception to the general decline in stomach cancer in the Americas.

Mortality from stomach cancer in Chile and Costa Rica was very high in the 1960s, around 140 per 100 000 in males and 80 per 100 000 in females, levels similar to those seen in Japan at the same period. Fortunately, the decline has also been similar to that observed in other parts of the world. Truncated rates fell by about half in the 20 years up to 1985 in both countries, and recent trends in Chile have been for a further decline of about 20% per five-year period in both sexes: the cumulative risk (30-74 years) for the 1940 birth cohort is likely to be only a quarter of that for the 1915 birth cohort for males (1.7%), and an eighth for females (0.6%). The rates of decline in mortality in Venezuela, Uruguay and Puerto Rico are all similar to those recorded elsewhere in South America: only in Panama is the rate of decline noticeably less, although a recent linear trend could not be calculated because of missing data for the period 1975-87.

Comment

The world-wide decline in gastric cancer has been aptly described[134] as an 'unplanned triumph'. This review suggested that the decline was mainly due to a fall in the incidence of the intestinal type of adenocarcinoma, most closely linked to environmental differences, and that dietary changes were largely responsible. These included an increase in consumption of fresh fruit and vegetables containing vitamins C, E and A, and widespread refrigeration of stored food, retaining its nutritional quality more effectively and reducing the need for salting and pickling to preserve food. In Sweden, however, where the decline in gastric cancer is as large as elsewhere in Europe, pathological review of a sample of cases diagnosed during the period 1950-80 revealed no discernible trend in the relative frequency of intestinal and diffuse adenocarcinomas[171]. The increase in adenocarcinoma at the cardia and in the lower oesophagus in the UK and the USA has been mentioned (see Chapter 9). The fall in stomach cancer incidence in all age groups in Sweden during 1960-84 has been well described with age-cohort models[122], showing a slight deceleration in the rapid rate of decline for cohorts born around 1930 and later.

The onset of the decline in stomach cancer mortality in Spain in the 1960s, some 10-15 years later than in all other EC countries except Portugal, has been attributed to greater availability of fresh fruit

continued page 220

STOMACH (ICD-9 151)

AMERICAS (except USA), INCIDENCE

MALES	Best model	Goodness of fit	1970 Rate	1970 Cases	1985 Rate	1985 Cases	Cumulative risk 1915	Cumulative risk 1940	Recent trend
BRAZIL									
Sao Paulo	A3P2C4	2.61	78.9	451	*240.5*	*1737*	35.2	*59.7*	–
CANADA									
Alberta	A2D	1.19	25.6	78	19.0	84	13.8	8.4	*-4.5*
British Columbia	A2D	0.99	27.6	129	18.4	134	14.1	7.2	-10.3
Maritime Provinces	A2D	-1.41	27.9	89	23.5	86	15.8	11.9	*-5.7*
Newfoundland	A2C2	-0.39	60.6	52	41.1	47	32.3	13.6	-10.0
Quebec	A8P4C9	0.56	26.6	286	25.9	375	16.8	14.2	*-0.2*
COLOMBIA									
Cali	A2P3	0.96	80.9	50	60.1	82	45.4	25.4	-13.2
CUBA	A3C2	3.68	24.3	349	15.5	325	11.5	*7.4*	–
PUERTO RICO	A2C3	-0.45	43.6	198	24.3	172	20.6	7.8	-18.3

FEMALES	Best model	Goodness of fit	1970 Rate	1970 Cases	1985 Rate	1985 Cases	Cumulative risk 1915	Cumulative risk 1940	Recent trend
BRAZIL									
Sao Paulo	A2P2	-0.28	31.7	211	*116.3*	*1062*	16.6	*25.4*	–
CANADA									
Alberta	A2D	0.04	10.2	29	7.7	36	5.5	3.5	*-5.8*
British Columbia	A3D	0.16	11.9	57	7.4	60	5.9	2.7	-17.0
Maritime Provinces	A3D	0.14	15.0	50	8.4	35	7.2	2.7	-11.2
Newfoundland	A8C9	0.74	28.6	23	15.8	18	10.7	7.6	*-11.2*
Quebec	A3D	1.44	12.0	145	10.8	187	7.2	6.1	*-3.7*
COLOMBIA									
Cali	A2C2	1.71	46.2	35	34.1	51	26.3	12.1	-16.1
CUBA	A1C2	4.86	12.2	151	8.3	173	5.9	*4.2*	–
PUERTO RICO	A2D	-0.05	18.7	85	11.5	90	9.2	4.1	-15.6

* : not enough cases for reliable estimation
– : incomplete or missing data
Best model: polynomial of the given degree in age (A), period (P) or cohort (C), or linear drift (D) model.
Goodness of fit: the normalised likelihood ratio chi-square for the best model (see Method).
Rate: world-standardised truncated rate per 100 000 per year (30-74 years) and number of **cases** are both estimated from the best-fitting model for the single years cited.
Cumulative risk per 1000 (30-74 years) is estimated from the best-fitting *age-cohort* model for cohorts of central birth year cited.
Recent trend: estimated mean percentage change per five-year period in the age-specific rates (30-74 years) over the period 1973-1987.
Italics denote recent trends not significant at 5 per cent level, or other figures which should be interpreted with caution (see Method).

STOMACH (ICD-9 151)

AMERICAS (except USA), INCIDENCE

MALES

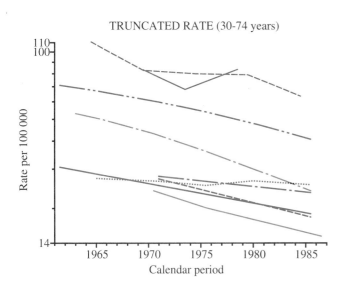

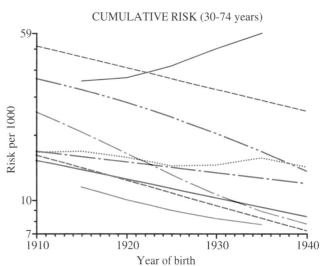

FEMALES

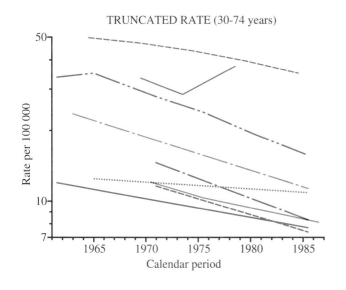

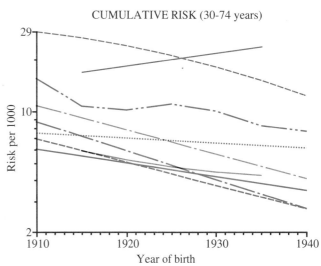

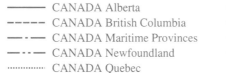

CANADA Alberta
CANADA British Columbia
CANADA Maritime Provinces
CANADA Newfoundland
CANADA Quebec
CUBA
PUERTO RICO
BRAZIL Sao Paulo
COLOMBIA Cali

STOMACH (ICD-9 151)

AMERICAS (USA), INCIDENCE

MALES	Best model	Goodness of fit	1970 Rate	1970 Cases	1985 Rate	1985 Cases	Cumulative risk 1915	Cumulative risk 1940	Recent trend
USA									
Bay Area, Black	A2	1.82	33.9	18	33.9	27	21.3	21.3	*-5.4*
Bay Area, Chinese	A2	-1.17	19.4	4	*19.4*	*9*	11.9	*11.9*	–
Bay Area, White	A2D	-0.42	19.4	115	16.8	106	11.5	9.0	-6.6
Connecticut	A8P5C9	0.26	24.2	160	18.4	150	13.3	6.5	-7.2
Detroit, Black	A2	-0.67	28.8	38	28.8	50	17.7	17.7	*-7.1*
Detroit, White	A2D	0.89	19.6	143	16.6	121	11.5	8.7	*-5.0*
Iowa	A2D	-0.32	14.4	98	11.4	81	8.1	5.5	*-4.0*
New Orleans, Black	A1D	1.18	*56.6*	*29*	27.1	16	25.0	7.4	-21.4
New Orleans, White	A2	1.23	*14.3*	*20*	14.3	22	8.9	8.9	*12.3*
Seattle	A2D	0.40	*17.4*	*84*	13.7	92	9.6	6.4	-7.2

FEMALES	Best model	Goodness of fit	1970 Rate	1970 Cases	1985 Rate	1985 Cases	Cumulative risk 1915	Cumulative risk 1940	Recent trend
USA									
Bay Area, Black	A1	1.20	10.9	6	10.9	11	7.0	7.0	*-13.1*
Bay Area, Chinese	A1	0.81	9.7	1	*9.7*	*5*	6.0	*6.0*	–
Bay Area, White	A3C3	-1.95	10.4	76	7.0	51	4.7	3.5	*-8.0*
Connecticut	A3D	-0.15	10.1	79	6.4	62	5.1	2.4	-12.2
Detroit, Black	A1C3	-1.05	14.7	21	11.0	24	7.3	5.4	*-3.3*
Detroit, White	A2P2	0.58	10.0	83	6.8	59	4.7	2.8	*-1.3*
Iowa	A2D	0.57	6.0	48	4.5	38	3.3	2.0	*-3.6*
New Orleans, Black	A1	0.29	*13.2*	*8*	13.2	10	8.8	8.8	*-9.3*
New Orleans, White	A1	-1.35	*5.8*	*11*	5.8	11	3.6	3.6	*-5.1*
Seattle	A2	1.76	*6.0*	*34*	6.0	45	3.8	3.8	*-3.6*

* : not enough cases for reliable estimation
– : incomplete or missing data
Best model: polynomial of the given degree in age (A), period (P) or cohort (C), or linear drift (D) model.
Goodness of fit: the normalised likelihood ratio chi-square for the best model (see Method).
Rate: world-standardised truncated rate per 100 000 per year (30-74 years) and number of **cases** are both estimated from the best-fitting model for the single years cited.
Cumulative risk per 1000 (30-74 years) is estimated from the best-fitting *age-cohort* model for cohorts of central birth year cited.
Recent trend: estimated mean percentage change per five-year period in the age-specific rates (30-74 years) over the period 1973-1987.
Italics denote recent trends not significant at 5 per cent level, or other figures which should be interpreted with caution (see Method).

STOMACH (ICD-9 151)

AMERICAS (USA), INCIDENCE

MALES

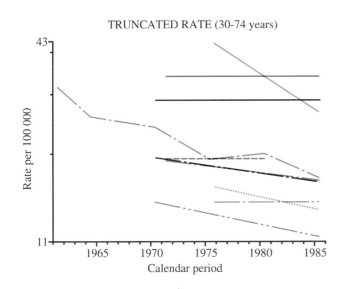

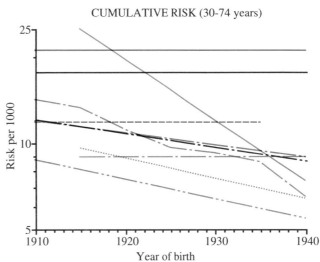

FEMALES

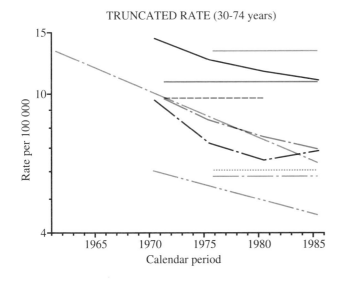

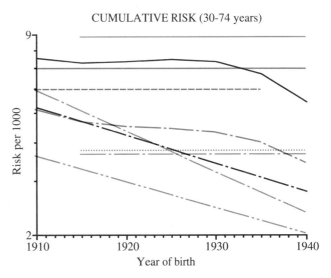

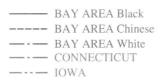

—————— BAY AREA Black	·············· SEATTLE
– – – – BAY AREA Chinese	—————— NEW ORLEANS Black
– · — · – BAY AREA White	– · — · – NEW ORLEANS White
– ·· — ·· – CONNECTICUT	—————— DETROIT Black
– ··· — ··· – IOWA	– ·· — ·· – DETROIT White

STOMACH (ICD-9 151)

AMERICAS (except USA), INCIDENCE
Percentage change per five-year period, 1973-1987

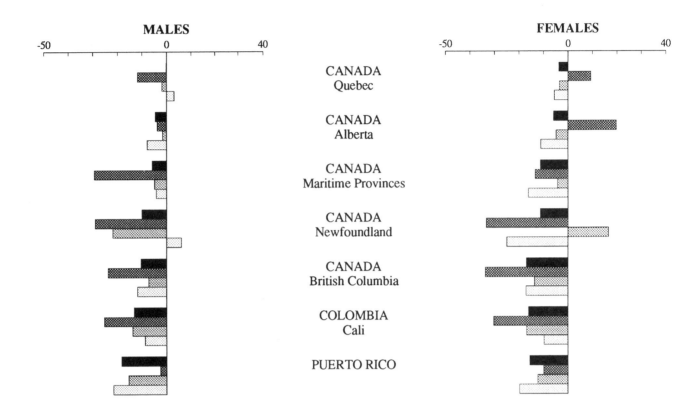

MALES	FEMALES
CANADA Quebec	
CANADA Alberta	
CANADA Maritime Provinces	
CANADA Newfoundland	
CANADA British Columbia	
COLOMBIA Cali	
PUERTO RICO	

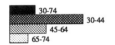

30-74
30-44
45-64
65-74

from page 215

and vegetables following industrialisation, and to food refrigeration[31]. Mortality in Spain is lower in coastal provinces[217]: variation in the mortality trends was linked to large-scale migration from rural to urban areas in the 1960s and 1970s, and improvements in transportation of fresh food. Mortality fell significantly in Northern Ireland at 4-5% per year in the 10 years to 1988[224], slightly faster than in England and Wales. The rate of decline in incidence in Slovakia[237], around 16% every five years in the decade to 1988, is very similar to the rate of decline in incidence[80] and mortality (reported here) in the former Czechoslovakia as a whole.

In six republics of the former Soviet Union (Belarus, Estonia, Georgia, Latvia, Lithuania and Moldavia) where stomach cancer ranks second in males and females, there was apparently a three-fold range in incidence, and a significant decline of some 25% in all the republics in the period 1971-87[310]. Incidence rates in Belarus and Lithua-

nia are comparable with the highest in Europe.

Stomach cancer mortality increased substantially in Henan Province (China) between 1974 and 1985[169], world-standardised rates rising from 36 to 54 per 100 000 per year in males and from 20 to 27 in females. Although data for 1974-76 covered the whole province, while data for 1983-85 came from 12 county and city registries covering about 10% of the population, there seems little reason to doubt this unusual trend. Stomach cancer mortality rates in urban areas of the province were some 40% lower than in rural areas. Mortality from oesophageal cancer (which is twice as frequent as stomach cancer in Henan) fell slightly during the period, but misclassification of oesophageal cancer to the stomach at death certification would need to have been very substantial for the two trends to be spurious, and the trends in stomach cancer in Shanghai and Henan are clearly in opposite directions.

The decline in stomach cancer mortality in Japan

continued page 224

STOMACH (ICD-9 151)

AMERICAS (USA), INCIDENCE
Percentage change per five-year period, 1973-1987

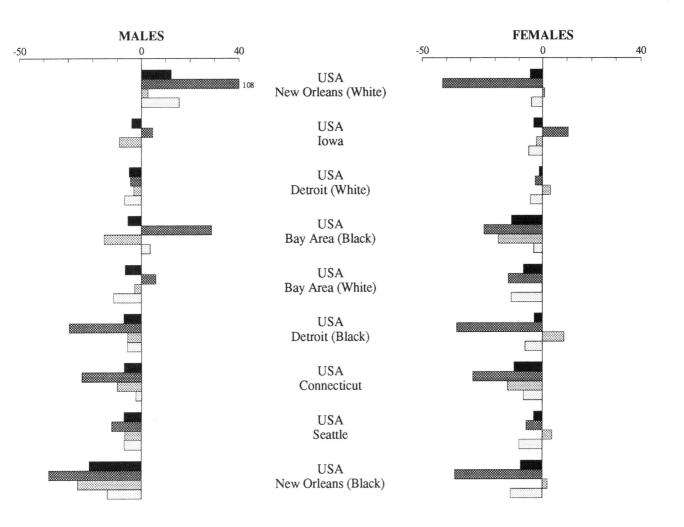

STOMACH (ICD-9 151)

AMERICAS, MORTALITY

MALES	Best model	Goodness of fit	1965 Rate	1965 Deaths	1985 Rate	1985 Deaths	Cumulative risk 1900	Cumulative risk 1940	Recent trend
CANADA	A2C6	-0.40	30.1	1142	14.5	852	20.8	4.8	-17.4
CHILE	A8P6C9	0.39	111.0	1262	63.2	1108	74.9	16.9	-18.4
COSTA RICA	A2P4C2	2.69	*114.8*	*173*	66.2	205	*68.1*	22.5	-8.7
PANAMA	A2D	-0.43	27.9	40	20.3	58	17.9	9.6	–
PUERTO RICO	A2P4C3	-0.32	44.7	182	19.2	84	*34.2*	4.0	-21.6
URUGUAY	A2P4C4	0.45	62.9	370	29.3	217	42.9	11.4	-19.4
USA	A5P6C5	4.91	17.5	7510	9.7	5486	11.8	3.5	-9.9
VENEZUELA	A2P4C9	3.76	61.9	510	*37.0*	*587*	43.0	15.3	–

FEMALES	Best model	Goodness of fit	1965 Rate	1965 Deaths	1985 Rate	1985 Deaths	Cumulative risk 1900	Cumulative risk 1940	Recent trend
CANADA	A4C6	2.56	12.9	513	6.3	419	9.1	2.2	-15.8
CHILE	A2P3C3	-0.51	68.9	866	23.3	485	47.5	5.5	-23.4
COSTA RICA	A2P3	-1.02	*55.1*	*64*	30.8	75	*35.9*	10.7	*-4.4*
PANAMA	A4D	-0.59	14.3	19	11.6	32	8.9	5.9	–
PUERTO RICO	A4D	3.17	19.9	81	8.5	46	*13.9*	2.6	-21.7
URUGUAY	A2P2C3	-0.87	27.4	168	11.9	100	18.5	5.3	-20.2
USA	A4P5C6	0.21	8.4	4121	4.2	2820	5.7	1.4	-12.8
VENEZUELA	A2P2C4	0.85	38.4	346	*17.0*	*275*	25.6	6.5	–

* : not enough deaths for reliable estimation
– : incomplete or missing data
Best model: polynomial of the given degree in age (A), period (P) or cohort (C), or linear drift (D) model.
Goodness of fit: the normalised likelihood ratio chi-square for the best model (see Method).
Rate: world-standardised truncated rate per 100 000 per year (30-74 years) and number of **deaths** are both estimated from the best-fitting model for the single years cited.
Cumulative risk per 1000 (30-74 years) is estimated from the best-fitting *age-cohort* model for cohorts of central birth year cited.
Recent trend: estimated mean percentage change per five-year period in the age-specific rates (30-74 years) over the period 1975-1988.
Italics denote recent trends not significant at 5 per cent level, or other figures which should be interpreted with caution (see Method).

STOMACH (ICD-9 151)

AMERICAS, MORTALITY

MALES

TRUNCATED RATE (30-74 years)

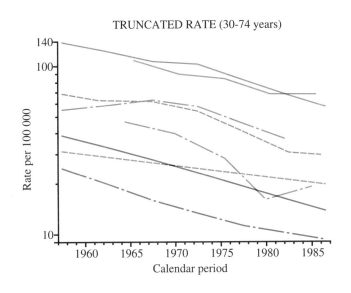

CUMULATIVE RISK (30-74 years)

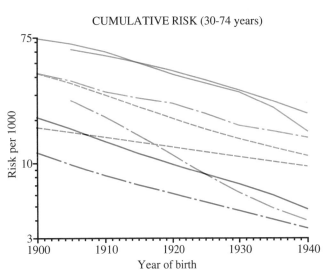

FEMALES

TRUNCATED RATE (30-74 years)

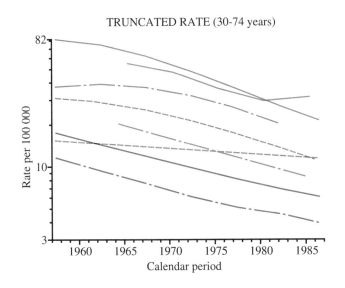

CUMULATIVE RISK (30-74 years)

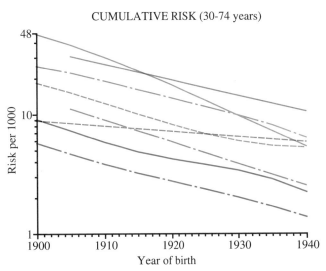

—— CANADA   —·—· PUERTO RICO
—··—·· USA   —— CHILE
—— COSTA RICA   ----- URUGUAY
----- PANAMA   —·—· VENEZUELA

STOMACH (ICD-9 151)

AMERICAS, MORTALITY
Percentage change per five-year period, 1975-1988

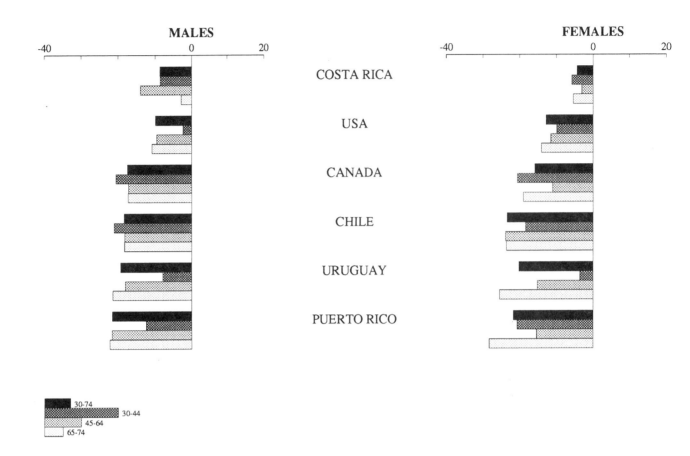

MALES — FEMALES

COSTA RICA
USA
CANADA
CHILE
URUGUAY
PUERTO RICO

30-74
30-44
45-64
65-74

from page 220

has been associated with westernisation of the diet on the basis of time-lagged correlations between mortality rates and intakes of food and nutrients derived from routine national surveys[287]. The mortality trend appears unlikely to be due to screening[273]. The decline is similar to that seen elsewhere, but more than two million persons were screened for stomach cancer each year in Japan around 1970, and more than five million a year in the 1980s[273], and this suggests that the lack of decline in recorded incidence is due to registration of lesions which are biologically more benign than those recorded in the past. A shift to more proximal tumours has also been noted in Japan[138]. Trends in incidence and mortality in New Zealand by ethnic group and sex have been reported[81], showing parallel declines in incidence of around 1% per year between 1948 and 1984.

Incidence of stomach cancer in Kingston and St Andrew (Jamaica) has declined substantially since 1964 in both sexes, as for oesophageal cancer[42]. In Ontario (Canada), the decline of 7% and 15% in the age-standardised rates in males and females, respectively, in the two quinquennia up to 1988[182] resembles the pattern in British Columbia, and is faster than the decline in Quebec.

The continuing decline in incidence and mortality from stomach cancer in most parts of the world for which data have been analysed here is evidence that the unidentified changes in dietary or environmental influences likely to be responsible are still in operation. Stomach cancer remains one of the most frequent and lethal malignancies in the world, however, and it is still the most common cancer in Japan. The increase in mortality in Henan Province in China gives cause for concern. The deceleration in the rate of decline in many areas implies the need for continued surveillance, and for further investigations into the specific causes of stomach cancer.

Chapter 11

COLON AND RECTUM

Cancers of the large bowel are the third most frequent in the world in both sexes, after cancers of the lung and stomach in males and after those of breast and cervix in females[286]. In developed countries, large bowel cancer ranks second: age-standardised rates are about four times higher than in developing countries, and about two-thirds of the estimated world total of 572 000 new cases a year in 1980 occurred in the developed world, which includes only a quarter of the world population[219].

Tumours of the colon and rectum are considered together here, as in many previous studies of cancer trends, despite the loss of information which this entails. It can be difficult to determine the precise anatomical origin of tumours arising at or near the rectosigmoid junction, and thus to assign a tumour unequivocally either to the sigmoid colon or to the rectosigmoid junction, which is classified with the rectum at the three-digit level (154) of the eighth and ninth revisions of the International Classification of Diseases; further, clinicians often use the terms 'sigmoid colon' and 'rectosigmoid junction' interchangeably[247]. This is important because in many populations up to half the large bowel tumours arise in this part of the bowel[196]. There has also been a shift in the distribution of cancers between the various anatomical sub-sites of the colon in some populations, with tumours of the descending and sigmoid colon becoming relatively more frequent. Consideration of tumours of the colon and rectum as a single group avoids the potential difficulty of comparing trends between populations in which the degree of misclassification between the two sites may differ, or vary at different rates over time, as in the USA[77]. Further, tumours of 'large bowel', not otherwise specified, are assigned to the colon. The geographical patterns of colon and rectal cancer are also similar, though not identical, and although the causes of both tumours are essentially unknown, environmental and particularly dietary factors are likely to predominate in both[101,303]. An important difference between cancers of the colon and rectum is the sex ratio (male-to-female), which is now generally around unity for colon cancer, but around 1.5 or greater for rectal cancer. Colon cancer is rather more common than rectal cancer in most populations.

Europe

Europe has seen a widespread increase in the incidence of colorectal cancer, more marked in eastern than in western populations, and the increases in the UK and Denmark have been slight. There has been no significant decrease in incidence in the past 15 years in any of the populations reported here. By contrast, there has been a general plateau or decline in mortality, particularly in the northern countries. The mortality trends show a marked geographical gradient, starting in the north in the 1960s (UK and Denmark), affecting south and west Europe in the 1970s (rest of EC) and Greece after 1980. A major exception to the European trend is provided by four eastern European nations, namely Czechoslovakia, Hungary, Poland and Yugoslavia. In these countries, mortality has recently been increasing at 11-15% every five years in males and at 5-8% in females, and mortality in both sexes has now overtaken that in most other European countries. Romania provides one exception in eastern Europe, where mortality has remained relatively low by European standards. Norway stands out as the exception from northern Europe, although the incidence rates and trends are similar for Jews in Israel. Not only has incidence increased more in Norway than in the other Nordic countries and the European Community, but mortality has also been increasing steadily at 13% and 4% every five years in males and females, respectively, in sharp contrast to the general decline in mortality elsewhere in the north and west of Europe. There are signs of an impending deceleration in the rate of increase in incidence and mortality in Norway, however, at least among males.

Asia and Oceania

There is a ten-fold range in the incidence of colorectal cancer across Asia and Oceania. There have been increases among Japanese and Chinese populations and little change or a decline in Indian populations.

The largest rises are seen in Japan, where initially low rates in the 1960s have given way to rates comparable with those seen among Chinese in Singapore and Hong Kong, and in other developed countries, around 50-60 per 100 000 in males and 30-40 in females. The cumulative risk (30-74 years) in Japan-

225

continued page 246

EUROPE (non-EC), INCIDENCE

MALES	Best model	Goodness of fit	1970		1985		Cumulative risk		Recent trend
			Rate	Cases	Rate	Cases	1915	1940	
FINLAND	A3C2	1.55	27.9	284	38.0	454	23.5	32.3	14.5
HUNGARY									
County Vas	A2P2	1.60	36.1	29	66.7	50	37.2	122.2	13.9
Szabolcs-Szatmar	A2P3C4	1.04	14.8	19	41.0	57	21.1	34.5	27.0
ISRAEL									
All Jews	A2C2	2.36	40.0	171	63.9	333	38.6	66.7	14.4
Non-Jews	A1	0.35	13.1	4	13.1	7	7.7	7.7	*5.7*
NORWAY	A2C5	0.94	39.3	437	64.2	786	35.9	67.3	17.5
POLAND									
Warsaw City	A2P3C2	-0.13	29.4	83	36.4	139	24.4	21.2	*-0.1*
ROMANIA									
Cluj	A2D	0.45	*19.7*	*31*	27.3	49	14.6	25.0	12.7
SWEDEN	A3C5	-0.26	44.9	1120	50.0	1362	32.1	31.6	4.0
SWITZERLAND									
Geneva	A4P2	0.79	51.3	40	60.8	55	41.1	41.9	*-5.9*
YUGOSLAVIA									
Slovenia	A2D	2.83	31.2	116	47.3	203	26.1	51.5	15.0

FEMALES	Best model	Goodness of fit	1970		1985		Cumulative risk		Recent trend
			Rate	Cases	Rate	Cases	1915	1940	
FINLAND	A4C2	2.18	25.0	344	30.5	486	17.6	26.2	4.9
HUNGARY									
County Vas	A4D	2.48	27.7	25	49.7	45	24.6	63.8	13.8
Szabolcs-Szatmar	A4C2	-1.09	17.0	26	31.3	55	16.4	34.5	14.9
ISRAEL									
All Jews	A2C2	0.18	39.4	176	56.2	349	32.3	48.1	11.6
Non-Jews	A1C2	-0.37	7.9	3	15.3	9	7.5	15.8	38.5
NORWAY	A3P5C3	-0.05	36.6	450	55.4	737	29.1	53.9	12.3
POLAND									
Warsaw City	A2P3	0.86	24.8	108	28.4	151	17.4	20.1	*0.0*
ROMANIA									
Cluj	A1	-0.35	*18.8*	*34*	18.8	39	11.4	11.4	*9.5*
SWEDEN	A3C5	0.68	38.5	1023	42.7	1237	25.7	26.5	4.6
SWITZERLAND									
Geneva	A2	-0.94	43.1	45	43.1	49	27.2	27.2	*1.2*
YUGOSLAVIA									
Slovenia	A2C2	-0.22	25.2	124	33.8	197	19.6	27.6	11.8

* : not enough cases for reliable estimation
– : incomplete or missing data
Best model: polynomial of the given degree in age (A), period (P) or cohort (C), or linear drift (D) model.
Goodness of fit: the normalised likelihood ratio chi-square for the best model (see Method).
Rate: world-standardised truncated rate per 100 000 per year (30-74 years) and number of **cases** are both estimated from the best-fitting model for the single years cited.
Cumulative risk per 1000 (30-74 years) is estimated from the best-fitting *age-cohort* model for cohorts of central birth year cited.
Recent trend: estimated mean percentage change per five-year period in the age-specific rates (30-74 years) over the period 1973-1987.
Italics denote recent trends not significant at 5 per cent level, or other figures which should be interpreted with caution (see Method).

COLON AND RECTUM (ICD-9 153-154)

EUROPE (non-EC), INCIDENCE

MALES

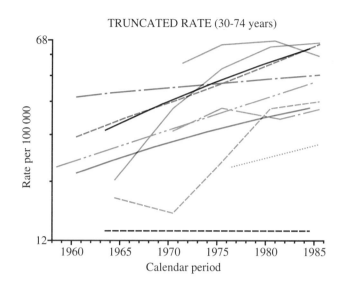
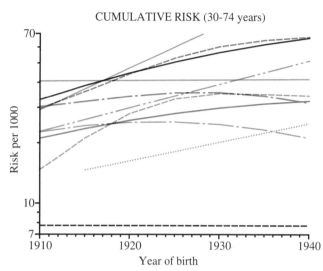

FEMALES

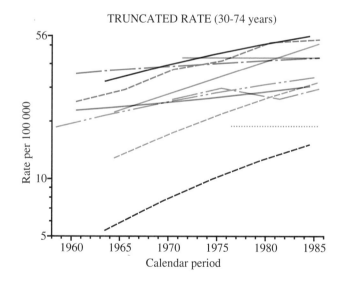
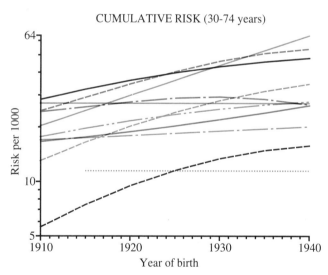

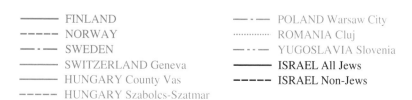

——— FINLAND	—·— POLAND Warsaw City
----- NORWAY	··········· ROMANIA Cluj
—··— SWEDEN	—··— YUGOSLAVIA Slovenia
——— SWITZERLAND Geneva	——— ISRAEL All Jews
——— HUNGARY County Vas	----- ISRAEL Non-Jews
----- HUNGARY Szabolcs-Szatmar	

EUROPE (EC), INCIDENCE

MALES	Best model	Goodness of fit	1970 Rate	1970 Cases	1985 Rate	1985 Cases	Cumulative risk 1915	Cumulative risk 1940	Recent trend
DENMARK	A2C6	0.28	58.7	805	65.5	973	41.0	42.9	3.3
FRANCE									
Bas-Rhin	A4D	0.86	*69.3*	*170*	86.6	174	52.8	75.6	9.0
Doubs	A2P2	0.84	*2.6*	*1*	68.0	74	40.9	57.2	*8.2*
GERMANY (FRG)									
Hamburg	A2D	2.09	43.6	245	*63.7*	*237*	37.6	*69.4*	–
Saarland	A2P2	0.86	55.8	161	72.5	203	45.2	64.6	*2.7*
GERMANY (GDR)	A3P4C6	3.62	38.7	1802	53.2	1966	31.1	52.4	9.7
ITALY									
Varese	A2	0.18	*66.4*	*76*	66.4	137	42.3	42.3	*3.7*
SPAIN									
Navarra	A2C2	0.13	*33.9*	*42*	44.0	62	22.7	73.4	13.2
Zaragoza	A2P3	-0.17	22.0	41	40.9	98	17.0	35.6	35.0
UK									
Birmingham	A2P3	0.76	58.5	788	66.0	993	39.2	46.3	6.7
Scotland	A2P2C2	0.45	51.7	707	60.9	857	38.4	45.5	3.7
South Thames	A2C9	2.87	45.3	1147	47.6	931	30.1	29.9	*-0.2*

FEMALES	Best model	Goodness of fit	1970 Rate	1970 Cases	1985 Rate	1985 Cases	Cumulative risk 1915	Cumulative risk 1940	Recent trend
DENMARK	A6C3	-0.35	51.5	787	53.7	898	34.3	31.4	2.6
FRANCE									
Bas-Rhin	A2D	-0.77	*38.3*	*118*	52.2	134	28.2	46.8	11.8
Doubs	A2	0.40	*42.7*	*30*	42.7	53	26.5	26.5	*9.1*
GERMANY (FRG)									
Hamburg	A2D	1.86	39.3	313	*48.7*	*274*	28.5	*40.6*	–
Saarland	A4P2	-0.05	45.8	178	53.2	209	32.4	39.6	*-0.1*
GERMANY (GDR)	A3P2C2	5.92	34.5	2370	43.4	2488	26.3	32.7	6.5
ITALY									
Varese	A2	0.75	*46.5*	*68*	46.5	120	28.5	28.5	*-0.2*
SPAIN									
Navarra	A1	-0.41	*27.7*	*38*	27.7	43	17.0	17.0	*8.1*
Zaragoza	A1P3	0.21	13.6	30	28.3	77	12.1	23.2	*10.6*
UK									
Birmingham	A4P5C2	2.03	43.4	682	45.2	753	27.8	25.3	*0.7*
Scotland	A3C2	-0.96	45.8	791	47.6	818	30.4	26.9	*-0.4*
South Thames	A3C4	5.48	39.3	1248	39.5	910	25.0	21.8	*-2.0*

* : not enough cases for reliable estimation
– : incomplete or missing data
Best model: polynomial of the given degree in age (A), period (P) or cohort (C), or linear drift (D) model.
Goodness of fit: the normalised likelihood ratio chi-square for the best model (see Method).
Rate: world-standardised truncated rate per 100 000 per year (30-74 years) and number of **cases** are both estimated from the best-fitting model for the single years cited.
Cumulative risk per 1000 (30-74 years) is estimated from the best-fitting *age-cohort* model for cohorts of central birth year cited.
Recent trend: estimated mean percentage change per five-year period in the age-specific rates (30-74 years) over the period 1973-1987.
Italics denote recent trends not significant at 5 per cent level, or other figures which should be interpreted with caution (see Method).

COLON AND RECTUM (ICD-9 153-154)

EUROPE (EC), INCIDENCE

MALES

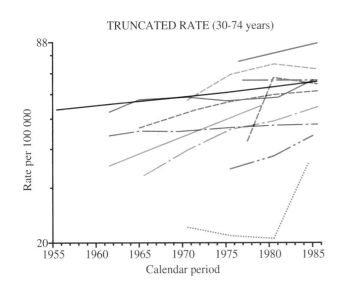

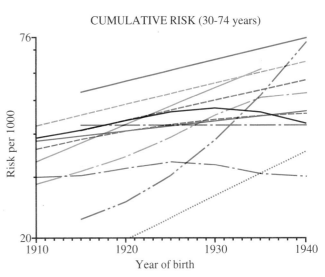

FEMALES

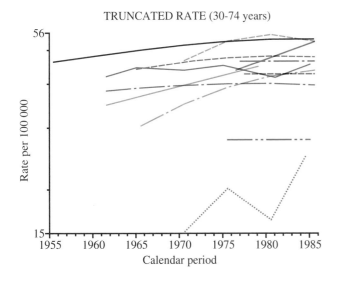

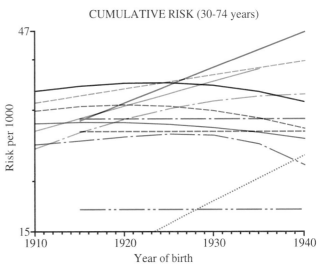

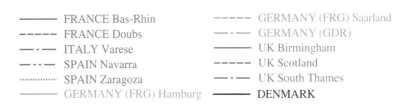

—— FRANCE Bas-Rhin	------ GERMANY (FRG) Saarland
------ FRANCE Doubs	—·—·— GERMANY (GDR)
—·—·— ITALY Varese	—— UK Birmingham
—··—··— SPAIN Navarra	------ UK Scotland
············ SPAIN Zaragoza	—·—·— UK South Thames
—— GERMANY (FRG) Hamburg	—— DENMARK

COLON AND RECTUM (ICD-9 153-154)

EUROPE (non-EC), INCIDENCE
Percentage change per five-year period, 1973-1987

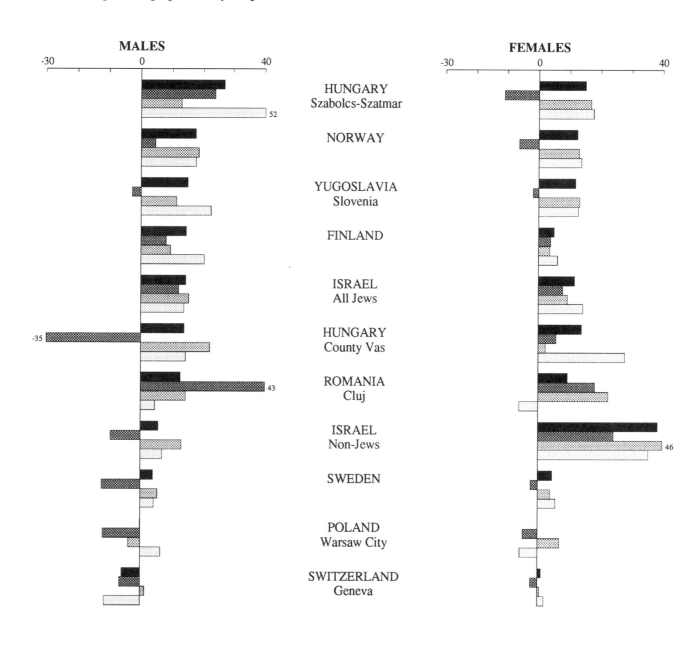

MALES | FEMALES

-30   0   40

HUNGARY
Szabolcs-Szatmar

NORWAY

YUGOSLAVIA
Slovenia

FINLAND

ISRAEL
All Jews

HUNGARY
County Vas

ROMANIA
Cluj

ISRAEL
Non-Jews

SWEDEN

POLAND
Warsaw City

SWITZERLAND
Geneva

30-74
30-44
45-64
65-74

COLON AND RECTUM (ICD-9 153-154)

EUROPE (EC), INCIDENCE
Percentage change per five-year period, 1973-1987

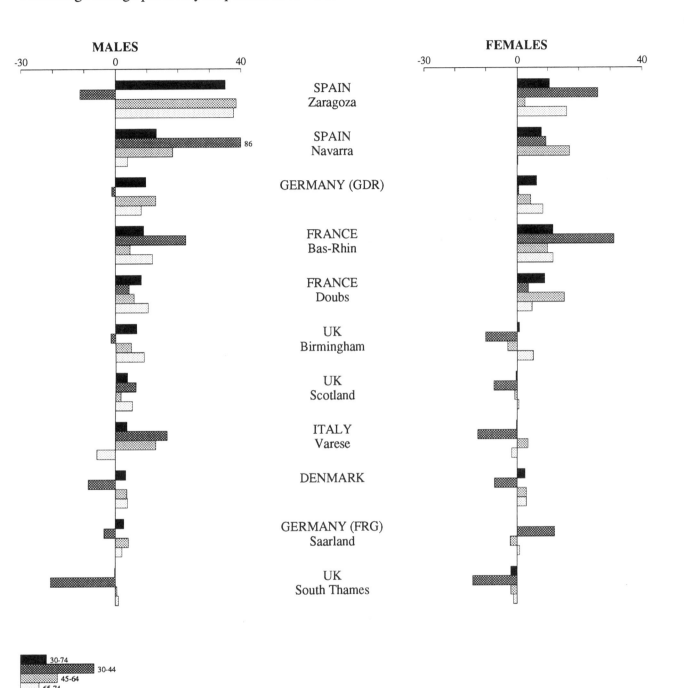

COLON AND RECTUM (ICD-9 153-154)

EUROPE (non-EC), MORTALITY

MALES	Best model	Goodness of fit	1965 Rate	Deaths	1985 Rate	Deaths	Cumulative risk 1900	1940	Recent trend
AUSTRIA	A2P4C6	0.72	31.2	625	35.0	659	22.7	28.7	-4.6
CZECHOSLOVAKIA	A2P5C5	4.39	29.1	1018	48.9	1808	20.2	51.4	11.2
FINLAND	A1C2	0.79	16.3	148	18.0	215	11.1	12.2	*-2.0*
HUNGARY	A4P5C5	0.35	24.4	633	44.2	1243	16.9	48.9	12.8
NORWAY	A2C6	0.35	21.4	224	28.9	363	14.6	20.6	12.7
POLAND	A2P3C4	2.76	12.4	731	24.2	1866	8.6	27.1	10.0
ROMANIA	A4P4	2.92	13.2	530	*13.3*	*698*	7.2	13.5	–
SWEDEN	A2P5C4	-0.63	24.7	579	22.5	623	17.1	13.2	-7.1
SWITZERLAND	A3D	1.20	30.2	433	27.4	488	20.7	17.0	*-2.8*
YUGOSLAVIA	A4P3C2	3.81	9.9	357	21.9	1063	6.8	28.0	14.2

FEMALES	Best model	Goodness of fit	1965 Rate	Deaths	1985 Rate	Deaths	Cumulative risk 1900	1940	Recent trend
AUSTRIA	A8P6C9	0.49	23.1	641	23.6	634	15.7	16.2	-6.1
CZECHOSLOVAKIA	A8P6C9	1.33	18.2	793	28.0	1300	12.2	24.7	7.1
FINLAND	A3P4	0.20	15.7	198	13.7	226	9.8	8.7	*-3.6*
HUNGARY	A4P3	0.45	21.3	684	28.8	1047	14.2	25.4	4.7
NORWAY	A8C9	1.08	18.3	214	24.7	343	11.9	23.6	*4.1*
POLAND	A2P3C4	2.96	10.4	794	17.6	1772	7.0	17.4	6.7
ROMANIA	A2D	2.86	11.3	548	*12.3*	*780*	7.1	8.4	–
SWEDEN	A3C4	0.80	21.1	534	18.5	559	13.6	8.7	-5.8
SWITZERLAND	A2P3	-0.42	19.1	343	16.9	358	13.1	9.7	-6.0
YUGOSLAVIA	A2P2C2	2.64	8.5	368	15.3	927	5.6	15.5	8.2

* : not enough deaths for reliable estimation
– : incomplete or missing data
Best model: polynomial of the given degree in age (A), period (P) or cohort (C), or linear drift (D) model.
Goodness of fit: the normalised likelihood ratio chi-square for the best model (see Method).
Rate: world-standardised truncated rate per 100 000 per year (30-74 years) and number of **deaths** are both estimated from the best-fitting model for the single years cited.
Cumulative risk per 1000 (30-74 years) is estimated from the best-fitting *age-cohort* model for cohorts of central birth year cited.
Recent trend: estimated mean percentage change per five-year period in the age-specific rates (30-74 years) over the period 1975-1988.
Italics denote recent trends not significant at 5 per cent level, or other figures which should be interpreted with caution (see Method).

COLON AND RECTUM (ICD-9 153-154)

EUROPE (non-EC), MORTALITY

MALES

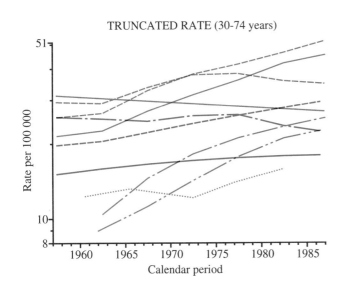

TRUNCATED RATE (30-74 years)

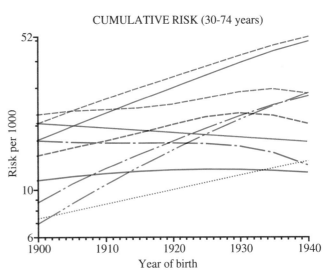

CUMULATIVE RISK (30-74 years)

FEMALES

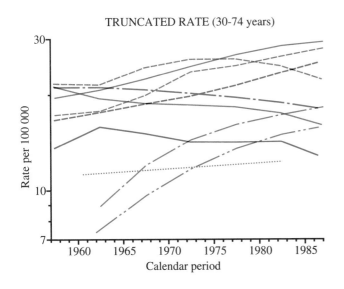

TRUNCATED RATE (30-74 years)

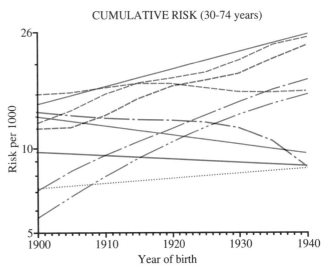

CUMULATIVE RISK (30-74 years)

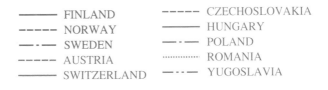

——— FINLAND	- - - - CZECHOSLOVAKIA
- - - - NORWAY	——— HUNGARY
—·—·— SWEDEN	—·—·— POLAND
- - - - AUSTRIA	·········· ROMANIA
——— SWITZERLAND	—··—··— YUGOSLAVIA

COLON AND RECTUM (ICD-9 153-154)

EUROPE (EC), MORTALITY

MALES	Best model	Goodness of fit	1965 Rate	1965 Deaths	1985 Rate	1985 Deaths	Cumulative risk 1900	Cumulative risk 1940	Recent trend
BELGIUM	A2P2C3	-1.74	32.8	877	30.1	829	21.9	17.5	*-3.3*
DENMARK	A2C5	-0.05	36.4	473	36.5	549	23.9	22.3	*0.5*
FRANCE	A4P5C8	7.53	30.2	3739	27.1	3834	21.2	15.6	-6.9
GERMANY (FRG)	A4P4C8	13.27	29.5	4581	32.9	5255	21.6	28.2	-5.8
GREECE	A2C2	-0.15	9.0	170	9.6	268	*5.9*	5.5	*-4.4*
IRELAND	A2C3	1.42	33.6	252	38.5	314	21.7	28.3	*2.1*
ITALY	A3P5C4	5.34	23.3	2837	23.7	3734	15.6	18.7	-5.3
NETHERLANDS	A3P2C3	1.03	26.7	756	28.4	1021	17.8	19.8	*-2.0*
PORTUGAL	A3P6C4	0.69	21.5	389	19.3	496	14.0	18.5	-6.3
SPAIN	A8P6	0.28	14.4	993	16.8	1638	9.6	15.4	-4.8
UK ENGLAND & WALES	A8P6C9	0.63	34.2	4422	33.2	4882	23.1	19.8	-1.9
UK SCOTLAND	A2C3	1.73	40.2	524	34.5	490	26.1	17.8	-3.6

FEMALES	Best model	Goodness of fit	1965 Rate	1965 Deaths	1985 Rate	1985 Deaths	Cumulative risk 1900	Cumulative risk 1940	Recent trend
BELGIUM	A3P2C5	0.69	27.4	878	21.9	717	17.2	10.8	-8.6
DENMARK	A4C3	0.07	30.7	444	28.3	479	19.5	14.7	*-2.3*
FRANCE	A4P5C2	5.49	21.4	3446	16.1	2690	14.2	9.1	-9.4
GERMANY (FRG)	A4P4C9	8.67	23.9	5159	25.2	5790	16.1	18.1	-6.8
GREECE	A2P4C2	0.31	8.8	192	8.5	271	*6.1*	4.9	-9.0
IRELAND	A3P4	2.18	30.3	232	26.3	229	19.5	16.8	-9.2
ITALY	A8P6C9	4.27	17.8	2661	15.6	2944	11.8	12.4	-10.1
NETHERLANDS	A3P2C3	0.22	25.0	795	21.7	912	16.0	11.6	-4.8
PORTUGAL	A2P6C9	1.85	20.5	483	11.7	365	13.3	9.1	-16.7
SPAIN	A8P6C9	1.38	13.1	1104	12.0	1370	9.2	8.9	-15.3
UK ENGLAND & WALES	A8P4C3	1.52	28.8	4682	23.9	4090	18.5	11.6	-5.1
UK SCOTLAND	A2C3	-0.40	34.6	589	26.3	461	22.1	11.2	-8.5

* : not enough deaths for reliable estimation
− : incomplete or missing data
Best model: polynomial of the given degree in age (A), period (P) or cohort (C), or linear drift (D) model.
Goodness of fit: the normalised likelihood ratio chi-square for the best model (see Method).
Rate: world-standardised truncated rate per 100 000 per year (30-74 years) and number of **deaths** are both estimated from the best-fitting model for the single years cited.
Cumulative risk per 1000 (30-74 years) is estimated from the best-fitting *age-cohort* model for cohorts of central birth year cited.
Recent trend: estimated mean percentage change per five-year period in the age-specific rates (30-74 years) over the period 1975-1988.
Italics denote recent trends not significant at 5 per cent level, or other figures which should be interpreted with caution (see Method).

COLON AND RECTUM (ICD-9 153-154)

EUROPE (EC), MORTALITY

MALES

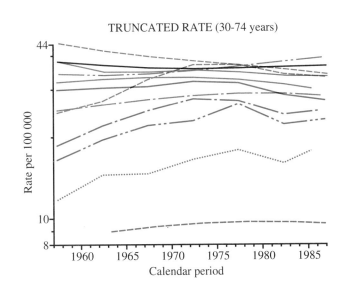

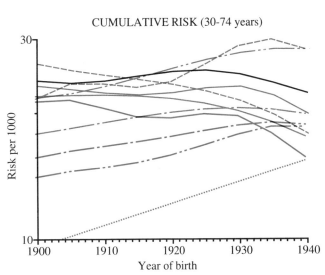

FEMALES

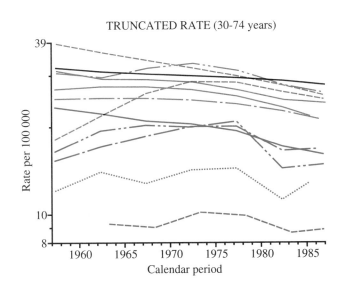

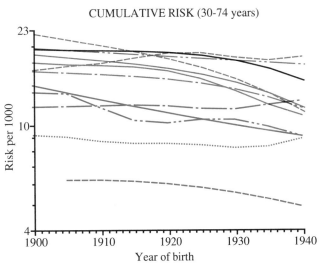

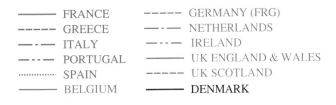

——— FRANCE   ----- GERMANY (FRG)
----- GREECE   —·— NETHERLANDS
—··— ITALY   —···— IRELAND
—···— PORTUGAL   ——— UK ENGLAND & WALES
········· SPAIN   ----- UK SCOTLAND
——— BELGIUM   ——— DENMARK

COLON AND RECTUM (ICD-9 153-154)

EUROPE (non-EC), MORTALITY
Percentage change per five-year period, 1975-1988

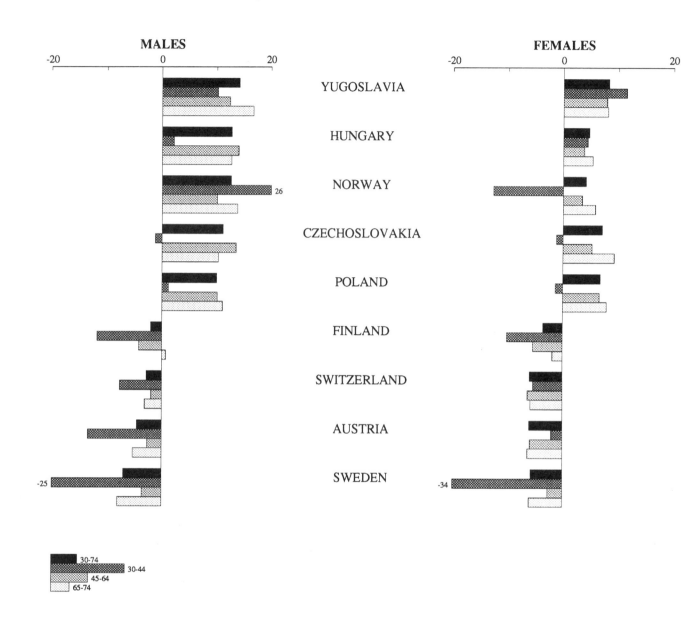

COLON AND RECTUM (ICD-9 153-154)

EUROPE (EC), MORTALITY
Percentage change per five-year period, 1975-1988

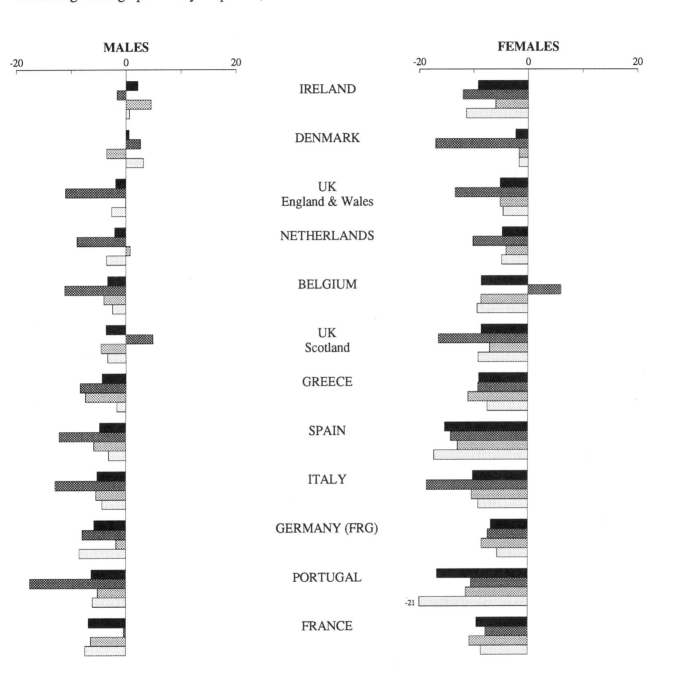

MALES

FEMALES

-20　　　　0　　　　20

-20　　　　0　　　　20

IRELAND

DENMARK

UK
England & Wales

NETHERLANDS

BELGIUM

UK
Scotland

GREECE

SPAIN

ITALY

GERMANY (FRG)

PORTUGAL

FRANCE

30-74
30-44
45-64
65-74

ASIA, INCIDENCE

MALES	Best model	Goodness of fit	1970		1985		Cumulative risk		Recent trend
			Rate	Cases	Rate	Cases	1915	1940	
CHINA									
Shanghai	A5C4	0.49	_23.6_	_265_	33.1	570	19.8	24.2	_4.2_
HONG KONG	A4C3	0.07	_38.9_	_188_	60.5	698	30.9	66.5	14.3
INDIA									
Bombay	A8P4	0.51	13.7	104	10.8	131	6.6	4.5	_0.1_
JAPAN									
Miyagi	A2P2C6	1.09	23.0	80	52.8	280	23.9	102.8	34.9
Nagasaki	A2D	0.10	_40.5_	_32_	69.4	73	35.0	83.8	19.9
Osaka	A8C3	0.64	22.7	282	47.7	895	24.0	84.4	28.0
SINGAPORE									
Chinese	A5D	-0.83	43.5	88	65.4	200	35.2	68.2	12.4
Indian	A1	2.86	26.6	6	26.6	10	17.5	17.5	_10.3_
Malay	A4	1.14	21.6	6	21.6	10	13.7	13.7	_13.8_

FEMALES	Best model	Goodness of fit	1970		1985		Cumulative risk		Recent trend
			Rate	Cases	Rate	Cases	1915	1940	
CHINA									
Shanghai	A2P2C3	-0.70	_14.0_	_167_	30.5	549	15.9	21.5	10.4
HONG KONG	A4C3	-0.45	_31.4_	_167_	46.8	541	23.1	47.6	14.3
INDIA									
Bombay	A4P2	-1.38	10.0	49	9.5	87	5.6	4.8	_0.6_
JAPAN									
Miyagi	A2C3	-0.52	20.2	82	40.2	253	18.7	59.5	26.7
Nagasaki	A2P2C3	1.24	_59.4_	_62_	41.6	55	19.8	43.4	14.3
Osaka	A2C3	-0.44	16.6	236	30.2	678	14.3	42.1	22.6
SINGAPORE									
Chinese	A2P2	1.01	30.5	69	53.4	187	27.4	61.9	15.8
Indian	A1D	2.41	36.9	2	26.0	4	19.3	10.8	_-4.4_
Malay	A3D	-0.36	13.2	3	23.6	11	11.3	29.4	_13.5_

* : not enough cases for reliable estimation
− : incomplete or missing data
Best model: polynomial of the given degree in age (A), period (P) or cohort (C), or linear drift (D) model.
Goodness of fit: the normalised likelihood ratio chi-square for the best model (see Method).
Rate: world-standardised truncated rate per 100 000 per year (30-74 years) and number of **cases** are both estimated from the best-fitting model for the single years cited.
Cumulative risk per 1000 (30-74 years) is estimated from the best-fitting _age-cohort_ model for cohorts of central birth year cited.
Recent trend: estimated mean percentage change per five-year period in the age-specific rates (30-74 years) over the period 1973-1987.
Italics denote recent trends not significant at 5 per cent level, or other figures which should be interpreted with caution (see Method).

COLON AND RECTUM (ICD-9 153-154)

ASIA, INCIDENCE

MALES

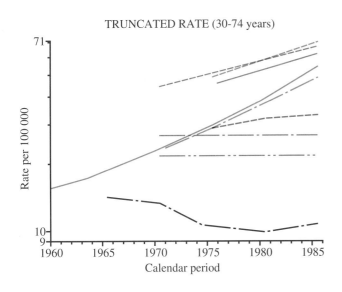

TRUNCATED RATE (30-74 years)

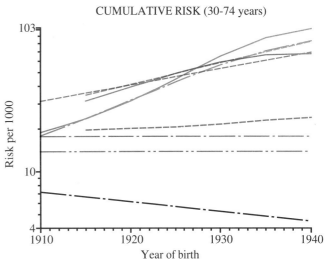

CUMULATIVE RISK (30-74 years)

FEMALES

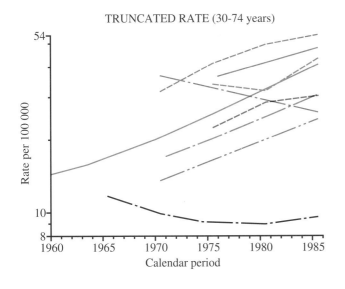

TRUNCATED RATE (30-74 years)

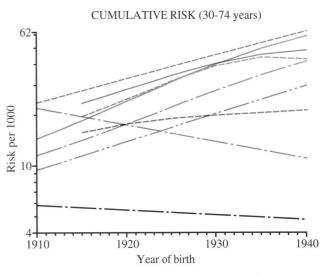

CUMULATIVE RISK (30-74 years)

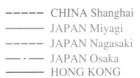

----- CHINA Shanghai
—— JAPAN Miyagi
----- JAPAN Nagasaki
—·— JAPAN Osaka
—— HONG KONG

----- SINGAPORE Chinese
—·— SINGAPORE Indian
—··— SINGAPORE Malay
—··— INDIA Bombay

COLON AND RECTUM (ICD-9 153-154)

OCEANIA, INCIDENCE

MALES	Best model	Goodness of fit	1970 Rate	1970 Cases	1985 Rate	1985 Cases	Cumulative risk 1915	Cumulative risk 1940	Recent trend
AUSTRALIA									
New South Wales	A2C5	-0.21	*50.5*	*519*	79.9	1066	42.3	79.2	14.1
South	A4C3	-0.14	*85.0*	*106*	73.7	259	40.8	60.0	*5.0*
HAWAII									
Caucasian	A4C2	-0.84	67.4	22	80.5	50	54.4	47.1	*7.7*
Chinese	A2C2	-0.04	91.6	9	60.6	10	50.9	15.2	*-4.8*
Filipino	A2C4	0.28	51.8	14	58.7	21	31.4	98.8	*-0.5*
Hawaiian	A8P4	0.20	40.7	5	80.6	20	31.9	72.2	45.9
Japanese	A2C2	-2.20	72.0	35	108.2	96	60.8	87.4	17.0
NEW ZEALAND									
Maori	A1D	0.18	26.6	5	48.6	15	26.0	69.1	*9.6*
Non-Maori	A2P2C6	3.45	71.8	403	93.4	655	49.6	63.1	10.0

FEMALES	Best model	Goodness of fit	1970 Rate	1970 Cases	1985 Rate	1985 Cases	Cumulative risk 1915	Cumulative risk 1940	Recent trend
AUSTRALIA									
New South Wales	A3C6	-1.60	*51.6*	*691*	59.9	845	30.4	63.4	12.0
South	A3C3	-2.29	*66.0*	*91*	58.5	219	30.8	47.0	*5.1*
HAWAII									
Caucasian	A2P3C2	0.45	62.9	21	58.6	36	37.1	21.4	17.2
Chinese	A1C3	-0.93	46.7	4	53.2	10	37.0	13.7	*6.4*
Filipino	A1	-0.68	35.0	2	35.0	9	22.0	22.0	*16.3*
Hawaiian	A2	1.16	36.2	5	36.2	10	22.2	22.2	*-8.0*
Japanese	A2C2	-1.25	50.1	25	54.5	55	34.6	29.4	*0.6*
NEW ZEALAND									
Maori	A2	1.79	29.8	5	29.8	10	17.8	17.8	*4.0*
Non-Maori	A3P3C6	1.38	64.9	395	81.1	614	42.9	51.9	6.1

* : not enough cases for reliable estimation
− : incomplete or missing data
Best model: polynomial of the given degree in age (A), period (P) or cohort (C), or linear drift (D) model.
Goodness of fit: the normalised likelihood ratio chi-square for the best model (see Method).
Rate: world-standardised truncated rate per 100 000 per year (30-74 years) and number of **cases** are both estimated from the best-fitting model for the single years cited.
Cumulative risk per 1000 (30-74 years) is estimated from the best-fitting *age-cohort* model for cohorts of central birth year cited.
Recent trend: estimated mean percentage change per five-year period in the age-specific rates (30-74 years) over the period 1973-1987.
Italics denote recent trends not significant at 5 per cent level, or other figures which should be interpreted with caution (see Method).

COLON AND RECTUM (ICD-9 153-154)

OCEANIA, INCIDENCE

MALES

TRUNCATED RATE (30-74 years)

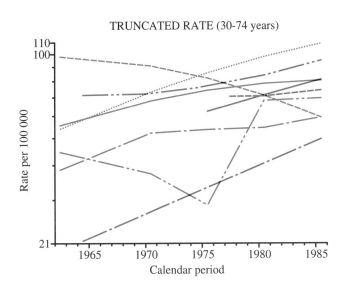

CUMULATIVE RISK (30-74 years)

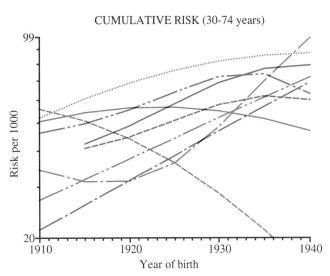

FEMALES

TRUNCATED RATE (30-74 years)

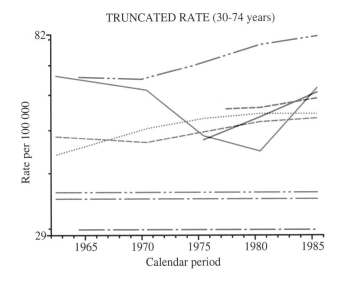

CUMULATIVE RISK (30-74 years)

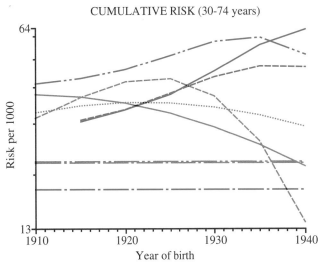

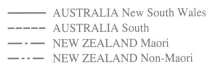

—— AUSTRALIA New South Wales	----- HAWAII Chinese
----- AUSTRALIA South	—·— HAWAII Filipino
—·—· NEW ZEALAND Maori	—··— HAWAII Hawaiian
—··—· NEW ZEALAND Non-Maori	············ HAWAII Japanese
—— HAWAII Caucasian	

COLON AND RECTUM (ICD-9 153-154)

ASIA, INCIDENCE
Percentage change per five-year period, 1973-1987

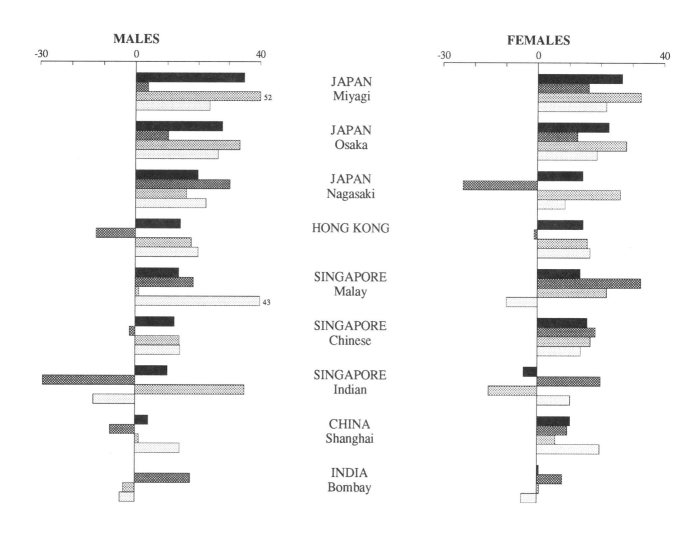

COLON AND RECTUM (ICD-9 153-154)

OCEANIA, INCIDENCE
Percentage change per five-year period, 1973-1987

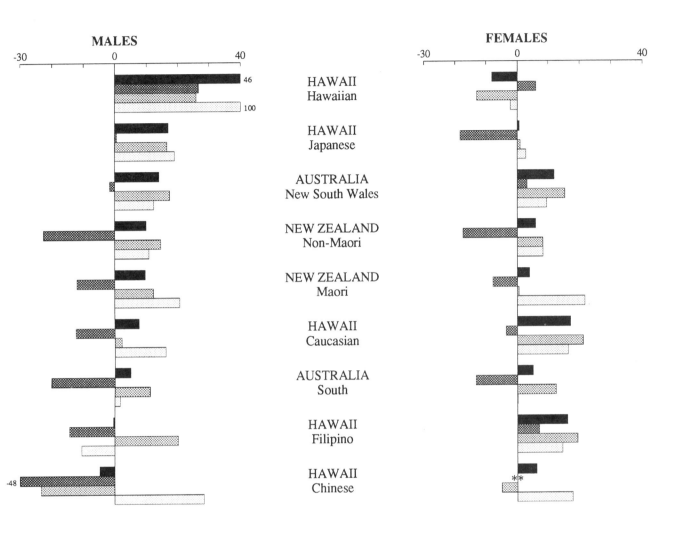

MALES

-30   0   40

46
100

FEMALES

-30   0   40

HAWAII
Hawaiian

HAWAII
Japanese

AUSTRALIA
New South Wales

NEW ZEALAND
Non-Maori

NEW ZEALAND
Maori

HAWAII
Caucasian

AUSTRALIA
South

HAWAII
Filipino

HAWAII
Chinese

-48

**

30-74
30-44
45-64
65-74

243

COLON AND RECTUM (ICD-9 153-154)

ASIA and OCEANIA, MORTALITY

MALES	Best model	Goodness of fit	1965 Rate	1965 Deaths	1985 Rate	1985 Deaths	Cumulative risk 1900	Cumulative risk 1940	Recent trend
AUSTRALIA	A2P3C6	4.19	30.2	727	36.5	1351	20.1	26.0	3.2
HONG KONG	A1C2	0.71	19.4	75	24.0	210	*12.3*	17.2	*2.3*
JAPAN	A4P4C9	5.83	13.6	2439	22.6	6626	9.1	24.7	10.7
MAURITIUS	A1D	-0.24	*13.8*	*9*	7.4	8	*9.4*	2.7	-26.9
NEW ZEALAND	A2P6C6	1.06	32.1	171	47.5	349	23.1	37.5	*1.8*
SINGAPORE	A4P3	2.32	*26.5*	*33*	32.1	62	*20.1*	29.7	–

FEMALES	Best model	Goodness of fit	1965 Rate	1965 Deaths	1985 Rate	1985 Deaths	Cumulative risk 1900	Cumulative risk 1940	Recent trend
AUSTRALIA	A4C4	0.14	27.6	746	26.6	1068	17.0	15.6	*-1.0*
HONG KONG	A4D	-0.18	13.5	65	18.1	159	*8.2*	14.7	*4.8*
JAPAN	A4P4C4	2.70	12.0	2412	15.4	5423	7.8	13.4	3.9
MAURITIUS	A1	1.44	*7.0*	*5*	7.0	8	*4.4*	4.4	*-1.1*
NEW ZEALAND	A2C6	0.41	34.3	202	37.4	301	21.1	22.8	*-4.4*
SINGAPORE	A5P3	5.85	*18.9*	*21*	26.3	53	*15.5*	28.2	–

* : not enough deaths for reliable estimation
– : incomplete or missing data
Best model: polynomial of the given degree in age (A), period (P) or cohort (C), or linear drift (D) model.
Goodness of fit: the normalised likelihood ratio chi-square for the best model (see Method).
Rate: world-standardised truncated rate per 100 000 per year (30-74 years) and number of **deaths** are both estimated from the best-fitting model for the single years cited.
Cumulative risk per 1000 (30-74 years) is estimated from the best-fitting *age-cohort* model for cohorts of central birth year cited.
Recent trend: estimated mean percentage change per five-year period in the age-specific rates (30-74 years) over the period 1975-1988.
Italics denote recent trends not significant at 5 per cent level, or other figures which should be interpreted with caution (see Method).

COLON AND RECTUM (ICD-9 153-154)

ASIA and OCEANIA, MORTALITY

MALES

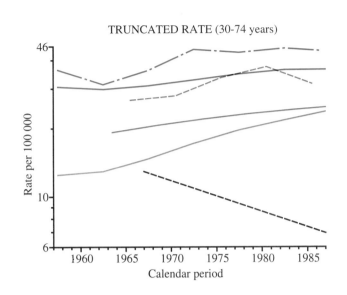
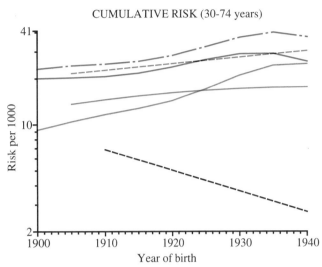

FEMALES

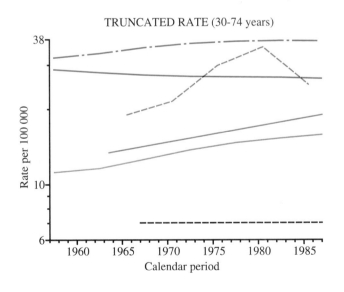
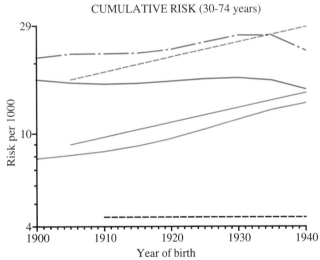

—— AUSTRALIA	—— HONG KONG
—·—· NEW ZEALAND	----- SINGAPORE
—— JAPAN	----- MAURITIUS

COLON AND RECTUM (ICD-9 153-154)

ASIA and OCEANIA, MORTALITY
Percentage change per five-year period, 1975-1988

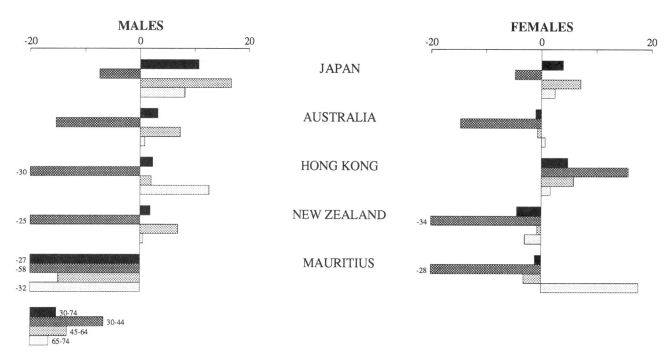

from page 225

ese males has risen two- to three-fold between successive cohorts born in 1915 and 1940, to around 9%, and the rise in females has been scarcely less dramatic, to 4-6%. Incidence is still increasing at 20-30% every five years in both sexes. The greatest increases in both incidence and mortality have occurred in the age range 45-64 years for both sexes, with the least increase in the youngest (30-44 years), and in Osaka the rates in the 15-29 year age group are declining (data not shown). Rates among Japanese living in Hawaii have also been rising, and males in this population now have one of the highest incidence rates of colorectal cancer in the world (102 per 100 000), increasing further at about 17% every five years.

There have been divergent trends in Chinese populations. Among Chinese in Singapore, incidence rates have increased significantly in both sexes, to around 65 per 100 000 in males and 50 in females, and cumulative risks for the 1940 birth cohort have reached an estimated 6-7%. Incidence has been increasing steadily in Hong Kong. Among Hawaii Chinese, by contrast, there has been a significant overall decline in males; estimated cumulative risks for the 1940 birth cohort are now less than 2%. The trend among Chinese females in Hawaii is unstable, and the cohort risk curve probably exaggerates the underlying trend, since there have been few cases among females younger than 45 years. Colorectal cancer remains very uncommon in Bom-

bay (India), occurring at about one-fifth of the rates elsewhere in this region of the world.

Colorectal cancer mortality has increased by about 25% in Japan as a whole since 1965, but less rapidly than incidence in Miyagi, Nagasaki and Osaka. In both Japan and Hong Kong the increase is essentially due to changes in persons aged 45 and over. There has been little change in 30-44 year-olds, and a decline at younger ages (data not shown), suggesting that the current rate of increase is likely to decelerate soon, as for incidence: this can be seen as a flattening of the cumulative risk curves for these populations, especially that of Japan, for cohorts born around 1930 and later.

In Australia, incidence has been rising by 12-14% every five years among both sexes in New South Wales, and less rapidly in South Australia: both data sets are well fitted by cohort models which suggest a plateau in risk for persons born around 1935-40, however, and there are declines among 30-44 year-olds of both sexes in South Australia. The pattern of age-specific trends is more marked for mortality, and there is already a small decline among females, which is likely to accelerate. Incidence among non-Maoris in New Zealand is 10-20% higher than among Australians, but the cohort trends are more marked, with a decline in risk for those born since 1935 in both sexes, suggesting that the plateau now seen for mortality in New Zealand in both sexes heralds an imminent decline in the death rates.

246

Americas

In Central and South America, the incidence of colorectal cancer is rising steadily in most populations, with the exception of males in Cali (Colombia). In Puerto Rico, truncated rates increased by 50% or more during the 1970s, and the recent rate of increase has been significantly high at 19% every five years (eight standard errors) in males and 11% (five standard errors) in females. Colorectal cancer incidence rates in Puerto Rico were less than a quarter of those in the rest of North America in the 1960s, but they are now approaching those rates, and for males born in 1940, the cumulative risk up to the age of 74 is likely to be only 30% lower than in North America. Incidence in Cuba and São Paulo (Brazil) has also been increasing in both sexes, but less rapidly than in Puerto Rico.

In the Chinese population of the San Francisco Bay Area (USA), the estimated rates of 65 and 45 per 100 000 in males and females, respectively, around 1985 were very similar to those among Chinese in Singapore, and much lower than in most North American populations, but unlike the steady increase seen in Singapore, there has been no significant change in the risk among Chinese in the Bay Area; cumulative risks for the 1940 birth cohort are estimated at 3-4%.

In the USA, there have been increases in risk in most of the male populations, but increases have generally been less marked among females. Most data sets were well fitted by simple age-cohort or age-drift models, suggesting that interpretation of risk trends in successive birth cohorts is reasonable. Incidence rates are broadly similar among blacks and whites, but the rates of increase since 1975 have been more rapid among blacks, particularly black males (about 10% every five years). The longest data series is from Connecticut, where incidence would appear to have been higher than in the other populations studied here for a number of years, with a continuing increase; these data show a marked deceleration and plateau of the rates among males in the 1980s, and a significant decline among females since the late 1970s. This can be seen as a gradual decline in cohort risk for females born after the turn of the century, and for males born after 1925. There is a suggestion of similar declines in cohort risk in other parts of the country, and age-specific trends in 30-44 year-olds show a decline in half of the US populations studied. In Detroit, however, the increasing trends have been sharply irregular in both sexes among blacks and whites, requiring period effects for satisfactory description, and suggesting that there may have been some deficit of registration during 1973-77.

The incidence rates and trends of colorectal cancer are much more homogeneous in Canada than in

the USA. Significant recent increases of 10-20% every five years have been occurring among males in all five provinces studied, although increases among females have been much less marked; evidence of deceleration or decline in cohort risks among females is also much less clear than in the USA.

Mortality from colorectal cancer in North America is falling significantly and steadily at around 10% every five years in females and about half that rate in males. In the USA and Canada, but also in Uruguay, where mortality rates and trends in both sexes are remarkably similar to those in North America, truncated rates for colorectal cancer mortality in women have fallen by almost 50% since the 1960s, and the quickest rates of decline are seen among 30-44 year-olds. Mortality elsewhere in Central and South America is around one-third of the levels in North America, but there have been clear declines in cohort mortality among both sexes in Chile and Venezuela.

Comment

In general, the incidence of colorectal cancer is rising, although there are a few notable exceptions. Mortality is not rising as rapidly as incidence, and in some countries it is falling steadily, particularly in developed countries such as Canada, USA, Sweden and European Community member states, where the recent decline of 6-9% every five years is remarkably consistent, particularly for females.

Many authors have examined incidence and mortality trends in cancers of the colon and rectum, either separately or, more often, combined. In Spain, the plateau in mortality from colorectal cancer after 1980, following a rapid increase between 1951 and 1980, has been attributed to improved survival[31]. Reversal of the male-to-female ratio was also noted, the female excess in the 1950s being replaced by rough equality or a male excess. The sharp increase in incidence in Doubs (France) since the late 1970s has been reported previously[260], with 18% and 10% increases in males and females, respectively, but there was virtually no change in incidence in Côte-d'Or (France) in the same 10-year period[236], although a shift from rectal to left-sided colon cancers was noted. The increase in incidence in Vaud (Switzerland) was also negligible during this period[164]. Mortality trends in Ireland[139] and Northern Ireland[224] have shown a recent increase in colon cancer, particularly among males, and a decline in rectal cancer. Changes in death certification practice may be partly responsible. The decline in bowel cancer mortality in England and Wales since 1960 and the decline among those born since 1920 were both more marked among

continued page 256

COLON AND RECTUM (ICD-9 153-154)

AMERICAS (except USA), INCIDENCE

MALES	Best model	Goodness of fit	1970 Rate	1970 Cases	1985 Rate	1985 Cases	Cumulative risk 1915	Cumulative risk 1940	Recent trend
BRAZIL									
Sao Paulo	A2D	1.25	28.2	142	*43.2*	*265*	23.6	*47.3*	–
CANADA									
Alberta	A5C3	-2.75	49.9	152	66.4	294	39.3	51.9	10.9
British Columbia	A2P2C5	2.04	73.4	343	73.0	532	45.1	54.8	8.9
Maritime Provinces	A2P2	-0.05	59.9	192	80.5	296	44.4	77.4	15.5
Newfoundland	A2D	1.71	57.8	50	87.7	100	46.6	91.2	19.2
Quebec	A2P3C2	3.02	49.8	537	81.3	1183	46.2	77.6	15.9
COLOMBIA									
Cali	A4	1.14	13.8	8	13.8	19	8.5	8.5	*0.7*
CUBA	A4C5	3.11	18.5	269	21.2	437	11.6	*20.0*	–
PUERTO RICO	A2P3C7	-0.17	18.8	85	37.2	251	17.4	40.2	18.8

FEMALES	Best model	Goodness of fit	1970 Rate	1970 Cases	1985 Rate	1985 Cases	Cumulative risk 1915	Cumulative risk 1940	Recent trend
BRAZIL									
Sao Paulo	A4P2	0.13	30.1	189	*81.8*	*705*	20.4	*32.2*	–
CANADA									
Alberta	A3C2	0.39	48.4	142	51.7	245	31.9	32.0	*3.2*
British Columbia	A4P2	1.62	66.6	323	56.5	451	35.3	30.6	*2.1*
Maritime Provinces	A3C2	1.52	61.9	203	59.8	244	38.9	29.3	*0.5*
Newfoundland	A2D	0.48	48.6	40	74.6	87	37.2	74.5	16.5
Quebec	A6P4C2	-1.47	49.3	598	66.8	1146	37.0	49.7	10.7
COLOMBIA									
Cali	A2D	-0.36	12.7	9	15.7	25	8.9	12.6	*8.3*
CUBA	A8D	0.29	21.4	265	24.5	511	15.7	*19.6*	–
PUERTO RICO	A4P2	-0.85	20.5	94	29.4	228	15.5	29.7	10.7

* : not enough cases for reliable estimation
– : incomplete or missing data
Best model: polynomial of the given degree in age (A), period (P) or cohort (C), or linear drift (D) model.
Goodness of fit: the normalised likelihood ratio chi-square for the best model (see Method).
Rate: world-standardised truncated rate per 100 000 per year (30-74 years) and number of **cases** are both estimated from the best-fitting model for the single years cited.
Cumulative risk per 1000 (30-74 years) is estimated from the best-fitting *age-cohort* model for cohorts of central birth year cited.
Recent trend: estimated mean percentage change per five-year period in the age-specific rates (30-74 years) over the period 1973-1987.
Italics denote recent trends not significant at 5 per cent level, or other figures which should be interpreted with caution (see Method).

COLON AND RECTUM (ICD-9 153-154)

AMERICAS (except USA), INCIDENCE

MALES

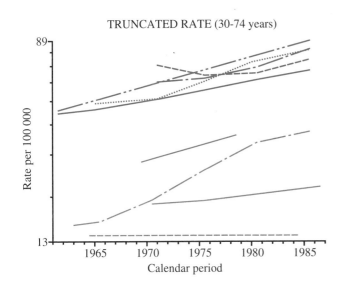

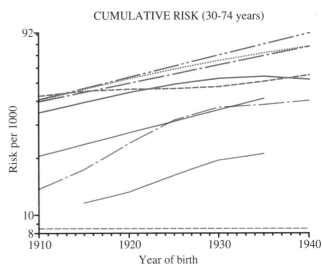

FEMALES

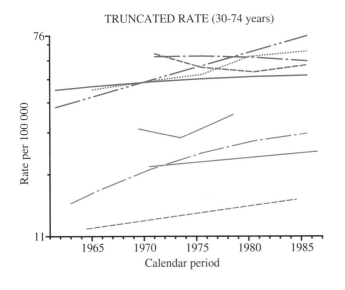

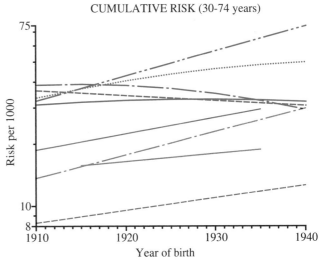

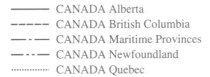

——— CANADA Alberta
- - - - CANADA British Columbia
—·—· CANADA Maritime Provinces
—··—·· CANADA Newfoundland
················ CANADA Quebec

——— CUBA
—·—· PUERTO RICO
——— BRAZIL Sao Paulo
- - - - COLOMBIA Cali

COLON AND RECTUM (ICD-9 153-154)

AMERICAS (USA), INCIDENCE

MALES	Best model	Goodness of fit	1970 Rate	1970 Cases	1985 Rate	1985 Cases	Cumulative risk 1915	Cumulative risk 1940	Recent trend
USA									
Bay Area, Black	A2C5	1.97	63.2	33	83.0	67	48.9	56.3	11.5
Bay Area, Chinese	A1	0.85	64.9	13	*64.9*	*34*	44.6	*44.6*	–
Bay Area, White	A3D	1.05	75.4	445	81.9	522	51.9	59.4	3.6
Connecticut	A3P2C2	-0.01	84.1	551	91.2	752	60.1	58.3	*2.4*
Detroit, Black	A2P3	0.18	74.9	100	82.8	147	47.0	64.0	9.8
Detroit, White	A2P3	1.38	79.0	578	87.1	637	52.9	67.2	6.9
Iowa	A2C2	-0.15	67.7	462	85.5	616	52.5	63.3	8.5
New Orleans, Black	A2D	1.16	*59.2*	*31*	84.2	51	48.0	84.6	12.7
New Orleans, White	A2	-0.99	*79.6*	*115*	79.6	125	50.7	50.7	*5.0*
Seattle	A5C3	1.28	*69.3*	*340*	81.6	556	48.6	65.6	7.7

FEMALES	Best model	Goodness of fit	1970 Rate	1970 Cases	1985 Rate	1985 Cases	Cumulative risk 1915	Cumulative risk 1940	Recent trend
USA									
Bay Area, Black	A2D	-1.37	50.6	30	71.6	71	38.2	67.1	11.8
Bay Area, Chinese	A2	1.55	45.9	8	*45.9*	*25*	28.5	*28.5*	–
Bay Area, White	A3	0.58	60.9	440	60.9	453	38.7	38.7	*-0.8*
Connecticut	A4C2	1.33	67.7	529	62.9	616	42.6	31.2	-2.9
Detroit, Black	A8C8	-0.37	56.8	83	67.8	148	35.8	40.8	7.3
Detroit, White	A2P3C5	-0.10	57.5	480	61.1	537	36.2	35.2	4.6
Iowa	A2C2	0.46	61.3	481	67.4	562	41.3	42.4	3.0
New Orleans, Black	A2	0.91	*64.9*	*42*	64.9	51	40.1	40.1	*8.8*
New Orleans, White	A2D	-0.73	*44.4*	*89*	61.7	121	35.4	60.3	11.7
Seattle	A2C3	-0.03	*61.2*	*357*	60.8	461	38.4	34.4	*0.7*

* : not enough cases for reliable estimation
– : incomplete or missing data
Best model: polynomial of the given degree in age (A), period (P) or cohort (C), or linear drift (D) model.
Goodness of fit: the normalised likelihood ratio chi-square for the best model (see Method).
Rate: world-standardised truncated rate per 100 000 per year (30-74 years) and number of **cases** are both estimated from the best-fitting model for the single years cited.
Cumulative risk per 1000 (30-74 years) is estimated from the best-fitting *age-cohort* model for cohorts of central birth year cited.
Recent trend: estimated mean percentage change per five-year period in the age-specific rates (30-74 years) over the period 1973-1987.
Italics denote recent trends not significant at 5 per cent level, or other figures which should be interpreted with caution (see Method).

COLON AND RECTUM (ICD-9 153-154)

AMERICAS (USA), INCIDENCE

MALES

TRUNCATED RATE (30-74 years)

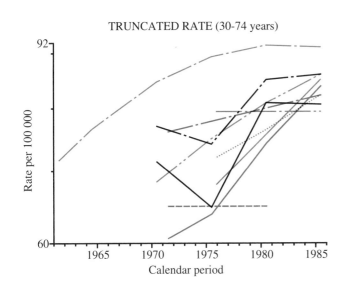

CUMULATIVE RISK (30-74 years)

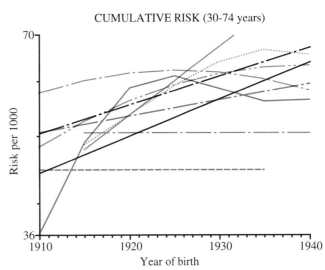

FEMALES

TRUNCATED RATE (30-74 years)

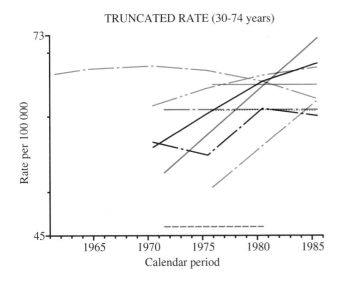

CUMULATIVE RISK (30-74 years)

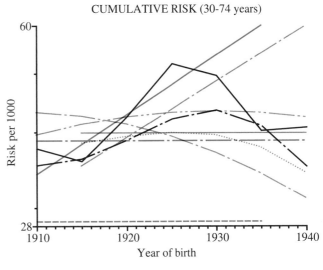

——— BAY AREA Black
– – – BAY AREA Chinese
–·– BAY AREA White
–··– CONNECTICUT
–···– IOWA

··········· SEATTLE
——— NEW ORLEANS Black
–·– NEW ORLEANS White
——— DETROIT Black
–··– DETROIT White

COLON AND RECTUM (ICD-9 153-154)

AMERICAS (except USA), INCIDENCE
Percentage change per five-year period, 1973-1987

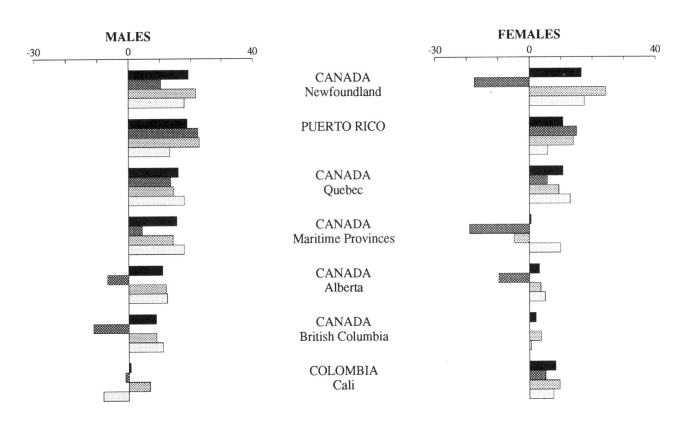

COLON AND RECTUM (ICD-9 153-154)

AMERICAS (USA), INCIDENCE
Percentage change per five-year period, 1973-1987

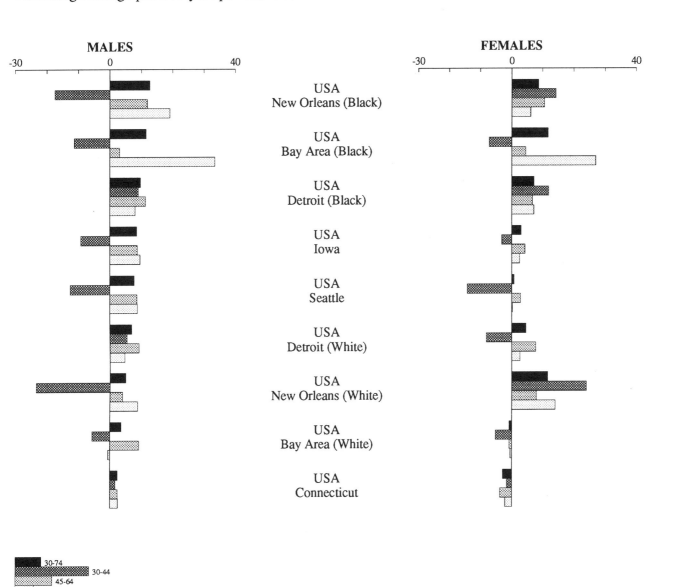

COLON AND RECTUM (ICD-9 153-154)

AMERICAS, MORTALITY

MALES	Best model	Goodness of fit	1965 Rate	1965 Deaths	1985 Rate	1985 Deaths	Cumulative risk 1900	Cumulative risk 1940	Recent trend
CANADA	A3P4C4	0.39	34.5	1312	29.5	1733	23.0	16.5	-6.8
CHILE	A2C2	1.86	10.4	119	10.9	191	6.8	*6.2*	–
COSTA RICA	A1	-0.19	8.7	13	8.7	27	*5.5*	*5.5*	–
PANAMA	–	–	–	–	–	–	–	–	–
PUERTO RICO	A2P2	0.85	9.7	39	14.9	71	*5.8*	*13.2*	–
URUGUAY	A2D	0.77	*33.8*	*199*	27.0	200	*22.1*	*14.1*	–
USA	A4P5C6	5.13	32.3	13807	29.6	16980	21.5	16.5	-3.8
VENEZUELA	A8P4C9	0.13	8.5	70	*5.3*	*85*	5.4	*6.2*	–

FEMALES	Best model	Goodness of fit	1965 Rate	1965 Deaths	1985 Rate	1985 Deaths	Cumulative risk 1900	Cumulative risk 1940	Recent trend
CANADA	A3P4C3	1.57	32.0	1263	21.5	1432	20.7	8.8	-12.4
CHILE	A2C3	-1.72	11.4	144	9.9	206	7.6	*5.3*	–
COSTA RICA	A1	-0.61	9.5	11	9.5	23	*6.1*	*6.1*	–
PANAMA	–	–	–	–	–	–	–	–	–
PUERTO RICO	A8	0.34	9.3	38	9.3	53	*5.5*	*5.5*	–
URUGUAY	A2D	-0.06	*32.0*	*196*	23.0	195	*20.9*	*10.8*	–
USA	A8P3C7	5.42	27.9	13651	20.8	14236	18.4	8.6	-8.2
VENEZUELA	A2P3C2	0.50	10.0	91	*6.5*	*105*	6.7	*3.3*	–

∗ : not enough deaths for reliable estimation
– : incomplete or missing data
Best model: polynomial of the given degree in age (A), period (P) or cohort (C), or linear drift (D) model.
Goodness of fit: the normalised likelihood ratio chi-square for the best model (see Method).
Rate: world-standardised truncated rate per 100 000 per year (30-74 years) and number of **deaths** are both estimated from the best-fitting model for the single years cited.
Cumulative risk per 1000 (30-74 years) is estimated from the best-fitting *age-cohort* model for cohorts of central birth year cited.
Recent trend: estimated mean percentage change per five-year period in the age-specific rates (30-74 years) over the period 1975-1988.
Italics denote recent trends not significant at 5 per cent level, or other figures which should be interpreted with caution (see Method).

COLON AND RECTUM (ICD-9 153-154)

AMERICAS, MORTALITY

MALES

TRUNCATED RATE (30-74 years)

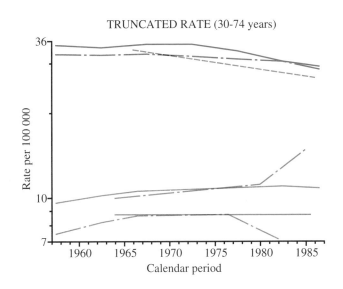

CUMULATIVE RISK (30-74 years)

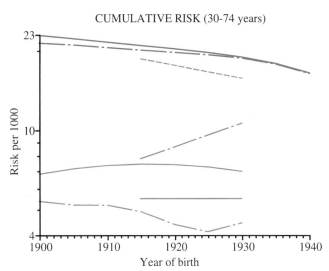

FEMALES

TRUNCATED RATE (30-74 years)

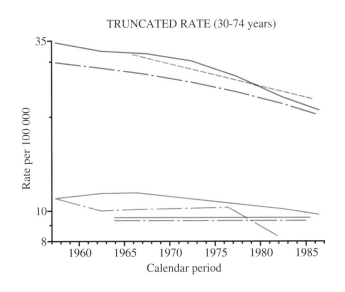

CUMULATIVE RISK (30-74 years)

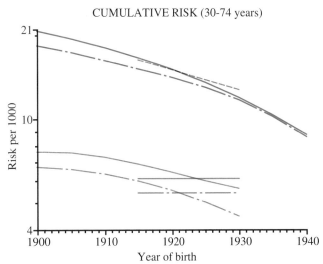

—— CANADA	—— CHILE
—·— USA	---- URUGUAY
—— COSTA RICA	—·—· VENEZUELA
—·— PUERTO RICO	

COLON AND RECTUM (ICD-9 153-154)

AMERICAS, MORTALITY
Percentage change per five-year period, 1975-1988

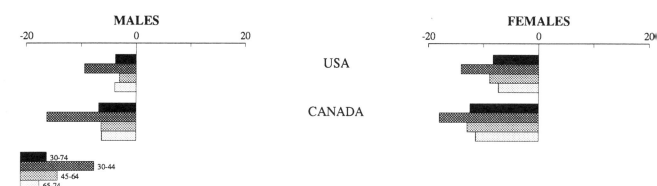

from page 247

females[212], as observed here for many countries, both for colorectal cancer and for cancers of the stomach and oesophagus, implying that women may have been changing their diets in a more beneficial way than men[213]. A similar effect is seen in France[128].

The rapid increase in incidence among Chinese in Singapore has been attributed to changes in diet[154]. Mortality in Henan province (China) between 1974 and 1985 was stable in males, but has declined substantially in females[169].

The increase in incidence in Ontario (Canada) between 1979 and 1988 was confined to males, and principally to cancer of the colon; cancer of the rectum became less frequent among females[182]. In the USA, incidence in the areas covered by the SEER programme has been analysed by race and sex for the period 1976-87[54]. Incidence rose more rapidly among blacks than whites, and more among males than females. The increases were attributed in part to a rise in the percentage of dietary energy intake from fat during this century. A trend towards diagnosis at earlier stages was noted, as well as an increase in relative survival at five years, from 50% to 56% for whites and from 44% to 46% for blacks. The cross-over from female to male excess in the incidence of colon cancer since the 1960s has also been noted for the USA[77].

The general increase in the incidence of colorectal cancer seen in the analyses reported here, coupled with a general decline in mortality, could be taken to imply that the increases in incidence are largely artefactual, due to widespread improvement in diagnostic techniques, particularly the availability of flexible endoscopes, and perhaps to improved registration of cancer, in particular of tumours that either would not have been diagnosed previously, or are biologically benign. The decrease in mortality would then reflect more accurately the underlying trends in colorectal cancer. However, the geographical patterns are not consistent with

this explanation. Trends are variable in both eastern European countries[218] and in western Europe. Norway provides a striking exception to the pattern seen in other Nordic countries, in that both incidence and mortality are increasing. Warsaw City (Poland) shows no sign of the increase in incidence seen in Hungary and Slovenia, although mortality in Poland as a whole has increased in line with that in other eastern European countries. These patterns run counter to what would be expected from a general improvement in diagnosis and registration. Secondly, the increases in incidence have generally been more marked among the elderly than in the young[76], whereas changes in diagnostic intensity might be expected to affect all ages similarly, or the young more than the old, at least in the age range 30-74 years. Likewise, the rate of reduction in mortality has generally been greater in 30-44 year-olds than in older age-groups, or, in eastern Europe, the rates of increase have been smaller than in older age groups. Finally, there are clear-cut differences in trend among different ethnic groups in the same area, as in New Zealand, Hawaii, the USA and Singapore, and between the various Chinese populations around the Pacific rim; there are similarities, however, in the trends among Indians in Bombay and in Singapore. These patterns suggest changes in cultural and dietary patterns of exposure rather than changes in diagnostic practices and cancer registration.

Such arguments do not rule out the possibility that artefact is responsible for the increase in incidence of colorectal cancer, but they suggest that much of the observed international pattern of variation in incidence over time does reflect the true underlying changes fairly well, and that the changes in mortality must to some extent reflect improvements in earlier diagnosis and more successful treatment. Evidence for this is seen in improved survival rates[27,54].

256

Chapter 12

PANCREAS

Cancer of the pancreas accounted for about 2% of all new cancers in the world around 1980[219], with about 140 000 new cases a year. Incidence is generally higher in developed regions of the world, especially Japan, North America and northern Europe, where it accounts for around 3% of all cancers. Diagnosis of cancer of the pancreas remains difficult, mainly because the clinical features are frequently non-specific. Non-invasive imaging techniques such as ultrasound and magnetic resonance have led to improvement in diagnostic accuracy, which could give rise to a spurious increase in incidence in successive calendar periods in regions where these techniques are widely available. Cancer of the pancreas is also said to be recorded particularly inaccurately on death certificates[286], but in the USA, at least, in the areas covered by the Surveillance, Epidemiology and End Results (SEER) programme between 1973 and 1986, accuracy appeared acceptable[229]. Among death certificates showing cancer of the pancreas as the underlying cause of death, 90% had been microscopically confirmed as such at registration, and conversely 91% of cases registered in 1974-75 with microscopic confirmation and dying of cancer by 1986 were certified as dying from cancer of the pancreas. The quality of cancer registration and death certification is certainly higher in the USA than in many other parts of the world, however.

The extremely poor survival from cancer of the pancreas, typically less than 5% at five years after diagnosis, suggests that in any given country, trends in incidence and mortality should be similar, although variations in incidence trends between areas covered by different cancer registries within a country may still arise. The highest incidence rates of pancreatic cancer during the period covered by these analyses have been seen among New Zealand Maoris and Hawaiians, and in black populations in the USA, with truncated rates (30-74 years) of up to 30 per 100 000 or more in males and 15-20 per 100 000 in females. Asian and Caucasian populations in various parts of the world have lower rates, generally in the range 10-20 for males and 3-10 for females. Mortality and incidence rates have been of similar magnitude in all countries for which both types of data were available.

The observed trends in incidence and mortality from cancer of the pancreas are generally cohe-rent, but there is wide variation in the trends between different regions of the world. Both significant increases and decreases have been occurring within the same geographical region, and in some areas the trends also differ between the sexes.

Europe

The Nordic countries (Denmark, Finland, Iceland, Norway and Sweden) have generally had the highest incidence and mortality rates in Europe. There has been a slight but consistent increase in both sexes, more marked in females, and the recent increase is significant for females in Denmark (6% every five years) and Sweden (4%). Among males, mortality in Hungary, Poland, Czechoslovakia and Yugoslavia is increasing more rapidly, by 10% or more every five years, and has either overtaken the mortality among males in the Nordic countries, or can be expected to do so in the near future. This is because the recent increases in risk among males in the Nordic countries show signs of deceleration or reversal, in that the increases are either smaller or reversed (decreases) among the youngest age group (30-44 year-olds). By contrast, there is little evidence of this among females in the Nordic countries. Their position at the top of the European risk table for cancer of the pancreas appears likely to be challenged only by females in Czechoslovakia. Although mortality is increasing rapidly in Yugoslavia in both sexes, at around 15% per five-year period, the truncated rates are still much lower than in northern Europe, and similar to the levels in the rest of southern Europe (Greece, Italy and Spain) at about 6 per 100 000.

In all the countries of eastern and southern Europe, mortality is increasing substantially in both sexes, and the available incidence data are consistent with this pattern. Although it is not obvious from examination of the cross-sectional data (truncated rates) or the recent linear trends, the geographical gradient for pancreas cancer, with high rates in the north and west of Europe and low rates in the south and east[269], appears to be undergoing an inversion. This is best seen by comparison of the various curves for the cumulative risk in successive birth cohorts. Mortality appears to have peaked in the Nordic countries and to be already declining in Scotland and Nor-

 continued page 278

PANCREAS (ICD-9 157)

EUROPE (non-EC), INCIDENCE

MALES	Best model	Goodness of fit	1970 Rate	1970 Cases	1985 Rate	1985 Cases	Cumulative risk 1915	Cumulative risk 1940	Recent trend
FINLAND	A3D	-0.61	17.1	174	18.7	222	11.7	13.7	*2.5*
HUNGARY									
County Vas	A2	0.32	14.4	11	14.4	10	9.3	9.3	*15.3*
Szabolcs-Szatmar	A2P3	1.04	4.3	5	12.6	17	5.8	17.7	24.5
ISRAEL									
All Jews	A4P2	0.11	16.6	72	14.5	77	10.3	10.4	-7.3
Non-Jews	A1C5	-0.56	6.7	2	5.8	2	4.6	0.1	*19.0*
NORWAY	A2P2	-0.71	14.5	162	15.1	186	10.1	12.7	*-1.0*
POLAND									
Warsaw City	A2D	-0.79	15.8	44	16.9	65	10.4	11.6	*-1.8*
ROMANIA									
Cluj	A2	-0.56	*11.5*	*18*	11.5	20	7.2	7.2	*14.1*
SWEDEN	A2P2	0.32	15.1	381	14.9	403	10.0	11.3	-2.6
SWITZERLAND									
Geneva	A2D	0.38	19.2	15	14.7	13	10.6	6.8	*0.4*
YUGOSLAVIA									
Slovenia	A2D	-0.68	9.7	36	13.9	59	7.5	13.6	17.9

FEMALES	Best model	Goodness of fit	1970 Rate	1970 Cases	1985 Rate	1985 Cases	Cumulative risk 1915	Cumulative risk 1940	Recent trend
FINLAND	A2D	1.07	9.7	137	11.4	189	7.3	9.6	*3.1*
HUNGARY									
County Vas	A2	-0.09	10.1	9	10.1	9	6.6	6.6	*13.8*
Szabolcs-Szatmar	A2D	-0.28	3.9	6	5.8	10	3.3	6.5	22.7
ISRAEL									
All Jews	A4	1.12	10.4	44	10.4	63	6.8	6.8	-6.7
Non-Jews	A1	1.48	3.4	1	3.4	2	2.2	2.2	*-31.1*
NORWAY	A2D	0.21	8.1	104	10.1	142	6.3	9.0	*2.8*
POLAND									
Warsaw City	A2	1.32	9.2	40	9.2	49	5.9	5.9	*0.5*
ROMANIA									
Cluj	A1	0.69	*5.8*	*10*	5.8	12	3.8	3.8	*12.6*
SWEDEN	A2P2	-0.38	9.6	265	10.8	327	7.0	9.4	3.6
SWITZERLAND									
Geneva	A2	-3.13	8.6	9	8.6	10	6.0	6.0	*-1.2*
YUGOSLAVIA									
Slovenia	A2C2	-0.34	5.9	29	7.3	43	4.7	5.2	*0.9*

* : not enough cases for reliable estimation
− : incomplete or missing data
Best model: polynomial of the given degree in age (A), period (P) or cohort (C), or linear drift (D) model.
Goodness of fit: the normalised likelihood ratio chi-square for the best model (see Method).
Rate: world-standardised truncated rate per 100 000 per year (30-74 years) and number of **cases** are both estimated from the best-fitting model for the single years cited.
Cumulative risk per 1000 (30-74 years) is estimated from the best-fitting *age-cohort* model for cohorts of central birth year cited.
Recent trend: estimated mean percentage change per five-year period in the age-specific rates (30-74 years) over the period 1973-1987.
Italics denote recent trends not significant at 5 per cent level, or other figures which should be interpreted with caution (see Method).

PANCREAS (ICD-9 157)

EUROPE (non-EC), INCIDENCE

MALES

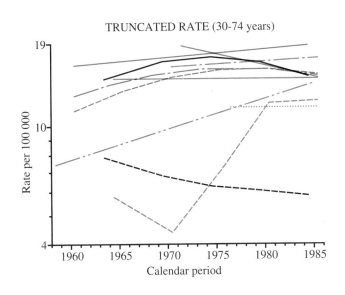

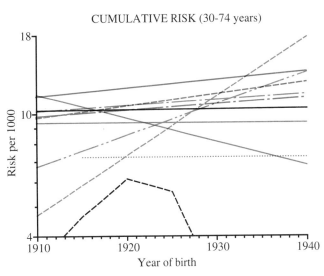

FEMALES

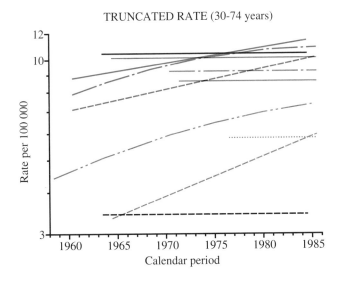

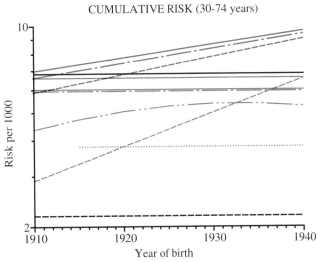

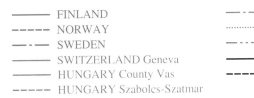

——— FINLAND	—·— POLAND Warsaw City
——— NORWAY	·········· ROMANIA Cluj
—·—·— SWEDEN	—··— YUGOSLAVIA Slovenia
——— SWITZERLAND Geneva	——— ISRAEL All Jews
——— HUNGARY County Vas	------- ISRAEL Non-Jews
------- HUNGARY Szabolcs-Szatmar	

PANCREAS (ICD-9 157)

EUROPE (EC), INCIDENCE

MALES	Best model	Goodness of fit	1970 Rate	1970 Cases	1985 Rate	1985 Cases	Cumulative risk 1915	Cumulative risk 1940	Recent trend
DENMARK	A2P6	0.11	18.3	251	17.7	261	11.1	14.5	*-2.4*
FRANCE									
Bas-Rhin	A8	1.20	*12.9*	*28*	12.9	26	7.5	7.5	16.7
Doubs	A2	-0.65	*8.9*	*6*	8.9	9	5.1	5.1	*-15.5*
GERMANY (FRG)									
Hamburg	A4	2.14	14.6	81	*14.6*	*55*	9.4	*9.4*	–
Saarland	A2D	-0.77	10.9	31	13.4	37	7.8	11.1	17.3
GERMANY (GDR)	A2P2	1.41	12.1	557	14.7	537	8.7	12.5	5.5
ITALY									
Varese	A2	0.51	*15.0*	*17*	15.0	31	9.7	9.7	*13.7*
SPAIN									
Navarra	A2D	-0.73	*5.7*	*6*	12.5	17	6.6	24.0	30.4
Zaragoza	A2D	-0.16	6.6	12	10.8	25	5.6	12.6	*5.3*
UK									
Birmingham	A2P2	0.64	14.4	195	13.7	205	9.1	9.7	*-3.4*
Scotland	A4P2C2	0.09	15.1	207	14.6	205	10.2	8.0	*-4.2*
South Thames	A8C9	1.33	14.1	359	14.7	291	10.1	10.5	-4.4

FEMALES	Best model	Goodness of fit	1970 Rate	1970 Cases	1985 Rate	1985 Cases	Cumulative risk 1915	Cumulative risk 1940	Recent trend
DENMARK	A2P2	1.08	10.5	164	12.5	211	7.9	11.7	6.2
FRANCE									
Bas-Rhin	A1D	0.45	*2.7*	*8*	6.1	16	3.3	12.9	28.7
Doubs	A3	-0.75	*4.1*	*2*	4.1	5	2.7	2.7	*0.2*
GERMANY (FRG)									
Hamburg	A2	-0.32	8.0	65	*8.0*	*46*	5.3	*5.3*	–
Saarland	A1D	0.75	5.3	21	7.0	28	4.4	6.9	*11.5*
GERMANY (GDR)	A2P3	1.28	6.8	492	8.4	486	5.2	7.8	7.3
ITALY									
Varese	A1	0.77	*7.2*	*8*	7.2	19	4.9	4.9	*4.4*
SPAIN									
Navarra	A2	-0.72	*4.7*	*6*	4.7	7	3.2	3.2	*12.0*
Zaragoza	A1	-0.99	3.5	8	3.5	10	2.4	2.4	*17.1*
UK									
Birmingham	A3C6	2.13	7.6	122	8.4	147	5.7	3.3	*1.2*
Scotland	A2C2	0.43	8.5	150	10.6	186	6.7	7.6	5.0
South Thames	A2D	0.67	8.2	272	9.4	224	5.9	7.5	*1.5*

* : not enough cases for reliable estimation
– : incomplete or missing data
Best model: polynomial of the given degree in age (A), period (P) or cohort (C), or linear drift (D) model.
Goodness of fit: the normalised likelihood ratio chi-square for the best model (see Method).
Rate: world-standardised truncated rate per 100 000 per year (30-74 years) and number of **cases** are both estimated from the best-fitting model for the single years cited.
Cumulative risk per 1000 (30-74 years) is estimated from the best-fitting *age-cohort* model for cohorts of central birth year cited.
Recent trend: estimated mean percentage change per five-year period in the age-specific rates (30-74 years) over the period 1973-1987.
Italics denote recent trends not significant at 5 per cent level, or other figures which should be interpreted with caution (see Method).

PANCREAS (ICD-9 157)

EUROPE (EC), INCIDENCE

MALES

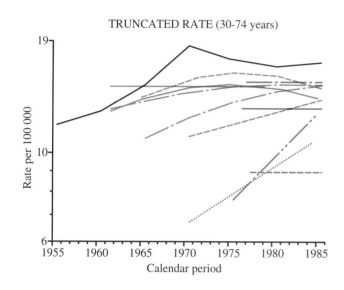
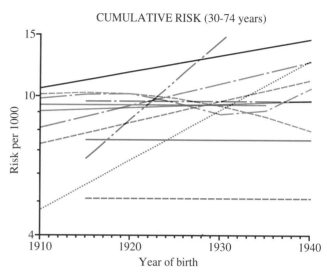

FEMALES

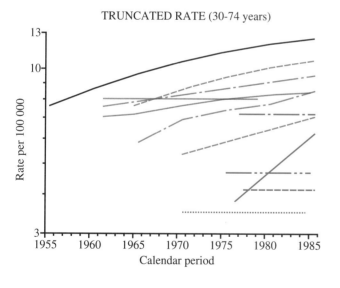
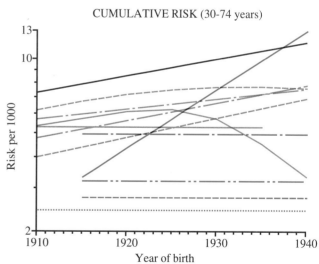

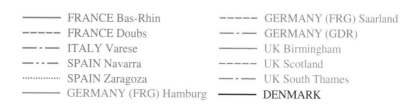

—— FRANCE Bas-Rhin	– – – GERMANY (FRG) Saarland
– – – FRANCE Doubs	–·–·– GERMANY (GDR)
–·–·– ITALY Varese	—— UK Birmingham
–··–··– SPAIN Navarra	– – – UK Scotland
·········· SPAIN Zaragoza	–·–·– UK South Thames
—— GERMANY (FRG) Hamburg	—— DENMARK

PANCREAS (ICD-9 157)

EUROPE (non-EC), INCIDENCE
Percentage change per five-year period, 1973-1987

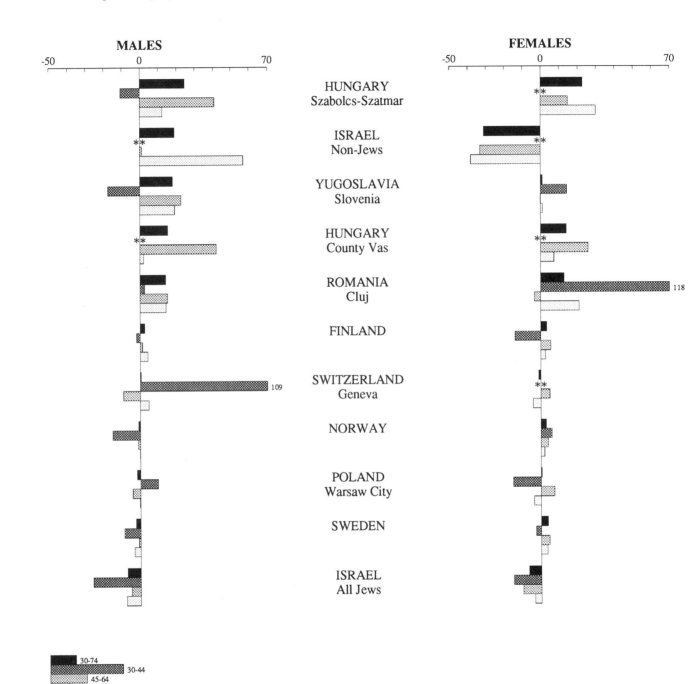

PANCREAS (ICD-9 157)

EUROPE (EC), INCIDENCE
Percentage change per five-year period, 1973-1987

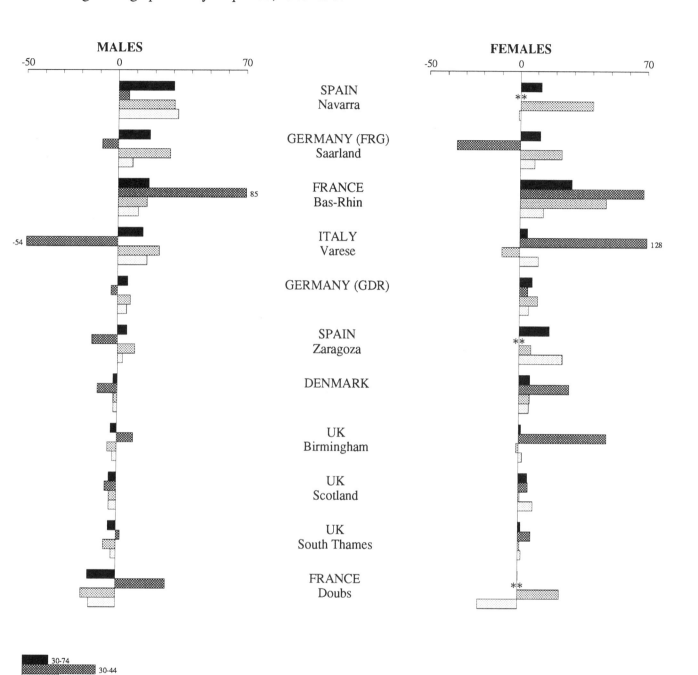

263

PANCREAS (ICD-9 157)

EUROPE (non-EC), MORTALITY

MALES	Best model	Goodness of fit	1965 Rate	1965 Deaths	1985 Rate	1985 Deaths	Cumulative risk 1900	Cumulative risk 1940	Recent trend
AUSTRIA	A2P2C5	0.27	14.2	282	16.2	299	9.3	14.9	*2.0*
CZECHOSLOVAKIA	A2P2C4	2.45	12.4	436	19.4	706	7.9	22.1	10.0
FINLAND	A4P3C4	0.45	16.6	153	17.1	201	10.7	12.0	*-2.8*
HUNGARY	A2D	0.58	*11.6*	*301*	18.4	509	*7.3*	18.2	12.6
NORWAY	A2C2	0.74	12.7	133	14.1	177	8.5	8.3	*-1.3*
POLAND	A3P3C4	2.80	7.6	456	15.3	1183	4.8	*19.2*	–
ROMANIA	–	–	–	–	–	–	–	–	–
SWEDEN	A3P2C6	0.35	14.6	342	14.9	407	10.0	8.8	*-3.1*
SWITZERLAND	A2C2	0.87	11.3	161	13.4	235	7.4	8.6	*-3.2*
YUGOSLAVIA	A3D	2.85	5.8	208	11.6	574	3.6	14.3	19.2

FEMALES	Best model	Goodness of fit	1965 Rate	1965 Deaths	1985 Rate	1985 Deaths	Cumulative risk 1900	Cumulative risk 1940	Recent trend
AUSTRIA	A2D	1.16	8.4	239	9.8	269	5.7	7.7	*3.5*
CZECHOSLOVAKIA	A2P3	0.57	7.3	321	9.9	461	4.7	9.9	6.0
FINLAND	A2P2C2	0.89	8.7	109	10.4	174	5.9	7.5	*1.5*
HUNGARY	A2D	1.99	*8.4*	*270*	10.1	366	*5.6*	8.0	4.4
NORWAY	A2D	0.14	6.9	81	9.3	132	4.7	8.4	7.7
POLAND	A2P4C3	0.66	5.7	439	8.7	879	3.6	*8.2*	–
ROMANIA	–	–	–	–	–	–	–	–	–
SWEDEN	A2P2	0.39	9.0	232	11.4	345	6.0	10.2	5.2
SWITZERLAND	A4C3	1.17	7.0	126	8.3	179	4.9	6.4	*4.7*
YUGOSLAVIA	A2C2	0.13	3.5	153	6.3	379	2.3	6.5	13.1

* : not enough deaths for reliable estimation
– : incomplete or missing data
Best model: polynomial of the given degree in age (A), period (P) or cohort (C), or linear drift (D) model.
Goodness of fit: the normalised likelihood ratio chi-square for the best model (see Method).
Rate: world-standardised truncated rate per 100 000 per year (30-74 years) and number of **deaths** are both estimated from the best-fitting model for the single years cited.
Cumulative risk per 1000 (30-74 years) is estimated from the best-fitting *age-cohort* model for cohorts of central birth year cited.
Recent trend: estimated mean percentage change per five-year period in the age-specific rates (30-74 years) over the period 1975-1988.
Italics denote recent trends not significant at 5 per cent level, or other figures which should be interpreted with caution (see Method).

PANCREAS (ICD-9 157)

EUROPE (non-EC), MORTALITY

MALES

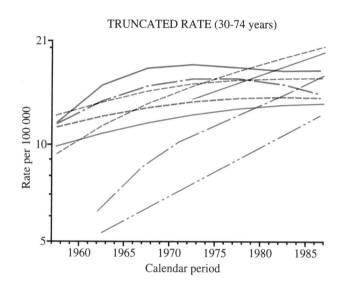

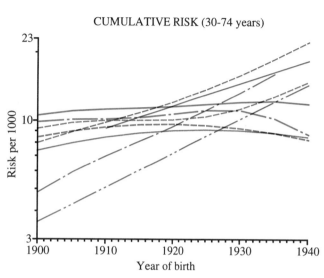

FEMALES

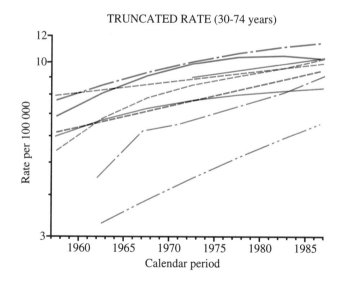

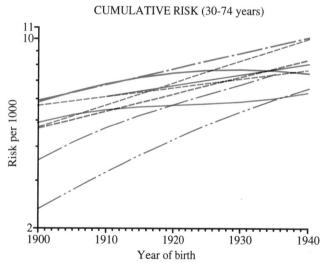

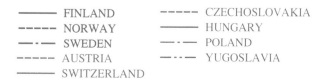

—— FINLAND	----- CZECHOSLOVAKIA
----- NORWAY	—— HUNGARY
—·—· SWEDEN	—·—· POLAND
----- AUSTRIA	—··—·· YUGOSLAVIA
—— SWITZERLAND	

PANCREAS (ICD-9 157)

EUROPE (EC), MORTALITY

MALES	Best model	Goodness of fit	1965 Rate	1965 Deaths	1985 Rate	1985 Deaths	Cumulative risk 1900	Cumulative risk 1940	Recent trend
BELGIUM	A4P2C2	0.36	10.6	279	13.6	369	6.8	10.8	-5.5
DENMARK	A2P2C2	1.34	14.9	192	16.1	239	9.7	10.5	*-1.6*
FRANCE	A3P3C6	1.78	9.2	1138	12.9	1798	6.2	12.1	3.5
GERMANY (FRG)	A3P4C8	4.19	11.5	1771	14.9	2362	7.2	12.8	7.8
GREECE	A2P4	-0.98	*2.5*	*47*	10.6	290	*3.4*	13.0	15.6
IRELAND	A2C2	0.24	13.5	100	16.1	132	8.9	9.3	*-1.0*
ITALY	A3P3C3	3.06	7.6	923	12.9	2003	4.7	12.1	10.0
NETHERLANDS	A2P2C2	0.06	12.8	358	16.0	569	8.3	11.5	*-0.5*
PORTUGAL	–	–	–	–	–	–	–	–	–
SPAIN	A2P5C2	-0.99	4.9	336	9.4	912	2.9	10.3	17.8
UK ENGLAND & WALES	A2P3C2	0.17	13.5	1750	13.8	2024	8.8	8.7	-5.2
UK SCOTLAND	A2P2C3	-0.31	15.3	201	13.7	193	10.0	8.1	-9.4

FEMALES	Best model	Goodness of fit	1965 Rate	1965 Deaths	1985 Rate	1985 Deaths	Cumulative risk 1900	Cumulative risk 1940	Recent trend
BELGIUM	A2P2	0.57	5.8	189	7.2	236	3.9	7.2	*-3.6*
DENMARK	A2P4C3	1.19	9.4	137	12.6	216	6.1	8.9	*2.7*
FRANCE	A3P5	0.32	4.8	778	5.7	968	3.2	4.7	8.8
GERMANY (FRG)	A8P4C8	2.24	6.8	1487	8.5	1943	4.4	6.7	8.8
GREECE	A2D	0.22	*2.8*	*62*	5.3	170	*2.0*	6.7	12.8
IRELAND	A3P3C2	-1.17	9.4	72	9.4	84	6.5	5.4	-11.1
ITALY	A2C2	3.43	4.3	649	6.8	1305	2.9	6.3	13.6
NETHERLANDS	A2P2	-0.70	7.6	244	9.2	391	5.1	8.6	*-0.7*
PORTUGAL	–	–	–	–	–	–	–	–	–
SPAIN	A2P3C2	0.60	3.3	280	4.7	558	2.1	3.3	12.7
UK ENGLAND & WALES	A2P4C5	-0.17	7.8	1286	8.8	1524	5.1	5.6	*1.8*
UK SCOTLAND	A2D	1.09	9.2	159	9.9	175	6.0	7.1	*0.6*

* : not enough deaths for reliable estimation
– : incomplete or missing data
Best model: polynomial of the given degree in age (A), period (P) or cohort (C), or linear drift (D) model.
Goodness of fit: the normalised likelihood ratio chi-square for the best model (see Method).
Rate: world-standardised truncated rate per 100 000 per year (30-74 years) and number of **deaths** are both estimated from the best-fitting model for the single years cited.
Cumulative risk per 1000 (30-74 years) is estimated from the best-fitting *age-cohort* model for cohorts of central birth year cited.
Recent trend: estimated mean percentage change per five-year period in the age-specific rates (30-74 years) over the period 1975-1988.
Italics denote recent trends not significant at 5 per cent level, or other figures which should be interpreted with caution (see Method).

PANCREAS (ICD-9 157)

EUROPE (EC), MORTALITY

MALES

TRUNCATED RATE (30-74 years)

CUMULATIVE RISK (30-74 years)

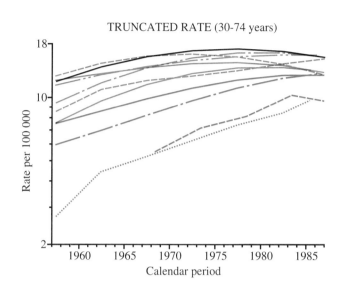
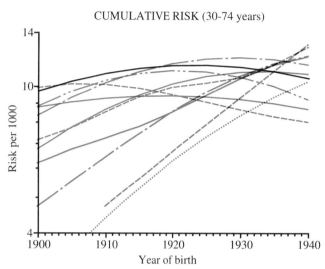

FEMALES

TRUNCATED RATE (30-74 years)

CUMULATIVE RISK (30-74 years)

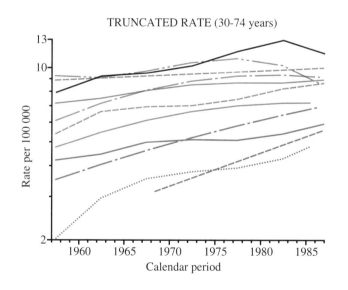
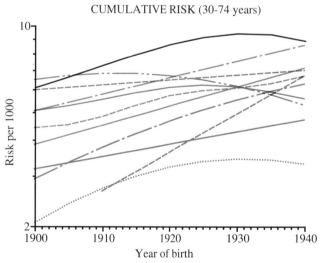

—— FRANCE	—·— NETHERLANDS
----- GREECE	—··— IRELAND
—·— ITALY	—— UK ENGLAND & WALES
·········· SPAIN	----- UK SCOTLAND
—— BELGIUM	—— DENMARK
----- GERMANY (FRG)	

PANCREAS (ICD-9 157)

EUROPE (non-EC), MORTALITY
Percentage change per five-year period, 1975-1988

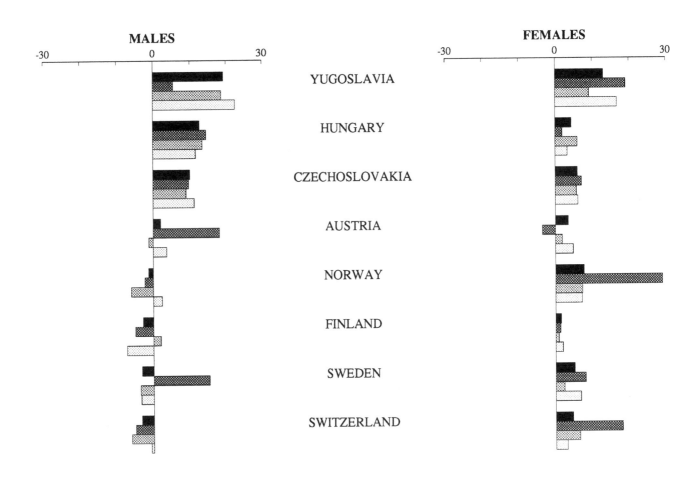

MALES

-30   0   30

FEMALES

-30   0   30

YUGOSLAVIA

HUNGARY

CZECHOSLOVAKIA

AUSTRIA

NORWAY

FINLAND

SWEDEN

SWITZERLAND

30-74
30-44
45-64
65-74

PANCREAS (ICD-9 157)

EUROPE (EC), MORTALITY
Percentage change per five-year period, 1975-1988

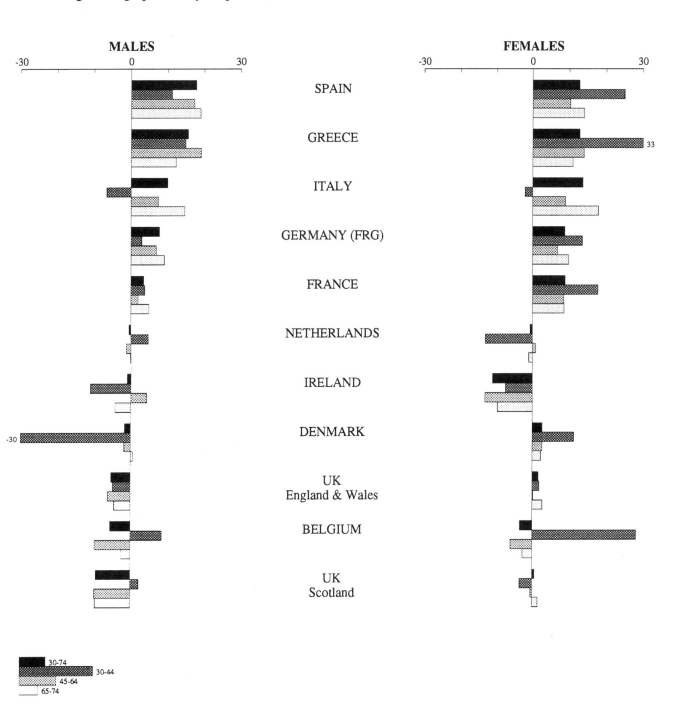

PANCREAS (ICD-9 157)

ASIA, INCIDENCE

MALES	Best model	Goodness of fit	1970 Rate	Cases	1985 Rate	Cases	Cumulative risk 1915	1940	Recent trend
CHINA									
Shanghai	A8D	0.49	*7.2*	*72*	9.3	159	4.7	7.1	11.4
HONG KONG	A2P2C2	0.05	*8.8*	*54*	8.2	93	4.6	8.3	21.7
INDIA									
Bombay	A2P2	1.35	3.6	24	4.5	50	2.5	3.4	14.7
JAPAN									
Miyagi	A2D	2.29	13.8	47	18.0	94	11.0	17.0	18.3
Nagasaki	A1	-0.02	*15.8*	*12*	15.8	16	10.1	10.1	*-4.7*
Osaka	A2P3C2	-1.67	12.5	152	16.4	300	9.3	15.0	20.4
SINGAPORE									
Chinese	A2D	-1.61	6.9	13	9.1	27	5.2	8.4	*9.4*
Indian	A1	-0.96	5.5	1	5.5	2	3.5	3.5	*49.7*
Malay	A1	1.07	4.1	1	4.1	2	2.6	2.6	*52.9*

FEMALES	Best model	Goodness of fit	1970 Rate	Cases	1985 Rate	Cases	Cumulative risk 1915	1940	Recent trend
CHINA									
Shanghai	A2P2	1.88	*2.0*	*22*	8.0	146	4.5	8.3	12.5
HONG KONG	A8C7	-0.25	*2.5*	*17*	4.7	53	2.0	2.2	19.0
INDIA									
Bombay	A2P2	-0.64	1.7	7	2.8	24	1.4	2.9	34.4
JAPAN									
Miyagi	A2C2	0.65	8.0	32	10.1	65	6.8	6.5	15.2
Nagasaki	A2D	0.20	*16.6*	*16*	6.8	9	6.8	1.5	-25.7
Osaka	A2C4	-0.10	5.3	74	8.7	194	5.7	7.1	13.8
SINGAPORE									
Chinese	A2D	0.98	3.3	7	5.8	20	3.1	8.0	20.8
Indian	A2C2	-2.89	*4.1*	*0*	*3.5*	*0*	3.2	0.0	*-55.0*
Malay	A1C4	-1.33	*2.4*	*0*	5.1	1	5.7	1.4	*22.0*

* : not enough cases for reliable estimation
– : incomplete or missing data
Best model: polynomial of the given degree in age (A), period (P) or cohort (C), or linear drift (D) model.
Goodness of fit: the normalised likelihood ratio chi-square for the best model (see Method).
Rate: world-standardised truncated rate per 100 000 per year (30-74 years) and number of **cases** are both estimated from the best-fitting model for the single years cited.
Cumulative risk per 1000 (30-74 years) is estimated from the best-fitting *age-cohort* model for cohorts of central birth year cited.
Recent trend: estimated mean percentage change per five-year period in the age-specific rates (30-74 years) over the period 1973-1987.
Italics denote recent trends not significant at 5 per cent level, or other figures which should be interpreted with caution (see Method).

PANCREAS (ICD-9 157)

ASIA, INCIDENCE

MALES

TRUNCATED RATE (30-74 years)

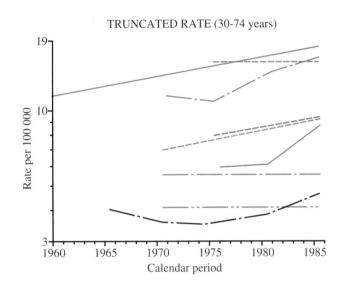

CUMULATIVE RISK (30-74 years)

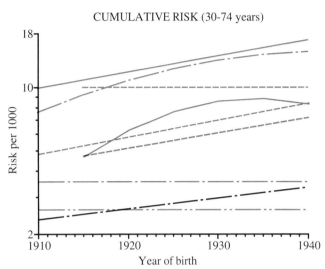

FEMALES

TRUNCATED RATE (30-74 years)

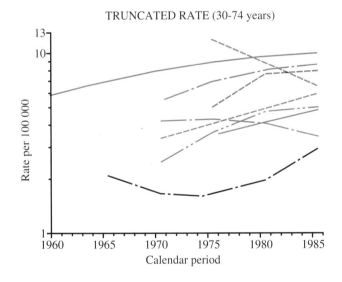

CUMULATIVE RISK (30-74 years)

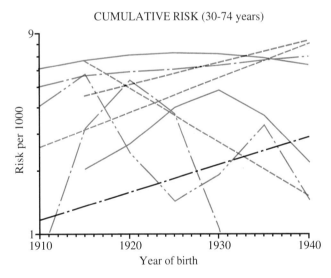

----- CHINA Shanghai
——— JAPAN Miyagi
----- JAPAN Nagasaki
—·—·— JAPAN Osaka
——— HONG KONG

----- SINGAPORE Chinese
—·—·— SINGAPORE Indian
—··—··— SINGAPORE Malay
—··—··— INDIA Bombay

PANCREAS (ICD-9 157)

OCEANIA, INCIDENCE

MALES	Best model	Goodness of fit	1970 Rate	Cases	1985 Rate	Cases	Cumulative risk 1915	1940	Recent trend
AUSTRALIA									
New South Wales	A2D	-0.67	*15.6*	*161*	12.8	172	8.9	6.4	-6.5
South	A2C2	0.67	*17.0*	*37*	11.8	42	11.5	2.1	-15.2
HAWAII									
Caucasian	A2	-0.93	16.0	5	16.0	9	10.2	10.2	*2.2*
Chinese	A1	-1.63	13.1	1	13.1	2	7.9	7.9	*11.9*
Filipino	A3	-0.90	8.7	2	8.7	3	5.6	5.6	*12.4*
Hawaiian	A1D	0.96	27.8	3	18.6	4	14.4	7.3	*3.2*
Japanese	A1	0.05	13.5	6	13.5	12	9.1	9.1	*3.7*
NEW ZEALAND									
Maori	A2D	1.17	29.8	5	21.1	6	15.4	8.7	*-6.6*
Non-Maori	A2P4C2	0.08	13.4	75	12.2	88	9.4	5.5	-10.6

FEMALES	Best model	Goodness of fit	1970 Rate	Cases	1985 Rate	Cases	Cumulative risk 1915	1940	Recent trend
AUSTRALIA									
New South Wales	A2	-1.04	*8.2*	*103*	8.2	122	5.4	5.4	*0.0*
South	A2	-0.57	*7.5*	*12*	7.5	29	5.0	5.0	*0.9*
HAWAII									
Caucasian	A3	1.74	11.9	3	11.9	7	8.1	8.1	*0.3*
Chinese	A1	0.12	10.8	1	10.8	2	7.2	7.2	*-5.4*
Filipino	A1	-0.23	*6.1*	*0*	6.1	1	4.0	4.0	*46.2*
Hawaiian	A1	0.70	15.1	2	15.1	4	10.1	10.1	*-4.7*
Japanese	A1	-1.15	7.6	3	7.6	7	5.2	5.2	*4.8*
NEW ZEALAND									
Maori	A1	-0.13	14.3	2	14.3	4	9.7	9.7	*-1.4*
Non-Maori	A2P3C2	-1.12	7.4	46	8.1	65	5.7	3.9	*-3.6*

* : not enough cases for reliable estimation
– : incomplete or missing data
Best model: polynomial of the given degree in age (A), period (P) or cohort (C), or linear drift (D) model.
Goodness of fit: the normalised likelihood ratio chi-square for the best model (see Method).
Rate: world-standardised truncated rate per 100 000 per year (30-74 years) and number of **cases** are both estimated from the best-fitting model for the single years cited.
Cumulative risk per 1000 (30-74 years) is estimated from the best-fitting *age-cohort* model for cohorts of central birth year cited.
Recent trend: estimated mean percentage change per five-year period in the age-specific rates (30-74 years) over the period 1973-1987.
Italics denote recent trends not significant at 5 per cent level, or other figures which should be interpreted with caution (see Method).

PANCREAS (ICD-9 157)

OCEANIA, INCIDENCE

MALES

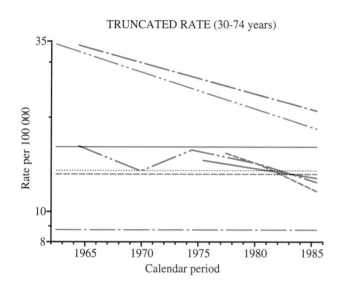

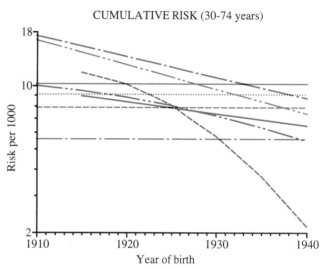

FEMALES

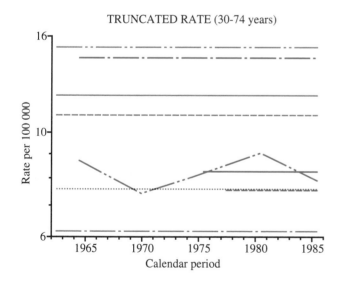

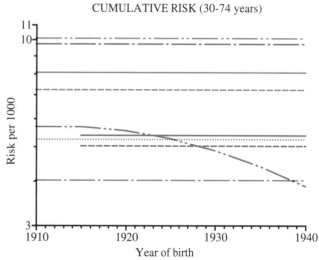

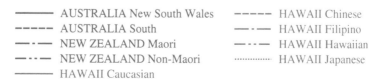

—— AUSTRALIA New South Wales	– – – – HAWAII Chinese
– – – AUSTRALIA South	–·—·— HAWAII Filipino
–·–·– NEW ZEALAND Maori	–··—··– HAWAII Hawaiian
–··–··– NEW ZEALAND Non-Maori	············ HAWAII Japanese
—— HAWAII Caucasian	

PANCREAS (ICD-9 157)

ASIA, INCIDENCE
Percentage change per five-year period, 1973-1987

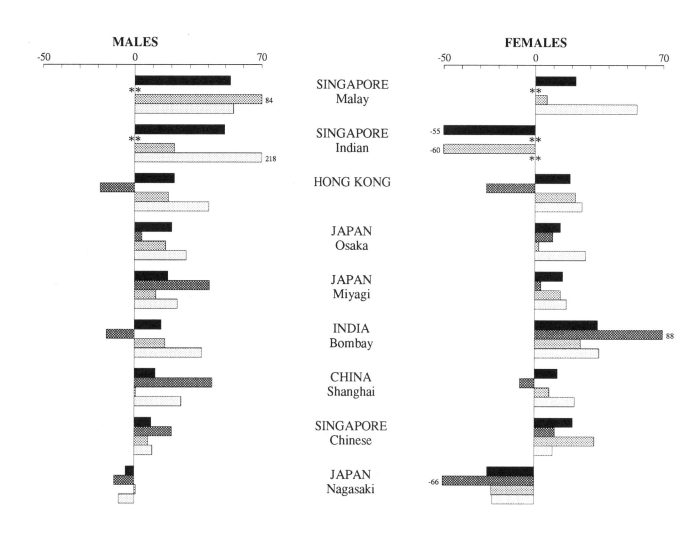

PANCREAS (ICD-9 157)

OCEANIA, INCIDENCE
Percentage change per five-year period, 1973-1987

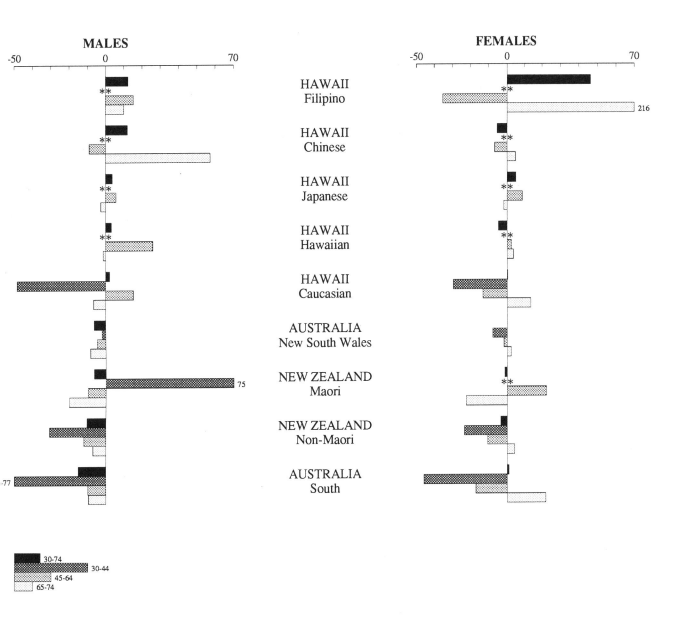

MALES

FEMALES

HAWAII
Filipino

HAWAII
Chinese

HAWAII
Japanese

HAWAII
Hawaiian

HAWAII
Caucasian

AUSTRALIA
New South Wales

NEW ZEALAND
Maori

NEW ZEALAND
Non-Maori

AUSTRALIA
South

30-74
30-44
45-64
65-74

ASIA and OCEANIA, MORTALITY

MALES	Best model	Goodness of fit	1965 Rate	1965 Deaths	1985 Rate	1985 Deaths	Cumulative risk 1900	Cumulative risk 1940	Recent trend
AUSTRALIA	A8P6C9	0.11	12.0	288	12.2	448	8.2	7.6	-7.7
HONG KONG	A2	0.44	*7.8*	*28*	7.8	70	*5.0*	5.0	*-0.6*
JAPAN	A8P6C9	1.71	8.5	1511	14.8	4266	5.3	12.2	9.5
MAURITIUS	A2	1.62	*6.5*	*4*	6.5	7	*4.0*	4.0	*9.6*
NEW ZEALAND	A2P5	-1.19	12.9	68	12.3	91	9.0	9.3	-12.0
SINGAPORE	A2D	-1.32	3.4	6	6.9	19	*1.5*	6.3	–

FEMALES	Best model	Goodness of fit	1965 Rate	1965 Deaths	1985 Rate	1985 Deaths	Cumulative risk 1900	Cumulative risk 1940	Recent trend
AUSTRALIA	A3P4C3	1.55	6.6	177	7.5	312	4.4	4.5	*0.8*
HONG KONG	A2C2	0.54	*3.5*	*17*	5.1	44	*2.1*	3.3	*-3.7*
JAPAN	A2P5C4	2.05	5.3	1054	7.8	2791	3.5	5.2	4.8
MAURITIUS	A1	2.00	*2.8*	*2*	2.8	3	*1.8*	1.8	*45.4*
NEW ZEALAND	A2C4	-0.58	7.3	43	8.1	69	4.6	3.6	*-5.8*
SINGAPORE	A2D	2.54	1.9	3	4.1	12	*0.8*	3.9	–

* : not enough deaths for reliable estimation
– : incomplete or missing data
Best model: polynomial of the given degree in age (A), period (P) or cohort (C), or linear drift (D) model.
Goodness of fit: the normalised likelihood ratio chi-square for the best model (see Method).
Rate: world-standardised truncated rate per 100 000 per year (30-74 years) and number of **deaths** are both estimated from the best-fitting model for the single years cited.
Cumulative risk per 1000 (30-74 years) is estimated from the best-fitting *age-cohort* model for cohorts of central birth year cited.
Recent trend: estimated mean percentage change per five-year period in the age-specific rates (30-74 years) over the period 1975-1988.
Italics denote recent trends not significant at 5 per cent level, or other figures which should be interpreted with caution (see Method).

PANCREAS (ICD-9 157)

ASIA and OCEANIA, MORTALITY

MALES

TRUNCATED RATE (30-74 years)

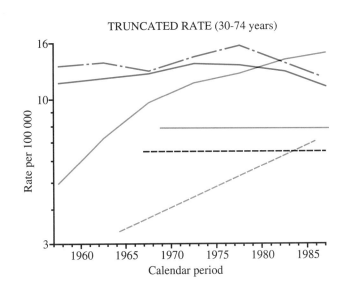

CUMULATIVE RISK (30-74 years)

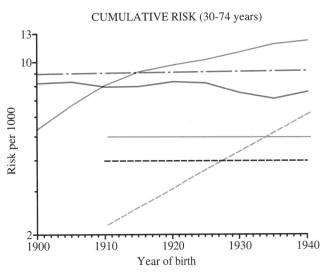

FEMALES

TRUNCATED RATE (30-74 years)

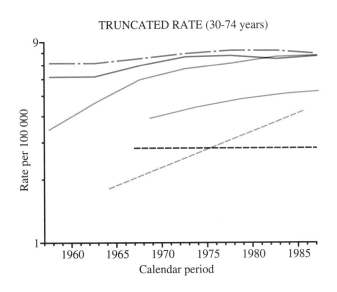

CUMULATIVE RISK (30-74 years)

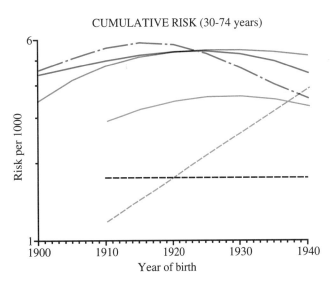

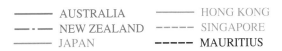

AUSTRALIA   HONG KONG
NEW ZEALAND   SINGAPORE
JAPAN   MAURITIUS

PANCREAS (ICD-9 157)

ASIA and OCEANIA, MORTALITY
Percentage change per five-year period, 1975-1988

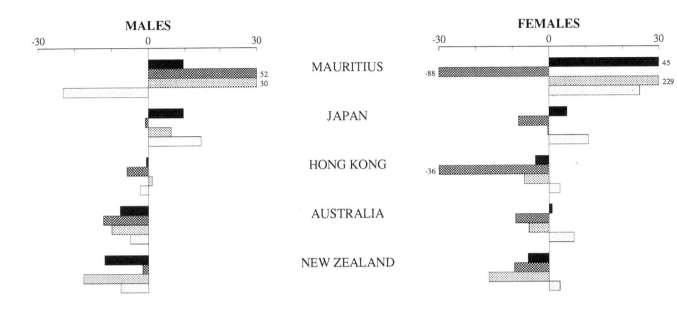

from page 257

thern Ireland. The current patterns of evolution of the cumulative risk suggest that the geographical gradient of pancreatic cancer in Europe will be completely inverted by the end of the first decade of the next century, when the 1940 birth cohort has reached the age of 70-74 years.

Asia and Oceania

The incidence of pancreatic cancer in Asian populations is relatively low on a global scale, but there have been substantial increases in most of the Asian populations examined for both sexes, particularly females. The rate of increase among females in Osaka and Miyagi prefectures (Japan) is now declining, and is likely to slow down further, since the recent increases in risk are due largely to the increase among the elderly. The increases in Japanese males — both in the Japanese prefectures and among Japanese in Hawaii — are also substantial, and mortality from cancer of the pancreas in Japan has also been rising quite quickly in both sexes. Females in the smaller population of Nagasaki provide a striking exception to the overall pattern in Japan, however:

there has been a steady fall in incidence of around 25% every five years since 1973, though the truncated rate of 6 per 100 000 is now similar to that in Osaka and Miyagi. The decline in Nagasaki cannot easily be explained by improved precision of diagnosis and registration, since although fewer than half of the pancreatic cancers were histologically confirmed during the decade 1973-82, there was little change in the levels of confirmation over this period, which were similar to those in Miyagi and Osaka. Mortality from cancer of the pancreas in Japan has risen substantially in both sexes, but is now levelling off, and the two to three-fold difference of 20-30 years ago with respect to mortality in Australia and New Zealand has now disappeared.

The small recent declines in mortality in Australia and New Zealand are more clear among females, and they furnish a good example of how examination of time trends using only cross-sectional data may be potentially misleading. For females in New Zealand, there is little change in the curve of truncated rates for the 30-74 years age range (no period effect) because the large decline in the rate among 30-44 year-olds is balanced by a small increase in the much larger rate among 65-74 year-olds (see histogram); the underlying change is reflected more clearly in the cumulative risk curve, which shows a rise from 4.6 per 1000 for the 1900 birth cohort to a peak of around 6 for the 1920 cohort and a decline to 3.6 per 1000 for the most recent cohort, born around 1940.

The very high incidence among male Maoris in New Zealand and in Hawaiian males in the 1960s, around 30 per 100 000, has fallen by almost half in the last 25 years, and rates similar to those occurring now in these populations (around 15-20 per 100 000), are also occurring among males in the two Japanese prefectures included here, in which incidence rates have been rising steadily over the same period.

Among Australian males and non-Maori males in New-Zealand, the incidence of cancer of the pancreas has been falling steadily by about 10% every five years.

Americas

Striking differences are seen by race, geography and sex for both the levels and the trends of incidence and mortality from cancer of the pancreas in North America. Incidence is higher for both sexes in blacks than in any of the white or mixed-race populations examined in the USA. There is a two- to three-fold range in incidence across Canada and the USA in both sexes, while levels of mortality at the national level are quite similar in the two countries, at around 15 and 10 per 100 000 in males and females, respectively. Examination of the truncated rates shows that mortality is still increasing slowly among females in both countries (more slowly in the USA), while among males it peaked in the 1970s (earlier in the USA), and is now declining; for both males and females, the truncated rates in each country are similar. In both countries, however, there is a clear downward trend in successive birth cohorts, more marked in males than in females, and more in the USA than in Canada, and this is reflected in the cumulative risk curves.

In the USA, the trends in incidence differ considerably by race and region. Incidence is falling slightly among black males, but increasing for black females, significantly so in Detroit. The trend in white females in Detroit is significantly upward (12% every five years), while among white females in New Orleans it is downward (15%). Incidence is still generally increasing in Canada, particularly in Quebec.

Incidence and mortality from cancer of the pancreas are several-fold lower in the South American populations for which data have been examined than in North America. Incidence is stable in Cuba and Puerto Rico, and falling in Cali (Colombia).

Comment

There is a general increase in cancer of the pancreas in European populations, but this is much less marked in North America. Previous analysis of incidence trends in the USA has suggested little continuing increase after the mid-1970s, when most of the data sets examined here became available. The slight decline in mortality from around 1970 was also noted[77]. At least part of the earlier increase was attributed to improvements in diagnosis and histological confirmation. The age-specific trends continue to suggest an imminent decline in age-adjusted mortality among US females. Increasing mortality from cancer of the pancreas in several developed countries up to 1976 has been attributed in part to improvement in diagnosis, especially of cancers that might previously have been assigned to the stomach[198]; the similarity with trends in mortality from colorectal cancers was also noted.

Incidence increased in Czechoslovakia at about 16% and 12% every five years in males and females, respectively, between 1968 and 1985[80], in line with mortality trends reported here. An increase in mortality from pancreatic cancer in the age range 40-84 years has also been noted for Taiwan in the period 1971-86[158], but there was a decline in risk for cohorts born after 1926.

PANCREAS (ICD-9 157)

AMERICAS (except USA), INCIDENCE

MALES	Best model	Goodness of fit	1970 Rate	1970 Cases	1985 Rate	1985 Cases	Cumulative risk 1915	Cumulative risk 1940	Recent trend
BRAZIL									
Sao Paulo	A1D	0.03	8.0	41	*14.8*	*94*	5.7	*16.0*	–
CANADA									
Alberta	A2D	1.01	12.7	38	15.9	70	9.6	14.0	*6.9*
British Columbia	A2D	0.26	16.0	74	14.3	103	9.6	7.9	*-0.7*
Maritime Provinces	A2P2	1.08	18.4	59	15.1	55	9.1	8.4	10.7
Newfoundland	A1	1.04	12.1	10	12.1	14	8.3	8.3	*8.0*
Quebec	A2C2	0.33	10.9	117	17.8	257	10.3	18.4	23.5
COLOMBIA									
Cali	A2	0.56	7.2	4	7.2	9	4.6	4.6	*-8.9*
CUBA	A2	3.24	8.1	119	8.1	168	5.4	*5.4*	–
PUERTO RICO	A2	-0.59	8.8	40	8.8	61	5.6	5.6	*-1.5*

FEMALES	Best model	Goodness of fit	1970 Rate	1970 Cases	1985 Rate	1985 Cases	Cumulative risk 1915	Cumulative risk 1940	Recent trend
BRAZIL									
Sao Paulo	A4	0.97	6.0	38	*6.0*	*52*	3.0	*3.0*	–
CANADA									
Alberta	A2D	1.44	7.8	22	10.3	49	6.3	10.0	15.7
British Columbia	A2	-1.45	9.8	47	9.8	80	6.4	6.4	*-2.3*
Maritime Provinces	A2P2C3	-0.35	8.1	27	9.7	40	5.4	7.8	19.6
Newfoundland	A1C3	-1.33	6.0	5	8.2	9	5.3	4.3	*5.8*
Quebec	A2D	-0.49	6.1	74	10.5	182	6.0	14.7	23.8
COLOMBIA									
Cali	A2C2	0.94	6.3	5	6.9	10	5.0	2.6	*20.2*
CUBA	A2	0.01	5.3	65	5.3	110	3.6	*3.6*	–
PUERTO RICO	A2C2	1.52	5.2	23	5.4	43	3.8	2.8	*7.9*

* : not enough cases for reliable estimation
– : incomplete or missing data
Best model: polynomial of the given degree in age (A), period (P) or cohort (C), or linear drift (D) model.
Goodness of fit: the normalised likelihood ratio chi-square for the best model (see Method).
Rate: world-standardised truncated rate per 100 000 per year (30-74 years) and number of **cases** are both estimated from the best-fitting model for the single years cited.
Cumulative risk per 1000 (30-74 years) is estimated from the best-fitting *age-cohort* model for cohorts of central birth year cited.
Recent trend: estimated mean percentage change per five-year period in the age-specific rates (30-74 years) over the period 1973-1987.
Italics denote recent trends not significant at 5 per cent level, or other figures which should be interpreted with caution (see Method).

PANCREAS (ICD-9 157)

AMERICAS (except USA), INCIDENCE

MALES

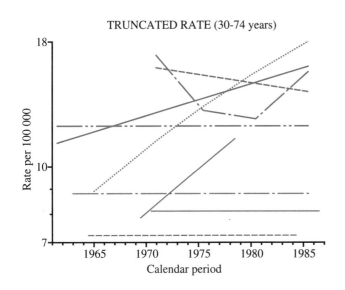

TRUNCATED RATE (30-74 years)

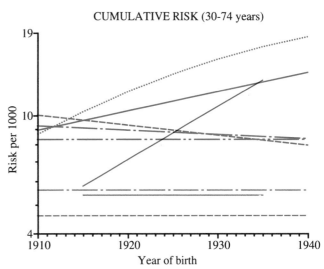

CUMULATIVE RISK (30-74 years)

FEMALES

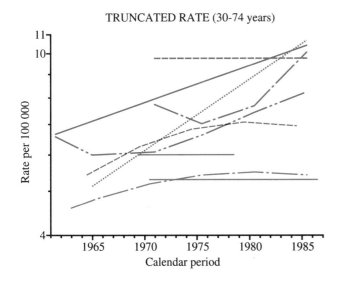

TRUNCATED RATE (30-74 years)

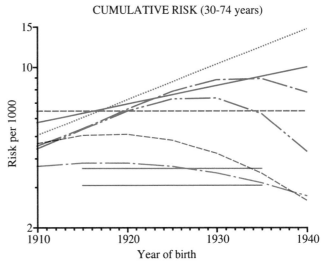

CUMULATIVE RISK (30-74 years)

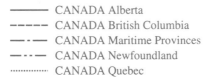

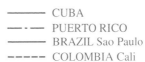

CANADA Alberta
CANADA British Columbia
CANADA Maritime Provinces
CANADA Newfoundland
CANADA Quebec
CUBA
PUERTO RICO
BRAZIL Sao Paulo
COLOMBIA Cali

PANCREAS (ICD-9 157)

AMERICAS (USA), INCIDENCE

MALES	Best model	Goodness of fit	1970 Rate	1970 Cases	1985 Rate	1985 Cases	Cumulative risk 1915	Cumulative risk 1940	Recent trend
USA									
Bay Area, Black	A2	0.13	28.7	14	28.7	23	18.6	18.6	-13.9
Bay Area, Chinese	A2	-0.46	14.4	3	*14.4*	*7*	8.8	*8.8*	–
Bay Area, White	A2D	0.21	18.1	107	15.3	97	10.6	8.0	-6.7
Connecticut	A2	1.25	15.7	103	15.7	127	10.1	10.1	-5.7
Detroit, Black	A2	0.15	24.0	32	24.0	42	14.7	14.7	*-4.0*
Detroit, White	A3	0.14	16.5	121	16.5	119	10.6	10.6	*3.0*
Iowa	A2D	1.36	15.4	105	14.9	106	9.6	9.1	*-2.1*
New Orleans, Black	A2	-1.76	*24.2*	*12*	24.2	14	14.7	14.7	*-10.8*
New Orleans, White	A2	1.20	*17.7*	*25*	17.7	27	11.2	11.2	*-8.6*
Seattle	A2	0.04	*14.7*	*70*	14.7	99	9.3	9.3	*-5.7*

FEMALES	Best model	Goodness of fit	1970 Rate	1970 Cases	1985 Rate	1985 Cases	Cumulative risk 1915	Cumulative risk 1940	Recent trend
USA									
Bay Area, Black	A2	1.01	18.5	10	18.5	18	11.4	11.4	*15.6*
Bay Area, Chinese	A1	-1.16	9.1	1	*9.1*	*5*	6.3	*6.3*	–
Bay Area, White	A2	-0.77	11.9	86	11.9	89	7.9	7.9	*0.7*
Connecticut	A8P5C9	0.27	10.9	85	11.4	113	7.6	5.9	*2.9*
Detroit, Black	A2D	0.17	14.5	20	18.4	40	10.7	16.0	*6.5*
Detroit, White	A2D	1.52	9.9	83	11.8	104	7.3	9.7	11.8
Iowa	A2	0.60	8.5	69	8.5	73	5.6	5.6	*-2.8*
New Orleans, Black	A2	-0.90	*13.7*	*8*	13.7	10	8.9	8.9	*21.3*
New Orleans, White	A2D	0.53	*15.4*	*30*	9.3	18	7.3	3.2	-15.4
Seattle	A2	1.82	*10.8*	*62*	10.8	82	6.9	6.9	*8.0*

* : not enough cases for reliable estimation
– : incomplete or missing data
Best model: polynomial of the given degree in age (A), period (P) or cohort (C), or linear drift (D) model.
Goodness of fit: the normalised likelihood ratio chi-square for the best model (see Method).
Rate: world-standardised truncated rate per 100 000 per year (30-74 years) and number of **cases** are both estimated from the best-fitting model for the single years cited.
Cumulative risk per 1000 (30-74 years) is estimated from the best-fitting *age-cohort* model for cohorts of central birth year cited.
Recent trend: estimated mean percentage change per five-year period in the age-specific rates (30-74 years) over the period 1973-1987.
Italics denote recent trends not significant at 5 per cent level, or other figures which should be interpreted with caution (see Method).

PANCREAS (ICD-9 157)

AMERICAS (USA), INCIDENCE

MALES

TRUNCATED RATE (30-74 years)

CUMULATIVE RISK (30-74 years)

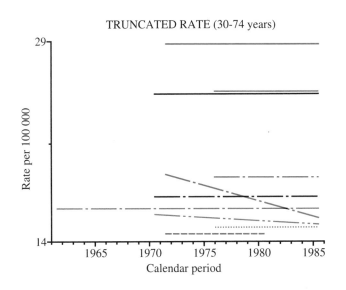
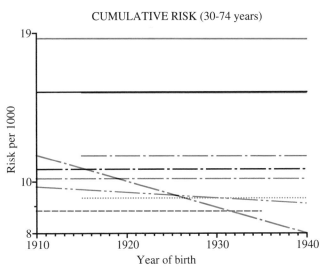

FEMALES

TRUNCATED RATE (30-74 years)

CUMULATIVE RISK (30-74 years)

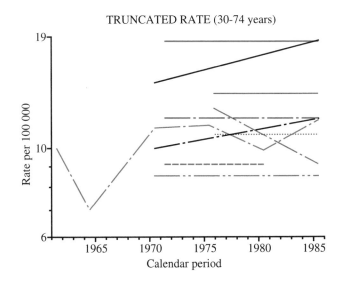
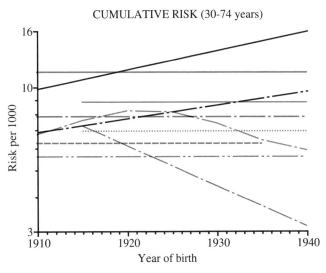

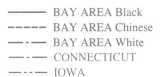

——— BAY AREA Black	·········· SEATTLE
------- BAY AREA Chinese	——— NEW ORLEANS Black
—·—·— BAY AREA White	—··—··— NEW ORLEANS White
—··—··— CONNECTICUT	——— DETROIT Black
—···—···— IOWA	—··—··— DETROIT White

PANCREAS (ICD-9 157)

AMERICAS (except USA), INCIDENCE
Percentage change per five-year period, 1973-1987

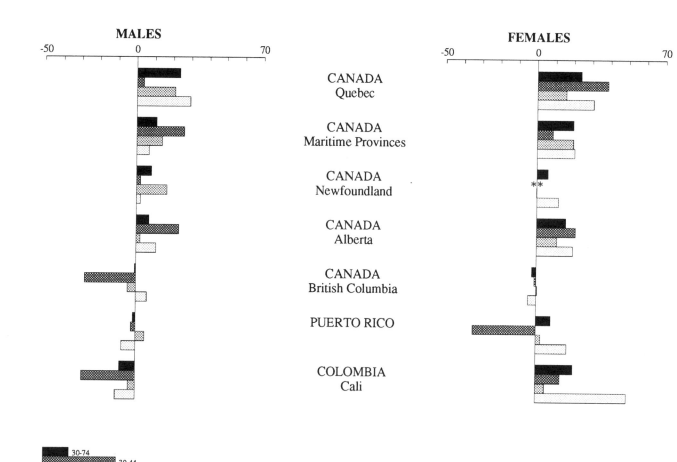

MALES

FEMALES

CANADA
Quebec

CANADA
Maritime Provinces

CANADA
Newfoundland

CANADA
Alberta

CANADA
British Columbia

PUERTO RICO

COLOMBIA
Cali

30-74
30-44
45-64
65-74

284

PANCREAS (ICD-9 157)

AMERICAS (USA), INCIDENCE
Percentage change per five-year period, 1973-1987

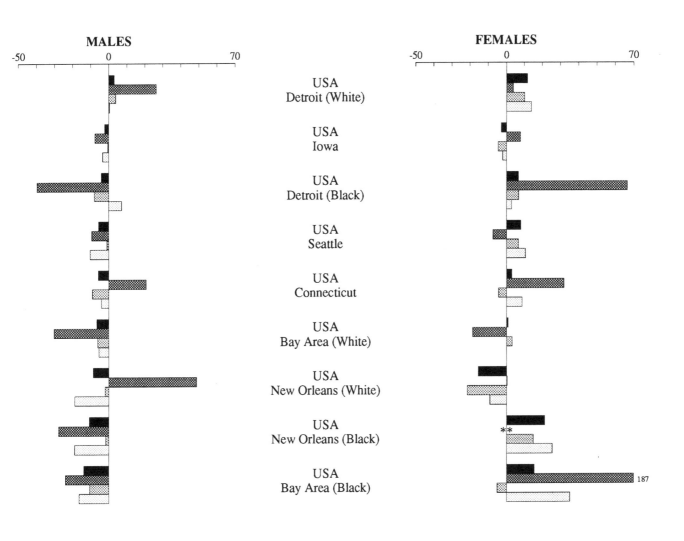

MALES

FEMALES

-50　　0　　70

-50　　0　　70

USA
Detroit (White)

USA
Iowa

USA
Detroit (Black)

USA
Seattle

USA
Connecticut

USA
Bay Area (White)

USA
New Orleans (White)

USA
New Orleans (Black)

USA
Bay Area (Black)

187

30-74
30-44
45-64
65-74

PANCREAS (ICD-9 157)

AMERICAS, MORTALITY

MALES	Best model	Goodness of fit	1965 Rate	1965 Deaths	1985 Rate	1985 Deaths	Cumulative risk 1900	Cumulative risk 1940	Recent trend
CANADA	A3P2C4	-1.94	15.4	584	15.2	892	10.1	9.6	-3.0
CHILE	A2D	0.92	6.7	77	*10.1*	*180*	4.2	*9.5*	–
COSTA RICA	–	–	–	–	–	–	–	–	–
PANAMA	–	–	–	–	–	–	–	–	–
PUERTO RICO	–	–	–	–	–	–	–	–	–
URUGUAY	–	–	–	–	–	–	–	–	–
USA	A3P5C6	2.59	16.1	6848	13.8	7806	10.3	7.2	-6.0
VENEZUELA	A2C2	-0.12	5.1	42	*7.2*	*109*	3.3	*5.1*	–

FEMALES	Best model	Goodness of fit	1965 Rate	1965 Deaths	1985 Rate	1985 Deaths	Cumulative risk 1900	Cumulative risk 1940	Recent trend
CANADA	A3C2	0.00	8.6	339	9.6	648	5.7	6.5	*-0.2*
CHILE	A2C2	1.84	6.2	77	*6.9*	*142*	4.3	2.9	–
COSTA RICA	–	–	–	–	–	–	–	–	–
PANAMA	–	–	–	–	–	–	–	–	–
PUERTO RICO	–	–	–	–	–	–	–	–	–
URUGUAY	–	–	–	–	–	–	–	–	–
USA	A3P5C4	0.06	9.0	4399	9.3	6385	5.8	5.3	*0.9*
VENEZUELA	A2D	-0.15	4.2	37	*5.8*	*98*	2.7	*5.1*	–

* : not enough deaths for reliable estimation
– : incomplete or missing data
Best model: polynomial of the given degree in age (A), period (P) or cohort (C), or linear drift (D) model.
Goodness of fit: the normalised likelihood ratio chi-square for the best model (see Method).
Rate: world-standardised truncated rate per 100 000 per year (30-74 years) and number of **deaths** are both estimated from the best-fitting model for the single years cited.
Cumulative risk per 1000 (30-74 years) is estimated from the best-fitting *age-cohort* model for cohorts of central birth year cited.
Recent trend: estimated mean percentage change per five-year period in the age-specific rates (30-74 years) over the period 1975-1988.
Italics denote recent trends not significant at 5 per cent level, or other figures which should be interpreted with caution (see Method).

PANCREAS (ICD-9 157)

AMERICAS, MORTALITY

MALES

TRUNCATED RATE (30-74 years)

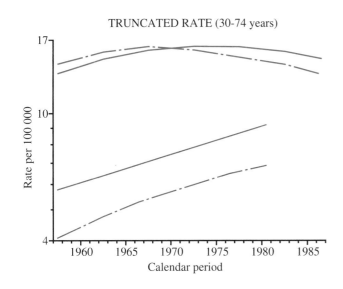

CUMULATIVE RISK (30-74 years)

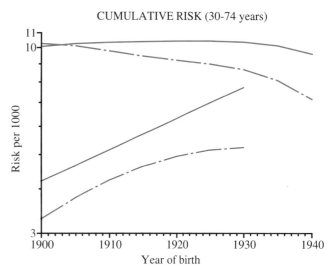

FEMALES

TRUNCATED RATE (30-74 years)

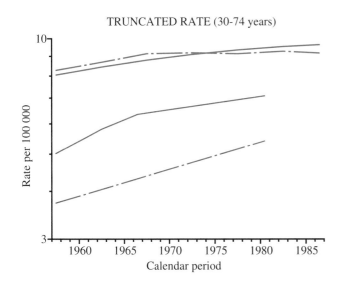

CUMULATIVE RISK (30-74 years)

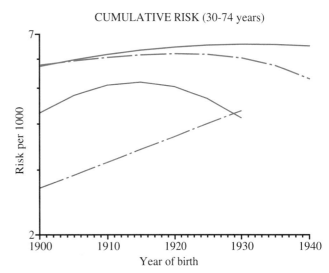

———— CANADA
—·—·— USA
———— CHILE
—··—··— VENEZUELA

PANCREAS (ICD-9 157)

AMERICAS, MORTALITY
Percentage change per five-year period, 1975-1988

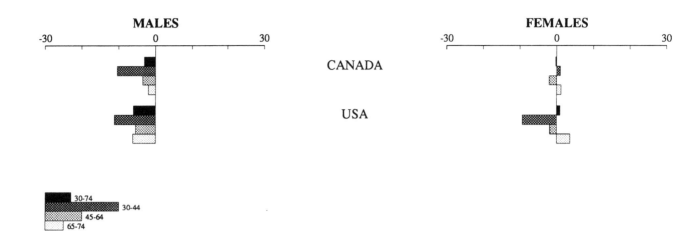

Chapter 13

LARYNX (MALES)

Cancer of the larynx is generally uncommon in males, and so rare in females that trends are not reported here. There were an estimated 120 000 new cases a year world-wide around 1980, with a male-to-female ratio of 6.5[219]. The lifetime risk (30-74 years) of larynx cancer in males was less than 1% in most countries for the generation born in 1915. The main exceptions arise in Italy, Spain and France, and among blacks in the San Francisco Bay Area (USA), where the risk was more than 1.5%. In Hungary, Warsaw City (Poland), Geneva (Switzerland), Hong Kong, Bombay (India), São Paulo (Brazil), Quebec (Canada), Cuba and among Caucasians in Hawaii, and in New Orleans and in black populations in the USA, the lifetime risk for the 1915 cohort was 1% or more.

The descriptive study of cancer of the larynx is complicated by the difficulty in distinguishing clinically between tumours of the supraglottis or epilarynx (ICD-9 161.1) and those of the hypopharynx (ICD-9 148), and by the international variation in the proportion of cancers of the glottis or endolarynx (including vocal cords) among all cancers of the larynx[289]. Survival from cancer of the endolarynx is fair (more than 50% at five years), whereas survival from cancer of the upper part of the larynx is poor, and similar to survival from cancer of the pharynx. As a consequence, mortality data for cancer of the larynx are difficult to interpret, the more so because cancer of the hypopharynx may be attributed to cancer of the larynx on the death certificate.

Tobacco smoking and alcohol are known risk factors for laryngeal cancer, and the two factors have a multiplicative effect[96]. The effect of alcohol is greater for cancers of the epilarynx. Overall mortality from larynx cancer is thus more closely related to alcohol than to tobacco consumption, and an increase or decrease in alcohol consumption is usually followed by a corresponding change in mortality from larynx cancer[288].

Europe

One striking feature of the trend in incidence of laryngeal cancer is the increase in the two Hungarian populations. The truncated rate has increased by more than three-fold over 20 years in County Vas, and by more than two-fold over 15 years in Szabolcs-Szatmar. The trends suggest that the risk

(30-74 years) for males born since 1940 in these areas will be more than 2.5%. The increase has also been substantial in Poland, Romania and Slovenia.

A second striking feature is the impressive decrease in risk which has occurred in successive birth cohorts in Finland; the lifetime risk for the 1915 birth cohort (about 8 per 1000) was six times that now estimated for the 1940 birth cohort. These two features of laryngeal cancer trends in Europe are consistent with trends in tobacco smoking, and with trends in the incidence of both lung cancer and cancers of the buccal cavity, pharynx and oesophagus. The marked increase in alcohol consumption in Finland up to 1985[116,189] appears to be at variance with the declines in alcohol-related cancers in this country. The risk for cancer of the larynx in Scandinavian countries was 3- to 5-fold less than in Finland for the 1910 cohort, but it has risen substantially; the increase has tended to stabilise in Sweden and Denmark. Incidence in Denmark is now higher than in Finland, and the lifetime risk for Danish males in the 1940 birth cohort now exceeds the risk seen in the 1915 cohort in Finland. The sudden change which occurred around 1975 in Sweden is difficult to explain. In Norway, the increase in incidence continues at around 12% every five years.

The 3- to 4-fold difference in incidence between Latin and English populations has not changed over the last 20 years. The risk in England is declining in successive cohorts born since 1925-30, but there is a strong suggestion of increasing risk in Scotland and Germany. The recent age-specific incidence trends in France and in Italy, although not significant, suggest a decreasing risk, which would be consistent with trends in other alcohol-related cancers and with the decrease in alcohol consumption in these countries[189].

The trends in mortality from cancer of the larynx are consistent with the high incidence in south-western Europe and with the decrease in Finland. The relationships between the trends in incidence and mortality in Norway and Sweden are not entirely consistent. A decline in recorded mortality has occurred in Norway, where incidence is increasing, and it is unlikely that this could be explained by better treatment in Norway than in Sweden and Denmark. The incidence-to-mortality ratio in 1985 was higher in Norway than in Finland, Sweden or Denmark. It is nevertheless possible that trends in survival depend in part on the aetiological factors responsible for the trend in incidence; survival trends

continued page 303

LARYNX (ICD-9 161)

EUROPE (non-EC), INCIDENCE

MALES	Best model	Goodness of fit	1970 Rate	1970 Cases	1985 Rate	1985 Cases	Cumulative risk 1915	Cumulative risk 1940	Recent trend
FINLAND	A5P3C5	0.48	13.9	141	9.0	106	7.8	1.3	-12.2
HUNGARY									
County Vas	A2P3	1.25	17.5	13	26.0	18	10.3	30.0	19.1
Szabolcs-Szatmar	A2C3	-1.22	11.8	15	24.7	34	8.4	25.6	24.3
ISRAEL									
All Jews	A3P2	0.26	12.0	56	9.5	54	6.4	5.4	-8.7
Non-Jews	A2C3	0.42	11.1	3	9.1	5	5.3	3.5	*-16.0*
NORWAY	A2D	-1.48	4.9	53	7.6	88	3.8	8.0	11.9
POLAND									
Warsaw City	A3P3	-0.37	13.5	38	22.6	90	11.9	18.6	*-4.0*
ROMANIA									
Cluj	A2C3	1.55	*27.3*	*42*	17.4	31	6.8	19.7	*7.9*
SWEDEN	A8P5C9	0.26	5.0	121	5.2	133	3.2	3.1	*-1.9*
SWITZERLAND									
Geneva	A2	-0.56	19.5	14	19.5	18	10.8	10.8	*-9.1*
YUGOSLAVIA									
Slovenia	A8P5C9	0.64	15.2	56	19.0	83	7.1	18.5	8.8

* : not enough cases for reliable estimation
– : incomplete or missing data
Best model: polynomial of the given degree in age (A), period (P) or cohort (C), or linear drift (D) model.
Goodness of fit: the normalised likelihood ratio chi-square for the best model (see Method).
Rate: world-standardised truncated rate per 100 000 per year (30-74 years) and number of **cases** are both estimated from the best-fitting model for the single years cited.
Cumulative risk per 1000 (30-74 years) is estimated from the best-fitting *age-cohort* model for cohorts of central birth year cited.
Recent trend: estimated mean percentage change per five-year period in the age-specific rates (30-74 years) over the period 1973-1987.
Italics denote recent trends not significant at 5 per cent level, or other figures which should be interpreted with caution (see Method).

MALES

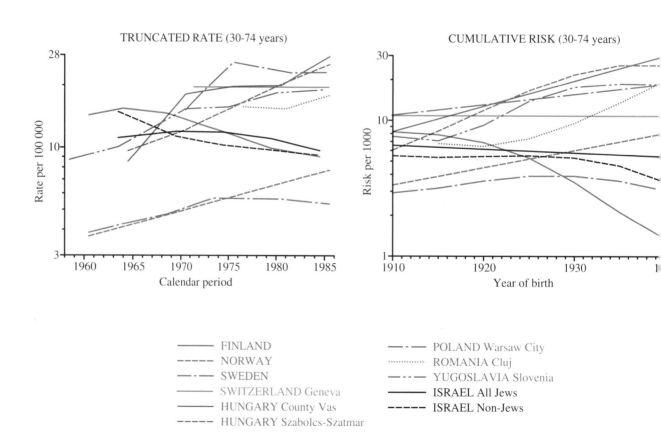

TRUNCATED RATE (30-74 years)

CUMULATIVE RISK (30-74 years)

——— FINLAND
- - - - - NORWAY
—·— SWEDEN
——— SWITZERLAND Geneva
——— HUNGARY County Vas
- - - - - HUNGARY Szabolcs-Szatmar
—·— POLAND Warsaw City
·········· ROMANIA Cluj
—··— YUGOSLAVIA Slovenia
——— ISRAEL All Jews
- - - - - ISRAEL Non-Jews

LARYNX (ICD-9 161)

EUROPE (non-EC), INCIDENCE
Percentage change per five-year period, 1973-1987

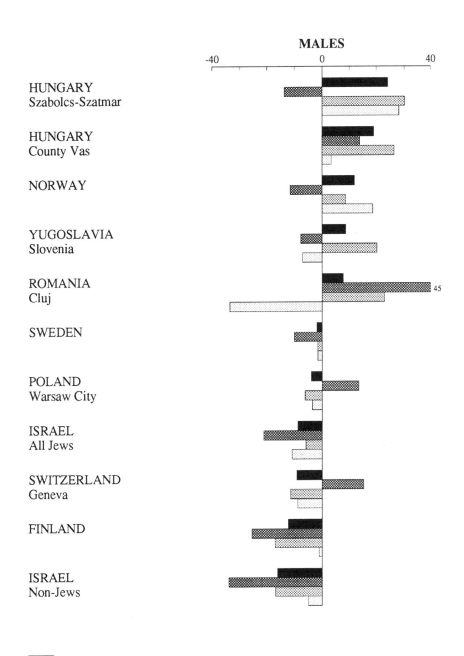

LARYNX (ICD-9 161)

EUROPE (EC), INCIDENCE

MALES	Best model	Goodness of fit	1970 Rate	Cases	1985 Rate	Cases	Cumulative risk 1915	1940	Recent trend
DENMARK	A8P6C9	-0.08	8.9	117	13.0	181	6.0	8.0	14.8
FRANCE									
Bas-Rhin	A3	-0.94	*26.9*	*57*	26.9	54	14.7	14.7	*7.3*
Doubs	A3	-0.14	*27.5*	*21*	27.5	29	15.2	15.2	*-15.4*
GERMANY (FRG)									
Hamburg	A2P2	0.20	9.6	51	*3.6*	*13*	4.6	2.9	–
Saarland	A4C2	-0.33	17.1	48	16.5	45	8.3	13.1	*3.2*
GERMANY (GDR)	A3P3	3.44	10.5	441	11.4	424	6.2	8.1	*1.7*
ITALY									
Varese	A2	-0.61	*34.0*	*51*	34.0	69	19.2	19.2	*-5.1*
SPAIN									
Navarra	A8C7	-1.04	*30.3*	*34*	38.9	52	16.1	18.3	11.5
Zaragoza	A2P3	0.21	27.8	51	35.1	80	15.7	29.1	22.6
UK									
Birmingham	A2C3	1.43	8.0	108	8.6	127	5.2	4.4	*1.2*
Scotland	A3D	-0.03	7.6	103	10.8	147	5.7	10.1	16.7
South Thames	A8C9	0.33	7.1	177	6.9	129	4.1	3.1	*-0.2*

* : not enough cases for reliable estimation
– : incomplete or missing data
Best model: polynomial of the given degree in age (A), period (P) or cohort (C), or linear drift (D) model.
Goodness of fit: the normalised likelihood ratio chi-square for the best model (see Method).
Rate: world-standardised truncated rate per 100 000 per year (30-74 years) and number of **cases** are both estimated from the best-fitting model for the single years cited.
Cumulative risk per 1000 (30-74 years) is estimated from the best-fitting *age-cohort* model for cohorts of central birth year cited.
Recent trend: estimated mean percentage change per five-year period in the age-specific rates (30-74 years) over the period 1973-1987.
Italics denote recent trends not significant at 5 per cent level, or other figures which should be interpreted with caution (see Method).

MALES

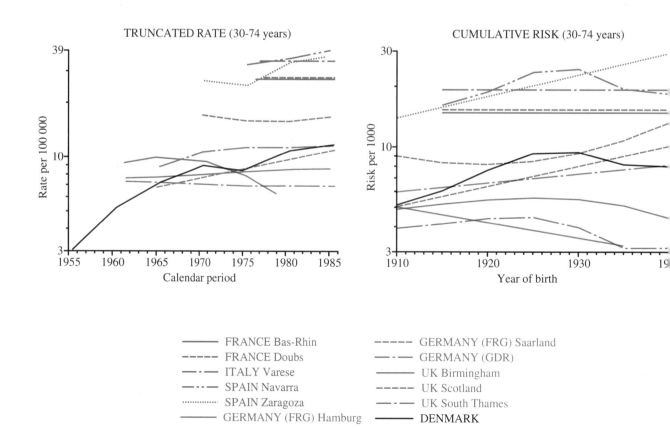

LARYNX (ICD-9 161)

EUROPE (EC), INCIDENCE
Percentage change per five-year period, 1973-1987

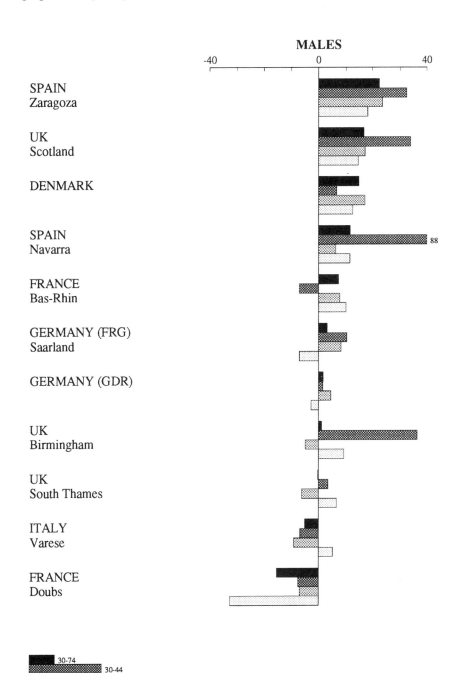

LARYNX (ICD-9 161)

EUROPE (non-EC), MORTALITY

MALES	Best model	Goodness of fit	1965 Rate	1965 Deaths	1985 Rate	1985 Deaths	Cumulative risk 1900	Cumulative risk 1940	Recent trend
AUSTRIA	A3P4C8	3.83	7.2	146	7.4	135	4.8	9.1	*-0.7*
CZECHOSLOVAKIA	A8P6C9	-0.01	6.1	216	10.4	370	4.1	15.5	14.0
FINLAND	A8P6C9	-0.37	6.0	55	3.7	43	4.1	0.7	-12.7
HUNGARY	A3P6C8	2.51	7.7	202	14.6	399	5.6	21.7	15.1
NORWAY	A2P2C2	-0.95	1.4	14	1.9	23	1.0	0.7	*4.8*
POLAND	A5P5C7	1.53	6.6	395	14.1	1098	3.3	20.7	22.0
ROMANIA	A4C5	4.44	10.9	437	*10.8*	*575*	6.7	6.9	–
SWEDEN	A2D	1.14	1.1	25	1.4	39	0.7	1.3	*-2.5*
SWITZERLAND	A2P3	3.34	6.1	87	4.8	83	4.0	2.7	-14.8
YUGOSLAVIA	A5P3C4	3.68	7.5	269	12.9	646	4.7	12.7	5.2

* : not enough deaths for reliable estimation
– : incomplete or missing data
Best model: polynomial of the given degree in age (A), period (P) or cohort (C), or linear drift (D) model.
Goodness of fit: the normalised likelihood ratio chi-square for the best model (see Method).
Rate: world-standardised truncated rate per 100 000 per year (30-74 years) and number of **deaths** are both estimated from the best-fitting model for the single years cited.
Cumulative risk per 1000 (30-74 years) is estimated from the best-fitting *age-cohort* model for cohorts of central birth year cited.
Recent trend: estimated mean percentage change per five-year period in the age-specific rates (30-74 years) over the period 1975-1988.
Italics denote recent trends not significant at 5 per cent level, or other figures which should be interpreted with caution (see Method).

MALES

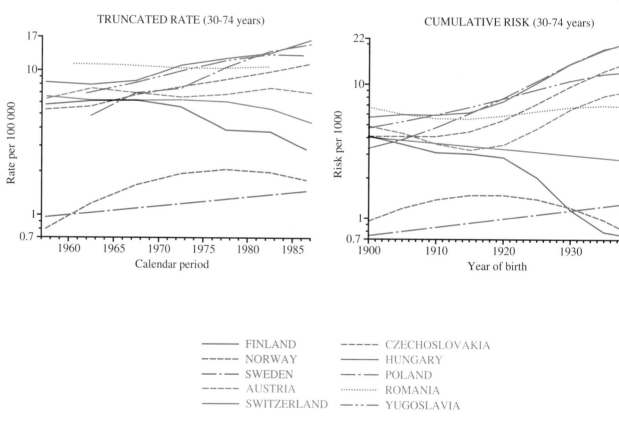

294

LARYNX (ICD-9 161)

EUROPE (non-EC), MORTALITY
Percentage change per five-year period, 1975-1988

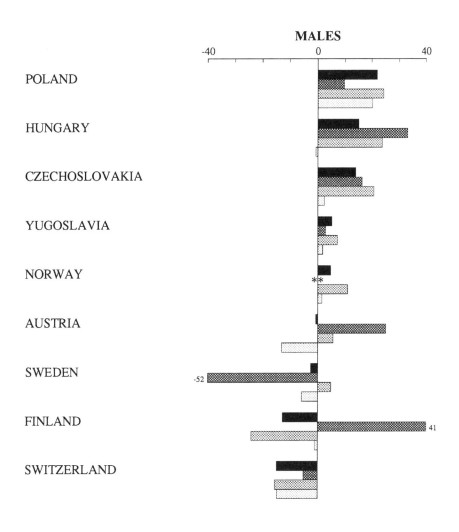

LARYNX (ICD-9 161)

EUROPE (EC), MORTALITY

MALES	Best model	Goodness of fit	1965		1985		Cumulative risk		Recent trend
			Rate	Deaths	Rate	Deaths	1900	1940	
BELGIUM	A3P3C3	0.01	9.4	247	8.9	240	5.8	7.0	*-3.9*
DENMARK	A2D	0.35	2.4	31	4.6	66	1.5	5.4	17.1
FRANCE	A4P6C8	12.95	23.4	2870	18.9	2579	14.2	11.5	-13.7
GERMANY (FRG)	A4P5C6	4.97	4.1	636	5.2	832	2.9	8.6	9.3
GREECE	A2C2	2.36	8.2	155	6.5	182	*5.4*	2.5	-10.7
IRELAND	A2P2C4	0.17	3.9	29	5.0	39	2.6	4.0	*9.7*
ITALY	A4P2C7	3.39	11.6	1413	12.7	1961	7.3	6.8	-4.3
NETHERLANDS	A2P2	0.77	3.0	84	3.1	110	2.0	2.4	*-4.9*
PORTUGAL	A3P5	0.17	11.8	215	12.6	315	6.3	7.2	*0.8*
SPAIN	A3P4C4	2.22	14.4	993	14.3	1371	8.4	9.7	-3.3
UK ENGLAND & WALES	A8P6C9	0.85	3.4	442	3.1	460	2.5	2.1	*2.3*
UK SCOTLAND	A3C4	-0.18	3.7	48	3.4	47	2.5	2.7	*4.6*

* : not enough deaths for reliable estimation
− : incomplete or missing data
Best model: polynomial of the given degree in age (A), period (P) or cohort (C), or linear drift (D) model.
Goodness of fit: the normalised likelihood ratio chi-square for the best model (see Method).
Rate: world-standardised truncated rate per 100 000 per year (30-74 years) and number of **deaths** are both estimated from the best-fitting model for the single years cited.
Cumulative risk per 1000 (30-74 years) is estimated from the best-fitting *age-cohort* model for cohorts of central birth year cited.
Recent trend: estimated mean percentage change per five-year period in the age-specific rates (30-74 years) over the period 1975-1988.
Italics denote recent trends not significant at 5 per cent level, or other figures which should be interpreted with caution (see Method).

MALES

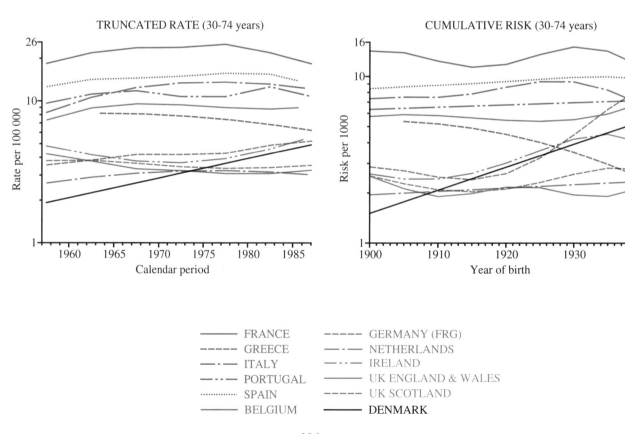

LARYNX (ICD-9 161)

EUROPE (EC), MORTALITY
Percentage change per five-year period, 1975-1988

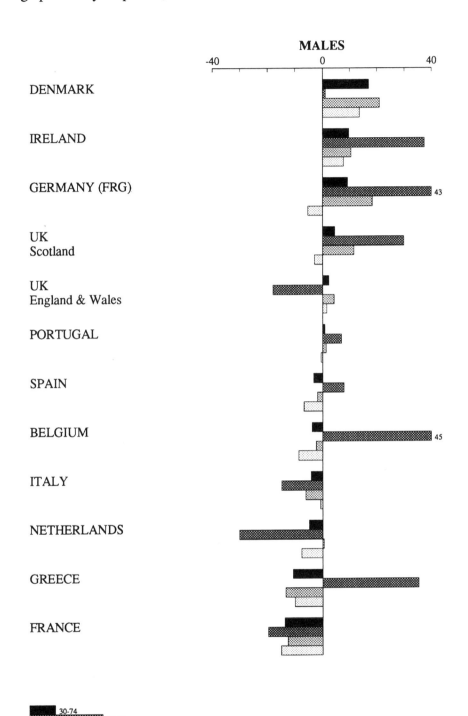

MALES

DENMARK

IRELAND

GERMANY (FRG)   43

UK
Scotland

UK
England & Wales

PORTUGAL

SPAIN

BELGIUM   45

ITALY

NETHERLANDS

GREECE

FRANCE

30-74
30-44
45-64
65-74

LARYNX (ICD-9 161)

ASIA, INCIDENCE

MALES	Best model	Goodness of fit	1970 Rate	1970 Cases	1985 Rate	1985 Cases	Cumulative risk 1915	Cumulative risk 1940	Recent trend
CHINA									
Shanghai	A4D	-1.04	*9.0*	*84*	5.6	97	4.4	2.0	-15.4
HONG KONG	A2C2	-0.22	*21.5*	*122*	18.1	208	13.5	5.8	-11.3
INDIA									
Bombay	A3P3C2	0.07	27.3	202	16.9	190	13.0	4.9	-12.1
JAPAN									
Miyagi	A2P2	-1.34	4.0	13	6.6	35	3.5	5.9	34.0
Nagasaki	A2	1.35	*9.2*	*7*	9.2	9	6.0	6.0	*13.5*
Osaka	A2P2	0.14	8.6	100	7.7	135	4.9	5.2	6.6
SINGAPORE									
Chinese	A8P3	0.48	14.4	29	11.7	34	8.4	6.1	*-8.2*
Indian	A2	0.83	12.1	3	12.1	4	7.8	7.8	*26.6*
Malay	A1	0.58	3.8	1	3.8	1	2.5	2.5	*-36.9*

* : not enough cases for reliable estimation
– : incomplete or missing data
Best model: polynomial of the given degree in age (A), period (P) or cohort (C), or linear drift (D) model.
Goodness of fit: the normalised likelihood ratio chi-square for the best model (see Method).
Rate: world-standardised truncated rate per 100 000 per year (30-74 years) and number of **cases** are both estimated from the best-fitting model for the single years cited.
Cumulative risk per 1000 (30-74 years) is estimated from the best-fitting *age-cohort* model for cohorts of central birth year cited.
Recent trend: estimated mean percentage change per five-year period in the age-specific rates (30-74 years) over the period 1973-1987.
Italics denote recent trends not significant at 5 per cent level, or other figures which should be interpreted with caution (see Method).

MALES

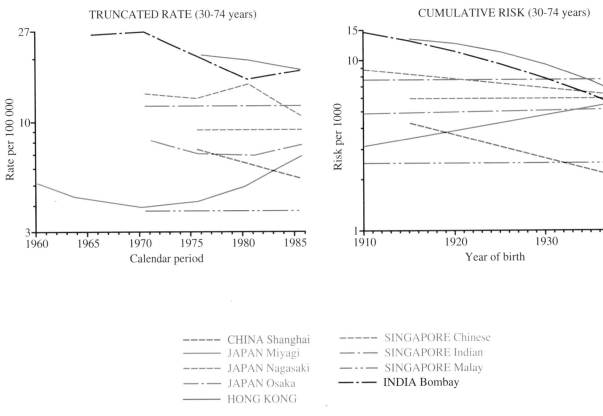

LARYNX (ICD-9 161)

ASIA, INCIDENCE
Percentage change per five-year period, 1973-1987

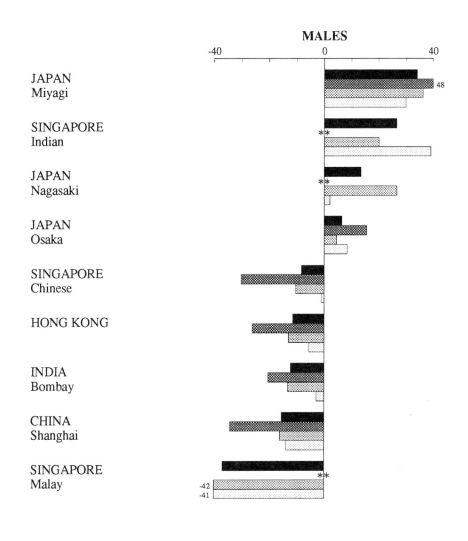

LARYNX (ICD-9 161)

OCEANIA, INCIDENCE

MALES	Best model	Goodness of fit	1970 Rate	1970 Cases	1985 Rate	1985 Cases	Cumulative risk 1915	Cumulative risk 1940	Recent trend
AUSTRALIA									
New South Wales	A4C3	-1.04	*10.2*	*106*	12.2	161	6.0	8.9	9.3
South	A2	-0.16	*10.4*	*20*	10.4	36	6.4	6.4	*16.1*
HAWAII									
Caucasian	A2	-0.84	20.6	7	20.6	12	12.5	12.5	21.2
Chinese	A1	-2.04	*3.7*	*0*	*3.7*	*0*	2.3	2.3	*14.8*
Filipino	A1	-0.89	4.4	1	4.4	1	2.7	2.7	*24.6*
Hawaiian	A2	-0.15	13.3	1	13.3	3	8.1	8.1	*20.0*
Japanese	A2	-2.32	6.5	3	6.5	6	4.3	4.3	*-16.7*
NEW ZEALAND									
Maori	A1	0.72	5.7	1	5.7	1	3.5	3.5	*13.7*
Non-Maori	A3C3	-0.47	7.2	40	8.7	61	5.2	4.4	*0.9*

* : not enough cases for reliable estimation
– : incomplete or missing data
Best model: polynomial of the given degree in age (A), period (P) or cohort (C), or linear drift (D) model.
Goodness of fit: the normalised likelihood ratio chi-square for the best model (see Method).
Rate: world-standardised truncated rate per 100 000 per year (30-74 years) and number of **cases** are both estimated from the best-fitting model for the single years cited.
Cumulative risk per 1000 (30-74 years) is estimated from the best-fitting *age-cohort* model for cohorts of central birth year cited.
Recent trend: estimated mean percentage change per five-year period in the age-specific rates (30-74 years) over the period 1973-1987.
Italics denote recent trends not significant at 5 per cent level, or other figures which should be interpreted with caution (see Method).

MALES

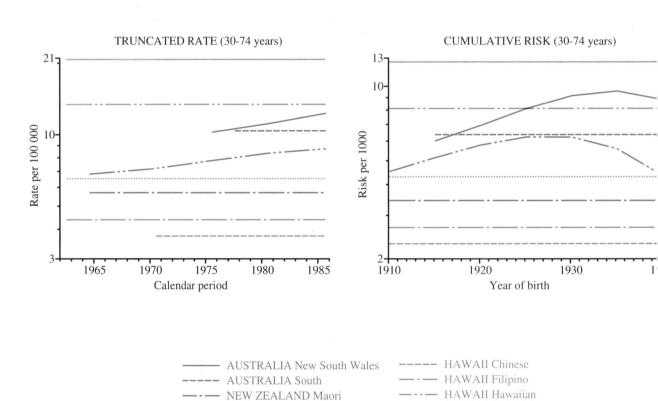

LARYNX (ICD-9 161)

OCEANIA, INCIDENCE
Percentage change per five-year period, 1973-1987

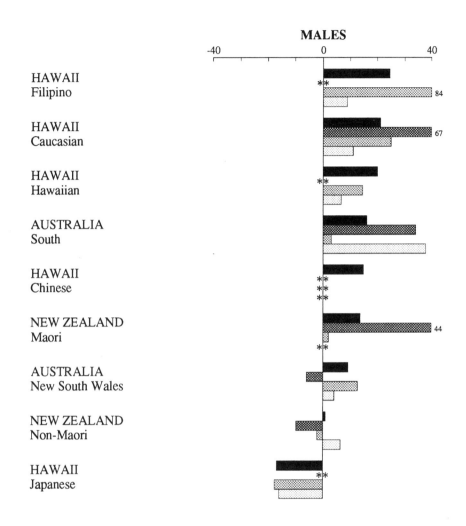

LARYNX (ICD-9 161)

ASIA and OCEANIA, MORTALITY

MALES	Best model	Goodness of fit	1965 Rate	1965 Deaths	1985 Rate	1985 Deaths	Cumulative risk 1900	Cumulative risk 1940	Recent trend
AUSTRALIA	A3P2C6	-0.48	3.4	82	4.3	157	2.1	2.6	*0.4*
HONG KONG	A3P4	0.63	2.9	10	5.7	52	*3.0*	6.3	-19.1
JAPAN	A8P6C9	0.27	2.8	482	1.7	480	2.2	0.5	-17.9
MAURITIUS	A2P2	1.39	3.7	2	5.6	5	*3.3*	6.0	*-20.3*
NEW ZEALAND	A2C3	-0.15	2.7	14	3.1	22	1.6	1.1	*8.1*
SINGAPORE	A2	-0.23	*5.6*	*9*	5.6	14	*2.9*	2.9	–

* : not enough deaths for reliable estimation
– : incomplete or missing data
Best model: polynomial of the given degree in age (A), period (P) or cohort (C), or linear drift (D) model.
Goodness of fit: the normalised likelihood ratio chi-square for the best model (see Method).
Rate: world-standardised truncated rate per 100 000 per year (30-74 years) and number of **deaths** are both estimated from the best-fitting model for the single years cited.
Cumulative risk per 1000 (30-74 years) is estimated from the best-fitting *age-cohort* model for cohorts of central birth year cited.
Recent trend: estimated mean percentage change per five-year period in the age-specific rates (30-74 years) over the period 1975-1988.
Italics denote recent trends not significant at 5 per cent level, or other figures which should be interpreted with caution (see Method).

MALES

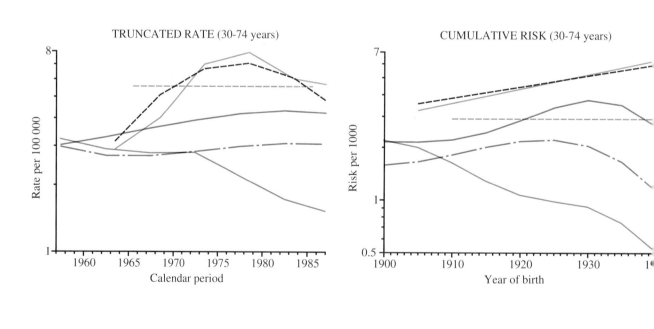

TRUNCATED RATE (30-74 years)

CUMULATIVE RISK (30-74 years)

———— AUSTRALIA ———— HONG KONG
—·—· NEW ZEALAND ----- SINGAPORE
———— JAPAN ----- MAURITIUS

LARYNX (ICD-9 161)

ASIA and OCEANIA, MORTALITY
Percentage change per five-year period, 1975-1988

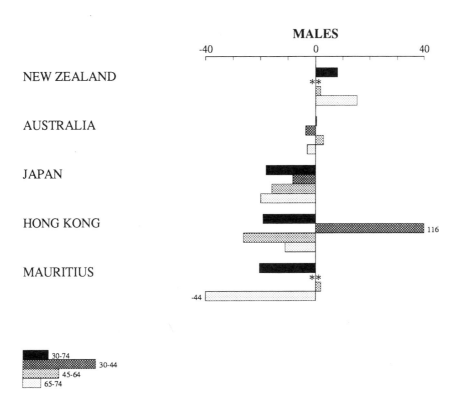

from page 289

could be affected by changes in the sub-site distri- bution of laryngeal cancer between cancers of the vocal cords and of the upper part of the larynx, which have a different aetiology and different survi- val, although no information is available to support or refute this possibility.

Another interesting feature of the mortality data is the parallel trend in France and Italy, with similar declines in risk for cohorts born since 1930, while a substantial increase in risk is occurring among younger males in Germany; this feature is seen consistently for all alcohol-related sites. Similar increases among younger males are occurring in Ireland and Scotland.

Asia and Oceania

There has been a fall in incidence of over 30% in Bombay (India) between 1970 and 1985. A similar recent rate of decline (11% every five years) is sug- gested by the data for Hong Kong, which are well fitted by a simple age-cohort model, although data are available only for a short period. A significant

fall in risk has also occurred in Shanghai (China) and among Singapore Chinese. By contrast, a per- iod-wise increase has been observed since the mid- 1970s in Miyagi and Osaka (Japan). Incidence has also increased in Nagasaki (Japan) in recent years, but not significantly.

The mortality trend in Hong Kong is not entirely consistent with the incidence data. There is a strong period effect, corresponding to a decrease in the overall death rate (30-74 years) of about 19% every five years since 1975, and this is similar to the over- all rate of decline in incidence. The rapid rate of recent increase in mortality among 30-44 year-old males, however, apparently more than doubling every five years, is due to an exceptionally high mortality rate in 1986-87, and it is not consistent with the decrease in incidence in this age group (26% decline every five years, 95% confidence interval -6% to -42%). Conversely, while mortality data for Japan show a similarly impressive rate of decline (18% every five years), this seems too rapid to be consistent with the overall increase in inci- dence in the prefectures of Miyagi and Osaka. The sudden decrease in mortality in Japan since 1975

continued page 309

LARYNX (ICD-9 161)

AMERICAS (except USA), INCIDENCE

MALES	Best model	Goodness of fit	1970 Rate	1970 Cases	1985 Rate	1985 Cases	Cumulative risk 1915	Cumulative risk 1940	Recent trend
BRAZIL									
Sao Paulo	A2D	2.33	25.5	169	*37.6*	*299*	13.8	*26.3*	–
CANADA									
Alberta	A2C2	1.58	6.9	21	9.5	41	5.3	5.8	*5.9*
British Columbia	A2	0.26	10.7	50	10.7	75	6.3	6.3	*1.6*
Maritime Provinces	A8P3C8	0.28	9.9	30	12.8	43	5.1	4.8	19.6
Newfoundland	A2D	2.67	8.0	7	12.7	13	5.5	11.7	*8.6*
Quebec	A2P3C2	-0.21	12.5	137	22.7	328	11.5	21.2	11.6
COLOMBIA									
Cali	A2D	0.04	11.5	6	8.1	10	6.0	3.3	*-14.4*
CUBA	A4D	2.90	16.3	241	19.2	391	11.5	*15.1*	–
PUERTO RICO	A2P2	-0.23	13.1	59	12.8	85	7.8	8.5	*-6.3*

* : not enough cases for reliable estimation
– : incomplete or missing data
Best model: polynomial of the given degree in age (A), period (P) or cohort (C), or linear drift (D) model.
Goodness of fit: the normalised likelihood ratio chi-square for the best model (see Method).
Rate: world-standardised truncated rate per 100 000 per year (30-74 years) and number of **cases** are both estimated from the best-fitting model for the single years cited.
Cumulative risk per 1000 (30-74 years) is estimated from the best-fitting *age-cohort* model for cohorts of central birth year cited.
Recent trend: estimated mean percentage change per five-year period in the age-specific rates (30-74 years) over the period 1973-1987.
Italics denote recent trends not significant at 5 per cent level, or other figures which should be interpreted with caution (see Method).

MALES

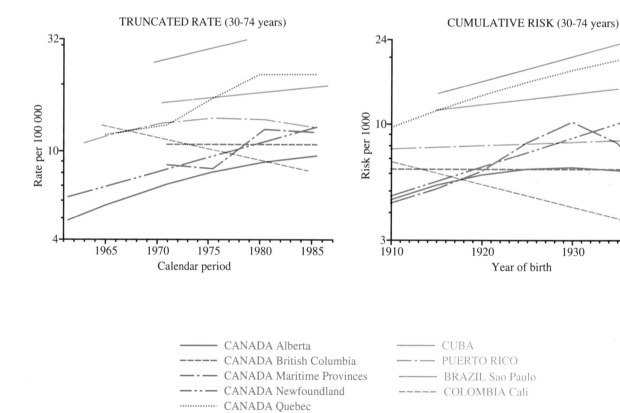

TRUNCATED RATE (30-74 years)

CUMULATIVE RISK (30-74 years)

——— CANADA Alberta
- - - - - CANADA British Columbia
— · — CANADA Maritime Provinces
— · · — CANADA Newfoundland
··············· CANADA Quebec

——— CUBA
— · — PUERTO RICO
——— BRAZIL Sao Paulo
- - - - - COLOMBIA Cali

LARYNX (ICD-9 161)

AMERICAS (except USA), INCIDENCE
Percentage change per five-year period, 1973-1987

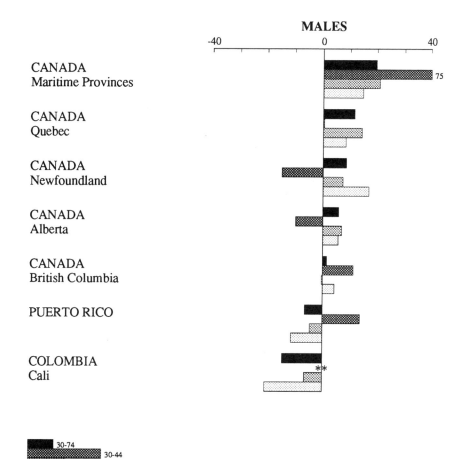

LARYNX (ICD-9 161)

AMERICAS (USA), INCIDENCE

MALES	Best model	Goodness of fit	1970 Rate	1970 Cases	1985 Rate	1985 Cases	Cumulative risk 1915	Cumulative risk 1940	Recent trend
USA									
Bay Area, Black	A2C2	-0.57	21.1	12	22.8	18	16.5	5.9	*3.2*
Bay Area, Chinese	A1P2	0.79	*0.1*	*0*	*0.1*	*0*	2.8	*12.6*	–
Bay Area, White	A2C3	0.33	15.0	89	14.0	86	8.9	5.2	*1.0*
Connecticut	A2P2	-0.06	17.0	112	16.0	125	9.7	10.2	-4.3
Detroit, Black	A2D	0.23	17.4	24	23.2	39	11.2	17.9	2.9
Detroit, White	A3	-0.48	16.8	125	16.8	120	10.1	10.1	*0.9*
Iowa	A3C2	1.18	12.7	84	15.6	106	8.9	9.4	6.4
New Orleans, Black	A8C7	-0.88	*16.0*	*8*	24.7	14	7.3	11.3	*0.4*
New Orleans, White	A4C2	0.84	*15.7*	*23*	22.2	34	13.8	9.0	7.5
Seattle	A2	0.62	*13.1*	*62*	13.1	86	7.8	7.8	*-0.3*

* : not enough cases for reliable estimation
– : incomplete or missing data
Best model: polynomial of the given degree in age (A), period (P) or cohort (C), or linear drift (D) model.
Goodness of fit: the normalised likelihood ratio chi-square for the best model (see Method).
Rate: world-standardised truncated rate per 100 000 per year (30-74 years) and number of **cases** are both estimated from the best-fitting model for the single years cited.
Cumulative risk per 1000 (30-74 years) is estimated from the best-fitting *age-cohort* model for cohorts of central birth year cited.
Recent trend: estimated mean percentage change per five-year period in the age-specific rates (30-74 years) over the period 1973-1987.
Italics denote recent trends not significant at 5 per cent level, or other figures which should be interpreted with caution (see Method).

MALES

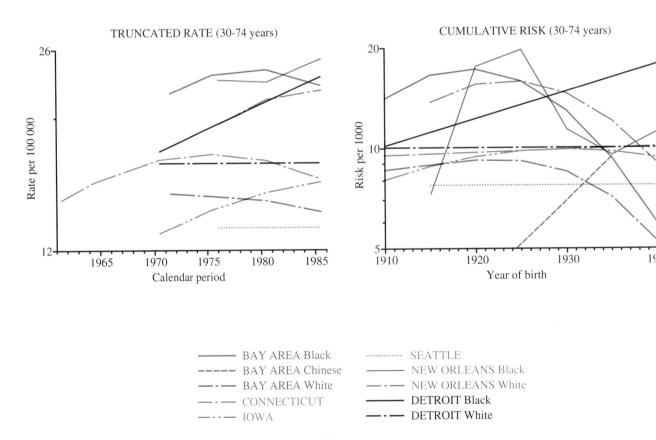

LARYNX (ICD-9 161)

AMERICAS (USA), INCIDENCE
Percentage change per five-year period, 1973-1987

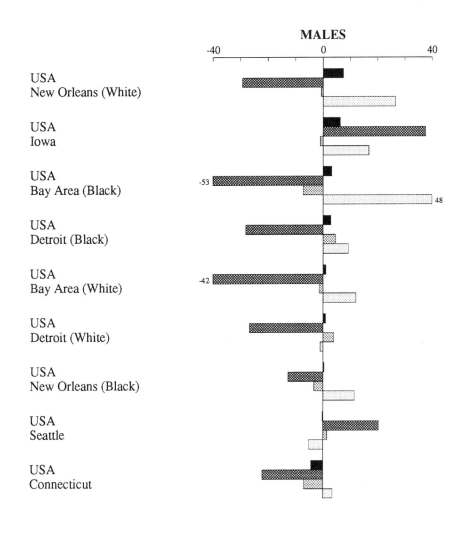

LARYNX (ICD-9 161)

AMERICAS, MORTALITY

MALES	Best model	Goodness of fit	1965 Rate	1965 Deaths	1985 Rate	1985 Deaths	Cumulative risk 1900	Cumulative risk 1940	Recent trend
CANADA	A3C6	1.38	3.7	141	4.9	285	2.4	2.9	*4.2*
CHILE	A3C2	2.19	3.4	39	4.2	74	2.0	2.0	-8.7
COSTA RICA	A2D	-0.24	*2.7*	*3*	4.1	12	*1.9*	4.4	*11.6*
PANAMA	A2	-0.56	3.7	5	3.7	10	2.5	2.5	–
PUERTO RICO	A3	0.96	8.7	35	8.7	42	*5.4*	5.4	-4.5
URUGUAY	A3D	0.66	14.0	83	15.4	112	8.2	10.0	*-0.3*
USA	A3P2C2	3.13	4.5	1912	4.0	2212	2.7	2.1	-7.0
VENEZUELA	A2C2	0.47	6.3	52	*4.7*	*69*	4.2	1.6	–

∗ : not enough deaths for reliable estimation
– : incomplete or missing data
Best model: polynomial of the given degree in age (A), period (P) or cohort (C), or linear drift (D) model.
Goodness of fit: the normalised likelihood ratio chi-square for the best model (see Method).
Rate: world-standardised truncated rate per 100 000 per year (30-74 years) and number of **deaths** are both estimated from the best-fitting model for the single years cited.
Cumulative risk per 1000 (30-74 years) is estimated from the best-fitting *age-cohort* model for cohorts of central birth year cited.
Recent trend: estimated mean percentage change per five-year period in the age-specific rates (30-74 years) over the period 1975-1988.
Italics denote recent trends not significant at 5 per cent level, or other figures which should be interpreted with caution (see Method).

MALES

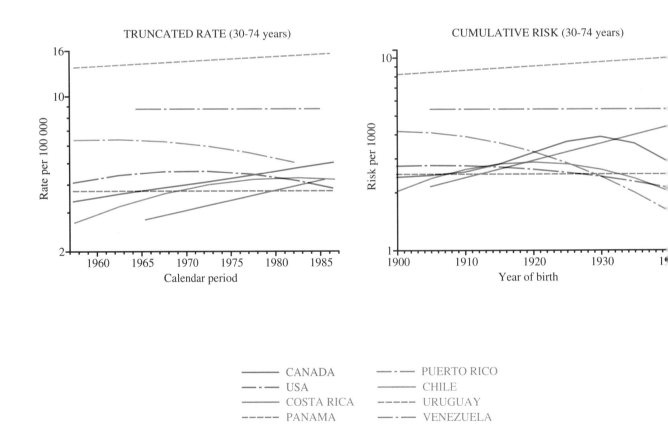

TRUNCATED RATE (30-74 years)

CUMULATIVE RISK (30-74 years)

CANADA
USA
COSTA RICA
PANAMA
PUERTO RICO
CHILE
URUGUAY
VENEZUELA

308

LARYNX (ICD-9 161)

AMERICAS, MORTALITY
Percentage change per five-year period, 1975-1988

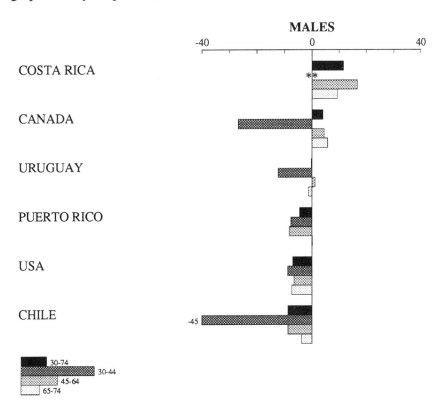

MALES

from page 303

and the complicated model needed to describe the trend need further explanation.

There has been an increase in incidence in New South Wales (Australia) and among non-Maoris in New Zealand. Age-cohort models fit well in both cases, and there is the suggestion of a decrease in risk for more recent generations. The pattern is consistent with that for other alcohol-related cancers. Mortality data for Australia and New Zealand are consistent with the trends in incidence. The high risk among Caucasians in Hawaii (1.3%) has not changed significantly, and the six-fold range of incidence between the various ethnic groups in Hawaii appears stable. The recent linear trend among Caucasians is of borderline significance, and is an example of how differences between denominators can occasionally lead to inconsistencies in the results (see Chapter 3).

Americas

There has been a general increase in the risk of laryngeal cancer in Canada, particularly in Quebec and the Maritime Provinces, but the increase is not significant in British Columbia and there has been a deceleration in the rate of increase among recent birth cohorts in most provinces. The risk is increasing in São Paulo (Brazil) and in Cuba, but decreasing in Cali (Colombia).

In the USA, incidence was highest in the three black populations of New Orleans (25 per 100 000), Detroit and San Francisco. The increase in risk among black males in Detroit appears to be continuing, and the risk for the 1940 birth cohort now exceeds 1.5%, while for blacks in New Orleans and San Francisco, the risk has been declining for males born after 1925. None of the recent trends is significant, but substantial rates of decline in incidence among 30-44 year-olds are seen in seven of the ten US populations studied, and there are signs of deceleration of some increasing trends or of actual decline in the risk for more recent birth cohorts.

The mortality data show a declining risk of death in the USA since 1975. There is a clear cohort effect in Canada, with a peak risk for the 1930 cohort and a decline in the youngest generations. In South America, the most striking observations are the steady increase in risk in Costa Rica, the high risk of death (1%) in Uruguay, also increasing slowly but steadily, and the declining risk among more recent birth cohorts in Chile and Venezuela.

309

Comment

Previous reports on trends in cancer of the larynx are mostly consistent with trends in other cancers associated with alcohol and tobacco in the same countries. Trends in the incidence of cancer of the larynx in males reported from Slovakia for the period 1979-88[237] and from the former Czechoslovakia as a whole for the period 1968-85[80] are comparable, increasing at about 7% every five years. These reports also show a male-to-female ratio of 10, and a 24% increase in incidence among females between the two quinquennia to 1988 in Slovakia, whereas virtually no change was recorded in Czechoslovakia as a whole. The trend data from Slovakia are likely to be more reliable. Although no data for laryngeal cancer in females are presented here, comparison of the mortality trends in the two sexes for other smoking-related cancers in Czechoslovakia suggests that a rapid increase in risk among females is plausible. The decline in age-standardised rates in Vaud (Switzerland) is similar in both sexes[164], and only slightly less than that observed here for Geneva. The 43% increase in mortality in Spain since 1951 was largely completed by 1969[31], and was reported as consistent with trends in cigarette consumption.

The irregular decline in mortality among successive birth cohorts in England and Wales and the decelerating decline in successive calendar periods, both shown here, have been previously reported[213]. These changes were not considered to correspond directly with trends in consumption of alcohol or tobacco, although the period effect was judged to be related to the decline in consumption of spirits. Improvements in treatment and survival were also considered contributory to the decline in mortality, both in England and Wales[213] and the USA[77]. Mor-

tality from cancer of the larynx in France increased on average by less than 1% a year in both sexes during the period 1950-85[128], but whereas the rate has declined recently in males, it is still rising in females; these changes are in keeping with sex-specific mortality trends for other cancers caused by alcohol and tobacco.

From the analyses reported here, the small (0.5%) average annual increase in age-standardised incidence previously reported among Singapore Chinese during the period 1968-82[154] appears to have reversed, and the rate for 1983-87 is the lowest since the registry in Singapore began operating in 1968. This is reflected by the recent non-significant decline of 8% every five years. The decline is most marked in younger males (30-44 years).

In Ontario (Canada), age-standardised laryngeal cancer incidence among males fell by 7% between the two quinquennia ending in 1988[182], in direct contrast to the trend in the five provinces examined here; this decline was based on over 300 cases a year. The corresponding change in females was a 20% increase (70 cases a year). The rate of increase of lung cancer in Ontario was also lower in both sexes than in the provinces studied here, whereas trends in alcohol-related sites were comparable with those in other provinces.

Previous analyses of laryngeal cancer trends in the USA have shown cohort effects in incidence and mortality among white males in five areas, including four of those studied here (Connecticut, Detroit, Iowa, San Francisco-Oakland and Atlanta)[77], with a decline among younger males in the early 1980s. Mortality trends showed a decline for white males born after 1925, while no decline was seen among non-white males[74]. The excess mortality among non-whites appeared in the 1960s.

Chapter 14

LUNG

Cancer of the lung is now the most frequent cancer in the world, but with wide geographical variation in risk. It is the most frequent cancer among males in many countries, but there are several exceptions: cancer of the stomach is still the most common cancer in Portugal and — by a two-fold margin in both sexes — in Japan; in India, cancers of the oral cavity rank first. The lifetime risk (30-74 years) of developing lung cancer varies widely: in developed countries alone it ranges from 3% to 14% in males, and from less than 1% to over 10% in females. The global range in risk among males is greater than ten-fold, from less than 1% among Indian populations in Bombay (India) and Singapore to more than 14% in the Maori population of New Zealand. Survival from lung cancer is poor (barely 10% at five years), and it has not improved; mortality data can be expected to provide a reliable picture of the frequency of the disease.

The main cause of lung cancer is tobacco smoking. The geographical distribution of lung cancer is largely explained by the prevalence of the tobacco habit, with the exception of some Chinese populations, where the rate of adenocarcinoma of the lung among non-smoking females is high. The level of tobacco consumption has changed markedly and in different directions in several countries in recent decades, and the geographical distribution of lung cancer is expected to change rapidly in the near future. This impending change can be seen today when lung cancer risk is analysed in terms of projected lifetime risk for the younger birth cohorts. Because tobacco smoking habits are generally established at an early age and are characteristic for a given birth cohort, trends in the occurrence of lung cancer have occurred in successive birth cohorts. It is therefore appropriate to examine carefully the trend in lifetime risk which has been observed or which may be predicted for successive birth cohorts.

Europe

The pattern of change over time of the risk of lung cancer in males can be summarised by dividing European males into three groups of populations in which major changes have occurred. Females are considered separately.

The populations in which the highest incidence rates were observed in the 1970s — UK, Finland and, to a lesser extent, Varese (Italy) and Geneva (Switzerland) — have achieved a substantial decrease in tobacco consumption[273,304], which can be seen to have led to a major reduction in the lifetime risk of lung cancer for the youngest generations, compared to that of their parents only 25 years earlier. In South Thames and Birmingham (UK), for example, the lifetime risk of the 1940 birth cohort is less than half that of the 1915 birth cohort (9%). In Scotland, the reduction in lifetime risk between these two generations is about 40%, but the decline in Scotland started slightly later, and the risk is now decreasing at the same rate as in the two English populations. In Finland, the risk fell from 9.3% to 3.7%, a reduction of almost two thirds. Varese (Italy) experienced a reduction in risk of about 20% between the two generations, but in Geneva (Switzerland), the reduction has only been 5%, and is mainly associated with a very recent decline.

The mortality data are consistent with this pattern in Scotland, England and Wales, Ireland and Finland. In Finland, the risk of death from lung cancer in the generation born in 1940 is now among the lowest in Europe, close to that of Sweden and Norway, a group of countries where the risk remains low despite a moderate increase over the period of the study. In contrast, no reduction in mortality has occurred in Switzerland or Italy, where the observed incidence trends among the populations covered by cancer registration cannot apparently be generalised to their respective countries; the two registries, Geneva and Varese, cover populations which are at high risk of lung cancer, but represent 5% or less of the national population as a whole, on average at lower risk. Switzerland has retained a moderate lifetime risk of about 5% for lung cancer mortality. In Italy, mortality from lung cancer doubled between the 1915 and 1940 birth cohorts, reaching an estimated average risk of death of about 9% for the 1940 birth cohort. The increase in mortality in Italy is partly explained by the rapid increase in incidence in the south of the country: while the truncated rate (35-64 years) fell between 1980 and 1985 in Varese and in Parma, in the north of Italy, it increased by 15% in Ragusa, in Sicily[202,221].

The second notable feature of the trends is the truly remarkable increase in lung cancer risk among males in eastern Europe, especially in

continued page 332

LUNG (ICD-9 162)

EUROPE (non-EC), INCIDENCE

MALES	Best model	Goodness of fit	1970 Rate	1970 Cases	1985 Rate	1985 Cases	Cumulative risk 1915	Cumulative risk 1940	Recent trend
FINLAND	A8P5C9	1.28	156.3	1606	122.1	1448	92.9	36.7	-7.1
HUNGARY									
County Vas	A2P3C4	2.66	84.5	70	133.2	98	60.9	*313.2*	15.0
Szabolcs-Szatmar	A2D	4.35	51.6	68	146.0	204	57.6	*285.8*	43.7
ISRAEL									
All Jews	A2P3C6	1.46	55.5	243	55.3	310	29.9	41.2	*-0.9*
Non-Jews	A2C3	1.79	48.9	15	50.0	25	30.6	24.6	-8.4
NORWAY	A8P5C9	0.94	46.6	515	71.8	871	39.1	52.0	13.9
POLAND									
Warsaw City	A2P3C5	-0.92	112.1	314	121.3	474	71.4	77.3	*-1.5*
ROMANIA									
Cluj	A2C3	1.44	*96.6*	*152*	79.4	144	36.9	86.6	*6.2*
SWEDEN	A3P2C7	0.23	45.1	1138	49.2	1315	29.9	37.9	1.5
SWITZERLAND									
Geneva	A2P2	0.83	107.1	83	125.0	114	79.0	75.4	-5.8
YUGOSLAVIA									
Slovenia	A3P2C8	4.04	100.6	378	124.3	537	58.6	109.5	4.5

FEMALES	Best model	Goodness of fit	1970 Rate	1970 Cases	1985 Rate	1985 Cases	Cumulative risk 1915	Cumulative risk 1940	Recent trend
FINLAND	A2C4	0.18	9.6	130	15.4	242	8.5	12.5	17.5
HUNGARY									
County Vas	A1P3C2	1.80	15.0	13	17.6	15	7.9	18.8	25.3
Szabolcs-Szatmar	A3D	0.16	7.5	11	19.1	32	7.8	36.5	22.5
ISRAEL									
All Jews	A4P3C3	0.86	18.8	83	18.6	118	10.8	11.0	*3.2*
Non-Jews	A2	-0.68	6.9	2	6.9	4	4.2	4.2	*4.7*
NORWAY	A3C3	0.59	8.5	100	20.1	250	8.3	32.5	37.3
POLAND									
Warsaw City	A4P3C8	-0.61	18.7	81	30.9	162	15.2	43.9	20.5
ROMANIA									
Cluj	A2	1.22	*12.4*	*22*	12.4	25	7.4	7.4	*1.8*
SWEDEN	A4C3	-0.51	10.0	260	19.1	519	8.6	25.5	27.5
SWITZERLAND									
Geneva	A2C3	-0.48	12.2	11	28.2	31	14.5	32.6	35.2
YUGOSLAVIA									
Slovenia	A2C3	0.88	10.3	50	14.7	84	7.4	13.3	*5.1*

* : not enough cases for reliable estimation
– : incomplete or missing data
Best model: polynomial of the given degree in age (A), period (P) or cohort (C), or linear drift (D) model.
Goodness of fit: the normalised likelihood ratio chi-square for the best model (see Method).
Rate: world-standardised truncated rate per 100 000 per year (30-74 years) and number of **cases** are both estimated from the best-fitting model for the single years cited.
Cumulative risk per 1000 (30-74 years) is estimated from the best-fitting *age-cohort* model for cohorts of central birth year cited.
Recent trend: estimated mean percentage change per five-year period in the age-specific rates (30-74 years) over the period 1973-1987.
Italics denote recent trends not significant at 5 per cent level, or other figures which should be interpreted with caution (see Method).

LUNG (ICD-9 162)

EUROPE (non-EC), INCIDENCE

MALES

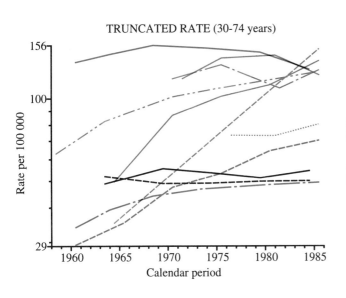

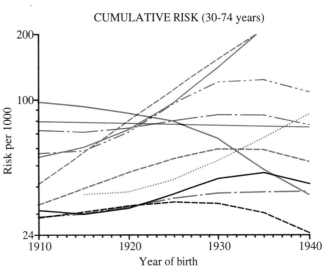

FEMALES

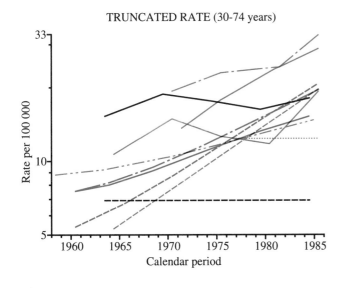

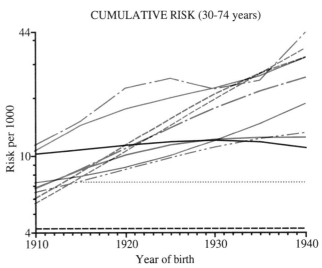

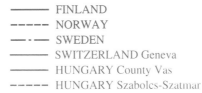

——— FINLAND	—·— POLAND Warsaw City
- - - NORWAY	············· ROMANIA Cluj
—··— SWEDEN	—···— YUGOSLAVIA Slovenia
——— SWITZERLAND Geneva	——— ISRAEL All Jews
——— HUNGARY County Vas	- - - - ISRAEL Non-Jews
- - - - - HUNGARY Szabolcs-Szatmar	

LUNG (ICD-9 162)

EUROPE (EC), INCIDENCE

MALES	Best model	Goodness of fit	1970 Rate	1970 Cases	1985 Rate	1985 Cases	Cumulative risk 1915	Cumulative risk 1940	Recent trend
DENMARK	A4P2C8	0.05	98.2	1348	114.7	1693	70.2	74.0	4.3
FRANCE									
Bas-Rhin	A3D	-1.17	*109.3*	*253*	136.7	274	74.4	106.2	9.3
Doubs	A2	0.41	*106.0*	*73*	106.0	115	62.7	62.7	*-0.1*
GERMANY (FRG)									
Hamburg	A3P3C4	0.32	132.3	755	*195.2*	*746*	74.3	*114.9*	–
Saarland	A2P2	4.41	141.3	409	138.3	388	88.2	83.3	-4.0
GERMANY (GDR)	A4P3C8	6.46	120.0	5663	121.3	4449	69.9	80.5	*-0.7*
ITALY									
Varese	A3C2	0.29	*128.5*	*188*	166.1	342	98.8	83.0	*4.8*
SPAIN									
Navarra	A2D	-0.37	*35.9*	*43*	86.8	124	43.6	176.1	34.9
Zaragoza	A2D	0.45	46.3	87	83.5	200	44.3	114.0	22.2
UK									
Birmingham	A4P5C7	3.44	163.0	2222	139.9	2140	98.2	41.6	-7.1
Scotland	A4P3C7	0.11	161.4	2221	166.9	2369	109.4	69.0	-2.4
South Thames	A4P5C5	2.16	150.7	3898	118.9	2386	87.8	40.1	-10.1

FEMALES	Best model	Goodness of fit	1970 Rate	1970 Cases	1985 Rate	1985 Cases	Cumulative risk 1915	Cumulative risk 1940	Recent trend
DENMARK	A3C6	0.46	18.6	274	47.8	736	18.5	73.7	39.5
FRANCE									
Bas-Rhin	A2D	-0.87	*5.7*	*17*	10.9	27	5.1	15.0	25.1
Doubs	A2D	0.33	*2.8*	*2*	9.5	11	3.5	26.1	51.2
GERMANY (FRG)									
Hamburg	A2P4	-0.10	18.5	142	*5.6*	*31*	13.2	*19.0*	–
Saarland	A2P3	0.33	12.7	48	15.3	57	7.6	11.9	18.5
GERMANY (GDR)	A8P4C9	-0.05	10.1	673	13.6	745	7.0	10.4	12.4
ITALY									
Varese	A2D	0.01	*8.0*	*12*	15.2	38	7.6	21.7	24.1
SPAIN									
Navarra	A8C7	0.48	*2.6*	*3*	6.6	9	2.2	18.6	*15.3*
Zaragoza	A1D	0.82	8.3	18	5.6	15	4.2	2.2	*2.2*
UK									
Birmingham	A2P4C7	0.34	24.3	370	38.6	644	21.2	19.9	17.5
Scotland	A2P3C4	0.74	29.3	475	63.5	1076	33.6	47.8	26.2
South Thames	A2P3C6	0.56	31.6	983	42.1	986	26.3	22.6	9.5

* : not enough cases for reliable estimation
– : incomplete or missing data
Best model: polynomial of the given degree in age (A), period (P) or cohort (C), or linear drift (D) model.
Goodness of fit: the normalised likelihood ratio chi-square for the best model (see Method).
Rate: world-standardised truncated rate per 100 000 per year (30-74 years) and number of **cases** are both estimated from the best-fitting model for the single years cited.
Cumulative risk per 1000 (30-74 years) is estimated from the best-fitting *age-cohort* model for cohorts of central birth year cited.
Recent trend: estimated mean percentage change per five-year period in the age-specific rates (30-74 years) over the period 1973-1987.
Italics denote recent trends not significant at 5 per cent level, or other figures which should be interpreted with caution (see Method).

LUNG (ICD-9 162)

EUROPE (EC), INCIDENCE

MALES

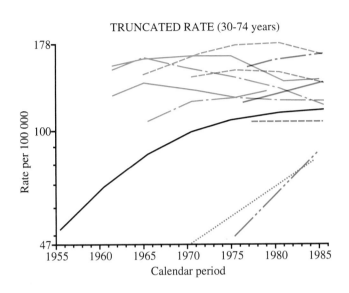

TRUNCATED RATE (30-74 years)

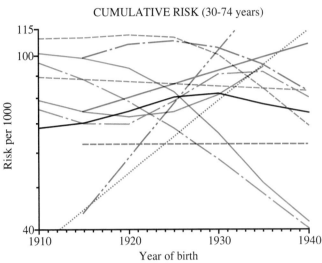

CUMULATIVE RISK (30-74 years)

FEMALES

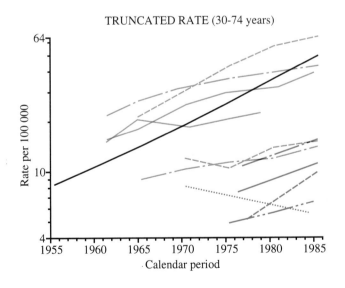

TRUNCATED RATE (30-74 years)

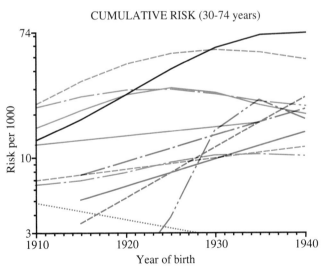

CUMULATIVE RISK (30-74 years)

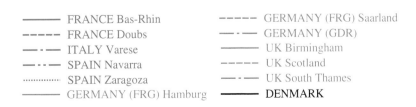

——— FRANCE Bas-Rhin	– – – GERMANY (FRG) Saarland
– – – FRANCE Doubs	–·–·– GERMANY (GDR)
–·–·– ITALY Varese	——— UK Birmingham
–··–··– SPAIN Navarra	– – – UK Scotland
············· SPAIN Zaragoza	–·–·– UK South Thames
——— GERMANY (FRG) Hamburg	▬▬▬ DENMARK

LUNG (ICD-9 162)

EUROPE (non-EC), INCIDENCE
Percentage change per five-year period, 1973-1987

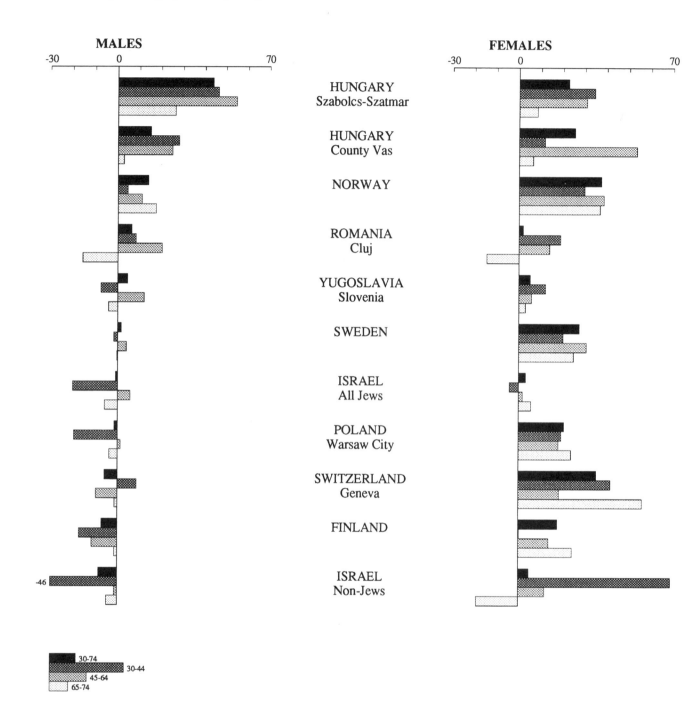

LUNG (ICD-9 162)

EUROPE (EC), INCIDENCE
Percentage change per five-year period, 1973-1987

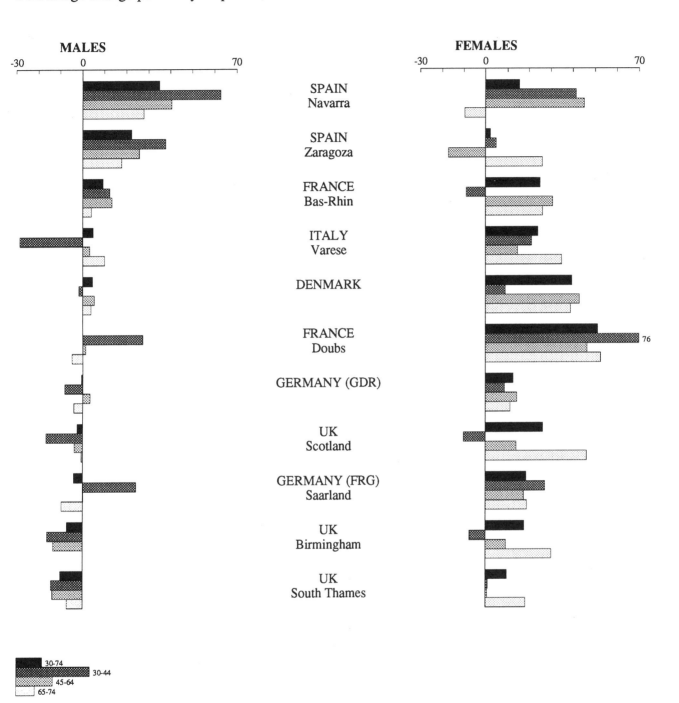

MALES		FEMALES
	SPAIN Navarra	
	SPAIN Zaragoza	
	FRANCE Bas-Rhin	
	ITALY Varese	
	DENMARK	
	FRANCE Doubs	76
	GERMANY (GDR)	
	UK Scotland	
	GERMANY (FRG) Saarland	
	UK Birmingham	
	UK South Thames	

30-74
30-44
45-64
65-74

LUNG (ICD-9 162)

EUROPE (non-EC), MORTALITY

MALES	Best model	Goodness of fit	1965 Rate	1965 Deaths	1985 Rate	1985 Deaths	Cumulative risk 1900	Cumulative risk 1940	Recent trend
AUSTRIA	A4P3C8	2.19	105.3	2145	87.3	1627	76.4	58.3	-6.2
CZECHOSLOVAKIA	A2P5C9	8.75	119.8	4273	149.0	5421	81.0	156.4	6.1
FINLAND	A8P6C9	0.09	129.3	1203	107.5	1269	83.0	31.0	-11.9
HUNGARY	A4P5C8	4.22	71.9	1892	137.3	3793	50.9	*217.9*	19.2
NORWAY	A2C6	0.66	31.8	329	58.3	715	21.9	49.5	13.3
POLAND	A8P4C8	10.47	56.9	3407	132.9	10303	37.9	174.9	17.6
ROMANIA	A7P4C4	10.55	63.5	2580	*61.5*	*3311*	37.3	87.7	–
SWEDEN	A8P6C9	1.09	34.2	801	43.0	1163	26.4	39.7	*-2.1*
SWITZERLAND	A3P3C8	2.40	75.4	1076	93.7	1634	49.3	50.8	-3.5
YUGOSLAVIA	A8P3C8	5.62	46.4	1678	89.7	4499	30.1	114.1	15.2

FEMALES	Best model	Goodness of fit	1965 Rate	1965 Deaths	1985 Rate	1985 Deaths	Cumulative risk 1900	Cumulative risk 1940	Recent trend
AUSTRIA	A2P2	2.51	11.5	315	15.6	408	7.4	12.4	11.3
CZECHOSLOVAKIA	A3P6C6	1.84	11.2	484	14.3	642	6.4	12.7	16.3
FINLAND	A2P2C6	-1.21	7.1	89	12.2	195	4.1	8.3	18.4
HUNGARY	A3P3C4	2.32	13.5	427	22.8	785	8.3	27.1	22.6
NORWAY	A3P2C3	-0.07	5.7	64	16.3	208	3.3	24.9	40.9
POLAND	A2P4C6	5.29	8.9	676	16.6	1644	5.3	17.5	20.4
ROMANIA	A3P4	0.84	12.3	592	*10.9*	*681*	6.5	7.8	–
SWEDEN	A8P6C9	0.44	7.3	181	17.3	472	4.6	21.6	24.4
SWITZERLAND	A2P3	1.17	6.0	102	12.8	256	3.9	14.1	26.6
YUGOSLAVIA	A2D	1.64	8.2	356	14.3	860	4.9	14.6	12.7

* : not enough deaths for reliable estimation
– : incomplete or missing data
Best model: polynomial of the given degree in age (A), period (P) or cohort (C), or linear drift (D) model.
Goodness of fit: the normalised likelihood ratio chi-square for the best model (see Method).
Rate: world-standardised truncated rate per 100 000 per year (30-74 years) and number of **deaths** are both estimated from the best-fitting model for the single years cited.
Cumulative risk per 1000 (30-74 years) is estimated from the best-fitting *age-cohort* model for cohorts of central birth year cited.
Recent trend: estimated mean percentage change per five-year period in the age-specific rates (30-74 years) over the period 1975-1988.
Italics denote recent trends not significant at 5 per cent level, or other figures which should be interpreted with caution (see Method).

LUNG (ICD-9 162)

EUROPE (non-EC), MORTALITY

MALES

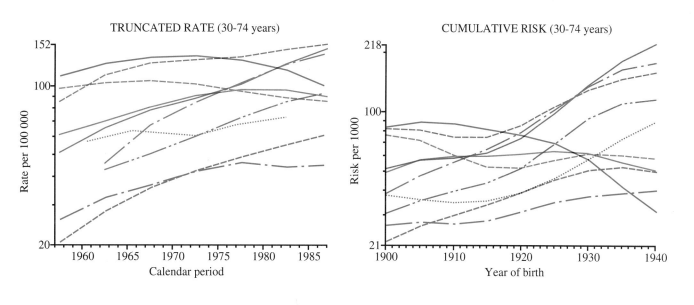

TRUNCATED RATE (30-74 years)

CUMULATIVE RISK (30-74 years)

FEMALES

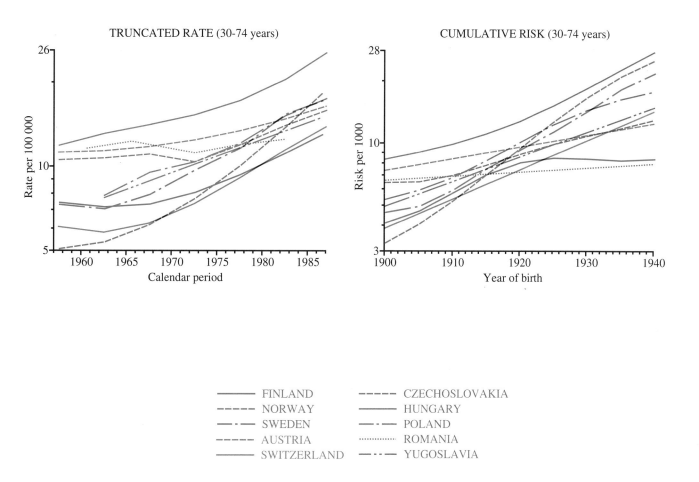

TRUNCATED RATE (30-74 years)

CUMULATIVE RISK (30-74 years)

—— FINLAND	----- CZECHOSLOVAKIA
----- NORWAY	—— HUNGARY
—·—· SWEDEN	—··— POLAND
----- AUSTRIA	·········· ROMANIA
—— SWITZERLAND	—···— YUGOSLAVIA

LUNG (ICD-9 162)

EUROPE (EC), MORTALITY

MALES	Best model	Goodness of fit	1965 Rate	1965 Deaths	1985 Rate	1985 Deaths	Cumulative risk 1900	Cumulative risk 1940	Recent trend
BELGIUM	A2P3C6	4.81	101.9	2714	148.6	4063	69.1	128.9	*1.4*
DENMARK	A4C8	0.20	75.3	972	103.7	1549	51.6	62.5	3.4
FRANCE	A3P6C8	12.55	56.4	6977	85.2	11789	35.8	87.0	7.8
GERMANY (FRG)	A8P6C9	21.76	86.4	13588	90.4	14267	59.7	72.3	*-0.6*
GREECE	A4P5C7	-0.31	60.9	1154	91.5	2527	*40.4*	93.4	6.0
IRELAND	A3C6	-0.73	70.3	512	94.9	775	46.0	48.3	*0.5*
ITALY	A4P6C7	22.98	64.5	7884	115.8	18020	41.0	94.8	10.1
NETHERLANDS	A2P2C9	1.75	112.5	3148	138.1	4958	74.5	76.9	-2.8
PORTUGAL	A2D	3.17	21.6	393	45.7	1158	13.4	58.4	18.6
SPAIN	A6P6C8	3.89	39.2	2711	74.6	7238	25.6	101.2	14.3
UK ENGLAND & WALES	A8P3C9	7.89	144.5	18841	116.5	17398	95.5	40.1	-10.1
UK SCOTLAND	A3P3C8	1.51	161.8	2138	144.8	2064	105.6	53.7	-7.8

FEMALES	Best model	Goodness of fit	1965 Rate	1965 Deaths	1985 Rate	1985 Deaths	Cumulative risk 1900	Cumulative risk 1940	Recent trend
BELGIUM	A3P2C3	1.20	8.2	250	13.8	433	4.8	11.2	16.0
DENMARK	A3C6	1.09	12.9	182	41.5	649	7.8	62.2	34.5
FRANCE	A4P5C5	5.27	6.8	1046	8.3	1330	4.0	5.6	15.4
GERMANY (FRG)	A2P4	12.10	9.6	2032	13.1	2870	5.6	10.5	18.8
GREECE	A2C2	-0.88	10.8	234	12.2	383	*6.3*	6.3	*-1.6*
IRELAND	A2P3C2	0.49	16.1	118	34.2	298	*10.3*	26.0	10.6
ITALY	A2P6C6	5.42	8.9	1298	12.6	2349	5.0	9.0	13.5
NETHERLANDS	A4P4C4	0.41	6.4	199	15.9	619	3.6	25.5	38.9
PORTUGAL	A2C2	-0.59	5.2	119	7.4	222	3.0	5.6	7.9
SPAIN	A3P2C8	-0.77	7.4	617	6.3	715	4.3	3.3	-8.4
UK ENGLAND & WALES	A2C7	5.51	20.7	3219	39.1	6600	11.7	21.7	14.0
UK SCOTLAND	A3C6	1.64	22.9	369	54.3	927	11.2	33.7	20.6

* : not enough deaths for reliable estimation
− : incomplete or missing data
Best model: polynomial of the given degree in age (A), period (P) or cohort (C), or linear drift (D) model.
Goodness of fit: the normalised likelihood ratio chi-square for the best model (see Method).
Rate: world-standardised truncated rate per 100 000 per year (30-74 years) and number of **deaths** are both estimated from the best-fitting model for the single years cited.
Cumulative risk per 1000 (30-74 years) is estimated from the best-fitting *age-cohort* model for cohorts of central birth year cited.
Recent trend: estimated mean percentage change per five-year period in the age-specific rates (30-74 years) over the period 1975-1988.
Italics denote recent trends not significant at 5 per cent level, or other figures which should be interpreted with caution (see Method).

LUNG (ICD-9 162)

EUROPE (EC), MORTALITY

MALES

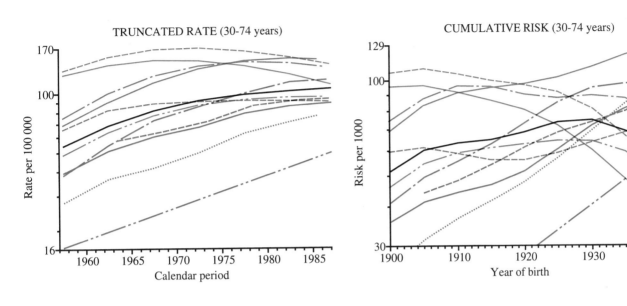

FEMALES

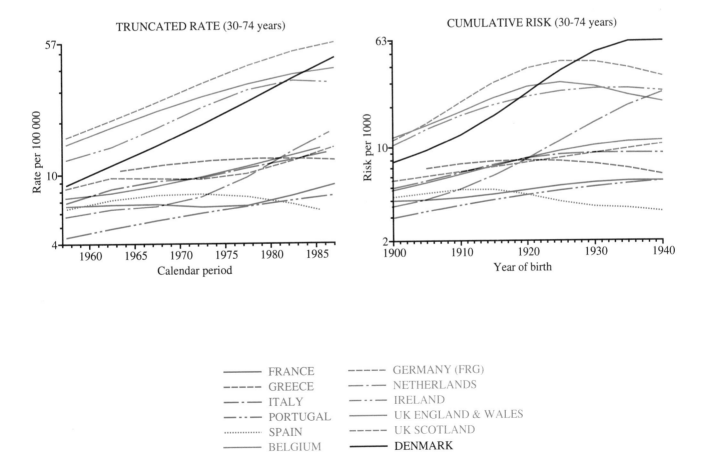

FRANCE	GERMANY (FRG)
GREECE	NETHERLANDS
ITALY	IRELAND
PORTUGAL	UK ENGLAND & WALES
SPAIN	UK SCOTLAND
BELGIUM	DENMARK

LUNG (ICD-9 162)

EUROPE (non-EC), MORTALITY
Percentage change per five-year period, 1975-1988

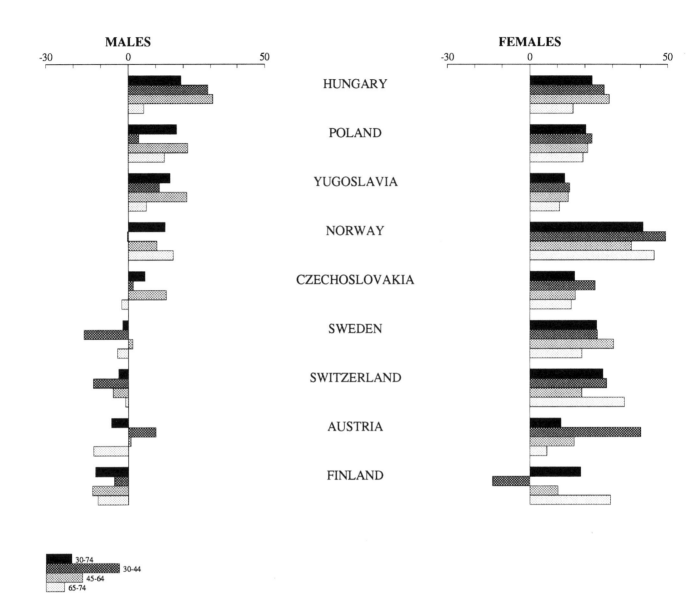

LUNG (ICD-9 162)

EUROPE (EC), MORTALITY
Percentage change per five-year period, 1975-1988

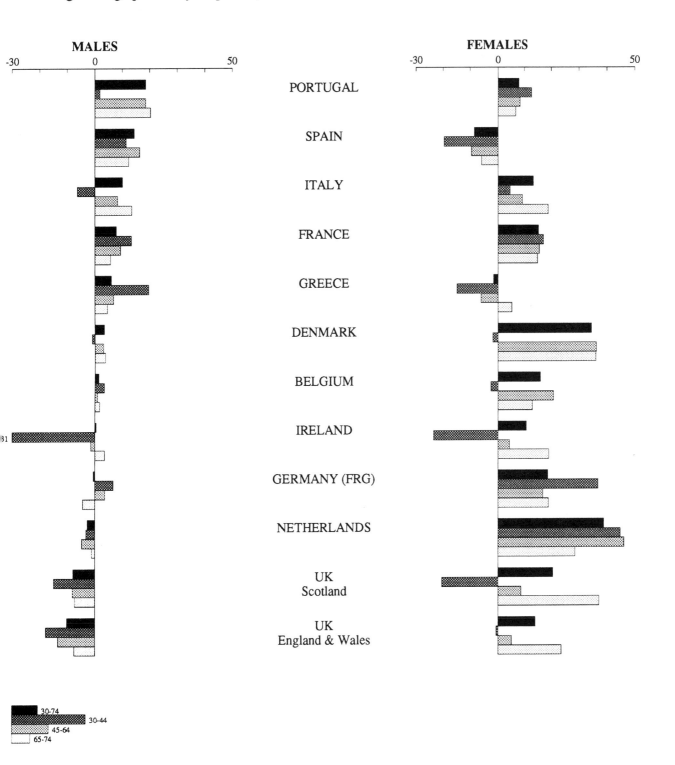

323

LUNG (ICD-9 162)

ASIA, INCIDENCE

MALES	Best model	Goodness of fit	1970 Rate	1970 Cases	1985 Rate	1985 Cases	Cumulative risk 1915	Cumulative risk 1940	Recent trend
CHINA									
Shanghai	A4P2C4	0.70	*70.7*	*678*	101.0	1741	69.4	59.4	-2.9
HONG KONG	A8P2C7	0.62	*98.3*	*580*	134.5	1546	64.1	126.8	18.2
INDIA									
Bombay	A3C6	0.52	25.1	177	27.7	303	17.3	15.0	*1.1*
JAPAN									
Miyagi	A2P2	1.78	37.2	125	64.7	338	38.3	88.2	22.3
Nagasaki	A2P2	-0.55	*127.0*	*101*	65.0	68	43.5	38.4	*-2.2*
Osaka	A3P3C3	4.16	40.1	474	69.3	1224	45.8	73.3	13.8
SINGAPORE									
Chinese	A2P2C7	0.91	109.6	222	130.5	385	84.2	76.4	*-1.8*
Indian	A2	1.94	33.8	8	33.8	13	21.8	21.8	*2.3*
Malay	A2P3	0.83	24.2	7	57.0	28	31.0	79.6	*9.5*

FEMALES	Best model	Goodness of fit	1970 Rate	1970 Cases	1985 Rate	1985 Cases	Cumulative risk 1915	Cumulative risk 1940	Recent trend
CHINA									
Shanghai	A4D	0.05	*37.3*	*421*	34.8	641	22.9	20.5	*-2.5*
HONG KONG	A2P2C2	1.60	*61.0*	*351*	57.0	669	32.5	53.3	17.6
INDIA									
Bombay	A2	1.29	6.2	29	6.2	55	3.7	3.7	-11.0
JAPAN									
Miyagi	A2D	0.00	13.3	53	18.8	119	10.7	19.1	21.8
Nagasaki	A1D	0.04	*29.4*	*30*	18.6	25	14.7	6.9	-14.5
Osaka	A2P2C2	0.94	11.9	166	19.9	446	12.6	19.1	10.8
SINGAPORE									
Chinese	A2C2	0.77	35.2	79	40.7	140	27.3	21.8	*3.0*
Indian	A1	0.19	*12.9*	*0*	12.9	2	8.8	8.8	*-18.8*
Malay	A1P2	0.61	17.2	3	21.7	9	11.9	30.9	44.6

* : not enough cases for reliable estimation
– : incomplete or missing data
Best model: polynomial of the given degree in age (A), period (P) or cohort (C), or linear drift (D) model.
Goodness of fit: the normalised likelihood ratio chi-square for the best model (see Method).
Rate: world-standardised truncated rate per 100 000 per year (30-74 years) and number of **cases** are both estimated from the best-fitting model for the single years cited.
Cumulative risk per 1000 (30-74 years) is estimated from the best-fitting *age-cohort* model for cohorts of central birth year cited.
Recent trend: estimated mean percentage change per five-year period in the age-specific rates (30-74 years) over the period 1973-1987.
Italics denote recent trends not significant at 5 per cent level, or other figures which should be interpreted with caution (see Method).

LUNG (ICD-9 162)

ASIA, INCIDENCE

MALES

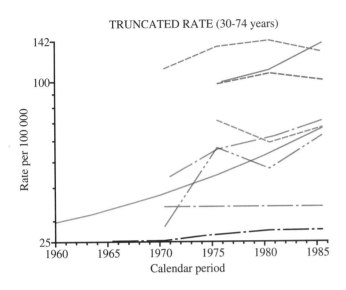

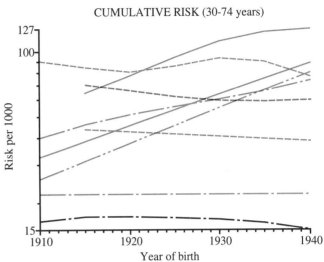

FEMALES

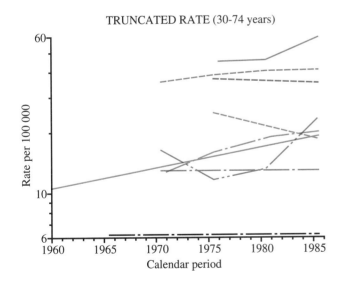

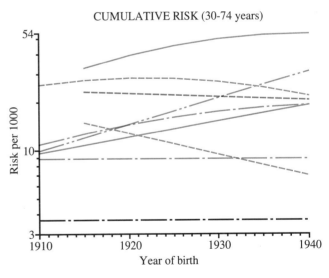

------- CHINA Shanghai
——— JAPAN Miyagi
------- JAPAN Nagasaki
—·—·— JAPAN Osaka
——— HONG KONG

------- SINGAPORE Chinese
—·—·— SINGAPORE Indian
—··—··— SINGAPORE Malay
——··— INDIA Bombay

LUNG (ICD-9 162)

OCEANIA, INCIDENCE

MALES	Best model	Goodness of fit	1970 Rate	Cases	1985 Rate	Cases	Cumulative risk 1915	1940	Recent trend
AUSTRALIA									
New South Wales	A2C3	-0.39	*102.2*	*1056*	101.7	1368	64.1	59.7	*-0.1*
South	A4C2	-0.94	*109.1*	*212*	91.5	329	68.0	27.7	-8.5
HAWAII									
Caucasian	A2C3	-0.76	101.9	36	138.0	84	78.5	77.3	8.2
Chinese	A2	0.54	58.2	6	58.2	10	36.4	36.4	*7.3*
Filipino	A2D	-0.11	36.9	9	63.9	21	29.5	72.0	21.5
Hawaiian	A5C2	0.80	163.2	22	190.9	45	121.7	77.7	*-1.2*
Japanese	A2D	-1.49	51.1	24	67.5	60	39.3	61.7	*9.4*
NEW ZEALAND									
Maori	A2C2	1.11	158.3	30	232.7	67	134.3	142.6	*1.4*
Non-Maori	A8C9	0.41	99.4	563	97.8	702	63.2	44.0	-3.5

FEMALES	Best model	Goodness of fit	1970 Rate	Cases	1985 Rate	Cases	Cumulative risk 1915	1940	Recent trend
AUSTRALIA									
New South Wales	A2C4	1.12	*13.7*	*156*	27.6	395	14.1	39.1	22.1
South	A2D	-1.15	*14.0*	*27*	25.0	94	12.4	32.3	22.7
HAWAII									
Caucasian	A4C4	-0.77	36.7	13	77.8	46	41.4	62.7	23.5
Chinese	A2	-0.02	34.6	3	34.6	6	20.7	20.7	*-11.8*
Filipino	A2	-0.39	31.5	2	31.5	8	18.8	18.8	*22.0*
Hawaiian	A5D	-0.97	56.0	8	85.5	24	41.1	81.3	*0.6*
Japanese	A2P2	-0.75	15.5	7	16.8	17	10.6	15.6	*-10.1*
NEW ZEALAND									
Maori	A2P3	1.04	70.5	12	132.4	42	68.7	138.5	*8.2*
Non-Maori	A2C2	1.02	18.0	110	32.4	251	17.6	28.3	15.5

* : not enough cases for reliable estimation
− : incomplete or missing data
Best model: polynomial of the given degree in age (A), period (P) or cohort (C), or linear drift (D) model.
Goodness of fit: the normalised likelihood ratio chi-square for the best model (see Method).
Rate: world-standardised truncated rate per 100 000 per year (30-74 years) and number of **cases** are both estimated from the best-fitting model for the single years cited.
Cumulative risk per 1000 (30-74 years) is estimated from the best-fitting *age-cohort* model for cohorts of central birth year cited.
Recent trend: estimated mean percentage change per five-year period in the age-specific rates (30-74 years) over the period 1973-1987.
Italics denote recent trends not significant at 5 per cent level, or other figures which should be interpreted with caution (see Method).

LUNG (ICD-9 162)

OCEANIA, INCIDENCE

MALES

TRUNCATED RATE (30-74 years)

CUMULATIVE RISK (30-74 years)

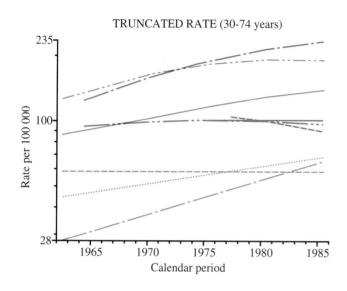
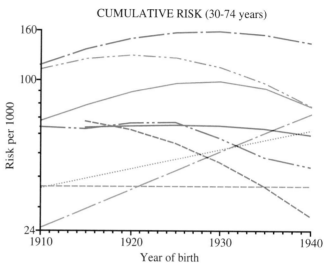

FEMALES

TRUNCATED RATE (30-74 years)

CUMULATIVE RISK (30-74 years)

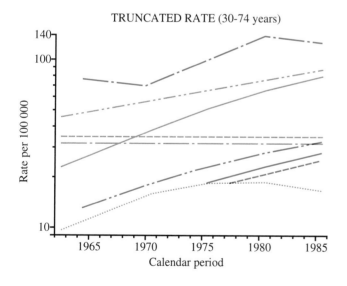
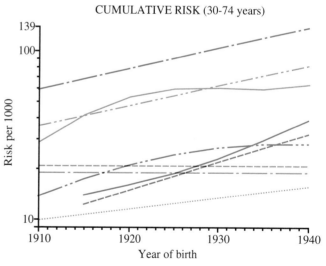

———— AUSTRALIA New South Wales
– – – – AUSTRALIA South
–·–·– NEW ZEALAND Maori
–··–··– NEW ZEALAND Non-Maori
———— HAWAII Caucasian
– – – – HAWAII Chinese
–·–·– HAWAII Filipino
–··–··– HAWAII Hawaiian
············· HAWAII Japanese

LUNG (ICD-9 162)

ASIA, INCIDENCE
Percentage change per five-year period, 1973-1987

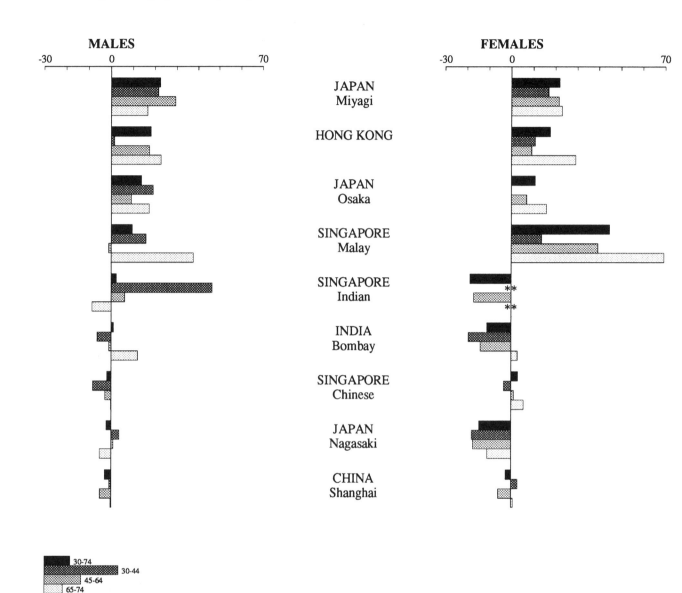

MALES   FEMALES

-30   0   70   -30   0   70

JAPAN
Miyagi

HONG KONG

JAPAN
Osaka

SINGAPORE
Malay

SINGAPORE
Indian

INDIA
Bombay

SINGAPORE
Chinese

JAPAN
Nagasaki

CHINA
Shanghai

30-74
30-44
45-64
65-74

LUNG (ICD-9 162)

OCEANIA, INCIDENCE
Percentage change per five-year period, 1973-1987

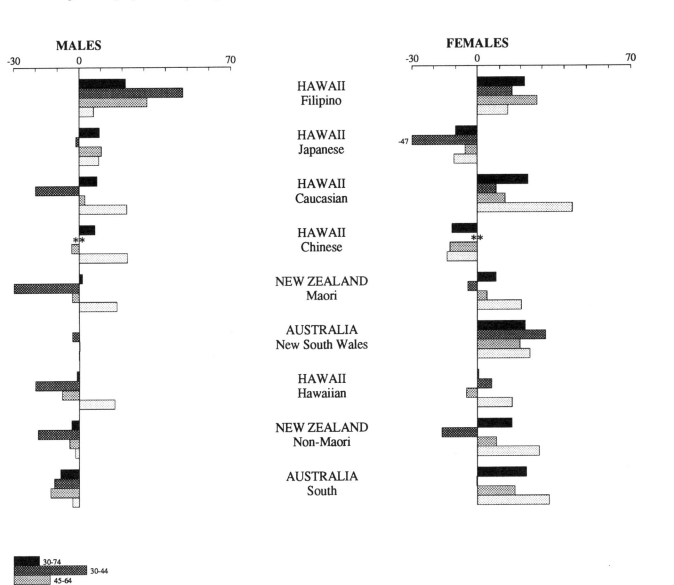

MALES   FEMALES

HAWAII
Filipino

HAWAII
Japanese

HAWAII
Caucasian

HAWAII
Chinese

NEW ZEALAND
Maori

AUSTRALIA
New South Wales

HAWAII
Hawaiian

NEW ZEALAND
Non-Maori

AUSTRALIA
South

30-74
30-44
45-64
65-74

LUNG (ICD-9 162)

ASIA and OCEANIA, MORTALITY

MALES	Best model	Goodness of fit	1965 Rate	1965 Deaths	1985 Rate	1985 Deaths	Cumulative risk 1900	Cumulative risk 1940	Recent trend
AUSTRALIA	A2P5C8	1.79	72.5	1740	87.8	3264	49.0	51.2	-2.4
HONG KONG	A2P2C2	1.82	56.7	222	105.6	942	*38.2*	81.8	*-0.9*
JAPAN	A8P6C9	7.43	25.6	4497	46.1	13214	18.7	43.9	9.8
MAURITIUS	A2D	1.46	18.2	12	30.5	34	*11.9*	33.0	17.4
NEW ZEALAND	A2P3C4	1.63	74.2	395	88.1	660	50.1	51.7	-4.5
SINGAPORE	A2P2C2	1.54	*50.0*	*89*	82.0	209	*25.4*	48.8	–

FEMALES	Best model	Goodness of fit	1965 Rate	1965 Deaths	1985 Rate	1985 Deaths	Cumulative risk 1900	Cumulative risk 1940	Recent trend
AUSTRALIA	A2P3C4	1.27	8.5	225	22.9	919	5.0	23.4	18.2
HONG KONG	A8P5C9	0.59	29.3	156	42.6	351	*22.3*	32.1	*-0.5*
JAPAN	A4P5C3	4.49	9.2	1839	13.4	4773	5.8	10.3	6.7
MAURITIUS	A3D	1.03	3.2	2	8.1	10	*1.9*	12.8	*11.6*
NEW ZEALAND	A2P2C3	-0.14	11.9	70	30.8	250	6.9	29.7	17.9
SINGAPORE	A3C2	1.98	*19.0*	*31*	26.1	65	*8.6*	12.1	–

* : not enough deaths for reliable estimation
– : incomplete or missing data
Best model: polynomial of the given degree in age (A), period (P) or cohort (C), or linear drift (D) model.
Goodness of fit: the normalised likelihood ratio chi-square for the best model (see Method).
Rate: world-standardised truncated rate per 100 000 per year (30-74 years) and number of **deaths** are both estimated from the best-fitting model for the single years cited.
Cumulative risk per 1000 (30-74 years) is estimated from the best-fitting *age-cohort* model for cohorts of central birth year cited.
Recent trend: estimated mean percentage change per five-year period in the age-specific rates (30-74 years) over the period 1975-1988.
Italics denote recent trends not significant at 5 per cent level, or other figures which should be interpreted with caution (see Method).

LUNG (ICD-9 162)

ASIA and OCEANIA, MORTALITY

MALES

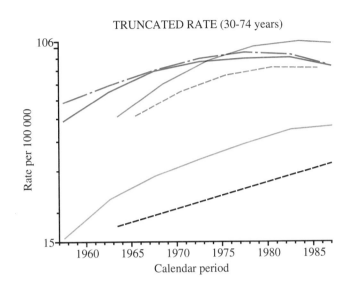

TRUNCATED RATE (30-74 years)

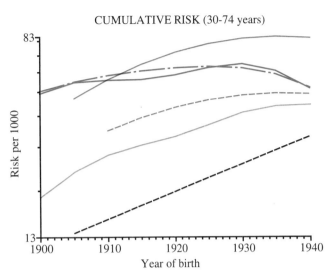

CUMULATIVE RISK (30-74 years)

FEMALES

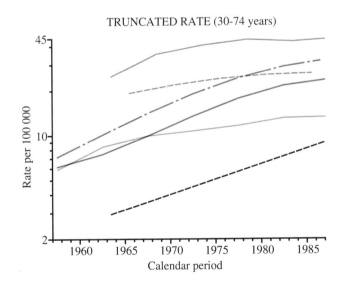

TRUNCATED RATE (30-74 years)

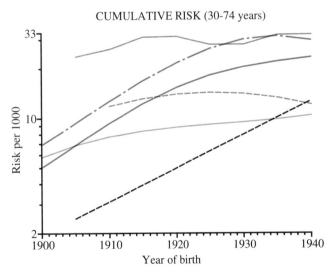

CUMULATIVE RISK (30-74 years)

——— AUSTRALIA   ——— HONG KONG
—·—·— NEW ZEALAND   ------- SINGAPORE
——— JAPAN   ------- MAURITIUS

LUNG (ICD-9 162)

ASIA and OCEANIA, MORTALITY
Percentage change per five-year period, 1975-1988

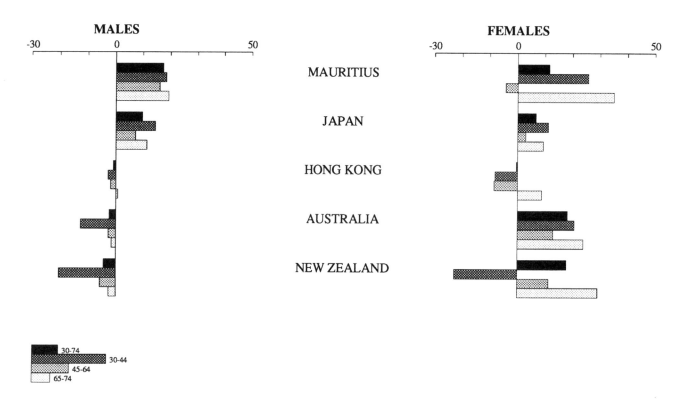

from page 311

Hungary. The lifetime risk (30-74 years) of death predicted for the 1940 birth cohort in Hungary now greatly exceeds 20%, a figure which has never been reached in western Europe, even for the generations which experienced the highest risk (11%). Furthermore, incidence and mortality trends in these countries are consistent, except in Warsaw City (Poland), which recorded only a small increase in risk in successive birth cohorts.

The third feature is the dramatic increase in risk among males in the countries of western Europe which experienced low death rates from lung cancer in the 1960s. Spain, Portugal, Italy and, to a lesser extent, France are the most notable examples of this pattern. The trend in Spain is particularly alarming: the risk has risen from 2.5% to 10% in little more than one generation, and this is clearly reflected by the rapid upward trends in incidence in Navarra and Zaragoza. In contrast, in Belgium, the Netherlands, Germany and Denmark, already at high or moderate risk of death from lung cancer, this risk has not declined or has even slightly increased. This is particularly striking for Belgium, which now ranks first in western Europe, both for truncated rates and the lifetime risk for the most recent birth cohorts. Examina-

tion of the recent linear trends suggests, however, that a reduction in risk may occur in the Netherlands and Denmark during the next decade.

The pattern of change of lung cancer risk among females in Europe is much simpler, and can be described as a general and rapid increase. The main exception is the decreasing risk of death in Spain, which is difficult to explain; there are opposite incidence trends in Navarra and in Zaragoza.

Asia and Oceania

In Asia, a clear distinction can be made between Chinese, Japanese and Indian populations.

Chinese populations have been at highest risk for both sexes, but there is a suggestion of a levelling off or even a decrease, as in Singapore. In Hong Kong, the incidence data suggest an increase, but the mortality data suggest stabilisation of the risk; the recent inclusion in the incidence data of cases registered solely from a death certificate may explain this apparent contradiction, since about 15% of lung cancer registrations for the period 1983-87 in Hong Kong were based only on death certificates, not included in earlier data sets. Interestingly, a decrease is also seen among females in Shanghai (China), who have an elevated risk of lung adenocarcinoma not related to tobacco smoking[108].

Incidence and mortality are increasing in Japan among both males and females, except in Nagasaki City, where the rate of lung cancer was higher than in the other Japanese populations around 1975, but has been similar in the last decade; this excess risk for the period 1973-77 in Nagasaki, with respect to the much larger populations covered by the prefectural registries of Miyagi and Osaka, is seen for almost all cancer sites.

The two Indian populations in Bombay (India) and Singapore have retained their low risk of lung cancer since the 1960s. Among females in Bombay there is even a slight decrease in risk.

In Oceania, the very high risk seen among Maoris of both sexes in New Zealand has started to decrease among males, but not females. A similar and more pronounced pattern holds for Hawaiians in Hawaii. The decreasing risk is also seen in non-Maori males in New Zealand, and the age-specific trends also strongly suggest an impending decrease in females. Although the incidence data from New South Wales and South Australia are not entirely consistent, an overall evaluation of the trend for Australia and New Zealand can be made with the help of the mortality data, which suggest that in both countries the risk has started to decrease in the youngest male cohorts and to reach a plateau in females. The trends among male and female Caucasians in Hawaii also follow this pattern. By contrast, the risk is increasing exponentially among Filipino and Japanese males in Hawaii.

Americas

In Canada and the USA, the trends are qualitatively similar, and suggest a decreasing risk in the youngest male birth cohorts and a stabilisation of the risk in females. This pattern is considerably more pronounced in the USA than in Canada, where the risk continues to increase in successive birth cohorts among males both in Alberta and in Quebec; the risk is higher among Canadian females, and the plateau is seen only in Newfoundland. This difference in incidence trends between the two countries can also be seen in the mortality trends: the trends in cumulative risk and the age-specific recent linear trends show that the situation is more encouraging in the USA than in Canada. The rate of decline in mortality among males aged 30-44 years is 16% every five years in the USA, but only 5% in Canada; the mortality

rate among young females is still increasing in Canada at 21% every five years, whereas it is decreasing in the USA (9%).

In South America, the available data suggest that little change has occurred except in São Paulo (Brazil), where a steady increase was seen up to 1978, but more recent data are unfortunately not available. Mortality trends for lung cancer in South America are remarkably diverse. Mortality in Uruguay has been similar to that observed in Canada and the USA, but it has increased steadily over the last two decades, and the risk in recent cohorts has not declined at all. In contrast, while the risk has been low in other South American countries, there has been a substantial rate of increase in males; rates are now similar to those observed in North America, and with the exception of Chile, no decrease is seen for the younger cohorts. Among females, the risk has not changed substantially, in stark contrast to the rapid increase seen in North American females since the 1960s. The only rapid increase in mortality among females has occurred in Panama, where the risk was very low in the 1960s, but lung cancer mortality in Panama has now reached the level observed in other South American countries.

Comment

Trends in lung cancer incidence and mortality have been reported from very many countries. Most authors relate the observed trends to sex-specific smoking habits in successive birth cohorts, sometimes separately by geographical region. Mortality trends in the UK have been closely related to cohort-specific measures of cumulative tar dose from cigarettes[157]. In Denmark, the 1930 birth cohorts are at peak risk for both lung and bladder cancer[268], with a decline for those born later. The dramatic increase in mortality among males in Spain up to 1985 has been reported[31]; the relatively small increase in mortality among females was attributed to smoking having become widespread only in the last 20 years, but the analyses reported here show that mortality rates are currently falling among females at all ages below 75 years.

Reports from eastern Europe generally confirm the large rates of increase reported here. Truncated incidence (30-74 years) rose sharply in Cracow (Poland) and Tallinn (Estonia) up to 1980, although there was an apparent decline in the city of Bratislava (Slovakia)[225]. In Slovakia as a whole, however, incidence increased by 11% and 14% in males and females, respectively, between the two quinquennia ending in 1988[237]. A report on trends in incidence in six republics of

continued page 338

AMERICAS (except USA), INCIDENCE

MALES	Best model	Goodness of fit	1970 Rate	1970 Cases	1985 Rate	1985 Cases	Cumulative risk 1915	Cumulative risk 1940	Recent trend
BRAZIL									
Sao Paulo	A2D	0.00	43.7	251	*75.7*	*530*	27.9	*68.4*	–
CANADA									
Alberta	A2C4	1.61	66.0	200	96.3	423	55.4	93.8	16.1
British Columbia	A3P3C3	-0.66	112.2	524	113.2	825	68.2	66.4	9.2
Maritime Provinces	A2C2	0.54	76.4	244	138.1	508	75.2	120.3	19.0
Newfoundland	A2C2	0.41	72.8	64	123.5	140	68.3	78.8	14.1
Quebec	A4P4C3	1.09	83.6	904	175.0	2537	89.2	*210.1*	24.6
COLOMBIA									
Cali	A2D	0.19	34.8	20	44.0	56	26.7	39.4	*7.6*
CUBA	A4C5	5.99	82.4	1213	73.4	1523	46.4	*61.0*	–
PUERTO RICO	A8C9	0.11	28.3	128	34.5	233	17.5	22.8	*3.6*

FEMALES	Best model	Goodness of fit	1970 Rate	1970 Cases	1985 Rate	1985 Cases	Cumulative risk 1915	Cumulative risk 1940	Recent trend
BRAZIL									
Sao Paulo	A2D	-1.93	8.8	62	*19.3*	*186*	5.8	*21.3*	–
CANADA									
Alberta	A3P3C3	-0.58	11.7	34	43.1	200	17.2	87.6	51.9
British Columbia	A3C2	0.52	21.3	101	54.7	427	25.2	80.0	38.0
Maritime Provinces	A3D	0.59	13.3	43	47.4	182	17.2	135.2	45.4
Newfoundland	A2C3	0.48	7.7	6	24.7	27	8.2	48.5	57.1
Quebec	A2P3C2	2.10	11.5	139	46.9	781	17.4	129.8	60.3
COLOMBIA									
Cali	A2D	-0.28	10.0	7	19.2	31	9.3	27.4	26.1
CUBA	A3P2C6	3.91	28.7	364	26.8	552	17.5	*18.8*	–
PUERTO RICO	A2C2	0.59	10.0	45	11.1	88	7.3	6.5	*1.7*

* : not enough cases for reliable estimation
– : incomplete or missing data
Best model: polynomial of the given degree in age (A), period (P) or cohort (C), or linear drift (D) model.
Goodness of fit: the normalised likelihood ratio chi-square for the best model (see Method).
Rate: world-standardised truncated rate per 100 000 per year (30-74 years) and number of **cases** are both estimated from the best-fitting model for the single years cited.
Cumulative risk per 1000 (30-74 years) is estimated from the best-fitting *age-cohort* model for cohorts of central birth year cited.
Recent trend: estimated mean percentage change per five-year period in the age-specific rates (30-74 years) over the period 1973-1987.
Italics denote recent trends not significant at 5 per cent level, or other figures which should be interpreted with caution (see Method).

LUNG (ICD-9 162)

AMERICAS (except USA), INCIDENCE

MALES

TRUNCATED RATE (30-74 years)

CUMULATIVE RISK (30-74 years)

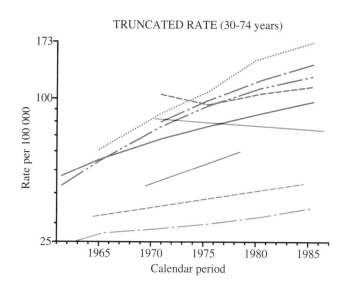
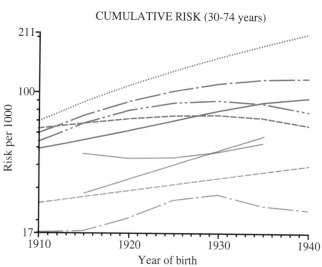

FEMALES

TRUNCATED RATE (30-74 years)

CUMULATIVE RISK (30-74 years)

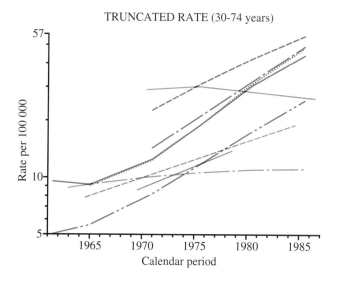
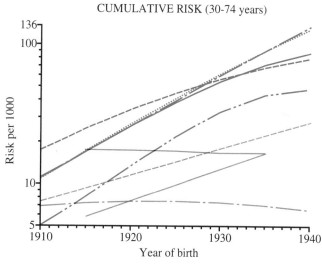

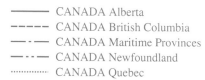

———	CANADA Alberta	———	CUBA
– – –	CANADA British Columbia	–·–·–	PUERTO RICO
–·–·–	CANADA Maritime Provinces	———	BRAZIL Sao Paulo
–··–··–	CANADA Newfoundland	– – – –	COLOMBIA Cali
··········	CANADA Quebec		

LUNG (ICD-9 162)

AMERICAS (USA), INCIDENCE

MALES	Best model	Goodness of fit	1970 Rate	1970 Cases	1985 Rate	1985 Cases	Cumulative risk 1915	Cumulative risk 1940	Recent trend
USA									
Bay Area, Black	A3C2	1.59	142.9	80	222.5	179	117.0	141.5	9.6
Bay Area, Chinese	A2	-0.12	106.8	22	*106.8*	*55*	66.4	*66.4*	–
Bay Area, White	A3P2C7	-0.58	120.0	713	123.7	777	76.3	60.0	-2.5
Connecticut	A2P2C6	1.93	110.0	722	127.1	1029	75.3	87.7	2.6
Detroit, Black	A3C2	0.66	163.1	225	222.9	390	118.2	144.5	7.4
Detroit, White	A5P3C5	-0.53	122.2	899	154.7	1129	87.2	98.7	8.8
Iowa	A3C4	-1.02	104.2	705	134.9	965	80.6	81.6	6.8
New Orleans, Black	A3C2	-1.16	*209.2*	*108*	237.0	141	138.0	105.6	*2.1*
New Orleans, White	A3C2	2.23	*155.9*	*226*	180.5	283	109.2	94.8	*3.0*
Seattle	A3C2	0.13	*123.7*	*594*	129.3	871	80.7	71.4	*1.0*

FEMALES	Best model	Goodness of fit	1970 Rate	1970 Cases	1985 Rate	1985 Cases	Cumulative risk 1915	Cumulative risk 1940	Recent trend
USA									
Bay Area, Black	A8D	0.35	35.8	22	77.1	72	28.0	96.8	26.5
Bay Area, Chinese	A3	-0.08	39.8	6	*39.8*	*22*	25.8	*25.8*	–
Bay Area, White	A3P3C2	-1.51	38.5	264	79.6	568	40.3	67.2	19.7
Connecticut	A2P3C3	-0.44	25.1	189	63.2	587	29.2	81.7	28.3
Detroit, Black	A3C2	1.07	30.3	46	76.8	162	32.4	91.1	30.0
Detroit, White	A4P2C3	1.81	22.8	188	71.8	601	30.4	105.6	34.8
Iowa	A2C2	0.66	16.9	122	47.8	380	21.0	65.6	40.2
New Orleans, Black	A2C2	-0.76	*33.4*	*20*	67.3	52	32.5	45.4	21.6
New Orleans, White	A3C2	0.90	*34.6*	*63*	72.4	139	37.4	60.0	25.6
Seattle	A3C2	-1.89	*33.5*	*171*	74.8	543	35.9	69.5	27.8

* : not enough cases for reliable estimation
– : incomplete or missing data
Best model: polynomial of the given degree in age (A), period (P) or cohort (C), or linear drift (D) model.
Goodness of fit: the normalised likelihood ratio chi-square for the best model (see Method).
Rate: world-standardised truncated rate per 100 000 per year (30-74 years) and number of **cases** are both estimated from the best-fitting model for the single years cited.
Cumulative risk per 1000 (30-74 years) is estimated from the best-fitting *age-cohort* model for cohorts of central birth year cited.
Recent trend: estimated mean percentage change per five-year period in the age-specific rates (30-74 years) over the period 1973-1987.
Italics denote recent trends not significant at 5 per cent level, or other figures which should be interpreted with caution (see Method).

LUNG (ICD-9 162)

AMERICAS (USA), INCIDENCE

MALES

TRUNCATED RATE (30-74 years)

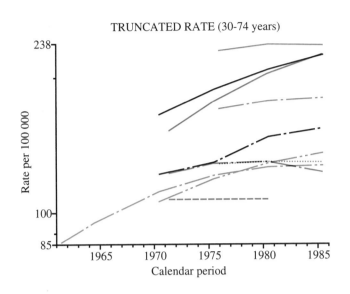

CUMULATIVE RISK (30-74 years)

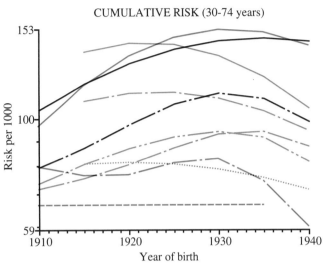

FEMALES

TRUNCATED RATE (30-74 years)

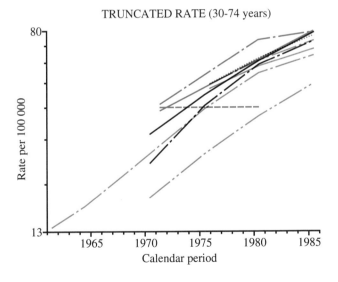

CUMULATIVE RISK (30-74 years)

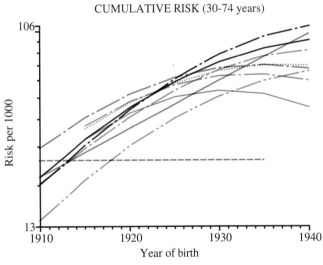

——— BAY AREA Black
- - - - BAY AREA Chinese
—·—· BAY AREA White
—··—·· CONNECTICUT
—···— IOWA

············· SEATTLE
——— NEW ORLEANS Black
—·—·— NEW ORLEANS White
——— DETROIT Black
—··—·· DETROIT White

LUNG (ICD-9 162)

AMERICAS (except USA), INCIDENCE
Percentage change per five-year period, 1973-1987

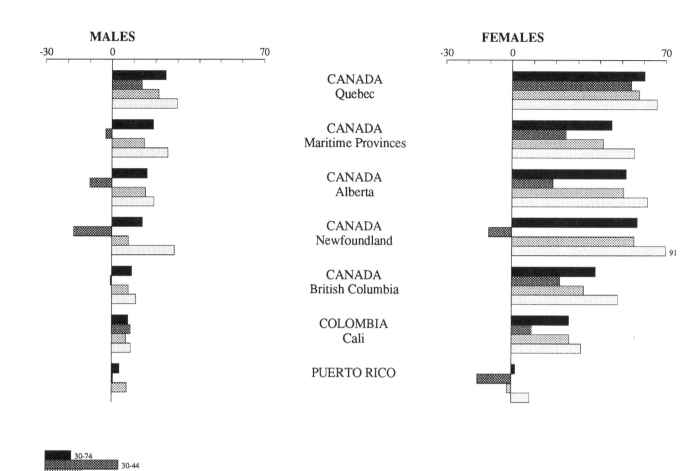

MALES

-30   0   70

CANADA
Quebec

CANADA
Maritime Provinces

CANADA
Alberta

CANADA
Newfoundland

CANADA
British Columbia

COLOMBIA
Cali

PUERTO RICO

FEMALES

-30   0   70

91

30-74
30-44
45-64
65-74

from page 333

the former Soviet Union (Belarus, Estonia, Georgia, Latvia, Lithuania, Moldavia) during the period 1971-87 suggests annual rates of increase ranging from 1.5% to 4.5% in males and up to 2.4% per year in females; this is remarkable for suggesting more rapid rates of increase in lung cancer incidence among males than females[310].

In Shanghai (China), over 70% of male controls in a large population-based case-control study were cigarette smokers. This study confirmed the relationship between smoking and lung cancer in both sexes, although smoking accounted for only about a quarter of cases in females, for whom adenocarcinoma was the predominant cell type[108]. Since lung cancer rates in Shanghai are three times higher than the national average in China,

the public health implications of the risk elsewhere in China approaching the levels seen in Shanghai would be enormous.

The incidence trends reported here for provinces in Canada are reflected in the mortality trends in each province up to 1986, with the highest rates among males in Quebec, a plateau in Ontario, and a decline in British Columbia[35]. Rates of change in incidence in Ontario in the 10 years up to 1988 were similar to those elsewhere in Canada, with an increase of 27% every five years in females, but less than 1% among males[182]. Mortality doubled among Canadian females between the 1970s and 1980s, and was expected to continue rising until after the turn of the century.

continued page 342

LUNG (ICD-9 162)

AMERICAS (USA), INCIDENCE
Percentage change per five-year period, 1973-1987

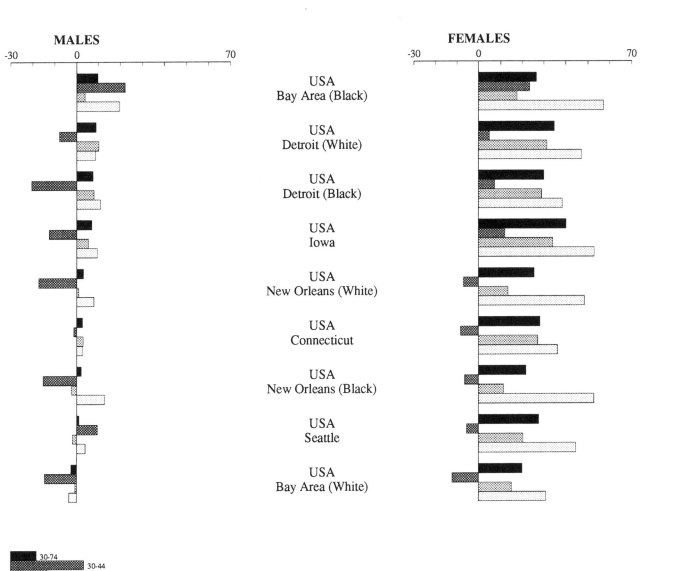

MALES

-30   0   70

FEMALES

-30   0   70

USA
Bay Area (Black)

USA
Detroit (White)

USA
Detroit (Black)

USA
Iowa

USA
New Orleans (White)

USA
Connecticut

USA
New Orleans (Black)

USA
Seattle

USA
Bay Area (White)

30-74
30-44
45-64
65-74

339

LUNG (ICD-9 162)

AMERICAS, MORTALITY

MALES	Best model	Goodness of fit	1965 Rate	1965 Deaths	1985 Rate	1985 Deaths	Cumulative risk 1900	Cumulative risk 1940	Recent trend
CANADA	A3P5C8	2.64	66.6	2521	105.4	6157	44.9	80.5	5.4
CHILE	A6C8	0.68	30.0	346	41.1	718	18.2	23.0	3.8
COSTA RICA	A2D	0.19	*13.4*	*19*	26.8	82	*9.2*	36.6	14.5
PANAMA	A2D	-0.81	18.9	27	27.3	78	11.9	24.5	–
PUERTO RICO	A2P3	-0.73	*20.2*	*82*	32.2	153	*14.6*	28.6	5.9
URUGUAY	A8C6	-0.32	80.9	476	105.2	765	50.9	91.6	6.9
USA	A8P5C9	20.45	81.3	34505	110.2	62092	51.0	68.4	1.8
VENEZUELA	A2P2C3	1.84	25.5	213	*28.2*	*445*	15.9	22.7	–

FEMALES	Best model	Goodness of fit	1965 Rate	1965 Deaths	1985 Rate	1985 Deaths	Cumulative risk 1900	Cumulative risk 1940	Recent trend
CANADA	A3P3C4	-0.28	9.5	373	35.6	2285	5.4	58.4	35.2
CHILE	A2C3	0.83	9.2	116	10.4	215	5.6	6.1	6.8
COSTA RICA	A2D	-2.89	*7.7*	*8*	10.1	23	*5.2*	9.0	*6.1*
PANAMA	A1D	0.12	4.0	5	7.7	21	2.6	9.5	–
PUERTO RICO	A2C3	-0.19	*8.5*	*34*	11.2	57	*5.4*	6.9	*-0.4*
URUGUAY	A4C2	3.21	6.5	39	7.2	59	4.1	5.9	*-4.1*
USA	A8P6C9	8.66	12.5	5916	44.5	28912	6.5	49.0	27.7
VENEZUELA	A2P2C2	0.36	11.5	104	*11.9*	*202*	6.8	8.1	–

* : not enough deaths for reliable estimation
– : incomplete or missing data
Best model: polynomial of the given degree in age (A), period (P) or cohort (C), or linear drift (D) model.
Goodness of fit: the normalised likelihood ratio chi-square for the best model (see Method).
Rate: world-standardised truncated rate per 100 000 per year (30-74 years) and number of **deaths** are both estimated from the best-fitting model for the single years cited.
Cumulative risk per 1000 (30-74 years) is estimated from the best-fitting *age-cohort* model for cohorts of central birth year cited.
Recent trend: estimated mean percentage change per five-year period in the age-specific rates (30-74 years) over the period 1975-1988.
Italics denote recent trends not significant at 5 per cent level, or other figures which should be interpreted with caution (see Method).

LUNG (ICD-9 162)

AMERICAS, MORTALITY

MALES

TRUNCATED RATE (30-74 years)

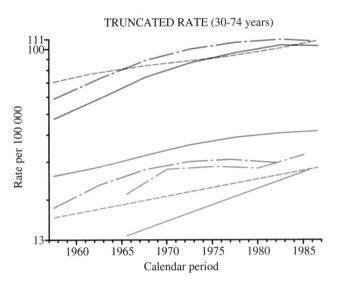

CUMULATIVE RISK (30-74 years)

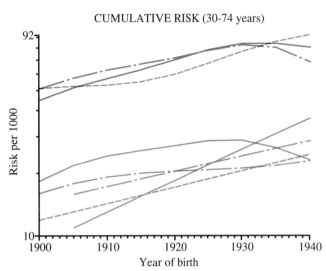

FEMALES

TRUNCATED RATE (30-74 years)

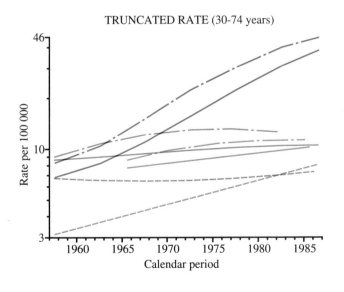

CUMULATIVE RISK (30-74 years)

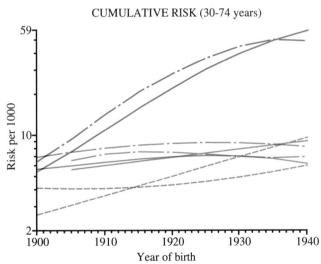

———— CANADA	—··— PUERTO RICO
—·—· USA	———— CHILE
———— COSTA RICA	——— URUGUAY
——— PANAMA	—··— VENEZUELA

LUNG (ICD-9 162)

AMERICAS, MORTALITY
Percentage change per five-year period, 1975-1988

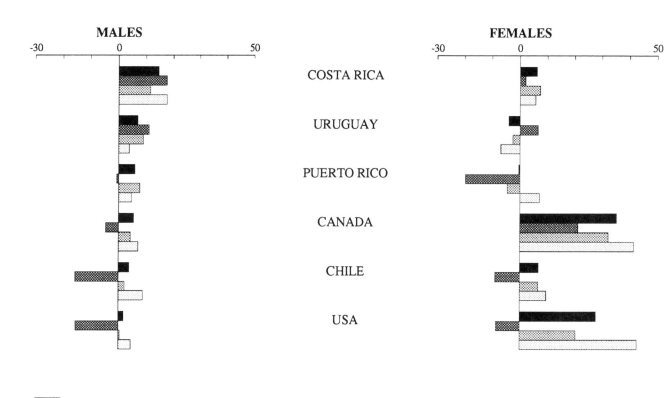

MALES

-30   0   50

FEMALES

-30   0   50

COSTA RICA

URUGUAY

PUERTO RICO

CANADA

CHILE

USA

30-74
30-44
45-64
65-74

from page 338

In the USA, cohort-based increases in mortality have been reported for both sexes, with males born around 1925-30 and females born around 1935-40 expected to have the highest mortality, and a downturn in mortality not expected until 1990 for males and 2000 for females[73]. Among females, lung cancer mortality exceeded breast cancer mortality as early as 1979 in Texas[43] and 1983 in California[142].

Except for Japan, lung cancer mortality among females was greatly exceeded by mortality from breast cancer in 14 of the most developed countries in the 1960s, but the ratio has declined rapidly since then, reaching unity in Scotland around 1985[306], and the incidence of lung cancer in females exceeded that of breast

cancer in the high-risk city of Glasgow (Scotland) in 1990[109].

Given the poor outcome of treatment, the rise of the twentieth century lung cancer epidemic in males and the early phase of its decline are clearly visible from both incidence and mortality data when these are examined by birth cohort. The widespread evidence of failure to prevent the lung cancer epidemic in females may be tempered by examination of the trends in lifetime risk and the recent linear trends in age-specific rates in the UK. These patterns suggest that the decrease in risk which has been observed in successive birth cohorts among males is now beginning to occur among females.

Chapter 15

BONE

Primary malignant neoplasms of the bones in adults aged 30 years or more comprise mainly osteosarcoma and chondrosarcoma; Ewing's sarcoma is largely confined to children and young adults. Incidence is bimodal, with a peak in adolescence, principally due to osteosarcoma; incidence increases again after the age of 30. Bone tumours are generally more frequent in males. Although osteosarcoma and chondrosarcoma are distinct clinical entities, data were not available to study trends in these two diseases separately. Both are coded to the same three-digit rubric in the International Classification of Diseases used for reporting mortality statistics to WHO, and while they can be distinguished by morphology codes in data from cancer registries, too few incidence data sets were available with this level of detail over the necessary time period to enable separate analyses of trends for the two types of sarcoma. Malignant bone tumours are therefore considered together as a single group. The aetiology of bone neoplasms is poorly understood. Ionising radiation is the only environmental agent known to cause bone cancers[103]. Malignant transformation of Paget's disease occurs in old age, especially in males.

A complication arises in the examination of trends, since bone is also a preferred site for metastasis of several common malignant tumours, such as cancers of the breast and prostate, themselves much more frequent than primary bone neoplasms. Relatively small misclassification rates of metastatic bone disease as primary malignant neoplasms of bone could therefore significantly distort comparison of rates between countries. If diagnostic accuracy in a given country were to change with the passage of time, this could affect the interpretation of observed trends. Further, since trends in diagnostic accuracy are unlikely to be similar in all countries, misclassification could also complicate the comparison of incidence trends between countries. The quality of the incidence data is therefore particularly important for the evaluation of trends in bone tumours. Histological confirmation of malignancy is more useful in distinguishing primary and secondary malignancy in bone than in, say, lung, because the most common primaries of bone are sarcomas, while the most common metastatic deposits in bone are from epithelial tumours, mainly adenocarcinomas and squamous cell tumours, which are readily distinguishable histologically from sarcomas. The percentage of bone tumours that were histologically confirmed is shown for each of the last three available incidence data sets in Table 15.1 by sex and broad age group (35-64, 65-74 years). Histological verification was available for 60% or less of bone tumours in Cluj (Romania), Bombay (India) and, for females only, in Warsaw City (Poland). In most other populations, the percentage of bone tumours confirmed by histology was 80% or more (frequently 90% or more) for at least the last 15 years of available data.

Europe

In Europe, incidence has generally been stable or declining. Truncated rates have decreased by half in both sexes since the 1960s in Finland, with consistently high levels of histological confirmation, and mortality has declined correspondingly. In Sweden, however, where incidence has changed very little in males and declined slightly in females, mortality has declined quickly in both sexes, at around 30% every five years, and the ratio of incidence to mortality is now about 1.6, similar to the ratio in Finland. There are some exceptions to the general pattern: in the last 15 years, incidence has increased slightly among females in Norway, Denmark and South Thames (UK). None of these recent increases is significant. In Norway, however, where over 90% of primary bone tumours are histologically verified, the overall trend is well fitted by an age-drift model, suggesting that the recent rate of increase of 2.3% every five years is a good estimate of the trend, and although the overall trend in mortality is not significant, age-specific mortality among females in Norway is also increasing, in contrast to the trend everywhere else in Europe.

Although some of the very rapid trends in incidence estimated for populations in Doubs (France), Varese (Italy) and in Spain are significant, they are all statistically unstable, and cannot be interpreted at face value. Incidence of bone tumours in Cluj (Romania) is twice as high as elsewhere in Europe in both sexes, at around 3 per 100 000; although there is some evidence of decline in age-specific rates, histological confirmation has also declined substantially. Mortality data for

Romania as a whole are incomplete, but national mortality rates appear stable, and are higher than incidence rates in Cluj. These data suggest that some cases of metastatic disease may be included among both incidence and mortality data in Romania. Mortality in Greece is also high, at about 5 and 3 per 100 000 in males and females, respectively, and it has changed very little since the 1970s, in contrast to the general decline elsewhere.

With the exceptions of Norway, where mortality is low but stable or increasing, and of Romania and Greece, where mortality may be artefactually high, the general decline in mortality from bone tumours in Europe is quite large (20% or more every five years), and it applies to both sexes and all age groups (30-74 years).

Asia and Oceania

Incidence rates are relatively high (2-3 per 100 000) in both sexes in Hong Kong and in Shanghai (China), with an upward tendency in both sexes in Shanghai. Rates are generally less than 1 per 100 000 in other Asian populations. The sharp decline in incidence in both sexes in Miyagi (Japan) in the 1960s may be partly due to improved diagnosis and exclusion of metastases in bone, particularly in males (see Table 15.1). More recent trends in Miyagi, Osaka and Nagasaki (Japan) are also downward, corresponding with a further marked increase in the percentage of bone tumours that were histologically verified. The decline in incidence in Bombay (India) is less easily explained, since while 60% or less of the tumours are histologically confirmed, there has been little change in the level of confirmation over time. Incidence in Australia and New Zealand is 1 per 100 000 or less, with no convincing evidence of change.

The persistently high incidence in Hong Kong is reflected in mortality rates which are also stable and almost as high, although it must be noted that less than half of the incident tumours are histologically confirmed. In contrast, there has been an 80% fall in recorded mortality from bone tumours in Japan in the 20 years to 1985, and incidence-to-mortality ratios in the three Japanese and two Australian populations included here are now 1.5- to 2-fold. A similar decline in mortality has occurred in Singapore, but the ratio of incidence to mortality there is close to unity. These changes suggest there may have been improvement in the quality of death certification in Japan, Singapore and Australia since the 1960s, rather than substantial declines in national mortality from bone tumours.

Americas

The incidence of bone tumours in Cuba has remained higher than elsewhere in the Americas, at around 2 per 100 000 in both sexes. These rates are based on more than 30 cases per year in the age range 30-74 years, and around two thirds of tumours are histologically verified. There has been a slight overall decline in the rate among males, associated with an increase in histological verification, but the true underlying incidence probably remains high. With the exception of Cuba, truncated incidence rates have generally been 1 per 100 000 or less, with irregular fluctuations over time in some populations. Perhaps the most notable change has been the increase in incidence in both sexes in Quebec (Canada), with recent linear trends of 20% or more every five years, also based on substantial numbers of cases each year; but the proportion of cases verified by histology has fallen steadily. Elsewhere in Canada, incidence has not changed substantially, and although Quebec covers about a quarter of the national population, mortality from bone tumours in Canada has been falling at around 18% every five years. The increase in incidence in Quebec may therefore be at least partly artefactual.

In the USA, incidence has been 1 per 100 000 or less; fewer than 10 cases are registered per year in the age range 30-74 years in each of the populations included here, and there is little or no evidence of change in incidence. Mortality in the USA has fallen substantially since 1965, from rates that must have exceeded incidence in most US populations to about half the incidence rates in 1985. A similar pattern of incidence and mortality trends occurred in Puerto Rico. Mortality in Chile, Uruguay and Venezuela has also declined substantially since 1965. The rapid increase among males in Costa Rica depends on very few recorded deaths, and is not reliable.

Comment

Few other reports on trends in bone cancer are available. Mortality declined steeply in both sexes in England and Wales during the period 1951-80[213], with steep falls in successive calendar periods and lesser rates of decline in successive birth cohorts. These were attributed to more accurate classification and the exclusion of secondary tumours, to improved survival, and possibly to decline in the incidence of Paget's disease. The widespread declines in mortality in Europe, with the exception of Greece, Yugoslavia and the countries of eastern Europe, have also been attri-

continued page 369

Table 15.1: Percentage of bone tumours histologically verified, by sex, age group (35-64, 65-74 years) and registry: Cancer Incidence in Five Continents, volumes IV-VI

	Males						Females					
	35-64			65-74			35-64			65-74		
	IV	V	VI	IV	V	VI	IV	V	VI	IV	V	VI
EUROPE (except European Community)												
Finland	96	99	96	81	94	99	95	99	96	84	90	93
Hungary												
County Vas	0	-	99	99	99	-	75	50	99	50	33	99
Szabolcs-Szatmar	99	60	80	20	60	-	88	29	99	99	0	67
Israel												
All Jews	84	83	99	99	33	92	95	82	87	71	64	89
Non-Jews	99	-	99	99	-	99	0	67	-	-	0	-
Norway	99	99	99	94	85	99	94	99	99	99	99	92
Poland												
Warsaw City	44	43	61	31	25	99	73	50	65	38	29	14
Romania												
County Cluj	78	87	62	99	75	33	99	46	38	80	50	44
Sweden	92	99	99	76	99	90	89	99	99	80	99	91
Switzerland												
Geneva	99	99	99	-	99	99	-	99	99	99	-	-
Yugoslavia												
Slovenia	88	88	99	60	99	99	50	99	99	20	99	99
EUROPE (European Community)												
Denmark	92	94	91	99	82	81	89	97	94	99	73	86
France												
Bas-Rhin	99	88	99	99	99	88	99	99	95	99	33	-
Doubs	-	75	99	99	67	99	99	99	-	99	67	99
Germany (FRG)												
Hamburg	83	80	..	58	67	..	61	71	..	71	0	..
Saarland	-	86	99	-	83	99	-	99	99	-	50	60
Germany (GDR)	93	95	96	83	82	89	93	97	93	81	79	82
Italy												
Varese	99	50	99	99	99	99	-	99	73	-	50	67
Spain												
Navarra	50	50	99	25	0	-	71	99	88	25	0	50
Zaragoza	86	93	99	60	89	0	99	83	75	91	71	0
United Kingdom												
Birmingham	89	99	90	78	71	88	80	99	72	79	86	78
Scotland	*	79	93	*	83	72	*	81	95	*	76	99
South Thames	92	88	78	86	83	56	95	81	81	72	93	67

Table 15.1 (cont.) :   Percentage of bone tumours histologically verified, by sex, age group (35-64, 65-74 years) and registry: Cancer Incidence in Five Continents, volumes IV-VI

	Males						Females					
	35-64			65-74			35-64			65-74		
	IV	V	VI	IV	V	VI	IV	V	VI	IV	V	VI
ASIA												
China												
Shanghai	45	26	33	67	8	8	36	27	27	99	13	6
Hong Kong	17	56	36	25	48	56	35	36	50	11	26	43
India												
Bombay	64	58	61	25	30	50	53	53	40	0	17	50
Japan												
Miyagi	68	62	94	38	58	64	17	54	92	80	50	99
Nagasaki	67	75	99	0	-	-	25	0	99	33	-	-
Osaka	50	57	87	33	21	63	42	58	88	27	31	63
Singapore												
Chinese	91	86	99	50	99	50	43	89	99	-	99	99
Indian	99	99	99	-	-	-	-	99	99	-	99	-
Malay	-	67	-	0	-	-	-	99	99	-	0	-
OCEANIA												
Australia												
New South Wales	96	99	95	99	99	89	99	99	97	99	99	99
South Australia	*	*	99	*	*	99	*	*	99	*	*	75
Hawaii												
Caucasian	99	99	99	99	99	-	99	-	99	-	-	-
Chinese	99	-	-	-	-	-	-	99	-	-	-	-
Filipino	-	99	-	-	-	99	-	99	-	-	-	-
Hawaiian	99	99	99	99	-	-	99	99	-	-	-	-
Japanese	-	99	99	99	-	-	-	99	-	99	-	-
New Zealand												
Maori	-	99	99	-	-	-	-	99	99	-	0	-
Non-Maori	-	99	99	-	99	93	-	63	99	-	79	92

Table 15.1 (cont.) : Percentage of bone tumours histologically verified, by sex, age group (35-64, 65-74 years) and registry: Cancer Incidence in Five Continents, volumes IV-VI

	Males						Females					
	35-64			65-74			35-64			65-74		
	IV	V	VI	IV	V	VI	IV	V	VI	IV	V	VI
AMERICAS (except USA)												
Brazil												
São Paulo	60	67	..	50	38	..	91	77	..	67	50	..
Canada												
Alberta	82	99	92	99	99	-	99	90	99	99	67	88
British Columbia	93	78	80	78	67	70	99	93	95	80	88	90
Maritime Provinces	99	99	99	99	88	-	99	99	99	99	99	99
Newfoundland	99	99	99	-	99	50	99	-	99	99	-	-
Quebec	80	77	69	88	55	59	91	72	63	71	68	42
Colombia												
Cali	80	99	75	50	99	-	56	0	71	99	99	17
Cuba	52	..	70	41	..	43	59	..	72	50	..	64
Puerto Rico	90	67	88	99	75	67	73	99	92	57	25	83
AMERICAS (USA)												
Bay Area, Black	99	99	99	99	99	-	0	99	99	0	99	99
Bay Area, Chinese	99	-	..	-	-	..	-	99	..	-	99	..
Bay Area, White	96	99	99	91	-	99	91	99	99	99	99	99
Connecticut	99	99	99	89	94	89	99	93	95	99	92	99
Detroit, Black	99	99	99	99	-	99	80	99	99	99	-	99
Detroit, White	99	99	96	75	78	99	99	99	99	75	99	99
Iowa	99	95	99	83	83	89	93	93	99	99	88	99
New Orleans, Black	99	99	67	-	-	-	99	99	99	99	99	-
New Orleans, White	99	99	67	99	99	99	99	99	99	99	99	99
Seattle	94	99	99	99	99	99	99	99	99	99	99	99

.. : data not presented in this volume
* : data presented, but histological verification figures not reported (Scotland: national data not reported)
- : histological verification figures reported, but no cases reported at this site
0 : one or more cases reported, but none histologically confirmed
99 : 99% or more

BONE (ICD-9 170)

EUROPE (non-EC), INCIDENCE

MALES	Best model	Goodness of fit	1970 Rate	1970 Cases	1985 Rate	1985 Cases	Cumulative risk 1915	Cumulative risk 1940	Recent trend
FINLAND	A3C2	-0.06	1.9	19	1.1	13	0.9	0.4	*-10.8*
HUNGARY									
County Vas	A1D	0.15	1.4	1	*0.3*	*0*	0.8	0.1	-65.6
Szabolcs-Szatmar	A1	1.20	1.3	1	1.3	1	0.7	0.7	-22.7
ISRAEL									
All Jews	A3D	1.04	1.2	5	1.1	6	0.6	0.6	*0.0*
Non-Jews	A2	-1.30	*0.7*	*0*	*0.7*	*0*	0.5	0.5	*-14.5*
NORWAY	A1P2	1.03	0.9	8	0.9	9	0.5	0.7	*-12.4*
POLAND									
Warsaw City	A1P2	1.25	1.0	2	1.1	4	0.9	0.6	-31.6
ROMANIA									
Cluj	A1	0.58	*3.7*	*5*	3.7	6	2.0	2.0	-24.0
SWEDEN	A1	-0.76	1.0	22	1.0	24	0.5	0.5	*0.7*
SWITZERLAND									
Geneva	A1	-0.58	*0.8*	*0*	*0.8*	*0*	0.4	0.4	*21.2*
YUGOSLAVIA									
Slovenia	A1D	-0.39	1.1	4	0.6	2	0.6	0.2	*-12.6*

FEMALES	Best model	Goodness of fit	1970 Rate	1970 Cases	1985 Rate	1985 Cases	Cumulative risk 1915	Cumulative risk 1940	Recent trend
FINLAND	A1C2	-1.46	1.2	14	0.6	8	0.6	0.2	*-14.4*
HUNGARY									
County Vas	A1	-0.36	1.2	1	1.2	1	0.7	0.7	*-5.2*
Szabolcs-Szatmar	A1	0.64	1.0	1	1.0	1	0.6	0.6	-28.5
ISRAEL									
All Jews	A1	0.69	1.0	5	1.0	7	0.5	0.5	*-13.1*
Non-Jews	A2	-0.96	*0.7*	*0*	*0.7*	*0*	0.5	0.5	-34.6
NORWAY	A1D	0.18	0.4	4	0.6	7	0.3	0.5	*2.3*
POLAND									
Warsaw City	A1D	0.68	0.5	2	1.0	5	0.5	1.3	*-4.0*
ROMANIA									
Cluj	A1	0.22	*2.6*	*4*	2.6	5	1.4	1.4	*-18.6*
SWEDEN	A1D	-0.49	0.8	17	0.7	15	0.4	0.3	-10.9
SWITZERLAND									
Geneva	A0	-0.79	*0.4*	*0*	*0.4*	*0*	0.2	0.2	*
YUGOSLAVIA									
Slovenia	A1P2	0.81	0.6	2	0.6	3	0.4	0.1	*-4.7*

* : not enough cases for reliable estimation
− : incomplete or missing data
Best model: polynomial of the given degree in age (A), period (P) or cohort (C), or linear drift (D) model.
Goodness of fit: the normalised likelihood ratio chi-square for the best model (see Method).
Rate: world-standardised truncated rate per 100 000 per year (30-74 years) and number of **cases** are both estimated from the best-fitting model for the single years cited.
Cumulative risk per 1000 (30-74 years) is estimated from the best-fitting *age-cohort* model for cohorts of central birth year cited.
Recent trend: estimated mean percentage change per five-year period in the age-specific rates (30-74 years) over the period 1973-1987.
Italics denote recent trends not significant at 5 per cent level, or other figures which should be interpreted with caution (see Method).

BONE (ICD-9 170)

EUROPE (non-EC), INCIDENCE

MALES

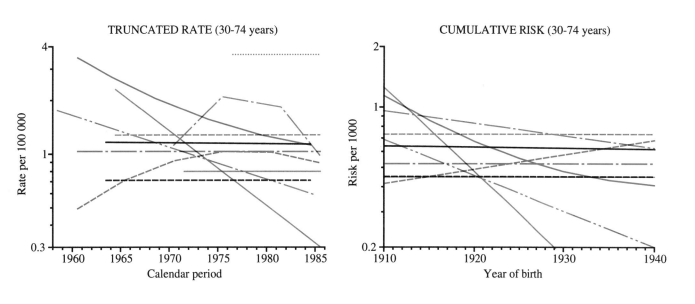

TRUNCATED RATE (30-74 years)

CUMULATIVE RISK (30-74 years)

FEMALES

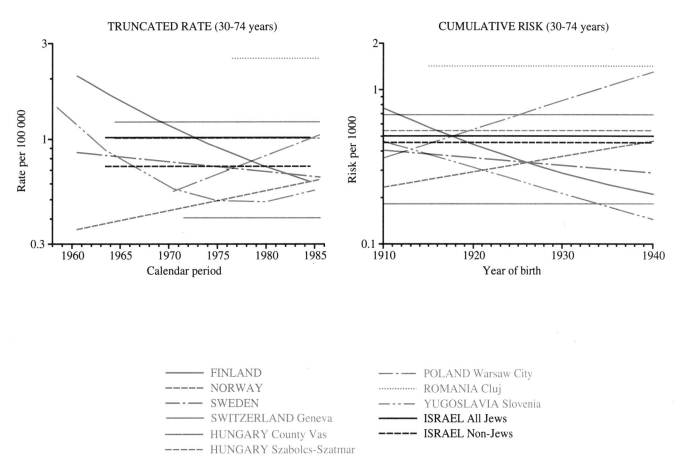

TRUNCATED RATE (30-74 years)

CUMULATIVE RISK (30-74 years)

——— FINLAND	—·— POLAND Warsaw City
– – – NORWAY	········ ROMANIA Cluj
–··– SWEDEN	–···– YUGOSLAVIA Slovenia
——— SWITZERLAND Geneva	——— ISRAEL All Jews
——— HUNGARY County Vas	– – – ISRAEL Non-Jews
– – – HUNGARY Szabolcs-Szatmar	

BONE (ICD-9 170)

EUROPE (EC), INCIDENCE

MALES	Best model	Goodness of fit	1970 Rate	1970 Cases	1985 Rate	1985 Cases	Cumulative risk 1915	Cumulative risk 1940	Recent trend
DENMARK	A5	1.26	1.1	13	1.1	15	0.6	0.6	*4.6*
FRANCE									
Bas-Rhin	A1	1.26	*1.9*	*4*	1.9	3	1.0	1.0	*16.1*
Doubs	A3C2	-0.11	*31.9*	*8*	1.6	1	1.5	0.9	-33.7
GERMANY (FRG)									
Hamburg	A1P2C3	-1.06	3.5	18	*0.2*	*0*	1.3	*0.5*	–
Saarland	A1P2	0.78	3.4	9	1.1	3	1.6	0.2	*-1.9*
GERMANY (GDR)	A3P3	-0.14	1.5	64	1.1	40	0.7	0.5	-6.4
ITALY									
Varese	A1	0.70	*1.0*	*1*	1.0	2	0.6	0.6	*13.7*
SPAIN									
Navarra	A1D	0.37	*6.1*	*6*	*0.4*	*0*	18.6	0.2	-61.5
Zaragoza	A1P3	0.65	5.8	10	0.6	1	2.6	0.3	-31.7
UK									
Birmingham	A4D	1.55	1.0	12	0.8	10	0.5	0.3	*-9.2*
Scotland	A1D	0.65	1.3	16	0.8	11	0.7	0.3	-21.5
South Thames	A2P3	0.07	1.3	29	1.0	17	0.6	0.4	*0.2*

FEMALES	Best model	Goodness of fit	1970 Rate	1970 Cases	1985 Rate	1985 Cases	Cumulative risk 1915	Cumulative risk 1940	Recent trend
DENMARK	A1	0.57	0.7	10	0.7	10	0.4	0.4	*6.5*
FRANCE									
Bas-Rhin	A0	0.88	*1.8*	*4*	1.8	4	0.8	0.8	*0.1*
Doubs	A1D	-1.32	*21.4*	*15*	0.2	0	185.8	0.1	-76.1
GERMANY (FRG)									
Hamburg	A1P3	0.24	1.9	13	*0.0*	*0*	0.8	*0.4*	–
Saarland	A1C3	0.36	2.4	8	0.4	1	3.2	0.1	*-28.8*
GERMANY (GDR)	A4D	-0.23	0.9	50	0.7	33	0.4	0.3	*-6.5*
ITALY									
Varese	A1D	-0.72	*0.0*	*0*	1.3	3	0.4	104.9	208.9
SPAIN									
Navarra	A1	-0.32	*1.4*	*1*	1.4	2	0.8	0.8	*-8.8*
Zaragoza	A1D	-0.34	2.9	6	1.0	2	1.4	0.3	*-31.6*
UK									
Birmingham	A2	0.53	0.5	7	0.5	7	0.3	0.3	*-19.4*
Scotland	A1D	-1.16	0.7	11	0.5	8	0.4	0.2	*-8.4*
South Thames	A1P3	-1.41	0.9	23	0.8	15	0.4	0.4	*15.0*

* : not enough cases for reliable estimation
– : incomplete or missing data
Best model: polynomial of the given degree in age (A), period (P) or cohort (C), or linear drift (D) model.
Goodness of fit: the normalised likelihood ratio chi-square for the best model (see Method).
Rate: world-standardised truncated rate per 100 000 per year (30-74 years) and number of **cases** are both estimated from the best-fitting model for the single years cited.
Cumulative risk per 1000 (30-74 years) is estimated from the best-fitting *age-cohort* model for cohorts of central birth year cited.
Recent trend: estimated mean percentage change per five-year period in the age-specific rates (30-74 years) over the period 1973-1987.
Italics denote recent trends not significant at 5 per cent level, or other figures which should be interpreted with caution (see Method).

BONE (ICD-9 170)

EUROPE (EC), INCIDENCE

MALES

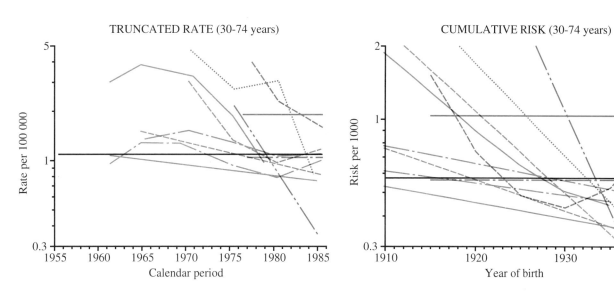

FEMALES

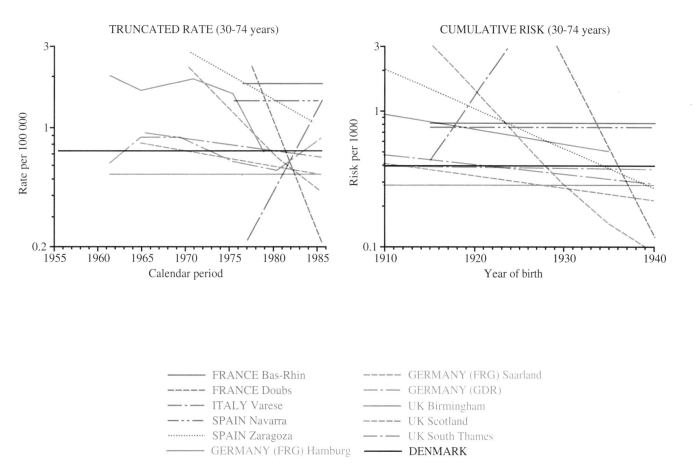

BONE (ICD-9 170)

EUROPE (non-EC), INCIDENCE
Percentage change per five-year period, 1973-1987

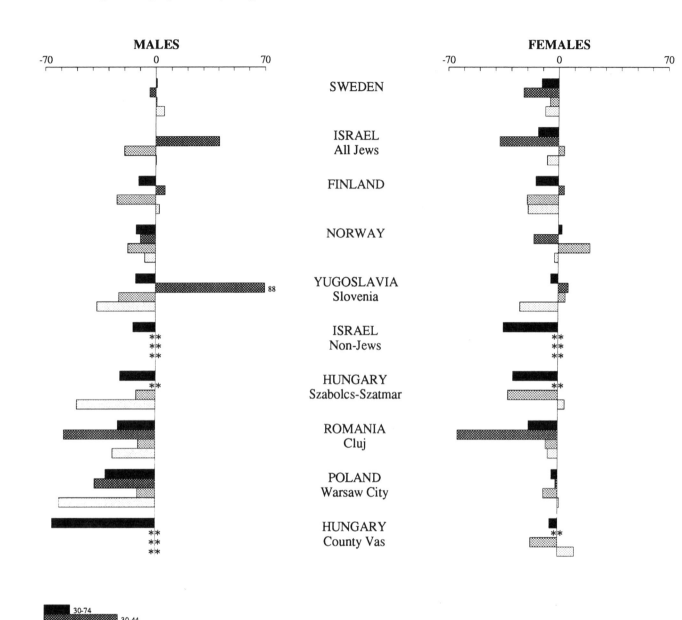

BONE (ICD-9 170)

EUROPE (EC), INCIDENCE
Percentage change per five-year period, 1973-1987

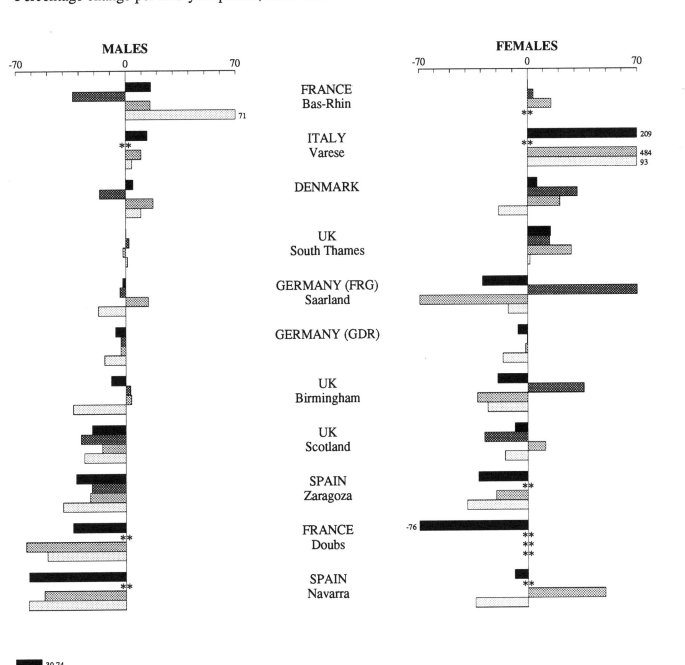

MALES

FEMALES

FRANCE
Bas-Rhin

ITALY
Varese

DENMARK

UK
South Thames

GERMANY (FRG)
Saarland

GERMANY (GDR)

UK
Birmingham

UK
Scotland

SPAIN
Zaragoza

FRANCE
Doubs

SPAIN
Navarra

30-74
30-44
45-64
65-74

BONE (ICD-9 170)

EUROPE (non-EC), MORTALITY

MALES	Best model	Goodness of fit	1965 Rate	Deaths	1985 Rate	Deaths	Cumulative risk 1900	1940	Recent trend
AUSTRIA	A8P6C9	0.94	2.7	52	1.0	17	1.9	0.6	-37.1
CZECHOSLOVAKIA	A8P6	1.28	3.3	114	1.9	68	2.2	0.9	-14.7
FINLAND	A3C3	1.12	2.2	20	0.7	8	2.1	0.2	*-10.3*
HUNGARY	A3P2	0.65	*3.3*	*85*	2.5	67	*2.7*	1.0	-22.0
NORWAY	A1	1.55	0.6	6	0.6	6	0.3	0.3	*-1.7*
POLAND	A8P5C9	0.62	2.9	174	3.3	256	1.8	2.3	*2.2*
ROMANIA	A3	2.40	*4.9*	*201*	*4.9*	*260*	*2.8*	2.8	–
SWEDEN	A2P4	1.86	1.4	30	0.6	15	1.3	0.2	-36.1
SWITZERLAND	A1P2C2	-0.14	1.9	27	0.4	7	1.5	0.2	-36.2
YUGOSLAVIA	A2P5	-0.58	3.7	134	3.4	168	2.0	2.6	-17.0

FEMALES	Best model	Goodness of fit	1965 Rate	Deaths	1985 Rate	Deaths	Cumulative risk 1900	1940	Recent trend
AUSTRIA	A1P4	-1.08	1.5	39	0.5	11	1.1	0.2	-36.9
CZECHOSLOVAKIA	A1D	3.39	2.1	86	1.1	50	1.4	0.4	-18.2
FINLAND	A1D	1.73	1.2	15	0.3	5	1.2	0.1	*-8.2*
HUNGARY	A2P2	-0.35	*2.2*	*68*	1.2	39	*1.9*	0.4	-25.8
NORWAY	A1	1.32	0.3	3	0.3	4	0.2	0.2	*26.0*
POLAND	A3P3	-1.09	1.9	142	1.4	139	1.1	0.8	-9.3
ROMANIA	A5	1.41	*2.7*	*128*	*2.7*	*164*	*1.5*	1.5	–
SWEDEN	A1P4C2	-0.04	0.9	21	0.4	11	0.9	0.1	-26.0
SWITZERLAND	A1D	0.00	1.0	16	0.3	5	0.9	0.1	-30.8
YUGOSLAVIA	A4P3C2	1.66	2.0	88	1.8	107	1.3	0.9	-21.1

* : not enough deaths for reliable estimation
– : incomplete or missing data
Best model: polynomial of the given degree in age (A), period (P) or cohort (C), or linear drift (D) model.
Goodness of fit: the normalised likelihood ratio chi-square for the best model (see Method).
Rate: world-standardised truncated rate per 100 000 per year (30-74 years) and number of **deaths** are both estimated from the best-fitting model for the single years cited.
Cumulative risk per 1000 (30-74 years) is estimated from the best-fitting *age-cohort* model for cohorts of central birth year cited.
Recent trend: estimated mean percentage change per five-year period in the age-specific rates (30-74 years) over the period 1975-1988.
Italics denote recent trends not significant at 5 per cent level, or other figures which should be interpreted with caution (see Method).

BONE (ICD-9 170)

EUROPE (non-EC), MORTALITY

MALES

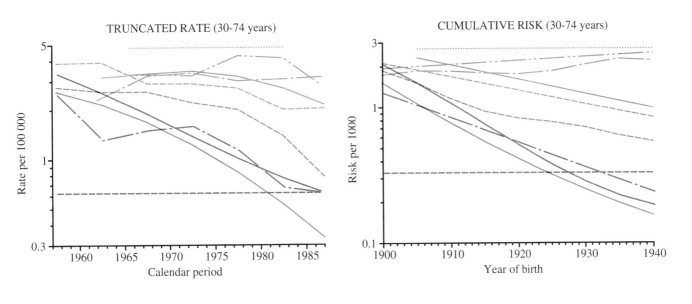

FEMALES

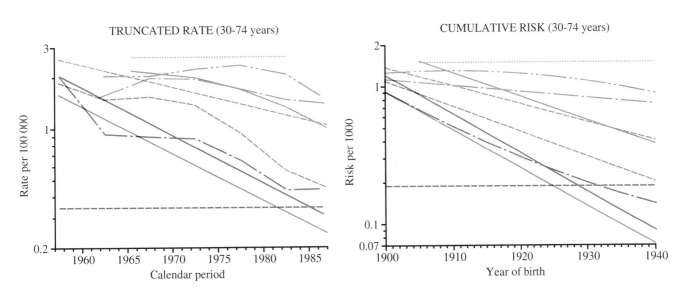

—— FINLAND	- - - - CZECHOSLOVAKIA		
- - - NORWAY	—— HUNGARY		
-·-·- SWEDEN	-·-·- POLAND		
- - - AUSTRIA	·········· ROMANIA		
—— SWITZERLAND	-··-··- YUGOSLAVIA		

BONE (ICD-9 170)

EUROPE (EC), MORTALITY

MALES	Best model	Goodness of fit	1965 Rate	1965 Deaths	1985 Rate	1985 Deaths	Cumulative risk 1900	Cumulative risk 1940	Recent trend
BELGIUM	A3P2	-1.87	3.1	81	1.5	38	1.9	0.7	-21.7
DENMARK	A1D	2.50	1.5	18	0.8	10	1.0	0.3	*-11.9*
FRANCE	A5P2C4	0.54	4.0	482	2.4	326	2.5	1.2	-14.6
GERMANY (FRG)	A3P6C4	1.15	3.1	469	1.1	170	1.9	0.5	-26.4
GREECE	A3C3	-1.11	*3.8*	*72*	4.7	129	*2.4*	3.2	*-3.7*
IRELAND	A1P2	0.93	3.4	24	0.9	6	2.3	0.3	-32.5
ITALY	A4P5C2	0.51	3.9	480	2.3	352	2.6	1.0	-19.9
NETHERLANDS	A1P4C3	-0.50	1.8	50	0.5	17	1.5	0.2	-22.3
PORTUGAL	A2D	0.30	*5.2*	*94*	2.7	67	*3.5*	1.0	-20.9
SPAIN	A3P6	1.69	3.2	222	2.5	235	2.0	1.9	-13.5
UK ENGLAND & WALES	A3P6C3	0.37	1.6	200	0.4	58	1.1	0.2	-33.2
UK SCOTLAND	A1D	1.47	2.1	26	0.7	9	1.7	0.2	-37.0

FEMALES	Best model	Goodness of fit	1965 Rate	1965 Deaths	1985 Rate	1985 Deaths	Cumulative risk 1900	Cumulative risk 1940	Recent trend
BELGIUM	A1D	0.33	1.7	53	0.9	26	1.2	0.3	-20.7
DENMARK	A1D	-1.26	0.9	11	0.5	7	0.6	0.2	*-14.2*
FRANCE	A4P2C3	1.38	2.0	297	0.8	117	1.4	0.3	-24.5
GERMANY (FRG)	A4P6C5	0.01	1.9	399	0.5	114	1.3	0.2	-26.1
GREECE	A2C2	-0.69	*2.6*	*56*	2.9	88	*1.4*	1.5	*1.5*
IRELAND	A1P2	0.75	2.1	15	0.6	5	1.4	0.2	-43.4
ITALY	A2P4	1.18	2.2	316	1.2	219	1.5	0.5	-20.1
NETHERLANDS	A1D	0.56	1.0	30	0.3	12	0.9	0.1	-21.4
PORTUGAL	A2D	-0.53	*4.9*	*112*	1.5	42	*4.3*	0.4	-24.4
SPAIN	A8P6C9	0.00	2.1	170	1.1	119	1.3	0.5	-26.1
UK ENGLAND & WALES	A3P4C3	-1.07	0.9	134	0.3	50	0.7	0.1	-27.1
UK SCOTLAND	A1P3	-0.37	0.9	15	0.2	3	1.1	0.1	-57.8

* : not enough deaths for reliable estimation
– : incomplete or missing data
Best model: polynomial of the given degree in age (A), period (P) or cohort (C), or linear drift (D) model.
Goodness of fit: the normalised likelihood ratio chi-square for the best model (see Method).
Rate: world-standardised truncated rate per 100 000 per year (30-74 years) and number of **deaths** are both estimated from the best-fitting model for the single years cited.
Cumulative risk per 1000 (30-74 years) is estimated from the best-fitting *age-cohort* model for cohorts of central birth year cited.
Recent trend: estimated mean percentage change per five-year period in the age-specific rates (30-74 years) over the period 1975-1988.
Italics denote recent trends not significant at 5 per cent level, or other figures which should be interpreted with caution (see Method).

BONE (ICD-9 170)

EUROPE (EC), MORTALITY

MALES

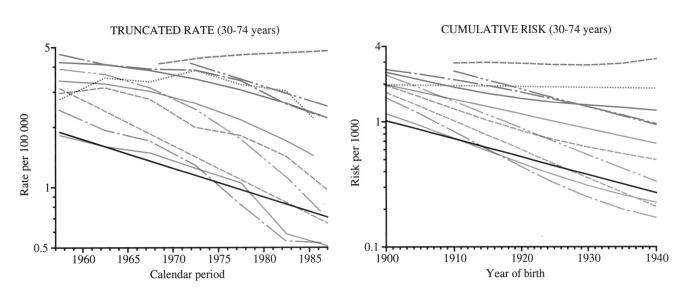

TRUNCATED RATE (30-74 years)

Rate per 100 000

Calendar period

CUMULATIVE RISK (30-74 years)

Risk per 1000

Year of birth

FEMALES

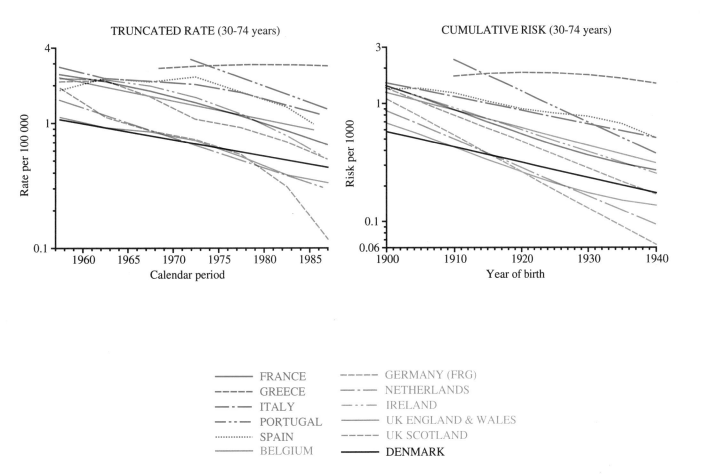

TRUNCATED RATE (30-74 years)

Rate per 100 000

Calendar period

CUMULATIVE RISK (30-74 years)

Risk per 1000

Year of birth

FRANCE	GERMANY (FRG)
GREECE	NETHERLANDS
ITALY	IRELAND
PORTUGAL	UK ENGLAND & WALES
SPAIN	UK SCOTLAND
BELGIUM	DENMARK

BONE (ICD-9 170)

EUROPE (non-EC), MORTALITY
Percentage change per five-year period, 1975-1988

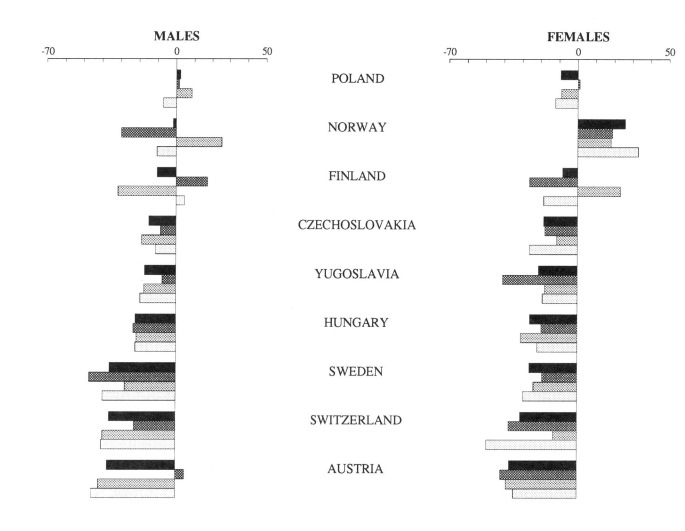

BONE (ICD-9 170)

EUROPE (EC), MORTALITY
Percentage change per five-year period, 1975-1988

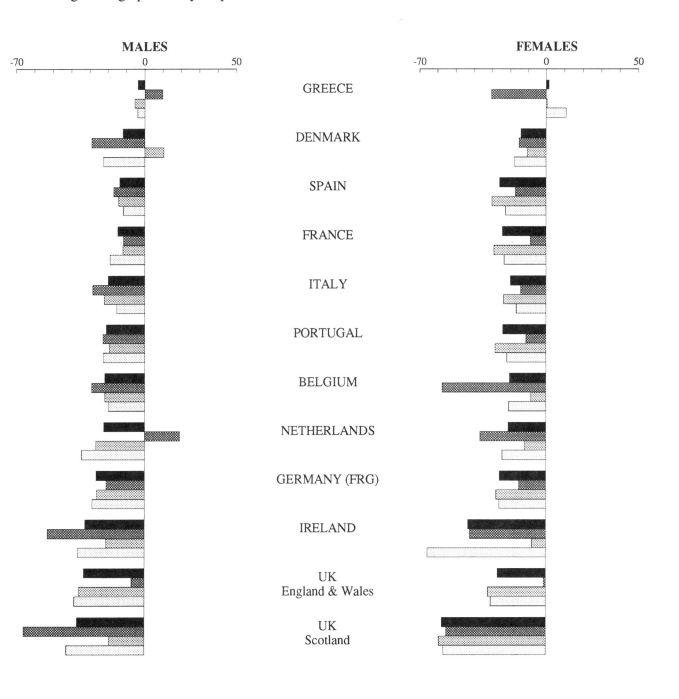

MALES

FEMALES

-70   0   50

-70   0   50

GREECE

DENMARK

SPAIN

FRANCE

ITALY

PORTUGAL

BELGIUM

NETHERLANDS

GERMANY (FRG)

IRELAND

UK
England & Wales

UK
Scotland

30-74
30-44
45-64
65-74

BONE (ICD-9 170)

ASIA, INCIDENCE

MALES	Best model	Goodness of fit	1970 Rate	1970 Cases	1985 Rate	1985 Cases	Cumulative risk 1915	Cumulative risk 1940	Recent trend
CHINA									
Shanghai	A3P2	0.57	*0.2*	*2*	3.3	57	1.8	3.3	*12.2*
HONG KONG	A1P2	-1.02	*17.2*	*98*	2.1	25	1.5	0.9	*-11.6*
INDIA									
Bombay	A3C3	-0.41	1.2	9	0.9	12	0.7	0.3	-21.1
JAPAN									
Miyagi	A1P3	0.00	1.0	3	1.1	5	0.8	0.4	*-15.3*
Nagasaki	A0	0.24	*0.6*	*0*	*0.6*	*0*	0.3	0.3	-50.2
Osaka	A1C2	0.37	1.8	22	0.8	16	0.7	0.3	-16.4
SINGAPORE									
Chinese	A0	-0.20	0.9	2	0.9	3	0.4	0.4	*-9.0*
Indian	A0	-1.45	*1.1*	*0*	*1.1*	*0*	0.5	0.5	*25.0*
Malay	*	..	..	..	..	..	..	..	..

FEMALES	Best model	Goodness of fit	1970 Rate	1970 Cases	1985 Rate	1985 Cases	Cumulative risk 1915	Cumulative risk 1940	Recent trend
CHINA									
Shanghai	A8P2	1.52	*0.1*	*0*	1.7	31	0.9	1.0	*5.5*
HONG KONG	A1	0.27	*1.6*	*9*	1.6	18	0.9	0.9	*8.1*
INDIA									
Bombay	A3C3	1.41	1.3	6	0.7	8	0.7	0.2	*-5.8*
JAPAN									
Miyagi	A1P3C2	-0.39	0.4	1	0.6	3	0.3	0.3	*-13.4*
Nagasaki	A0C3	-0.94	*4.5*	*5*	*0.3*	*0*	1.5	0.1	*-53.5*
Osaka	A1C3	1.09	0.9	12	0.5	11	0.5	0.1	-21.2
SINGAPORE									
Chinese	A0	0.45	0.6	1	0.6	2	0.3	0.3	*2.4*
Indian	*	..	..	..	..	..	..	..	..
Malay	A0	-1.84	*0.6*	*0*	*0.6*	*0*	0.3	0.3	*

* : not enough cases for reliable estimation
− : incomplete or missing data
Best model: polynomial of the given degree in age (A), period (P) or cohort (C), or linear drift (D) model.
Goodness of fit: the normalised likelihood ratio chi-square for the best model (see Method).
Rate: world-standardised truncated rate per 100 000 per year (30-74 years) and number of **cases** are both estimated from the best-fitting model for the single years cited.
Cumulative risk per 1000 (30-74 years) is estimated from the best-fitting *age-cohort* model for cohorts of central birth year cited.
Recent trend: estimated mean percentage change per five-year period in the age-specific rates (30-74 years) over the period 1973-1987.
Italics denote recent trends not significant at 5 per cent level, or other figures which should be interpreted with caution (see Method).

BONE (ICD-9 170)

ASIA, INCIDENCE

MALES

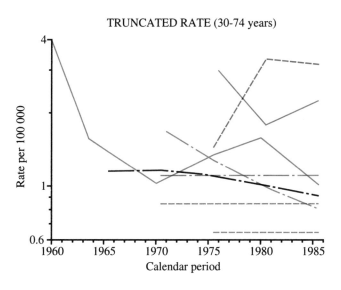

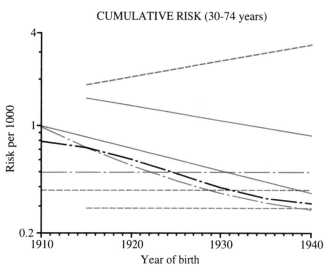

FEMALES

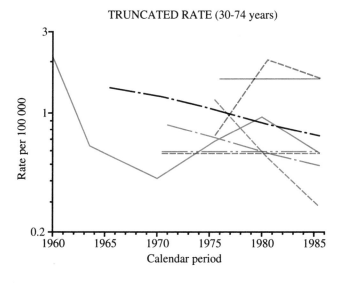

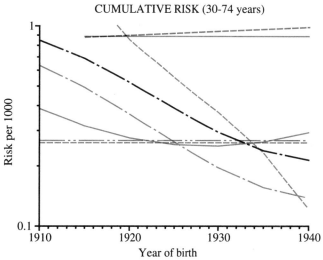

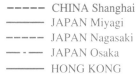

----- CHINA Shanghai
——— JAPAN Miyagi
----- JAPAN Nagasaki
—·—· JAPAN Osaka
——— HONG KONG

----- SINGAPORE Chinese
——— SINGAPORE Indian
—··—·· SINGAPORE Malay
—··— INDIA Bombay

BONE (ICD-9 170)

OCEANIA, INCIDENCE

MALES	Best model	Goodness of fit	1970 Rate	1970 Cases	1985 Rate	1985 Cases	Cumulative risk 1915	Cumulative risk 1940	Recent trend
AUSTRALIA									
New South Wales	A2	-0.95	*1.0*	*10*	1.0	13	0.5	0.5	*6.9*
South	A1	0.37	*1.0*	*1*	1.0	3	0.6	0.6	*-7.4*
HAWAII									
Caucasian	*	..	..	..	..	..	..	..	..
Chinese	*	..	..	..	..	..	..	..	..
Filipino	*	..	..	..	..	..	..	..	..
Hawaiian	A3	-1.92	*1.7*	*0*	*1.7*	*0*	1.1	1.1	*-62.7*
Japanese	A0	-2.00	*0.5*	*0*	*0.5*	*0*	0.2	0.2	*
NEW ZEALAND									
Maori	A0	-1.43	*1.2*	*0*	*1.2*	*0*	0.5	0.5	*62.3*
Non-Maori	A1P3	1.70	1.8	10	1.2	8	0.7	0.6	*5.2*

FEMALES	Best model	Goodness of fit	1970 Rate	1970 Cases	1985 Rate	1985 Cases	Cumulative risk 1915	Cumulative risk 1940	Recent trend
AUSTRALIA									
New South Wales	A1	-1.40	*0.7*	*8*	0.7	9	0.4	0.4	*10.8*
South	A1P2	-0.24	*	*	0.4	1	4.0	0.1	*-51.1*
HAWAII									
Caucasian	*	..	..	..	..	..	..	..	..
Chinese	*	..	..	..	..	..	..	..	..
Filipino	–	–	–	–	–	–	–	–	–
Hawaiian	*	..	..	..	..	..	..	..	..
Japanese	*	..	..	..	..	..	..	..	..
NEW ZEALAND									
Maori	*	..	..	..	..	..	..	..	..
Non-Maori	A8P4C9	-0.53	0.6	3	0.7	5	0.4	0.2	*-11.8*

* : not enough cases for reliable estimation
− : incomplete or missing data
Best model: polynomial of the given degree in age (A), period (P) or cohort (C), or linear drift (D) model.
Goodness of fit: the normalised likelihood ratio chi-square for the best model (see Method).
Rate: world-standardised truncated rate per 100 000 per year (30-74 years) and number of **cases** are both estimated from the best-fitting model for the single years cited.
Cumulative risk per 1000 (30-74 years) is estimated from the best-fitting *age-cohort* model for cohorts of central birth year cited.
Recent trend: estimated mean percentage change per five-year period in the age-specific rates (30-74 years) over the period 1973-1987.
Italics denote recent trends not significant at 5 per cent level, or other figures which should be interpreted with caution (see Method).

BONE (ICD-9 170)

OCEANIA, INCIDENCE

MALES

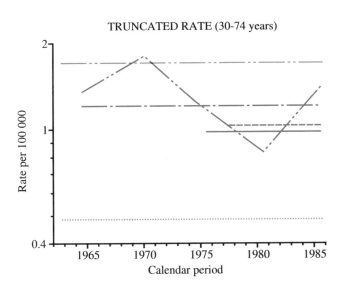

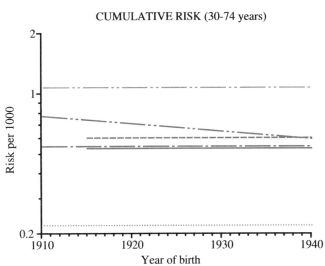

FEMALES

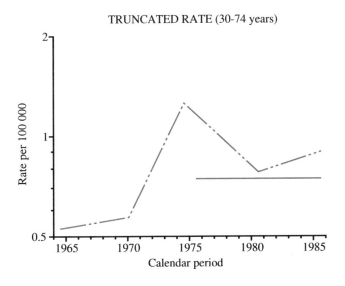

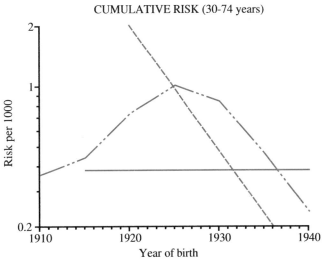

——————— AUSTRALIA New South Wales   ············· HAWAII Japanese
– – – – – AUSTRALIA South
– · – · – NEW ZEALAND Maori
– ·· – ·· – NEW ZEALAND Non-Maori
– ··· – ··· HAWAII Hawaiian

BONE (ICD-9 170)

ASIA, INCIDENCE
Percentage change per five-year period, 1973-1987

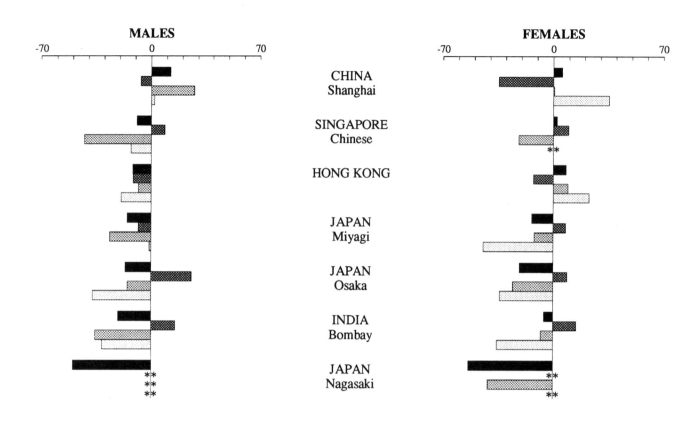

MALES

FEMALES

-70   0   70

-70   0   70

CHINA
Shanghai

SINGAPORE
Chinese

HONG KONG

JAPAN
Miyagi

JAPAN
Osaka

INDIA
Bombay

JAPAN
Nagasaki

30-74
30-44
45-64
65-74

BONE (ICD-9 170)

OCEANIA, INCIDENCE
Percentage change per five-year period, 1973-1987

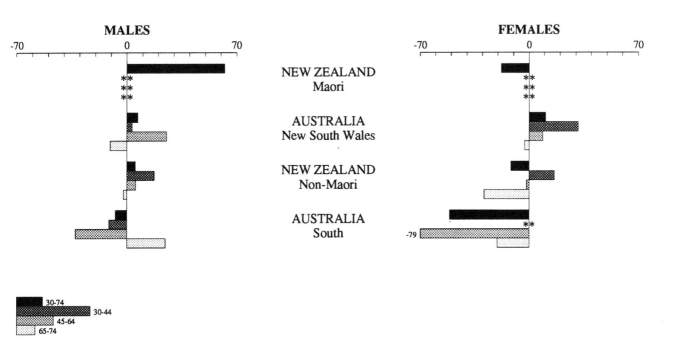

BONE (ICD-9 170)

ASIA and OCEANIA, MORTALITY

MALES	Best model	Goodness of fit	1965 Rate	1965 Deaths	1985 Rate	1985 Deaths	Cumulative risk 1900	Cumulative risk 1940	Recent trend
AUSTRALIA	A1P2C3	0.43	1.5	36	0.7	27	1.0	0.3	-23.9
HONG KONG	A1P3	-0.26	*8.2*	*33*	1.8	16	*0.8*	1.2	*8.3*
JAPAN	A3P5C3	-0.47	2.2	395	0.4	124	1.9	0.1	-36.4
MAURITIUS	A1	-0.20	*1.7*	*1*	1.7	2	*1.0*	1.0	*-22.3*
NEW ZEALAND	A1D	0.27	1.1	5	0.6	4	0.7	0.2	*-11.9*
SINGAPORE	A1D	0.81	1.9	3	0.9	2	*1.2*	0.3	–

FEMALES	Best model	Goodness of fit	1965 Rate	1965 Deaths	1985 Rate	1985 Deaths	Cumulative risk 1900	Cumulative risk 1940	Recent trend
AUSTRALIA	A1D	0.05	0.8	21	0.5	19	0.5	0.2	*-13.5*
HONG KONG	A1	0.07	*1.1*	*5*	1.1	9	*0.7*	0.7	*-1.7*
JAPAN	A3P5C3	-1.61	1.5	297	0.3	92	1.3	0.1	-34.1
MAURITIUS	A1	-0.39	*1.1*	*0*	1.1	1	*0.7*	0.7	*-17.3*
NEW ZEALAND	A4P3	1.11	0.5	2	0.7	5	0.4	0.4	*-12.8*
SINGAPORE	A2C2	-1.23	1.0	2	0.7	2	*0.3*	0.1	–

* : not enough deaths for reliable estimation
– : incomplete or missing data
Best model: polynomial of the given degree in age (A), period (P) or cohort (C), or linear drift (D) model.
Goodness of fit: the normalised likelihood ratio chi-square for the best model (see Method).
Rate: world-standardised truncated rate per 100 000 per year (30-74 years) and number of **deaths** are both estimated from the best-fitting model for the single years cited.
Cumulative risk per 1000 (30-74 years) is estimated from the best-fitting *age-cohort* model for cohorts of central birth year cited.
Recent trend: estimated mean percentage change per five-year period in the age-specific rates (30-74 years) over the period 1975-1988.
Italics denote recent trends not significant at 5 per cent level, or other figures which should be interpreted with caution (see Method).

BONE (ICD-9 170)

ASIA and OCEANIA, MORTALITY

MALES

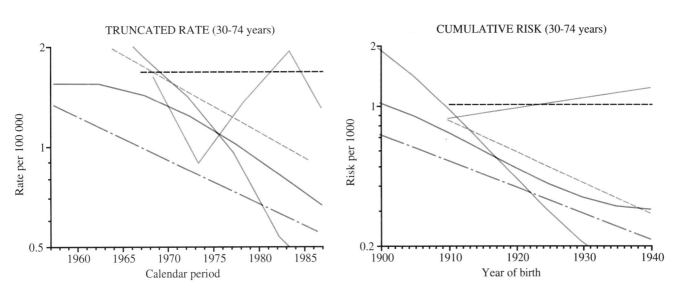

FEMALES

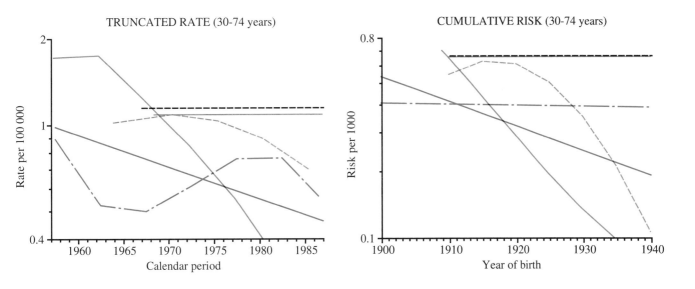

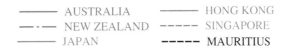

——— AUSTRALIA		——— HONG KONG	
—·—·— NEW ZEALAND		‑ ‑ ‑ ‑ SINGAPORE	
——— JAPAN		‑ ‑ ‑ ‑ MAURITIUS	

BONE (ICD-9 170)

ASIA and OCEANIA, MORTALITY
Percentage change per five-year period, 1975-1988

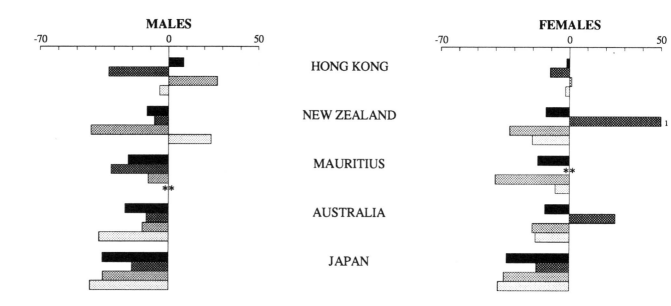

from page 344

buted to improvement (or the lack of it) in the quality of death certification[146].

The incidence of bone tumours in New York State did not change significantly in the 33-year period 1955-87 in adults aged 30 or more, although at younger ages there were increases during this period of 54% and 44% in males and females, respectively[174]. This report showed no differences in trend between areas with and without fluoridated public water supplies, and no significant trend in the incidence of osteosarcoma.

An international study of bone cancer trends in 40 cancer registries in 10 countries in North America, northern Europe, Australia and New Zealand and covering the period 1958-87 also found no evidence that the trends were associated with fluoridation of water supplies[105]. This study also showed that the ratio of incidence and mortality rates was less than unity in many populations in the early part of the period. The increase in the ratio in most populations was considered too great to be explained by the modest improvements in survival.

Mortality from bone tumours is declining in almost all countries studied, but trends in inci- dence are less consistent. In part, this is because truncated incidence rates in the age range 30-74 years are mostly around 1.0 per 100 000 per year; few registries record more than 15 malignant bone neoplasms a year for each sex in this age range, and the trends in the truncated incidence rates are often quite unstable as a result of ran- dom variation, whereas mortality rates are gene- rally based on larger (national) populations. Recent trends in incidence in many populations are not significantly different from zero. Many registries do record declining incidence of bone tumours, however, especially in Europe, despite having had consistently high proportions verified by histology (80% or more) for the last 15 years.

It seems likely that much of the apparent decline in mortality from bone tumours can be ascribed to improvements in cancer diagnosis during life, and a resultant decline in incorrect certification of the underlying cause of death as a primary bone neoplasm in cases of metastatic disease, but it is also possible that some of the improvements in mortality are due to true declines in incidence, as in Finland, and possibly to more successful treatment.

AMERICAS (except USA), INCIDENCE

MALES	Best model	Goodness of fit	1970		1985		Cumulative risk		Recent trend
			Rate	Cases	Rate	Cases	1915	1940	
BRAZIL									
Sao Paulo	A5P2	-0.16	1.6	14	*42.1*	*477*	0.6	*0.7*	–
CANADA									
Alberta	A1	0.77	0.8	2	0.8	3	0.4	0.4	*-21.1*
British Columbia	A2	-0.23	1.0	4	1.0	7	0.6	0.6	*-13.1*
Maritime Provinces	A1D	1.56	0.5	1	1.1	3	0.4	1.6	7.3
Newfoundland	A1	-0.12	1.5	1	1.5	1	0.9	0.9	*-18.9*
Quebec	A1D	1.42	1.6	17	2.0	30	1.0	1.5	19.7
COLOMBIA									
Cali	A1D	1.22	1.6	1	0.6	1	0.9	0.2	*-28.7*
CUBA	A1D	1.20	2.4	36	1.7	35	1.3	*0.7*	–
PUERTO RICO	A1	1.81	0.8	3	0.8	5	0.4	0.4	*6.4*

FEMALES	Best model	Goodness of fit	1970		1985		Cumulative risk		Recent trend
			Rate	Cases	Rate	Cases	1915	1940	
BRAZIL									
Sao Paulo	A1	-0.13	1.3	9	*1.3*	*13*	0.6	*0.6*	–
CANADA									
Alberta	A1	0.98	0.7	2	0.7	3	0.4	0.4	*16.1*
British Columbia	A1	3.08	0.7	3	0.7	5	0.4	0.4	*5.2*
Maritime Provinces	A1P2	0.07	*0.1*	*0*	0.4	1	0.2	0.5	*-18.2*
Newfoundland	A0	-0.81	*0.7*	*0*	*0.7*	*0*	0.3	0.3	*107.9*
Quebec	A1P4	0.93	0.9	11	1.6	26	0.6	1.0	28.7
COLOMBIA									
Cali	A1	0.19	*1.1*	*0*	1.1	1	0.6	0.6	*-13.2*
CUBA	A1	0.78	1.7	22	1.7	35	1.0	*1.0*	–
PUERTO RICO	A1	1.15	0.6	2	0.6	4	0.3	0.3	*-17.8*

* : not enough cases for reliable estimation
– : incomplete or missing data
Best model: polynomial of the given degree in age (A), period (P) or cohort (C), or linear drift (D) model.
Goodness of fit: the normalised likelihood ratio chi-square for the best model (see Method).
Rate: world-standardised truncated rate per 100 000 per year (30-74 years) and number of **cases** are both estimated from the best-fitting model for the single years cited.
Cumulative risk per 1000 (30-74 years) is estimated from the best-fitting *age-cohort* model for cohorts of central birth year cited.
Recent trend: estimated mean percentage change per five-year period in the age-specific rates (30-74 years) over the period 1973-1987.
Italics denote recent trends not significant at 5 per cent level, or other figures which should be interpreted with caution (see Method).

BONE (ICD-9 170)

AMERICAS (except USA), INCIDENCE

MALES

TRUNCATED RATE (30-74 years)

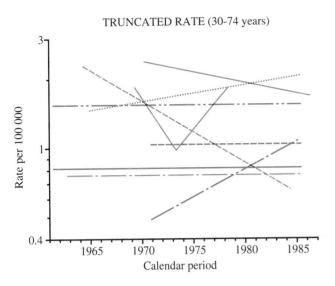

CUMULATIVE RISK (30-74 years)

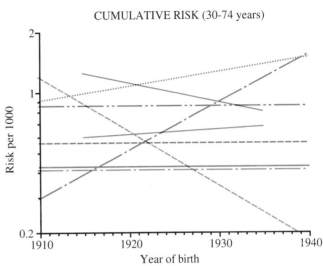

FEMALES

TRUNCATED RATE (30-74 years)

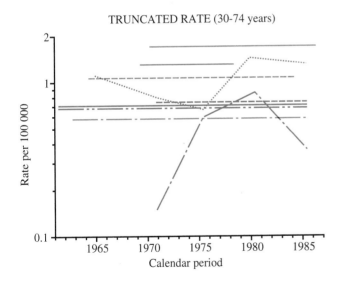

CUMULATIVE RISK (30-74 years)

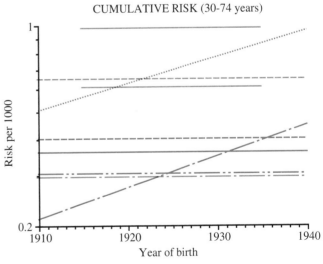

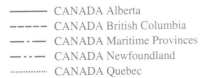

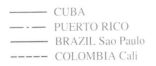

CANADA Alberta
CANADA British Columbia
CANADA Maritime Provinces
CANADA Newfoundland
CANADA Quebec

CUBA
PUERTO RICO
BRAZIL Sao Paulo
COLOMBIA Cali

BONE (ICD-9 170)

AMERICAS (USA), INCIDENCE

MALES	Best model	Goodness of fit	1970 Rate	1970 Cases	1985 Rate	1985 Cases	Cumulative risk 1915	Cumulative risk 1940	Recent trend
USA									
Bay Area, Black	A0	-0.74	*1.0*	*0*	*1.0*	*0*	0.4	0.4	*-25.5*
Bay Area, Chinese	A0	-1.17	*1.3*	*0*	*1.3*	*0*	0.6	*0.6*	*–*
Bay Area, White	A8P3	1.36	0.3	1	0.8	5	0.4	0.7	*-12.7*
Connecticut	A1C5	1.39	1.0	6	1.0	7	0.7	0.5	*-0.4*
Detroit, Black	A0D	0.32	*0.7*	*0*	*0.4*	*0*	0.4	0.2	*-9.1*
Detroit, White	A1	1.65	0.8	6	0.8	5	0.4	0.4	*19.3*
Iowa	A1C4	-0.38	1.0	6	1.0	6	0.6	0.3	*14.1*
New Orleans, Black	A0	-1.24	*1.1*	*0*	*1.1*	*0*	0.5	0.5	*15.2*
New Orleans, White	A1	-0.40	*0.9*	*1*	0.9	1	0.6	0.6	*-0.9*
Seattle	A1	3.12	*1.0*	*4*	1.0	6	0.5	0.5	*-14.7*

FEMALES	Best model	Goodness of fit	1970 Rate	1970 Cases	1985 Rate	1985 Cases	Cumulative risk 1915	Cumulative risk 1940	Recent trend
USA									
Bay Area, Black	A0	-1.13	*0.5*	*0*	*0.5*	*0*	0.2	0.2	*2.4*
Bay Area, Chinese	*	..	..	..	..	..	..	..	..
Bay Area, White	A1	-1.34	0.7	4	0.7	4	0.4	0.4	*11.6*
Connecticut	A1	1.55	0.8	5	0.8	6	0.4	0.4	32.8
Detroit, Black	A0	-0.76	*0.6*	*0*	0.6	1	0.3	0.3	*-12.6*
Detroit, White	A1	1.60	0.6	4	0.6	4	0.3	0.3	*21.9*
Iowa	A1	0.36	0.7	4	0.7	4	0.3	0.3	*-8.4*
New Orleans, Black	A0	-0.58	*0.7*	*0*	*0.7*	*0*	0.3	0.3	*-49.5*
New Orleans, White	A1	0.78	*0.7*	*1*	0.7	1	0.4	0.4	*81.1*
Seattle	A1	0.94	*0.8*	*4*	0.8	6	0.4	0.4	*30.0*

* : not enough cases for reliable estimation
− : incomplete or missing data
Best model: polynomial of the given degree in age (A), period (P) or cohort (C), or linear drift (D) model.
Goodness of fit: the normalised likelihood ratio chi-square for the best model (see Method).
Rate: world-standardised truncated rate per 100 000 per year (30-74 years) and number of **cases** are both estimated from the best-fitting model for the single years cited.
Cumulative risk per 1000 (30-74 years) is estimated from the best-fitting *age-cohort* model for cohorts of central birth year cited.
Recent trend: estimated mean percentage change per five-year period in the age-specific rates (30-74 years) over the period 1973-1987.
Italics denote recent trends not significant at 5 per cent level, or other figures which should be interpreted with caution (see Method).

372

BONE (ICD-9 170)

AMERICAS (USA), INCIDENCE

MALES

TRUNCATED RATE (30-74 years)

CUMULATIVE RISK (30-74 years)

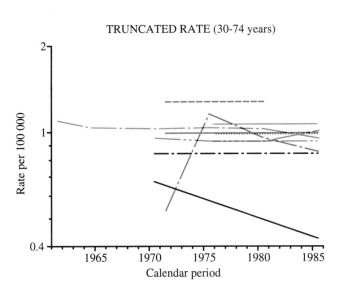
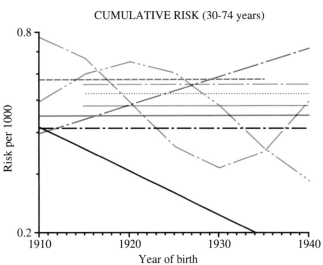

FEMALES

TRUNCATED RATE (30-74 years)

CUMULATIVE RISK (30-74 years)

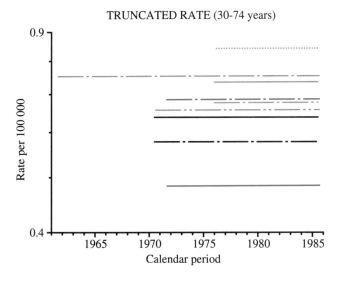
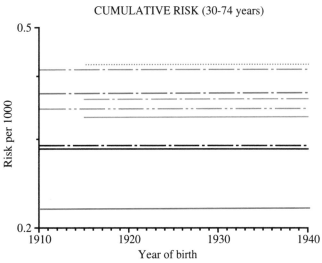

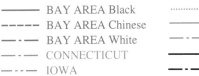

——— BAY AREA Black	·············· SEATTLE
- - - - BAY AREA Chinese	——— NEW ORLEANS Black
—·—· BAY AREA White	—·—· NEW ORLEANS White
—··— CONNECTICUT	——— DETROIT Black
—··— IOWA	—··— DETROIT White

BONE (ICD-9 170)

AMERICAS (except USA), INCIDENCE
Percentage change per five-year period, 1973-1987

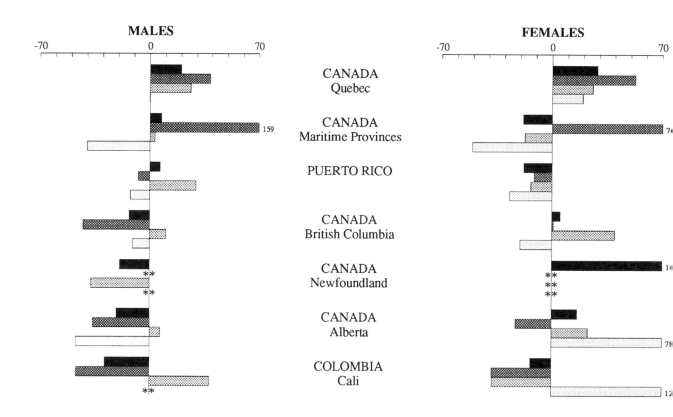

MALES

FEMALES

CANADA
Quebec

CANADA
Maritime Provinces

PUERTO RICO

CANADA
British Columbia

CANADA
Newfoundland

CANADA
Alberta

COLOMBIA
Cali

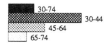
30-74
30-44
45-64
65-74

BONE (ICD-9 170)

AMERICAS (USA), INCIDENCE
Percentage change per five-year period, 1973-1987

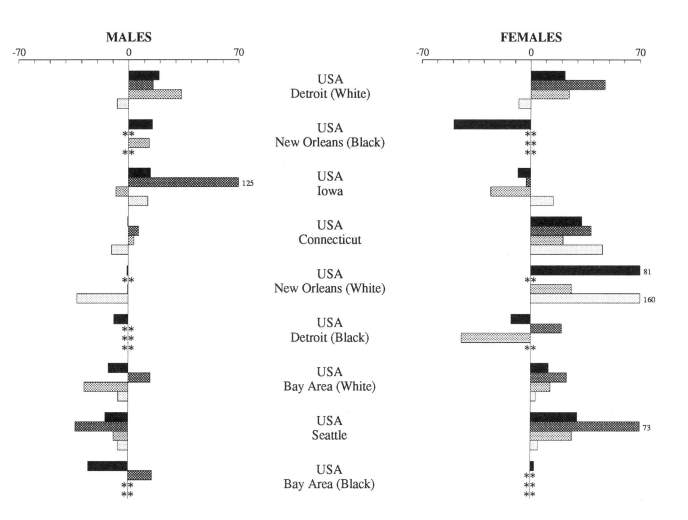

BONE (ICD-9 170)

AMERICAS, MORTALITY

MALES	Best model	Goodness of fit	1965 Rate	1965 Deaths	1985 Rate	1985 Deaths	Cumulative risk 1900	Cumulative risk 1940	Recent trend
CANADA	A3D	-0.47	1.5	58	0.8	44	1.1	0.3	-18.2
CHILE	A3P2C2	1.08	3.2	37	1.9	33	1.9	0.7	-24.7
COSTA RICA	A1P2	0.89	1.0	1	1.6	5	*0.2*	2.9	90.4
PANAMA	A1	-0.14	*0.7*	*1*	0.7	2	*0.5*	0.5	–
PUERTO RICO	A2P2	-0.23	1.7	6	1.0	4	*1.4*	0.5	-29.3
URUGUAY	A2D	-0.20	*4.3*	*25*	1.3	9	*3.6*	0.3	*-13.7*
USA	A4P5C5	2.43	1.4	580	0.5	268	1.1	0.2	-34.3
VENEZUELA	A3D	0.48	2.1	18	*1.1*	*20*	1.4	0.4	–

FEMALES	Best model	Goodness of fit	1965 Rate	1965 Deaths	1985 Rate	1985 Deaths	Cumulative risk 1900	Cumulative risk 1940	Recent trend
CANADA	A3D	-1.64	0.9	33	0.4	26	0.6	0.1	-18.3
CHILE	A2P2	-0.55	2.4	31	1.2	24	1.5	0.5	-21.1
COSTA RICA	A1	0.39	0.9	1	0.9	2	*0.5*	0.5	*19.7*
PANAMA	A1	0.21	*0.5*	*0*	0.5	1	*0.3*	0.3	–
PUERTO RICO	A2P4	-0.33	0.8	3	*0.1*	*0*	2.8	0.1	-80.0
URUGUAY	A1D	1.41	*2.3*	*14*	0.8	6	*1.9*	0.2	*-19.1*
USA	A4P5C3	1.14	0.8	406	0.3	187	0.7	0.1	-31.5
VENEZUELA	A2C2	0.59	2.0	19	*1.0*	*19*	1.4	0.4	–

* : not enough deaths for reliable estimation
– : incomplete or missing data
Best model: polynomial of the given degree in age (A), period (P) or cohort (C), or linear drift (D) model.
Goodness of fit: the normalised likelihood ratio chi-square for the best model (see Method).
Rate: world-standardised truncated rate per 100 000 per year (30-74 years) and number of **deaths** are both estimated from the best-fitting model for the single years cited.
Cumulative risk per 1000 (30-74 years) is estimated from the best-fitting *age-cohort* model for cohorts of central birth year cited.
Recent trend: estimated mean percentage change per five-year period in the age-specific rates (30-74 years) over the period 1975-1988.
Italics denote recent trends not significant at 5 per cent level, or other figures which should be interpreted with caution (see Method).

BONE (ICD-9 170)

AMERICAS, MORTALITY

MALES

TRUNCATED RATE (30-74 years)

CUMULATIVE RISK (30-74 years)

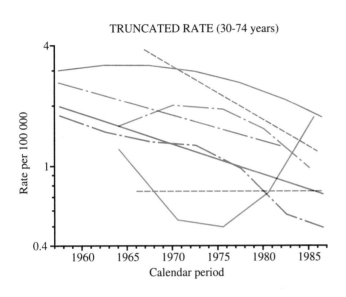
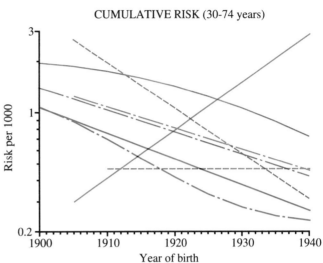

FEMALES

TRUNCATED RATE (30-74 years)

CUMULATIVE RISK (30-74 years)

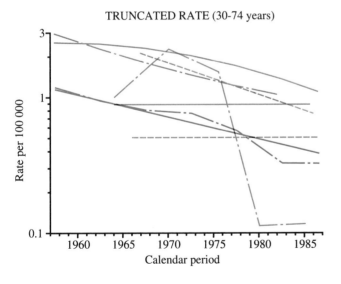
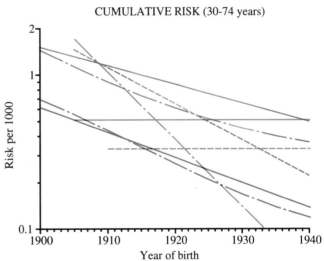

———— CANADA	—··— PUERTO RICO
—·—· USA	———— CHILE
———— COSTA RICA	------ URUGUAY
------ PANAMA	—··— VENEZUELA

BONE (ICD-9 170)

AMERICAS, MORTALITY
Percentage change per five-year period, 1975-1988

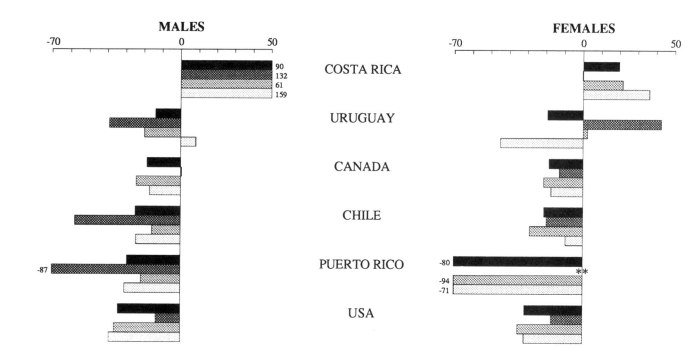

Chapter 16

MELANOMA OF THE SKIN

Malignant melanoma of the skin is generally infrequent, comprising less than 1% of all malignancies in most populations. Its importance lies in the rapid increase in incidence in the last 20-30 years in many Caucasian populations. In Australia, New Zealand, Norway and several areas of the USA, however, melanoma of the skin already comprised 2-8% of malignant tumours in females around 1975, and 2-5% in males[274]. By 1980, melanoma was one of the ten most frequent malignancies among females in 43 of the 137 populations included in volume V of *Cancer Incidence in Five Continents*, and among males as well in 20 of these populations, principally those of Australia, New Zealand, Canada, the USA and the Nordic countries, but also in Switzerland, France and Ireland[300]. In Australia, melanoma is now the third or fourth most frequent malignancy among females in every state, and it comprises more than 10% of all tumours in Queensland and Western Australia.

Incidence and mortality rates have increased substantially in the great majority of the 60 populations studied here. The increasing trends are greatest in predominantly Caucasian populations, particularly in North America, but substantial increases have also occurred in populations in which melanoma was previously much less common, including those of Cuba and Puerto Rico, and among Jews in Israel. In most populations, rates of increase are less marked for females than for males.

The rate of increase in incidence is between 30% and 50% every five years in many North American white populations and among Caucasians in Hawaii, who are of similar racial stock. Upward trends are only slightly less marked for most European populations, in the range of 15-50% every five years in northern Europe, but these are still substantial rates of increase.

Europe

In Europe, the consistency of the rapid increase in incidence is notable, particularly in EC member states, where it averages around 30% every five years in both sexes. The highest estimates of the cumulative risk of developing melanoma in the age range 30-74 years are seen for the 1940 birth cohort in Nordic countries (1-3%), with rates increasing at 20-30% every five years, while the corresponding risks of dying from melanoma are 0.2-0.6%, with rates increasing at around 10% every five years. The rates of increase decelerated during the 1980s, however, particularly for mortality.

The very large recent increase in incidence in both sexes in Zaragoza (Spain) is based on small numbers of cases in the earliest period for which data are available (1968-72), probably due at least in part to incomplete registration in that period, and incidence rates in Zaragoza are now similar to those in neighbouring Navarra. Zaragoza only includes 2% of the national population (see Table 2.8) and may not be representative of Spain as a whole, but the recent increase in mortality in Spain is also one of the largest in Europe, at around 50% every five years. Even so, incidence and mortality from malignant melanoma in Spain are still low by European standards. Similarly, the large early increases in incidence among Israeli Jews of both sexes and among females in Geneva (Switzerland) may also be partly artefactual, due to incomplete registration in the earliest period for each registry; this is suggested by the sharp change in the trend of the truncated rates, but current rates and recent trends in Israel (incidence) and Switzerland (mortality) are now well within the European range, and similar to those observed in the Nordic countries. The irregular trend for melanoma among males in Cluj (Romania) depends on few cases, and is probably an artefact of inconsistent registration: the values extrapolated for 1970 should be ignored (see Chapter 3).

In Poland, Hungary and Slovenia, incidence in both sexes is much lower than in other European countries, but it is now increasing at least as rapidly as in western Europe. Mortality has also been increasing rapidly in Czechoslovakia, Hungary, Poland, and Yugoslavia, and is now as high as in the Nordic countries.

Asia and Oceania

Melanoma incidence among the Indian, Chinese and Japanese populations of Asia and Oceania is up to an order of magnitude lower than in Caucasian populations, and there is very little evidence of change. Truncated rates among females in Osaka (Japan), for example, have increased

continued page 400

MELANOMA OF SKIN (ICD-9 172)

EUROPE (non-EC), INCIDENCE

MALES	Best model	Goodness of fit	1970 Rate	1970 Cases	1985 Rate	1985 Cases	Cumulative risk 1915	Cumulative risk 1940	Recent trend
FINLAND	A4D	-1.06	5.9	59	13.4	161	4.2	16.4	31.1
HUNGARY									
County Vas	A1D	-0.71	4.0	2	9.2	6	2.8	11.4	*24.8*
Szabolcs-Szatmar	A1P2	1.45	2.2	2	5.5	7	2.0	5.0	82.1
ISRAEL									
All Jews	A2P2	-1.26	5.9	28	13.2	83	4.1	20.3	24.7
Non-Jews	*	..	..	..	..	..	..	..	..
NORWAY	A2P3C3	-1.03	9.6	90	21.2	222	6.0	24.7	21.5
POLAND									
Warsaw City	A1P3	-0.24	3.6	10	5.6	22	2.5	5.0	*13.0*
ROMANIA									
Cluj	A1P2	2.47	*398.5*	*636*	3.4	6	4.8	1.1	-26.9
SWEDEN	A2C5	-0.82	8.3	180	18.6	436	6.2	20.4	30.9
SWITZERLAND									
Geneva	A1C2	2.42	9.7	7	16.7	15	7.3	14.4	*6.7*
YUGOSLAVIA									
Slovenia	A2P2	-0.03	2.8	10	7.1	32	2.1	7.3	46.6

FEMALES	Best model	Goodness of fit	1970 Rate	1970 Cases	1985 Rate	1985 Cases	Cumulative risk 1915	Cumulative risk 1940	Recent trend
FINLAND	A3D	-0.72	5.8	71	12.0	166	3.6	11.9	21.8
HUNGARY									
County Vas	A1D	-0.30	4.4	3	9.0	7	2.9	9.7	46.5
Szabolcs-Szatmar	A1	0.45	3.6	5	3.6	5	1.9	1.9	*20.9*
ISRAEL									
All Jews	A8P4	1.18	8.5	42	15.2	106	4.3	20.5	17.9
Non-Jews	*	..	..	..	..	..	..	..	..
NORWAY	A3P2C4	-1.05	10.8	103	25.8	274	6.0	29.2	26.8
POLAND									
Warsaw City	A2D	0.49	3.7	14	5.5	27	2.1	4.2	17.1
ROMANIA									
Cluj	A1	1.27	*4.1*	7	4.1	8	2.1	2.1	*3.4*
SWEDEN	A8P5	1.16	9.9	216	20.1	468	5.1	17.6	25.4
SWITZERLAND									
Geneva	A1P3	0.57	1.2	1	15.1	16	4.5	21.9	*15.1*
YUGOSLAVIA									
Slovenia	A3D	1.32	4.1	18	7.2	38	2.4	6.0	41.3

* : not enough cases for reliable estimation
− : incomplete or missing data
Best model: polynomial of the given degree in age (A), period (P) or cohort (C), or linear drift (D) model.
Goodness of fit: the normalised likelihood ratio chi-square for the best model (see Method).
Rate: world-standardised truncated rate per 100 000 per year (30-74 years) and number of **cases** are both estimated from the best-fitting model for the single years cited.
Cumulative risk per 1000 (30-74 years) is estimated from the best-fitting *age-cohort* model for cohorts of central birth year cited.
Recent trend: estimated mean percentage change per five-year period in the age-specific rates (30-74 years) over the period 1973-1987.
Italics denote recent trends not significant at 5 per cent level, or other figures which should be interpreted with caution (see Method).

MELANOMA OF SKIN (ICD-9 172)

EUROPE (non-EC), INCIDENCE

MALES

TRUNCATED RATE (30-74 years)

CUMULATIVE RISK (30-74 years)

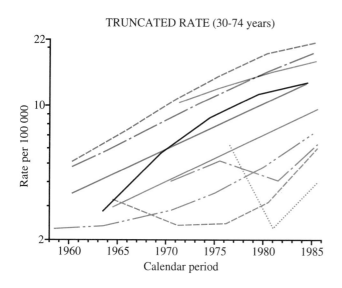 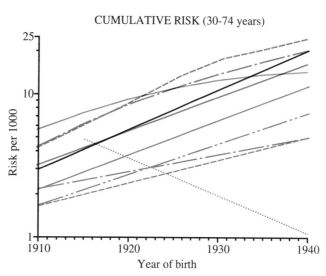

FEMALES

TRUNCATED RATE (30-74 years)

CUMULATIVE RISK (30-74 years)

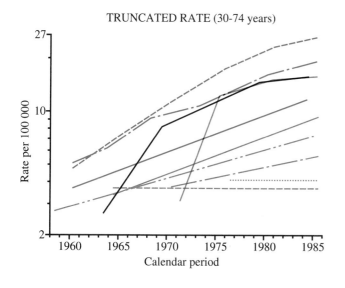 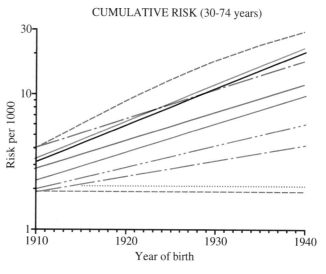

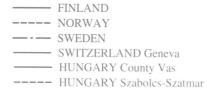 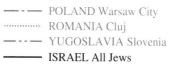

—————— FINLAND
— — — — NORWAY
— · — · — SWEDEN
—————— SWITZERLAND Geneva
—————— HUNGARY County Vas
— — — — HUNGARY Szabolcs-Szatmar

— · — · POLAND Warsaw City
· · · · · · · ROMANIA Cluj
— ·· — ·· YUGOSLAVIA Slovenia
—————— ISRAEL All Jews

MELANOMA OF SKIN (ICD-9 172)

EUROPE (EC), INCIDENCE

MALES	Best model	Goodness of fit	1970 Rate	1970 Cases	1985 Rate	1985 Cases	Cumulative risk 1915	Cumulative risk 1940	Recent trend
DENMARK	A3C3	-0.32	6.8	82	15.1	201	4.4	17.3	32.0
FRANCE									
Bas-Rhin	A1D	0.30	*3.0*	*6*	9.9	20	2.8	20.2	50.1
Doubs	A1	1.36	*6.5*	*5*	6.5	7	3.2	3.2	*39.7*
GERMANY (FRG)									
Hamburg	A2P2	-1.27	5.3	25	*73.7*	*300*	2.9	*14.5*	–
Saarland	A2D	-0.21	3.3	8	9.1	25	2.8	15.1	47.3
GERMANY (GDR)	A8P4C9	0.51	4.0	154	7.5	284	2.6	7.5	29.7
ITALY									
Varese	A1D	-0.01	*2.9*	*4*	8.2	16	2.4	13.8	41.3
SPAIN									
Navarra	A1D	0.41	*2.1*	*2*	5.7	7	2.1	11.0	41.5
Zaragoza	A1P2	0.79	*0.5*	*0*	4.5	9	1.4	29.1	53.8
UK									
Birmingham	A1P3	0.56	2.4	30	5.2	70	1.5	4.6	41.4
Scotland	A1D	0.42	2.4	30	7.7	97	2.1	14.6	54.0
South Thames	A2D	-1.54	2.9	64	6.5	109	1.8	6.9	28.8

FEMALES	Best model	Goodness of fit	1970 Rate	1970 Cases	1985 Rate	1985 Cases	Cumulative risk 1915	Cumulative risk 1940	Recent trend
DENMARK	A8P6C9	-0.09	10.9	137	19.6	272	5.5	16.8	23.6
FRANCE									
Bas-Rhin	A1D	0.13	*3.6*	*9*	12.2	28	3.3	25.2	53.5
Doubs	A3P2	-1.35	*0.0*	*0*	11.0	12	2.7	11.2	*33.7*
GERMANY (FRG)									
Hamburg	A3P2	0.35	4.5	27	*506.6*	*2398*	2.7	*38.8*	–
Saarland	A1D	1.17	3.9	13	9.0	29	2.5	10.2	34.4
GERMANY (GDR)	A8C9	-0.20	4.4	235	8.5	404	2.7	7.8	29.5
ITALY									
Varese	A8C7	-0.69	*5.8*	*13*	8.0	18	3.6	4.7	*9.2*
SPAIN									
Navarra	A0D	0.80	*2.2*	*2*	7.3	9	1.3	9.6	49.4
Zaragoza	A0D	-0.59	*0.6*	*1*	3.8	8	0.6	13.1	87.5
UK									
Birmingham	A1P3C3	0.89	4.1	53	10.4	143	2.3	10.1	54.2
Scotland	A3P2	2.04	4.3	61	12.9	180	3.0	17.9	52.0
South Thames	A8C9	0.21	5.6	136	10.9	199	3.0	7.8	24.4

* : not enough cases for reliable estimation
– : incomplete or missing data
Best model: polynomial of the given degree in age (A), period (P) or cohort (C), or linear drift (D) model.
Goodness of fit: the normalised likelihood ratio chi-square for the best model (see Method).
Rate: world-standardised truncated rate per 100 000 per year (30-74 years) and number of **cases** are both estimated from the best-fitting model for the single years cited.
Cumulative risk per 1000 (30-74 years) is estimated from the best-fitting *age-cohort* model for cohorts of central birth year cited.
Recent trend: estimated mean percentage change per five-year period in the age-specific rates (30-74 years) over the period 1973-1987.
Italics denote recent trends not significant at 5 per cent level, or other figures which should be interpreted with caution (see Method).

MELANOMA OF SKIN (ICD-9 172)

EUROPE (EC), INCIDENCE

MALES

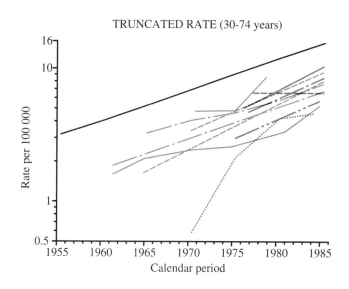

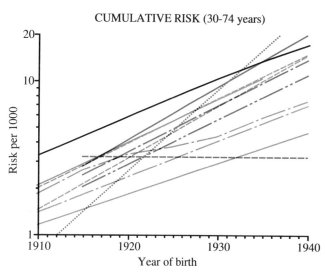

FEMALES

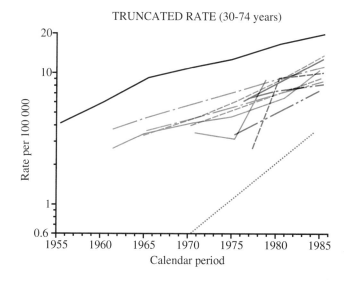

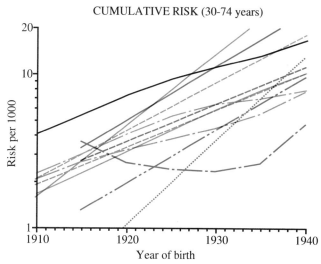

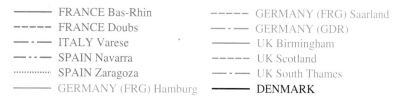

—————— FRANCE Bas-Rhin	------ GERMANY (FRG) Saarland
- - - - - FRANCE Doubs	—·—·— GERMANY (GDR)
—·—·— ITALY Varese	—————— UK Birmingham
—··—··— SPAIN Navarra	------ UK Scotland
············ SPAIN Zaragoza	—·—·— UK South Thames
—————— GERMANY (FRG) Hamburg	—————— DENMARK

MELANOMA OF SKIN (ICD-9 172)

EUROPE (non-EC), INCIDENCE
Percentage change per five-year period, 1973-1987

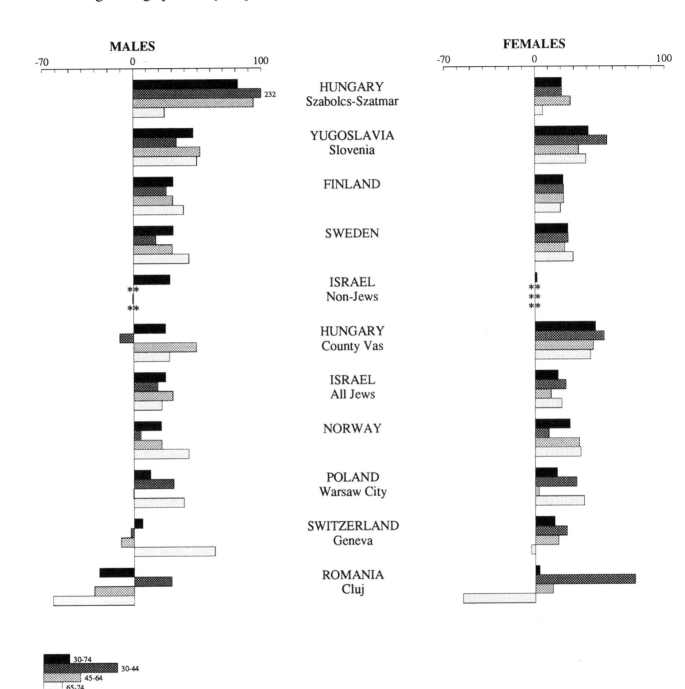

MELANOMA OF SKIN (ICD-9 172)

EUROPE (EC), INCIDENCE
Percentage change per five-year period, 1973-1987

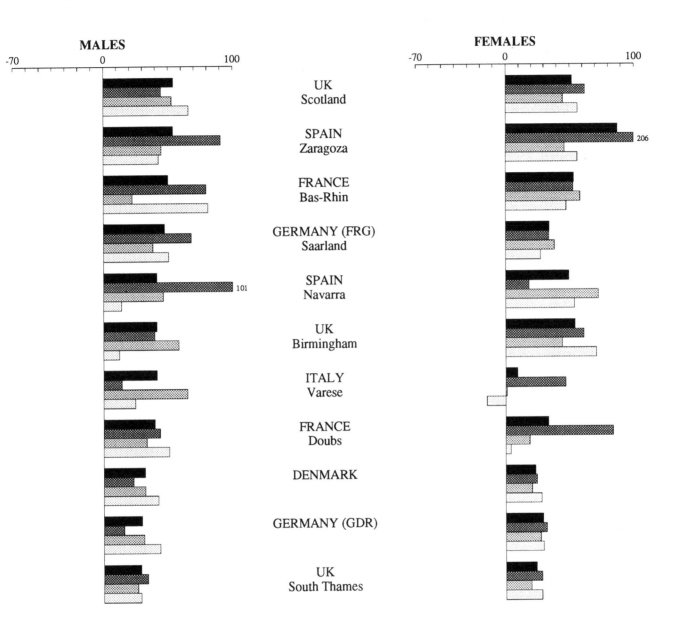

385

MELANOMA OF SKIN (ICD-9 172)

EUROPE (non-EC), MORTALITY

MALES	Best model	Goodness of fit	1965 Rate	1965 Deaths	1985 Rate	1985 Deaths	Cumulative risk 1900	Cumulative risk 1940	Recent trend
AUSTRIA	A4C2	-0.84	*2.5*	*42*	4.5	81	*1.0*	3.4	17.0
CZECHOSLOVAKIA	A2P2C4	2.11	1.4	48	4.7	168	0.5	6.0	20.2
FINLAND	A3P4	-2.60	2.2	21	3.8	45	1.2	3.9	*1.1*
HUNGARY	A1D	0.64	*1.4*	*35*	3.7	100	*0.7*	4.6	24.4
NORWAY	A2C3	-0.91	3.2	30	6.8	73	1.2	6.0	19.3
POLAND	A2P2C4	-1.10	0.7	45	2.5	203	0.3	*3.4*	–
ROMANIA	–	–	–	–	–	–	–	–	–
SWEDEN	A3C3	1.16	3.0	64	5.3	127	1.2	3.8	11.5
SWITZERLAND	A2C2	1.18	2.9	39	4.8	82	1.2	3.4	*-1.6*
YUGOSLAVIA	A2D	0.42	0.7	26	2.7	139	0.4	5.4	41.7

FEMALES	Best model	Goodness of fit	1965 Rate	1965 Deaths	1985 Rate	1985 Deaths	Cumulative risk 1900	Cumulative risk 1940	Recent trend
AUSTRIA	A3C2	-0.47	*2.1*	*44*	2.6	60	*0.8*	1.4	*8.5*
CZECHOSLOVAKIA	A3P2C2	-1.52	1.0	37	2.8	119	0.4	3.6	18.2
FINLAND	A1C2	1.59	1.8	20	2.4	34	0.8	1.5	*1.3*
HUNGARY	A3D	0.95	*1.3*	*37*	2.6	81	*0.6*	2.3	13.5
NORWAY	A1C3	0.80	2.1	20	4.1	46	0.8	3.7	16.1
POLAND	A2P2	1.59	0.7	54	2.1	196	0.3	*2.5*	–
ROMANIA	–	–	–	–	–	–	–	–	–
SWEDEN	A3P4	-0.20	2.2	50	3.3	81	0.9	2.6	*9.4*
SWITZERLAND	A3P2C2	2.30	1.9	30	3.2	60	0.8	2.4	*7.6*
YUGOSLAVIA	A3D	-0.38	0.6	24	1.8	105	0.3	2.9	30.8

* : not enough deaths for reliable estimation
– : incomplete or missing data
Best model: polynomial of the given degree in age (A), period (P) or cohort (C), or linear drift (D) model.
Goodness of fit: the normalised likelihood ratio chi-square for the best model (see Method).
Rate: world-standardised truncated rate per 100 000 per year (30-74 years) and number of **deaths** are both estimated from the best-fitting model for the single years cited.
Cumulative risk per 1000 (30-74 years) is estimated from the best-fitting *age-cohort* model for cohorts of central birth year cited.
Recent trend: estimated mean percentage change per five-year period in the age-specific rates (30-74 years) over the period 1975-1988.
Italics denote recent trends not significant at 5 per cent level, or other figures which should be interpreted with caution (see Method).

MELANOMA OF SKIN (ICD-9 172)

EUROPE (non-EC), MORTALITY

MALES

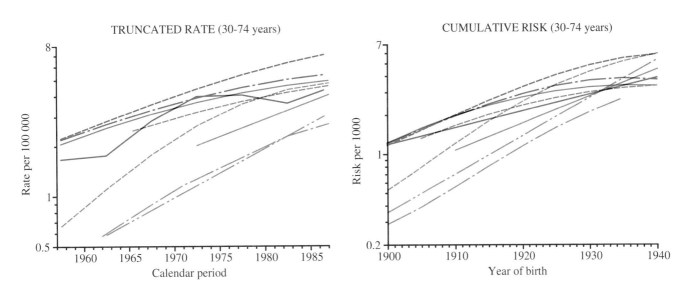

TRUNCATED RATE (30-74 years)   CUMULATIVE RISK (30-74 years)

FEMALES

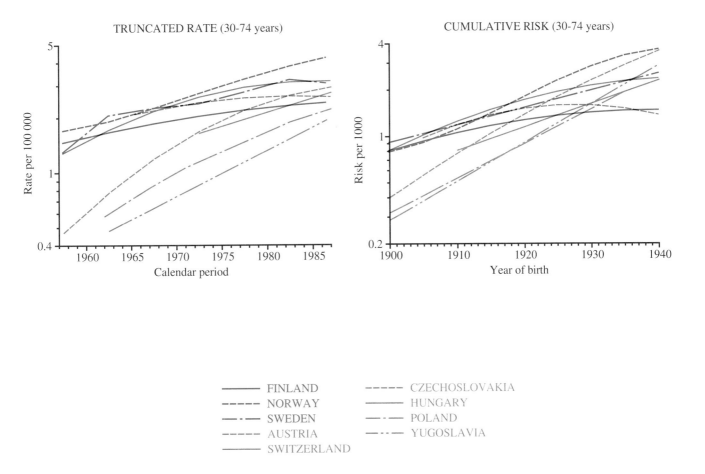

TRUNCATED RATE (30-74 years)   CUMULATIVE RISK (30-74 years)

——— FINLAND	------ CZECHOSLOVAKIA
-------- NORWAY	——— HUNGARY
—·—·— SWEDEN	—··—··— POLAND
-------- AUSTRIA	—··—··— YUGOSLAVIA
——— SWITZERLAND	

MELANOMA OF SKIN (ICD-9 172)

EUROPE (EC), MORTALITY

MALES	Best model	Goodness of fit	1965 Rate	1965 Deaths	1985 Rate	1985 Deaths	Cumulative risk 1900	Cumulative risk 1940	Recent trend
BELGIUM	A1P4	0.16	0.8	21	2.0	51	0.5	2.4	*9.2*
DENMARK	A2C4	-1.09	2.9	34	5.5	74	1.1	4.1	16.1
FRANCE	A2P6	0.30	0.8	89	1.9	254	0.3	3.3	26.9
GERMANY (FRG)	A3P3C2	5.57	*2.8*	*389*	3.4	540	*1.0*	2.2	11.0
GREECE	A1D	0.87	*0.4*	*8*	1.1	27	*0.2*	1.2	*11.5*
IRELAND	A1D	-0.28	1.1	7	2.1	15	0.5	1.8	38.6
ITALY	A2P5C6	0.17	0.9	110	2.9	422	0.3	3.0	30.9
NETHERLANDS	A2D	1.39	1.7	45	3.5	123	0.7	3.1	25.1
PORTUGAL	–	–	–	–	–	–	–	–	–
SPAIN	A1D	-0.02	0.2	11	1.4	126	0.1	5.8	55.5
UK ENGLAND & WALES	A5C5	1.05	1.3	159	2.7	348	0.5	2.3	14.2
UK SCOTLAND	A1C3	-0.21	1.3	16	2.4	31	0.6	2.1	22.5

FEMALES	Best model	Goodness of fit	1965 Rate	1965 Deaths	1985 Rate	1985 Deaths	Cumulative risk 1900	Cumulative risk 1940	Recent trend
BELGIUM	A1D	-0.57	0.8	23	1.5	44	0.4	1.4	*9.9*
DENMARK	A3C3	-1.35	2.8	35	4.2	59	1.1	2.7	*1.8*
FRANCE	A4P4	3.48	0.5	69	1.7	253	0.2	2.5	19.9
GERMANY (FRG)	A3C5	2.50	*1.9*	*347*	2.3	456	*0.7*	1.3	7.7
GREECE	A1D	-0.64	*0.3*	*6*	0.6	17	*0.1*	0.5	*16.1*
IRELAND	A1C2	0.59	1.4	9	2.6	20	0.6	2.0	*16.6*
ITALY	A8P6C9	2.79	0.8	107	1.8	311	0.3	1.9	28.0
NETHERLANDS	A1P2	1.09	1.5	44	2.4	92	0.7	2.0	*3.6*
PORTUGAL	–	–	–	–	–	–	–	–	–
SPAIN	A1P3	-1.15	0.1	7	0.8	85	0.1	4.6	43.7
UK ENGLAND & WALES	A3C6	-0.78	1.5	206	2.6	374	0.5	1.7	12.5
UK SCOTLAND	A1C2	-2.55	1.6	22	2.4	35	0.6	1.5	*5.5*

* : not enough deaths for reliable estimation
– : incomplete or missing data
Best model: polynomial of the given degree in age (A), period (P) or cohort (C), or linear drift (D) model.
Goodness of fit: the normalised likelihood ratio chi-square for the best model (see Method).
Rate: world-standardised truncated rate per 100 000 per year (30-74 years) and number of **deaths** are both estimated from the best-fitting model for the single years cited.
Cumulative risk per 1000 (30-74 years) is estimated from the best-fitting *age-cohort* model for cohorts of central birth year cited.
Recent trend: estimated mean percentage change per five-year period in the age-specific rates (30-74 years) over the period 1975-1988.
Italics denote recent trends not significant at 5 per cent level, or other figures which should be interpreted with caution (see Method).

MELANOMA OF SKIN (ICD-9 172)

EUROPE (EC), MORTALITY

MALES

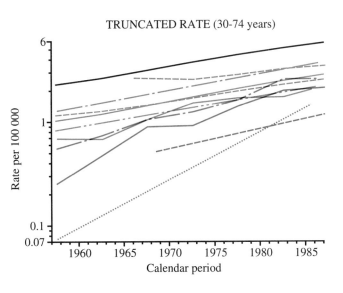

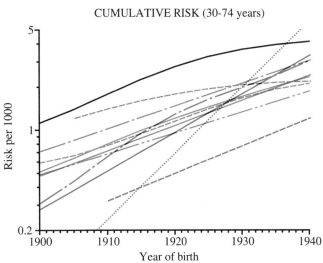

FEMALES

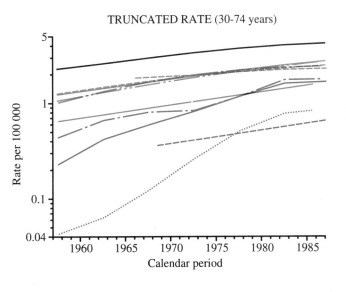

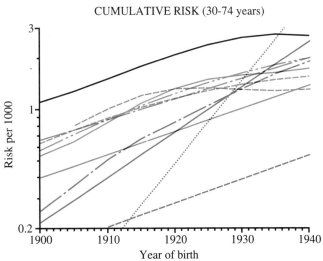

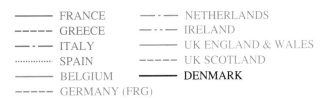

FRANCE — · — · NETHERLANDS

- - - - GREECE — · · — · · IRELAND

— · — · ITALY ——— UK ENGLAND & WALES

· · · · · · SPAIN - - - - UK SCOTLAND

——— BELGIUM ——— DENMARK

- - - - - GERMANY (FRG)

MELANOMA OF SKIN (ICD-9 172)

EUROPE (non-EC), MORTALITY
Percentage change per five-year period, 1975-1988

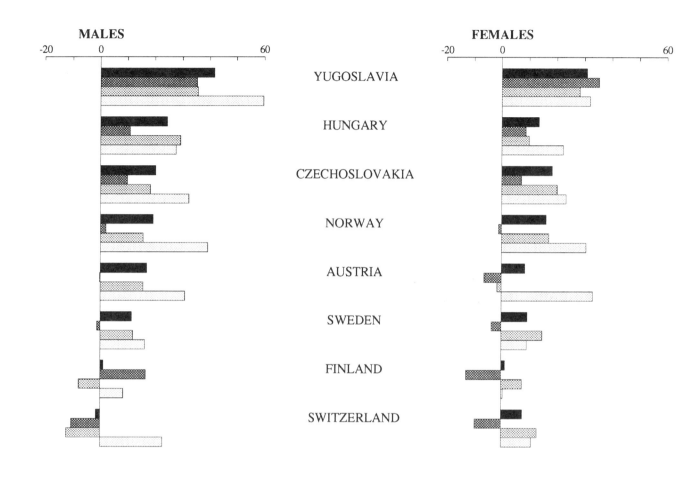

MELANOMA OF SKIN (ICD-9 172)

EUROPE (EC), MORTALITY
Percentage change per five-year period, 1975-1988

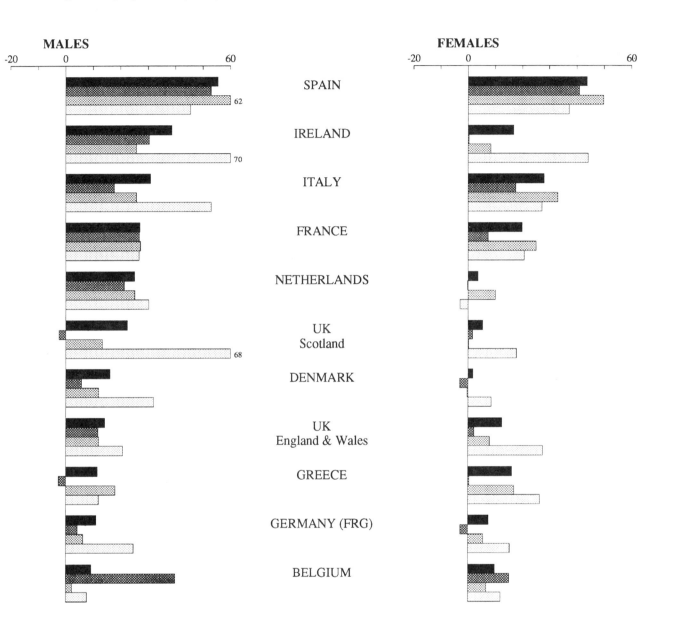

ASIA, INCIDENCE

MALES	Best model	Goodness of fit	1970 Rate	1970 Cases	1985 Rate	1985 Cases	Cumulative risk 1915	Cumulative risk 1940	Recent trend
CHINA									
Shanghai	A1	1.11	0.6	6	0.6	9	0.3	0.3	-9.4
HONG KONG	A2	-0.48	1.6	10	1.6	18	0.9	0.9	-15.5
INDIA									
Bombay	A2	1.02	0.4	3	0.4	5	0.2	0.2	10.7
JAPAN									
Miyagi	A1	-0.01	0.8	2	0.8	4	0.5	0.5	0.3
Nagasaki	A1	-0.08	0.7	0	0.7	0	0.4	0.4	19.4
Osaka	A1	0.02	0.4	5	0.4	7	0.2	0.2	9.2
SINGAPORE									
Chinese	A1	0.78	1.0	2	1.0	3	0.6	0.6	-13.4
Indian	*	..	..	..	..	..	..	..	..
Malay	A1	-1.41	1.2	0	1.2	0	0.8	0.8	1.5

FEMALES	Best model	Goodness of fit	1970 Rate	1970 Cases	1985 Rate	1985 Cases	Cumulative risk 1915	Cumulative risk 1940	Recent trend
CHINA									
Shanghai	A1	1.11	0.6	6	0.6	9	0.3	0.3	3.3
HONG KONG	A1P2	0.01	7.9	46	1.5	17	0.7	1.4	14.3
INDIA									
Bombay	A1	1.18	0.4	2	0.4	3	0.2	0.2	-3.9
JAPAN									
Miyagi	A1	0.06	0.5	2	0.5	3	0.3	0.3	-17.6
Nagasaki	A0	-0.32	0.6	0	0.6	0	0.2	0.2	-20.5
Osaka	A1D	0.41	0.2	3	0.4	9	0.2	0.5	21.1
SINGAPORE									
Chinese	A1	0.29	0.7	1	0.7	2	0.4	0.4	-34.4
Indian	A0	-2.09	0.9	0	0.9	0	0.4	0.4	*
Malay	–	–	–	–	–	–	–	–	–

* : not enough cases for reliable estimation
– : incomplete or missing data
Best model: polynomial of the given degree in age (A), period (P) or cohort (C), or linear drift (D) model.
Goodness of fit: the normalised likelihood ratio chi-square for the best model (see Method).
Rate: world-standardised truncated rate per 100 000 per year (30-74 years) and number of **cases** are both estimated from the best-fitting model for the single years cited.
Cumulative risk per 1000 (30-74 years) is estimated from the best-fitting *age-cohort* model for cohorts of central birth year cited.
Recent trend: estimated mean percentage change per five-year period in the age-specific rates (30-74 years) over the period 1973-1987.
Italics denote recent trends not significant at 5 per cent level, or other figures which should be interpreted with caution (see Method).

MELANOMA OF SKIN (ICD-9 172)

ASIA, INCIDENCE

MALES

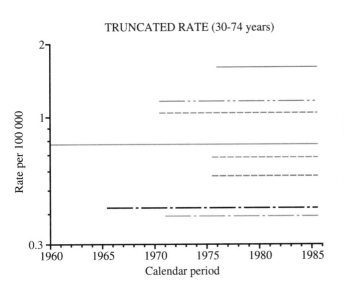

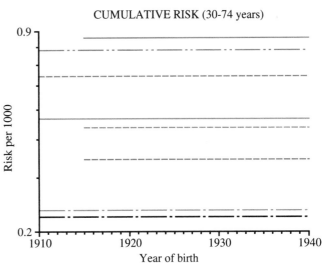

FEMALES

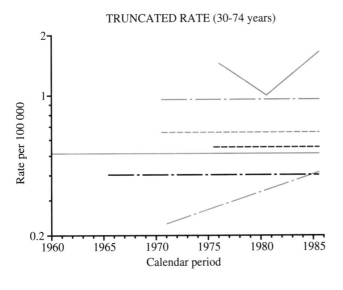

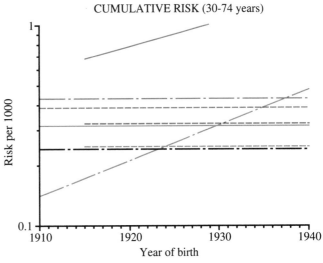

------ CHINA Shanghai
—— JAPAN Miyagi
- - - JAPAN Nagasaki
—·—· JAPAN Osaka
—— HONG KONG

------ SINGAPORE Chinese
—·—· SINGAPORE Indian
—··— SINGAPORE Malay
—··— INDIA Bombay

MELANOMA OF SKIN (ICD-9 172)

OCEANIA, INCIDENCE

MALES	Best model	Goodness of fit	1970 Rate	1970 Cases	1985 Rate	1985 Cases	Cumulative risk 1915	Cumulative risk 1940	Recent trend
AUSTRALIA									
New South Wales	A4P2C4	1.40	*45.0*	*469*	46.5	610	15.3	52.3	29.6
South	A1D	0.37	*15.8*	*35*	34.3	115	11.0	39.5	30.2
HAWAII									
Caucasian	A1P3	0.93	11.8	5	46.7	31	15.3	98.3	30.6
Chinese	*	..	..	..	..	..	..	..	..
Filipino	A1	-1.50	*1.8*	*0*	*1.8*	*0*	1.1	1.1	*-44.8*
Hawaiian	*	..	..	..	..	..	..	..	..
Japanese	*	..	..	..	..	..	..	..	..
NEW ZEALAND									
Maori	A2D	0.30	*3.5*	*0*	5.3	1	2.3	4.6	*-1.2*
Non-Maori	A1P3C2	-0.58	14.6	80	36.3	247	11.3	45.1	25.1

FEMALES	Best model	Goodness of fit	1970 Rate	1970 Cases	1985 Rate	1985 Cases	Cumulative risk 1915	Cumulative risk 1940	Recent trend
AUSTRALIA									
New South Wales	A3P2C3	-1.11	*62.6*	*659*	41.9	541	13.0	27.8	21.0
South	A3D	-0.33	*20.7*	*47*	37.9	130	11.6	31.4	24.1
HAWAII									
Caucasian	A1P4	-0.27	11.5	5	34.2	21	7.6	41.7	30.6
Chinese	–	–	–	–	–	–	–	–	–
Filipino	*	..	..	..	..	..	..	..	..
Hawaiian	A0C3	-1.19	*3.5*	*0*	*2.0*	*0*	0.5	2.3	*-26.1*
Japanese	*	..	..	..	..	..	..	..	..
NEW ZEALAND									
Maori	A1P2	0.36	*3.3*	*0*	5.4	1	2.6	2.6	*55.1*
Non-Maori	A3P4C2	1.71	20.8	116	42.4	298	12.9	39.6	13.7

* : not enough cases for reliable estimation
− : incomplete or missing data
Best model: polynomial of the given degree in age (A), period (P) or cohort (C), or linear drift (D) model.
Goodness of fit: the normalised likelihood ratio chi-square for the best model (see Method).
Rate: world-standardised truncated rate per 100 000 per year (30-74 years) and number of **cases** are both estimated from the best-fitting model for the single years cited.
Cumulative risk per 1000 (30-74 years) is estimated from the best-fitting *age-cohort* model for cohorts of central birth year cited.
Recent trend: estimated mean percentage change per five-year period in the age-specific rates (30-74 years) over the period 1973-1987.
Italics denote recent trends not significant at 5 per cent level, or other figures which should be interpreted with caution (see Method).

MELANOMA OF SKIN (ICD-9 172)

OCEANIA, INCIDENCE

MALES

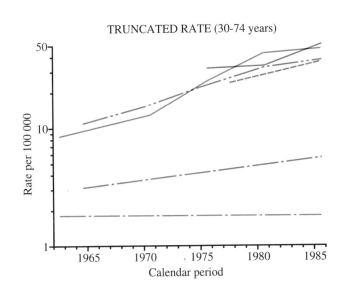

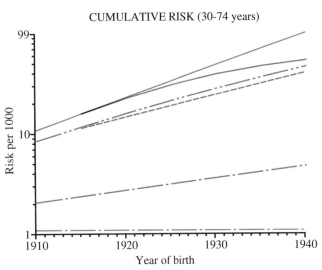

FEMALES

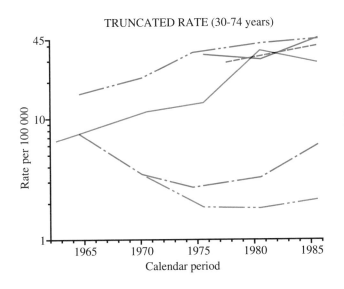

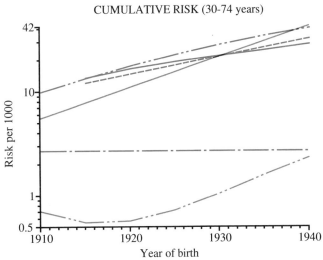

─────── AUSTRALIA New South Wales
─ ─ ─ ─ ─ AUSTRALIA South
─ · ─ · ─ NEW ZEALAND Maori
─ · · ─ · · NEW ZEALAND Non-Maori
─────── HAWAII Caucasian

─ · ─ · HAWAII Filipino
─ · · ─ · · HAWAII Hawaiian

MELANOMA OF SKIN (ICD-9 172)

ASIA, INCIDENCE
Percentage change per five-year period, 1973-1987

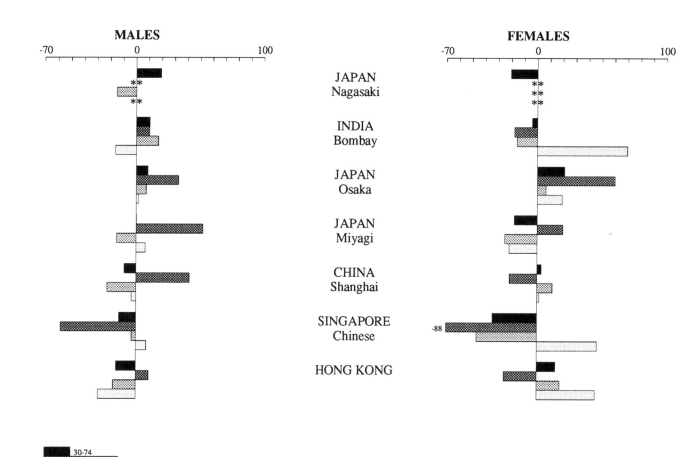

Legend:
30-74
30-44
45-64
65-74

MELANOMA OF SKIN (ICD-9 172)

OCEANIA, INCIDENCE
Percentage change per five-year period, 1973-1987

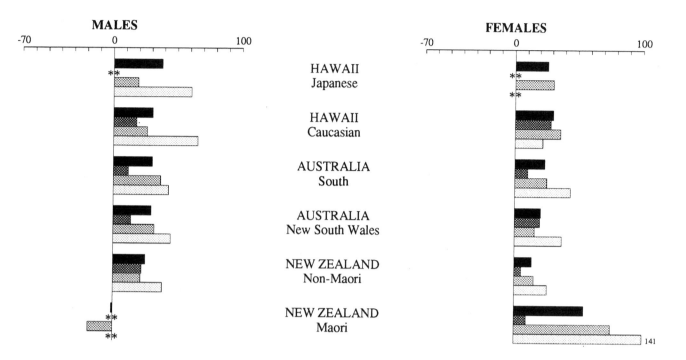

MELANOMA OF SKIN (ICD-9 172)

ASIA and OCEANIA, MORTALITY

MALES	Best model	Goodness of fit	1965 Rate	1965 Deaths	1985 Rate	1985 Deaths	Cumulative risk 1900	Cumulative risk 1940	Recent trend
AUSTRALIA	A1C4	-0.11	5.2	131	8.8	324	2.1	5.9	10.8
HONG KONG	A1	0.76	*0.4*	*1*	0.4	4	*0.3*	0.3	*9.9*
JAPAN	A2P2C3	1.02	0.2	40	0.4	112	0.1	0.3	*5.2*
MAURITIUS	*	..	..	..	..	..	..	..	..
NEW ZEALAND	A2C2	-0.78	4.6	25	9.8	70	1.9	8.7	12.7
SINGAPORE	A1	0.90	*0.4*	*0*	0.4	1	*0.2*	0.2	−

FEMALES	Best model	Goodness of fit	1965 Rate	1965 Deaths	1985 Rate	1985 Deaths	Cumulative risk 1900	Cumulative risk 1940	Recent trend
AUSTRALIA	A3C4	-1.31	3.6	92	4.7	178	1.5	2.6	6.6
HONG KONG	A1	-0.69	*0.2*	*1*	0.2	1	*0.1*	0.1	*-0.5*
JAPAN	A1P2C3	0.22	0.1	27	0.3	87	0.1	0.2	*4.1*
MAURITIUS	A0	-1.96	*0.2*	*0*	0.2	*0*	*0.1*	0.1	*
NEW ZEALAND	A3C2	-0.32	3.9	21	6.0	46	1.5	3.9	*8.1*
SINGAPORE	A1	0.29	*0.4*	*0*	0.4	1	*0.2*	0.2	−

* : not enough deaths for reliable estimation
− : incomplete or missing data
Best model: polynomial of the given degree in age (A), period (P) or cohort (C), or linear drift (D) model.
Goodness of fit: the normalised likelihood ratio chi-square for the best model (see Method).
Rate: world-standardised truncated rate per 100 000 per year (30-74 years) and number of **deaths** are both estimated from the best-fitting model for the single years cited.
Cumulative risk per 1000 (30-74 years) is estimated from the best-fitting *age-cohort* model for cohorts of central birth year cited.
Recent trend: estimated mean percentage change per five-year period in the age-specific rates (30-74 years) over the period 1975-1988.
Italics denote recent trends not significant at 5 per cent level, or other figures which should be interpreted with caution (see Method).

398

MELANOMA OF SKIN (ICD-9 172)

ASIA and OCEANIA, MORTALITY

MALES

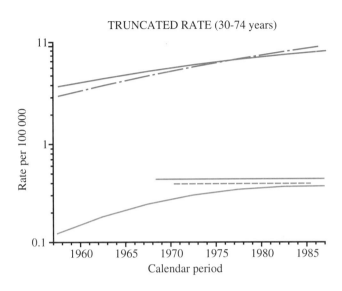

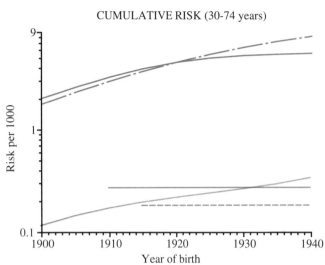

FEMALES

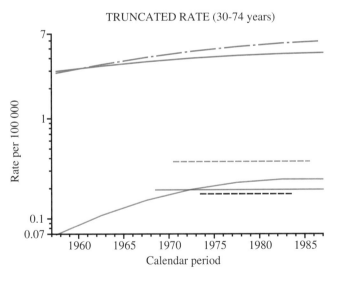

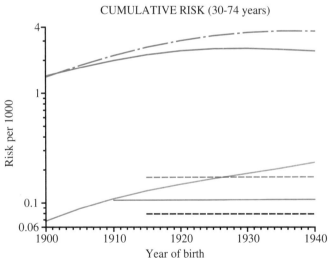

—— AUSTRALIA	—— HONG KONG
—·—· NEW ZEALAND	----- SINGAPORE
—— JAPAN	▬ ▬ ▬ MAURITIUS

MELANOMA OF SKIN (ICD-9 172)

ASIA and OCEANIA, MORTALITY
Percentage change per five-year period, 1975-1988

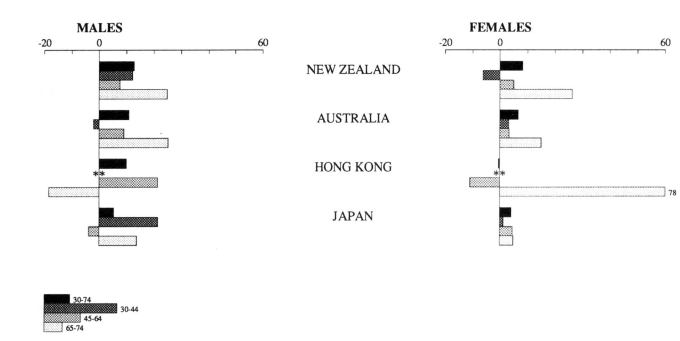

from page 379

significantly over the 18-year period 1970-87, but only from 0.2 to 0.4 per 100 000 per year. Incidence rates among Maoris in New Zealand are higher than in other non-Caucasian populations in Asia, around 5 per 100 000, and have also increased since 1962, but the population is small, and these rates are based on an average of only one case per year. In none of these populations does the risk of melanoma of the skin appear to have increased significantly in the last 10-15 years, in sharp contrast to the trends observed in predominantly Caucasian populations, both around the Pacific Ocean and elsewhere. These differences are largely reflected in the mortality trends. Mortality from melanoma in Japan has increased several-fold in both sexes since 1960, when it was extremely low (0.1 per 100 000), but increases since 1980 have been small.

Incidence rates and trends for malignant melanoma of the skin in both sexes are generally similar among the four Caucasian populations in Asia and Oceania which are included here. Lifetime risks (30-74 years) for the 1940 birth cohort are in the range 3-5%, and rates are increasing rapidly at 15-30% every five years. For non-Maoris in New Zealand, for example, the cumulative risk for

those born around 1940 is some 4% for males and females, and incidence rates have been increasing by about 25% and 14% every five years, respectively. These estimates are based on substantial numbers of cases (200 or more a year in each sex), and the estimated rates of increase are highly significant (more than six standard errors). For the same birth cohorts, the risk of dying from malignant melanoma in the New Zealand population as a whole, which is predominantly non-Maori, is around 0.9% in males and 0.4% in females, increasing by 13% and 8% per five years, respectively. These figures suggest that by the end of the first decade in the next century, at least one in 20 males and one in 25 females will have developed melanoma in this population by the age of 75, and unless the increasing trend begins to decelerate soon, even these figures will seem conservative.

Among Caucasians in Hawaii, the cumulative risks for the cohort born in 1940 are even higher than in New Zealand non-Maoris, and the rates of increase are also higher, at 31% every five years in both sexes. It is likely that the cumulative risks for Hawaii Caucasians are somewhat over-estimated, however, since an age-period model fits the data

400

best, and the age-cohort model used to estimate the cumulative risks is in fact an age-drift model, in which the linear term exaggerates the trend by year of birth.

Americas

Melanoma incidence has been increasing rapidly in both sexes since the late 1960s in each of the five Canadian provinces examined, at about 20-45% every five years; there is still a three-fold range in lifetime risk between British Columbia (2-3%) and Quebec (less than 1%). Melanoma rates are generally lower in the Caribbean than in North America, but incidence in Cuba and Puerto Rico has been increasing as rapidly as in North America in recent years: in Puerto Rico, the recent increases have been 42% every five years for males and 26% for females, and 81% (three standard errors) for females aged 30-44 years. Incidence in São Paulo (Brazil) and Cali (Colombia) is similar to that in Canada, but has not increased significantly since the late 1970s.

The large racial differences in melanoma risk between the various populations in the USA are widening further. Incidence in white or predominantly white populations is high (10-25 per 100 000) and increasing by 20-40% every five years, with lifetime risks for the 1940 birth cohort of around 2-3% in males and 1-2% in females. Incidence in black populations is 10-20 times lower, at around 1 per 100 000, and is generally stable. There is some evidence of deceleration of the rate of increase in most of the white populations in the USA (but not in Canada), particularly among males, for whom rates of increase are generally lower in the younger age groups. Mortality trends reflect these patterns, with the rates for Canada increasing more rapidly than those for the USA. The lifetime risks for the 1940 birth cohort in the two countries are very similar in both sexes, but the indications are that risks in Canada will shortly exceed those in the USA.

Mortality in Central and South America is 3-5 times lower than in North America: while increases have occurred in Chile and Venezuela, there has been no discernible trend in Costa Rica. In Puerto Rico, however, the rapid increase in incidence contrasts sharply with broadly stable mortality rates, and the ratio of incidence and mortality rates is 6- to 8-fold.

Comment

Increasing trends in incidence and mortality from malignant melanoma of the skin have been reported previously from many areas of the world[278], including Denmark[214-216], Sweden[284,285], the Nordic countries as a group[116], England and Wales[213], Scotland[173], Singapore[153,154], Switzerland[8,160], Japan[200], Canada[107] and the USA[9,44,77,90,110,133,240,261]. The remarkable changes in risk are clearly real; a meticulous review of several thousand pathological specimens from skin lesions diagnosed in nine countries around 1930, 1955 and 1980 has identified a tendency for increasing uniformity of diagnosis with the passage of time, and it strongly suggests that little (if any) of the observed increase in the incidence of malignant melanoma of the skin could be due to changes in diagnostic criteria for the classification of malignancy in pigmented skin lesions[290]. The data presented here extend these observations and enable quantitative comparison of the trends.

There has been a deceleration, or levelling off, of the rate of increase in melanoma risk among recent birth cohorts, especially in males, in several populations. Deceleration of rising cohort incidence trends is seen for predominantly Caucasian populations across the USA, in the San Francisco Bay Area, Iowa, Detroit and Connecticut, as well as in New South Wales (Australia), Sweden, Denmark and Geneva (Switzerland). A plateau or deceleration of increasing mortality trends can also be seen in the USA (more than in Canada) and Australia (more than in New Zealand), and in Germany, Switzerland, Italy and the Nordic countries. The marked flattening of the increase in incidence and mortality for cohorts born since 1930 in the USA has been noted previously[77,261]. Projection of mortality for the USA suggests that death rates will probably reach a maximum by about 2010, although the numbers of deaths will continue to increase for some decades, due to ageing of the population[261]. A plateau and eventual decline of age-standardised mortality has also been projected for Sweden[285], although the effect was more marked for males than females.

The generality of the increase in incidence and mortality from melanoma is so striking that the exceptions are worthy of comment. In Asia, there were no significant trends in incidence or mortality in any of the Indian, Chinese or Japanese populations, in which melanoma is rare. Similarly, in the black populations of Detroit, New Orleans and the San Francisco Bay Area (USA), melanoma remains extremely uncommon, and there has been virtually no change in incidence.

Mortality has increased less rapidly than incidence in most populations. This discrepancy is most notable for Finland, where mortality is stable while incidence continues to increase rapidly. The considerable recent increase in incidence of 31% per five years in males is not reflec-

continued page 410

MELANOMA OF SKIN (ICD-9 172)

AMERICAS (except USA), INCIDENCE

MALES	Best model	Goodness of fit	1970 Rate	1970 Cases	1985 Rate	1985 Cases	Cumulative risk 1915	Cumulative risk 1940	Recent trend
BRAZIL									
Sao Paulo	A1D	1.51	3.4	25	*7.9*	*74*	2.0	*8.1*	–
CANADA									
Alberta	A1C3	0.92	4.7	14	11.7	56	3.1	18.0	38.6
British Columbia	A1D	-0.95	5.8	26	18.0	127	4.9	31.8	47.2
Maritime Provinces	A1D	-0.28	3.2	9	11.1	39	2.9	22.3	47.9
Newfoundland	A1D	-0.06	2.9	2	6.3	7	2.2	8.0	37.7
Quebec	A1P3	1.40	2.1	23	5.9	88	1.9	7.4	32.2
COLOMBIA									
Cali	A3C5	0.70	4.0	3	4.6	6	2.3	4.4	*-2.0*
CUBA	A1D	0.57	0.8	12	2.1	42	0.8	*3.8*	–
PUERTO RICO	A1P2	-0.52	1.4	6	3.0	20	1.2	3.5	42.3

FEMALES	Best model	Goodness of fit	1970 Rate	1970 Cases	1985 Rate	1985 Cases	Cumulative risk 1915	Cumulative risk 1940	Recent trend
BRAZIL									
Sao Paulo	A1D	0.22	3.1	26	*10.8*	*123*	2.0	*16.0*	–
CANADA									
Alberta	A1P3	0.36	5.3	16	12.3	61	3.6	10.5	18.0
British Columbia	A1P3	1.72	9.8	44	20.4	149	4.7	20.4	37.9
Maritime Provinces	A1D	0.14	5.1	15	12.8	47	3.2	14.6	29.8
Newfoundland	A0C3	1.01	3.1	2	7.8	9	1.4	8.7	43.5
Quebec	A1C3	1.96	2.9	36	5.5	90	1.6	5.4	32.9
COLOMBIA									
Cali	A1	1.12	3.8	3	3.8	7	2.0	2.0	*11.5*
CUBA	A1D	0.62	0.6	8	1.6	33	0.6	*3.3*	–
PUERTO RICO	A1D	2.31	1.5	6	2.1	16	0.9	1.6	25.7

* : not enough cases for reliable estimation
– : incomplete or missing data
Best model: polynomial of the given degree in age (A), period (P) or cohort (C), or linear drift (D) model.
Goodness of fit: the normalised likelihood ratio chi-square for the best model (see Method).
Rate: world-standardised truncated rate per 100 000 per year (30-74 years) and number of **cases** are both estimated from the best-fitting model for the single years cited.
Cumulative risk per 1000 (30-74 years) is estimated from the best-fitting *age-cohort* model for cohorts of central birth year cited.
Recent trend: estimated mean percentage change per five-year period in the age-specific rates (30-74 years) over the period 1973-1987.
Italics denote recent trends not significant at 5 per cent level, or other figures which should be interpreted with caution (see Method).

MELANOMA OF SKIN (ICD-9 172)

AMERICAS (except USA), INCIDENCE

MALES

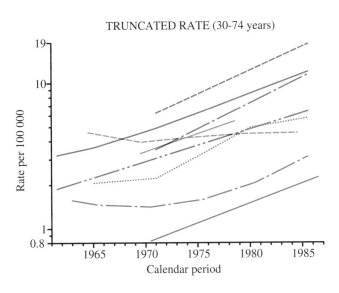

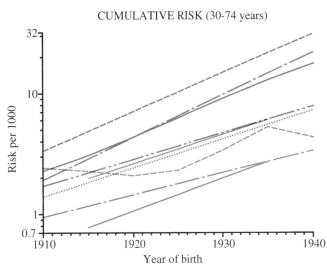

FEMALES

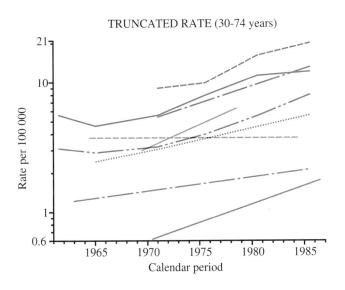

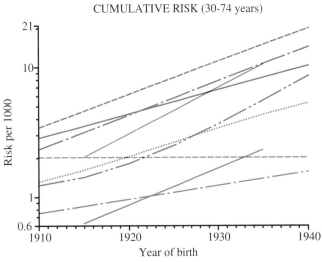

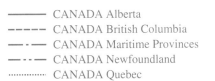

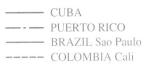

———— CANADA Alberta
– – – – CANADA British Columbia
–·–·– CANADA Maritime Provinces
–··–··– CANADA Newfoundland
·············· CANADA Quebec

———— CUBA
–·–·– PUERTO RICO
———— BRAZIL Sao Paulo
– – – – COLOMBIA Cali

AMERICAS (USA), INCIDENCE

MALES	Best model	Goodness of fit	1970 Rate	1970 Cases	1985 Rate	1985 Cases	Cumulative risk 1915	Cumulative risk 1940	Recent trend
USA									
Bay Area, Black	A1	-0.09	*1.0*	*0*	*1.0*	*0*	0.6	0.6	*-49.4*
Bay Area, Chinese	–	–	–	–	–	–	–	–	–
Bay Area, White	A1C2	0.62	10.9	64	26.1	165	7.9	30.9	26.0
Connecticut	A2C4	-0.32	9.1	59	19.7	152	6.9	20.3	24.1
Detroit, Black	A1	-0.19	0.8	1	0.8	1	0.5	0.5	*-38.3*
Detroit, White	A4P2C2	0.17	4.8	35	18.2	126	5.3	34.0	42.4
Iowa	A1C2	-0.02	6.2	37	15.9	103	4.5	20.4	33.4
New Orleans, Black	A1	-0.92	*1.8*	*0*	1.8	1	1.2	1.2	*-18.8*
New Orleans, White	A1P2	-1.39	*54.9*	*79*	12.9	20	5.9	8.6	*8.3*
Seattle	A2C2	1.90	*9.2*	*41*	21.4	144	6.3	23.8	30.3

FEMALES	Best model	Goodness of fit	1970 Rate	1970 Cases	1985 Rate	1985 Cases	Cumulative risk 1915	Cumulative risk 1940	Recent trend
USA									
Bay Area, Black	A3C3	-1.15	*0.6*	*0*	1.1	1	0.9	3.4	*49.8*
Bay Area, Chinese	–	–	–	–	–	–	–	–	–
Bay Area, White	A2D	1.64	11.2	70	20.9	138	5.2	14.5	19.5
Connecticut	A2P3C5	0.57	7.4	52	15.6	130	4.0	14.1	23.5
Detroit, Black	A1	0.96	1.0	1	1.0	2	0.5	0.5	*-27.6*
Detroit, White	A2P3	1.51	6.2	49	14.6	110	3.1	15.3	40.4
Iowa	A3P2	0.25	4.5	29	13.3	93	3.5	14.4	24.7
New Orleans, Black	A0	-0.66	*0.7*	*0*	*0.7*	*0*	0.3	0.3	*-2.7*
New Orleans, White	A0C2	-1.66	*7.5*	*12*	9.8	16	3.5	5.5	*8.2*
Seattle	A2D	1.52	*9.8*	*46*	16.9	119	4.8	11.9	20.1

* : not enough cases for reliable estimation
– : incomplete or missing data
Best model: polynomial of the given degree in age (A), period (P) or cohort (C), or linear drift (D) model.
Goodness of fit: the normalised likelihood ratio chi-square for the best model (see Method).
Rate: world-standardised truncated rate per 100 000 per year (30-74 years) and number of **cases** are both estimated from the best-fitting model for the single years cited.
Cumulative risk per 1000 (30-74 years) is estimated from the best-fitting *age-cohort* model for cohorts of central birth year cited.
Recent trend: estimated mean percentage change per five-year period in the age-specific rates (30-74 years) over the period 1973-1987.
Italics denote recent trends not significant at 5 per cent level, or other figures which should be interpreted with caution (see Method).

MELANOMA OF SKIN (ICD-9 172)

AMERICAS (USA), INCIDENCE

MALES

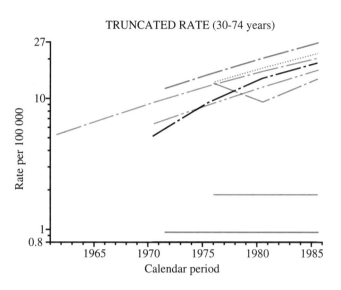
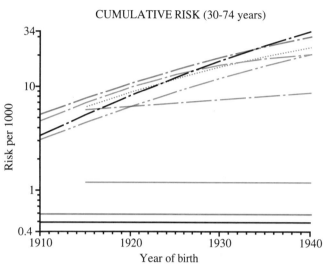

FEMALES

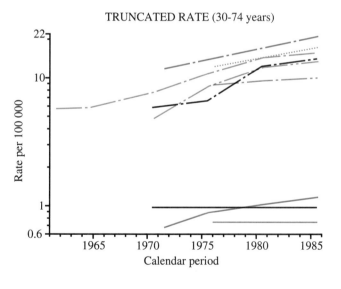
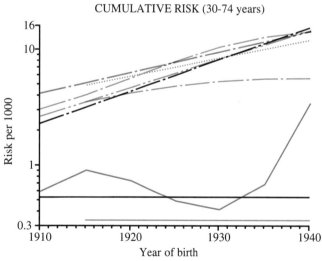

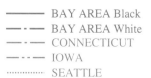

———— BAY AREA Black	———— NEW ORLEANS Black
—·—·— BAY AREA White	—·—·— NEW ORLEANS White
—··—··— CONNECTICUT	———— DETROIT Black
—···—··· IOWA	—··—··— DETROIT White
············ SEATTLE	

MELANOMA OF SKIN (ICD-9 172)

AMERICAS (except USA), INCIDENCE
Percentage change per five-year period, 1973-1987

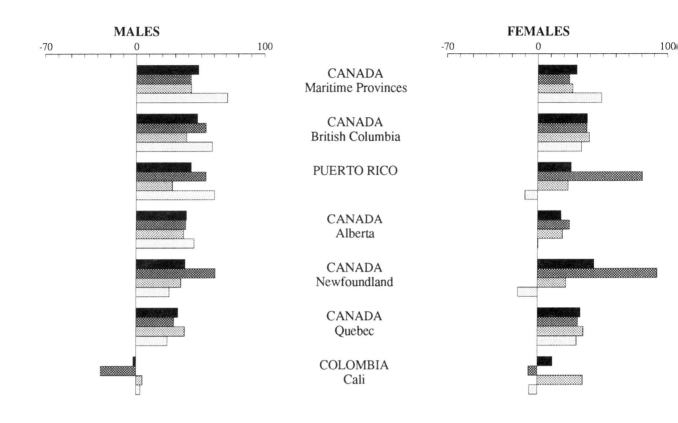

MELANOMA OF SKIN (ICD-9 172)

AMERICAS (USA), INCIDENCE
Percentage change per five-year period, 1973-1987

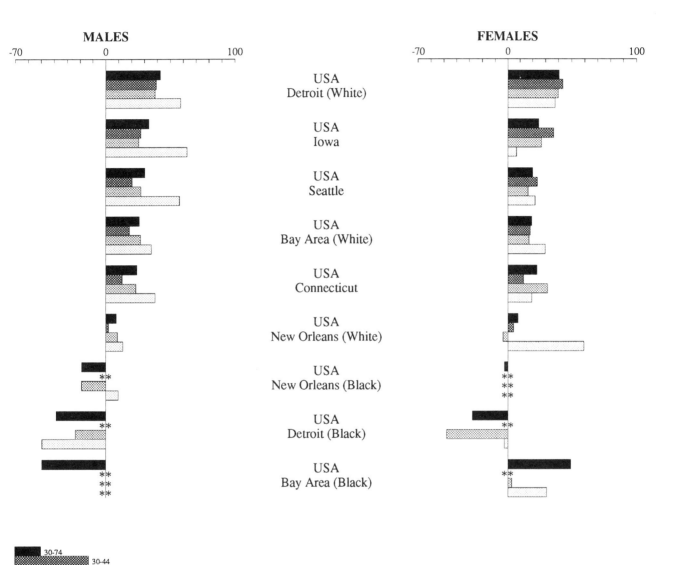

MALES

FEMALES

-70   0   100

USA
Detroit (White)

USA
Iowa

USA
Seattle

USA
Bay Area (White)

USA
Connecticut

USA
New Orleans (White)

USA
New Orleans (Black)

USA
Detroit (Black)

USA
Bay Area (Black)

30-74
30-44
45-64
65-74

MELANOMA OF SKIN (ICD-9 172)

AMERICAS, MORTALITY

MALES	Best model	Goodness of fit	1965 Rate	1965 Deaths	1985 Rate	1985 Deaths	Cumulative risk 1900	Cumulative risk 1940	Recent trend
CANADA	A2C3	-0.60	1.7	67	3.3	187	0.7	2.8	17.9
CHILE	A2P2	0.74	0.8	9	1.2	23	0.3	*1.1*	–
COSTA RICA	A1	-0.39	1.1	1	1.1	3	*0.7*	*0.7*	–
PANAMA	–	–	–	–	–	–	–	–	–
PUERTO RICO	A1	0.60	0.6	2	0.6	3	*0.3*	*0.3*	–
URUGUAY	A1	0.99	*1.2*	*7*	1.2	8	*0.7*	*0.7*	–
USA	A3P6C5	2.97	2.9	1193	4.5	2465	1.2	3.5	9.2
VENEZUELA	A1D	1.41	0.5	4	*0.7*	*12*	0.3	*0.7*	–

FEMALES	Best model	Goodness of fit	1965 Rate	1965 Deaths	1985 Rate	1985 Deaths	Cumulative risk 1900	Cumulative risk 1940	Recent trend
CANADA	A3P2	0.06	1.4	57	2.1	133	0.6	1.5	9.9
CHILE	A1P3	1.93	0.6	7	1.1	22	0.3	*1.3*	–
COSTA RICA	A1	0.35	*0.5*	*0*	0.5	1	*0.3*	*0.3*	–
PANAMA	–	–	–	–	–	–	–	–	–
PUERTO RICO	A1D	1.29	0.5	1	0.4	2	*0.3*	*0.2*	–
URUGUAY	A1	0.19	*0.7*	*4*	0.7	5	*0.4*	*0.4*	–
USA	A3P2C5	0.75	1.9	897	2.5	1519	0.9	1.6	2.6
VENEZUELA	A2P2	0.22	0.6	5	*0.3*	*5*	0.2	*0.4*	–

* : not enough deaths for reliable estimation
– : incomplete or missing data
Best model: polynomial of the given degree in age (A), period (P) or cohort (C), or linear drift (D) model.
Goodness of fit: the normalised likelihood ratio chi-square for the best model (see Method).
Rate: world-standardised truncated rate per 100 000 per year (30-74 years) and number of **deaths** are both estimated from the best-fitting model for the single years cited.
Cumulative risk per 1000 (30-74 years) is estimated from the best-fitting *age-cohort* model for cohorts of central birth year cited.
Recent trend: estimated mean percentage change per five-year period in the age-specific rates (30-74 years) over the period 1975-1988.
Italics denote recent trends not significant at 5 per cent level, or other figures which should be interpreted with caution (see Method).

MELANOMA OF SKIN (ICD-9 172)

AMERICAS, MORTALITY

MALES

TRUNCATED RATE (30-74 years)

CUMULATIVE RISK (30-74 years)

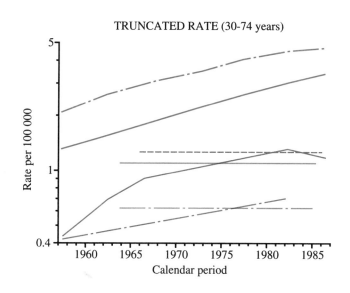
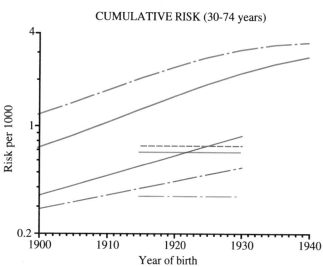

FEMALES

TRUNCATED RATE (30-74 years)

CUMULATIVE RISK (30-74 years)

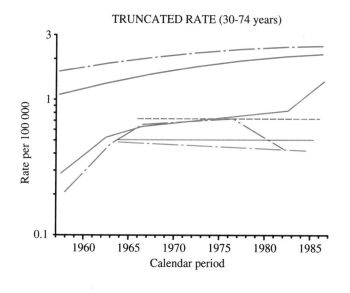
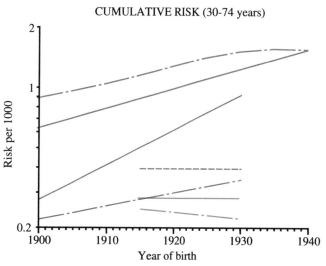

——— CANADA	——— CHILE
—·—· USA	– – – URUGUAY
——— COSTA RICA	—··— VENEZUELA
—·—· PUERTO RICO	

MELANOMA OF SKIN (ICD-9 172)

AMERICAS, MORTALITY
Percentage change per five-year period, 1975-1988

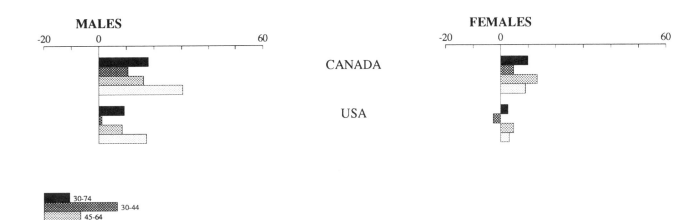

from page 401

ted at all in mortality, which appears to have reached a plateau: none of the age-specific trends nor the small overall rate of increase (1% every five years) is significant. Better survival for females and improvements in survival over time in both sexes[26,27,46,283,285] account for at least part of the divergence in incidence and mortality trends. In Sweden, for example, the hazard of death within 5 years of diagnosis fell by about 70% between 1960-64 and 1975-79: the improvement was larger and began earlier in females[283]. Greater awareness of the disease[44,283,284] and earlier diagnosis, reflected in an increase in the percentage of lesions less than 1.5mm in thickness[173,290], are probably responsible for much of this improvement.

More detailed analyses of trends in the incidence of malignant melanoma of the skin in different regions of the body have been carried out in Denmark[214,216], Sweden[284], Scotland[173], Canada[107] and the USA[90,261]. These studies have shown marked increases in melanoma of the skin of the trunk, particularly in males, and increases in melanoma of the leg and arm, particularly in females. The study of Connecticut data[90] covering the 50 years 1935-84 showed a 12- to 16-fold increase in melanoma of the skin of the upper arm and forearm in both sexes, but much smaller increases in melanoma of the hand. These variations in trend patterns for different regions of the skin in males and females can best be interpreted as being due to the local effects on the skin of different trends between the sexes in environmental exposure. Greater health awareness among women than men was also invoked to explain the difference in incidence trends between the sexes in Sweden[284].

Malignant melanoma remains relatively infrequent in most parts of the world, despite these increases, but in many populations it is now among the ten most frequent malignancies, especially for females. The causes of the widespread increase in melanoma remain uncertain. Use of oral contraceptives seems unlikely to increase the risk[121]. The role of exposure to ultra-violet light, particularly UV-B (280-320nm wavelength), has been of central interest[106]. In Spain, for example, melanoma mortality by province during the period 1975-83 was significantly correlated with solar radiation intensity during July and August but not with the mean annual intensity[191]. If depletion of the ozone layer since the 1980s and any consequent increase in exposure to UV-B is indeed a significant factor in melanoma incidence, which is not yet clear[261,272,278], it will be of considerable interest to know if the deceleration in the rate of increase in melanoma risk, seen in several countries for more recent birth cohorts, will in fact continue. If it does, this would suggest either that the nature of individuals' exposure to UV-B irradiation is changing so as to pose less of a hazard, and/or that some other protective factor is operating to reduce lifetime risk of melanoma, counterbalancing any effect of increased exposure to ultra-violet radiation.

410

Chapter 17

BREAST (FEMALES)

Cancer of the breast is the most frequent tumour in females world-wide. While cervix cancer is more frequent in some developing countries, breast cancer is often the commonest tumour by a wide margin in developed countries. The relative frequency of breast cancer among females varies widely from place to place, and is changing with time. In some regions of the world, where the prevalence of smoking among females has been high, lung cancer incidence is approaching that of breast cancer, or has overtaken it already, as in Glasgow (Scotland)[109]. Further, since survival from breast cancer is considerably higher, lung cancer mortality already exceeds mortality from breast cancer in several places. Wide geographical variation is observed for both incidence and mortality, but these two indices of breast cancer frequency do not rank the various countries in the same order, and consequently there is wide variability of the ratio of mortality to incidence. The populations at highest risk for breast cancer incidence are found in western Europe and in North America, and those at lowest risk in Asia. The highest risk is more than five-fold greater than the lowest. Even within western Europe, there is almost a two-fold difference between the highest incidence rate, seen in Geneva (Switzerland), and the lowest, in Spain. A similar range is seen in North America between white females in the San Francisco Bay Area (USA) and those in Newfoundland (Canada).

Several factors have been identified as potentially responsible for increasing breast cancer risk, but their mechanism of action is unclear. Early menarche, late first pregnancy, low parity and late menopause have all been associated with an increased risk of breast cancer in several studies[98,124,170], suggesting strongly that reproductive history plays a role as a determinant of the risk of this disease. The increase in risk has been attributed to the pattern of exposure to oestrogens, a notion which is supported by the protective effect of oophorectomy. Oral contraceptive use has been suspected of increasing the risk of breast cancer, especially after long-term use before age 25 or before the first pregnancy, but the evidence is still limited[281]. The interplay of hormonal factors is still difficult to assess from epidemiological data. Migrant studies have shown that the risk of the country of adoption is reached in several generations, a longer time than for colorectal cancer, sug-

gesting that events occurring in childhood may play a more important role for breast cancer than for colorectal cancer. The role of dietary factors has been carefully investigated in several ecological and case-control studies, and these suggest that diet, by influencing the pattern of oestrogen exposure, may also be an important determinant of the risk. Further, the risk of breast cancer is positively associated with socio-economic status, and it is difficult to assess the specific role of each of the potential risk factors, given their strong inter-correlation and the difficulty in adjusting for confounding. The well identified role of genetic predisposition and ionising radiation should also be noted, although these factors have little relevance in the interpretation of time trends.

Several other features of breast cancer epidemiology are relevant. Firstly, the cross-sectional age-incidence curve shows a change in the slope after age 45 years, which is usually the combined result of a real change in the age effect and of a birth cohort effect. Secondly, mass screening programmes have been implemented in several countries, and these have further modified the age curve by bringing forward the date of diagnosis of some tumours. Thirdly, the active search for breast tumours in most developed countries has increased the proportion of the less aggressive forms of the disease, leading to an artefactual increase in incidence[88], and to some uncertainty about the size of the improvement in survival. These factors make it difficult to describe time trends in incidence with simple age-period-cohort models, and it was expected that the combined interpretation of incidence and mortality trends would be far more complex than for other cancers.

Europe

The truncated incidence rate (30-74 years) has increased steadily everywhere in Europe over the period of the study, with the exception of Geneva (Switzerland) and Saarland (FRG). In Geneva, where the highest European rate was recorded, there has been a significant decrease in younger and middle-aged women, well described by an age-cohort model predicting a lower risk for the younger generations. Part of this decrease, however, may be explained by over-estimation of the rates around 1975 and 1980 because of under-estimation of the population by the Federal Office of

411

continued page 425

BREAST (ICD-9 174)

EUROPE (non-EC), INCIDENCE

FEMALES	Best model	Goodness of fit	1970 Rate	1970 Cases	1985 Rate	1985 Cases	Cumulative risk 1915	Cumulative risk 1940	Recent trend
FINLAND	A8D	0.83	74.0	926	113.1	1577	43.0	85.3	13.4
HUNGARY									
County Vas	A8D	0.73	55.4	45	92.7	76	33.4	77.2	26.9
Szabolcs-Szatmar	A7P2	1.75	40.2	58	61.7	96	21.9	39.6	20.1
ISRAEL									
All Jews	A8P2C4	3.69	117.1	584	136.9	905	63.2	83.0	4.0
Non-Jews	A3D	0.37	21.2	9	36.5	30	10.9	26.8	23.7
NORWAY	A7C4	2.21	94.6	1025	115.6	1316	51.9	67.9	4.6
POLAND									
Warsaw City	A3P3	3.05	65.7	264	77.8	393	36.4	45.5	*3.2*
ROMANIA									
Cluj	A3C2	1.79	*72.6*	*129*	67.9	133	31.3	38.8	*2.7*
SWEDEN	A8P5C9	1.82	111.4	2656	133.2	3337	60.5	76.3	6.2
SWITZERLAND									
Geneva	A6C2	-0.38	148.9	138	152.3	167	78.5	74.2	*-1.3*
YUGOSLAVIA									
Slovenia	A3P3C3	4.83	61.3	278	87.1	466	34.0	61.4	9.2

* : not enough cases for reliable estimation
– : incomplete or missing data
Best model: polynomial of the given degree in age (A), period (P) or cohort (C), or linear drift (D) model.
Goodness of fit: the normalised likelihood ratio chi-square for the best model (see Method).
Rate: world-standardised truncated rate per 100 000 per year (30-74 years) and number of **cases** are both estimated from the best-fitting model for the single years cited.
Cumulative risk per 1000 (30-74 years) is estimated from the best-fitting *age-cohort* model for cohorts of central birth year cited.
Recent trend: estimated mean percentage change per five-year period in the age-specific rates (30-74 years) over the period 1973-1987.
Italics denote recent trends not significant at 5 per cent level, or other figures which should be interpreted with caution (see Method).

FEMALES

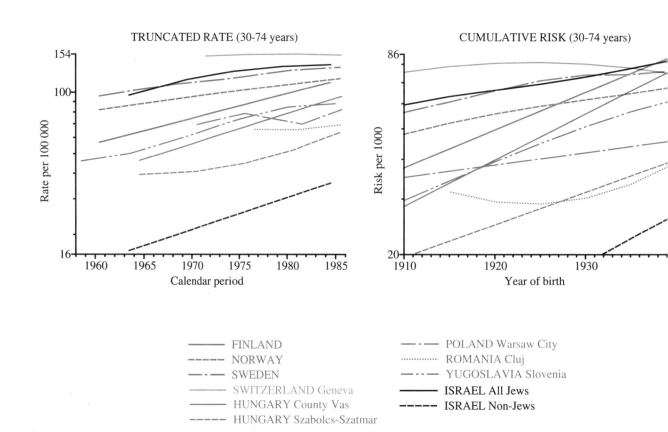

TRUNCATED RATE (30-74 years)

CUMULATIVE RISK (30-74 years)

——— FINLAND
----- NORWAY
—·— SWEDEN
——— SWITZERLAND Geneva
——— HUNGARY County Vas
----- HUNGARY Szabolcs-Szatmar
—·—· POLAND Warsaw City
·········· ROMANIA Cluj
—··— YUGOSLAVIA Slovenia
——— ISRAEL All Jews
----- ISRAEL Non-Jews

BREAST (ICD-9 174)

EUROPE (non-EC), INCIDENCE
Percentage change per five-year period, 1973-1987

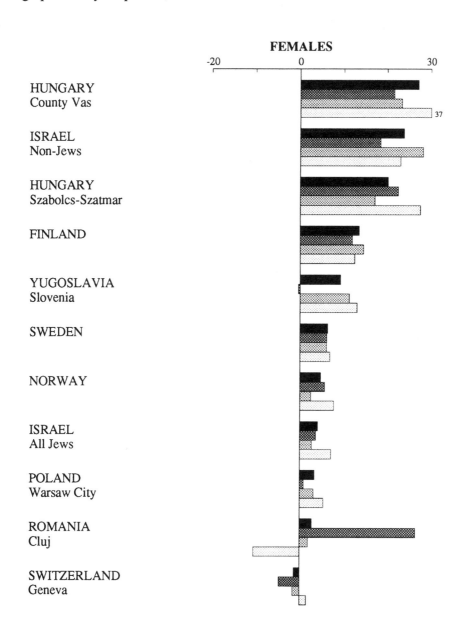

FEMALES

HUNGARY
County Vas

ISRAEL
Non-Jews

HUNGARY
Szabolcs-Szatmar

FINLAND

YUGOSLAVIA
Slovenia

SWEDEN

NORWAY

ISRAEL
All Jews

POLAND
Warsaw City

ROMANIA
Cluj

SWITZERLAND
Geneva

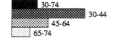

30-74
30-44
45-64
65-74

BREAST (ICD-9 174)

EUROPE (EC), INCIDENCE

FEMALES	Best model	Goodness of fit	1970 Rate	1970 Cases	1985 Rate	1985 Cases	Cumulative risk 1915	Cumulative risk 1940	Recent trend
DENMARK	A8P4C5	0.33	112.6	1522	145.8	2075	59.0	94.0	9.1
FRANCE									
Bas-Rhin	A8C7	-0.13	*152.3*	*510*	142.1	330	65.9	94.5	9.9
Doubs	A4	-0.02	*119.8*	*104*	119.8	137	58.7	58.7	*5.7*
GERMANY (FRG)									
Hamburg	A7D	1.38	101.1	643	*154.6*	*772*	56.6	*111.6*	–
Saarland	A3P2	3.36	106.1	366	120.5	411	57.2	67.8	*-0.7*
GERMANY (GDR)	A8C9	6.54	71.0	4034	99.3	4999	41.9	72.3	12.1
ITALY									
Varese	A3D	0.92	*108.7*	*187*	137.8	326	58.5	85.6	8.2
SPAIN									
Navarra	A3D	2.62	*70.7*	*86*	96.5	132	37.9	62.8	10.9
Zaragoza	A3P3C4	1.37	62.4	127	89.8	214	35.5	48.6	*5.1*
UK									
Birmingham	A8P5C4	1.43	113.5	1597	133.2	1935	60.2	71.0	5.6
Scotland	A8P4C5	2.27	102.3	1533	132.1	1916	56.0	83.9	5.0
South Thames	A8P5C9	8.20	104.3	2815	119.6	2316	57.7	67.2	2.8

* : not enough cases for reliable estimation
– : incomplete or missing data
Best model: polynomial of the given degree in age (A), period (P) or cohort (C), or linear drift (D) model.
Goodness of fit: the normalised likelihood ratio chi-square for the best model (see Method).
Rate: world-standardised truncated rate per 100 000 per year (30-74 years) and number of **cases** are both estimated from the best-fitting model for the single years cited.
Cumulative risk per 1000 (30-74 years) is estimated from the best-fitting *age-cohort* model for cohorts of central birth year cited.
Recent trend: estimated mean percentage change per five-year period in the age-specific rates (30-74 years) over the period 1973-1987.
Italics denote recent trends not significant at 5 per cent level, or other figures which should be interpreted with caution (see Method).

FEMALES

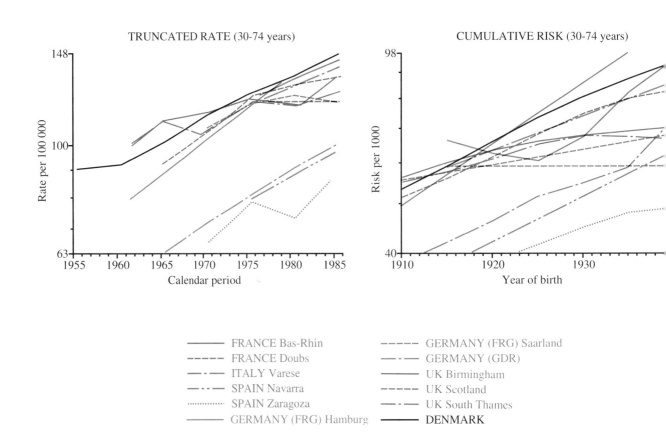

TRUNCATED RATE (30-74 years) — Rate per 100 000 vs Calendar period

CUMULATIVE RISK (30-74 years) — Risk per 1000 vs Year of birth

——— FRANCE Bas-Rhin
------- FRANCE Doubs
—·— ITALY Varese
—··— SPAIN Navarra
············ SPAIN Zaragoza
——— GERMANY (FRG) Hamburg
------- GERMANY (FRG) Saarland
—·— GERMANY (GDR)
——— UK Birmingham
------- UK Scotland
—·— UK South Thames
▬▬▬ DENMARK

BREAST (ICD-9 174)

EUROPE (EC), INCIDENCE
Percentage change per five-year period, 1973-1987

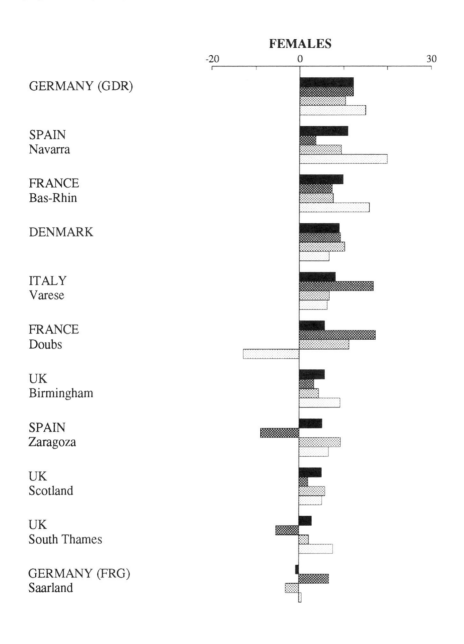

FEMALES

GERMANY (GDR)

SPAIN
Navarra

FRANCE
Bas-Rhin

DENMARK

ITALY
Varese

FRANCE
Doubs

UK
Birmingham

SPAIN
Zaragoza

UK
Scotland

UK
South Thames

GERMANY (FRG)
Saarland

30-74
30-44
45-64
65-74

BREAST (ICD-9 174)

EUROPE (non-EC), MORTALITY

FEMALES	Best model	Goodness of fit	1965 Rate	1965 Deaths	1985 Rate	1985 Deaths	Cumulative risk 1900	Cumulative risk 1940	Recent trend
AUSTRIA	A3P4C4	4.05	34.2	844	42.2	1000	17.3	26.7	7.5
CZECHOSLOVAKIA	A8P3C2	3.36	29.4	1184	39.5	1686	15.1	24.8	4.0
FINLAND	A3C2	-0.77	29.0	351	31.7	461	15.2	17.6	*2.8*
HUNGARY	A3P5C2	3.16	28.1	838	42.0	1382	14.5	31.5	6.2
NORWAY	A4C6	1.12	35.6	385	36.0	440	18.5	18.9	*-1.2*
POLAND	A8P5C9	1.15	21.3	1589	32.0	3018	9.6	23.4	5.2
ROMANIA	A3D	3.53	19.2	905	*27.9*	*1683*	9.1	19.0	–
SWEDEN	A4C6	3.17	38.3	913	36.3	957	20.9	18.6	-2.7
SWITZERLAND	A3C5	-0.36	44.7	738	47.7	920	24.2	25.9	*0.7*
YUGOSLAVIA	A4D	4.13	16.8	720	29.1	1729	7.9	23.3	12.6

* : not enough deaths for reliable estimation
– : incomplete or missing data
Best model: polynomial of the given degree in age (A), period (P) or cohort (C), or linear drift (D) model.
Goodness of fit: the normalised likelihood ratio chi-square for the best model (see Method).
Rate: world-standardised truncated rate per 100 000 per year (30-74 years) and number of **deaths** are both estimated from the best-fitting model for the single years cited.
Cumulative risk per 1000 (30-74 years) is estimated from the best-fitting *age-cohort* model for cohorts of central birth year cited.
Recent trend: estimated mean percentage change per five-year period in the age-specific rates (30-74 years) over the period 1975-1988.
Italics denote recent trends not significant at 5 per cent level, or other figures which should be interpreted with caution (see Method).

FEMALES

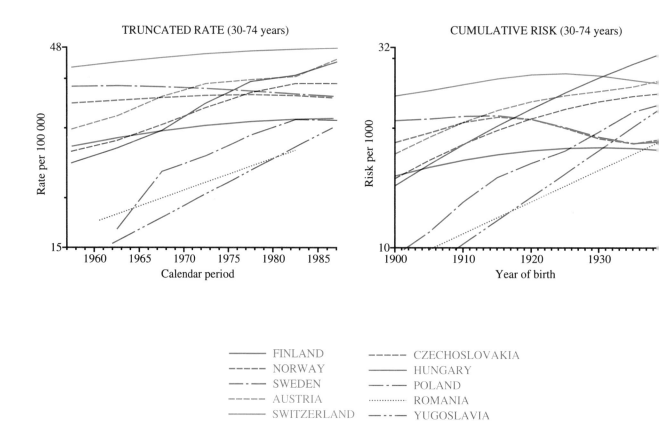

BREAST (ICD-9 174)

EUROPE (non-EC), MORTALITY
Percentage change per five-year period, 1975-1988

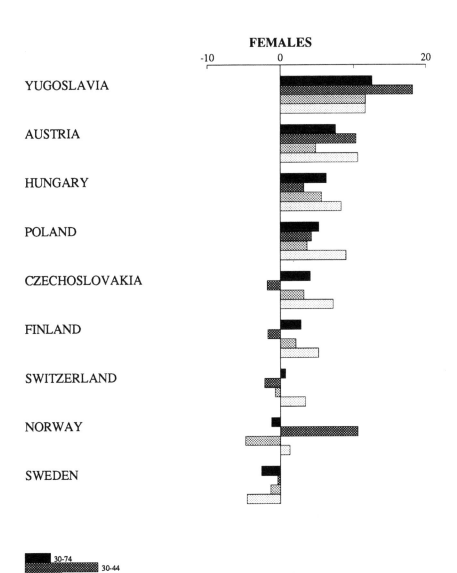

BREAST (ICD-9 174)

EUROPE (EC), MORTALITY

FEMALES	Best model	Goodness of fit	1965 Rate	Deaths	1985 Rate	Deaths	Cumulative risk 1900	1940	Recent trend
BELGIUM	A3P2C6	0.95	43.1	1226	54.8	1599	21.0	33.0	8.8
DENMARK	A4C3	2.54	48.2	655	54.8	819	25.4	32.3	4.6
FRANCE	A4P5C6	7.12	32.8	4639	39.0	5903	17.0	23.7	2.5
GERMANY (FRG)	A3P4C8	11.00	35.9	6987	44.7	8976	17.8	28.4	6.2
GREECE	A3P2C2	0.36	15.8	334	32.3	939	*7.0*	27.1	8.1
IRELAND	A3C3	1.12	45.7	320	55.7	431	22.2	32.3	*1.7*
ITALY	A3P6C9	8.50	32.6	4570	42.1	7255	15.8	24.8	5.9
NETHERLANDS	A4P5C6	2.82	50.9	1528	52.2	1999	25.5	27.5	*1.3*
PORTUGAL	A3C3	0.60	24.7	551	33.7	938	11.8	22.2	10.0
SPAIN	A3P5C6	1.29	18.9	1528	30.8	3186	8.0	26.3	8.6
UK ENGLAND & WALES	A8P3C4	7.25	50.7	7480	59.0	8746	25.4	33.5	2.6
UK SCOTLAND	A3C3	1.40	49.5	771	57.5	875	24.8	32.9	*2.1*

* : not enough deaths for reliable estimation
– : incomplete or missing data
Best model: polynomial of the given degree in age (A), period (P) or cohort (C), or linear drift (D) model.
Goodness of fit: the normalised likelihood ratio chi-square for the best model (see Method).
Rate: world-standardised truncated rate per 100 000 per year (30-74 years) and number of **deaths** are both estimated from the best-fitting model for the single years cited.
Cumulative risk per 1000 (30-74 years) is estimated from the best-fitting *age-cohort* model for cohorts of central birth year cited.
Recent trend: estimated mean percentage change per five-year period in the age-specific rates (30-74 years) over the period 1975-1988.
Italics denote recent trends not significant at 5 per cent level, or other figures which should be interpreted with caution (see Method).

FEMALES

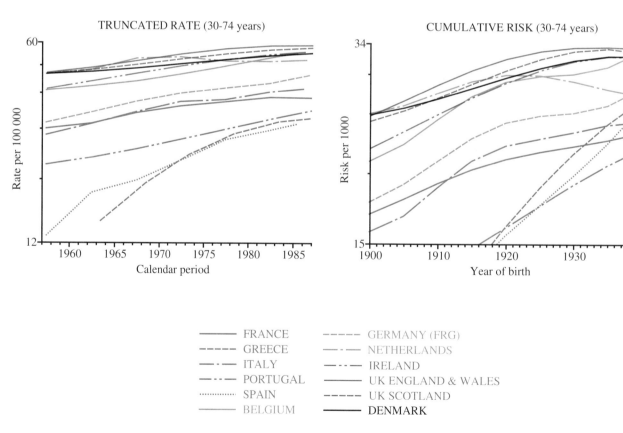

TRUNCATED RATE (30-74 years)

CUMULATIVE RISK (30-74 years)

—— FRANCE	----- GERMANY (FRG)
----- GREECE	—·— NETHERLANDS
—·— ITALY	—··— IRELAND
—··— PORTUGAL	—— UK ENGLAND & WALES
·········· SPAIN	----- UK SCOTLAND
—— BELGIUM	—— DENMARK

BREAST (ICD-9 174)

EUROPE (EC), MORTALITY
Percentage change per five-year period, 1975-1988

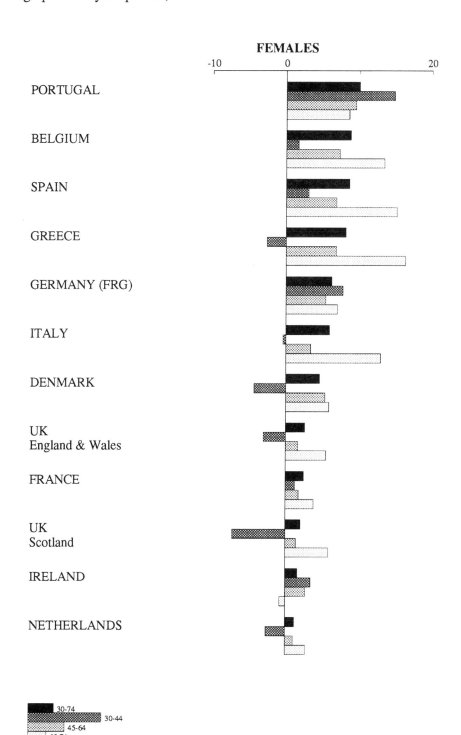

BREAST (ICD-9 174)

ASIA, INCIDENCE

FEMALES	Best model	Goodness of fit	1970 Rate	1970 Cases	1985 Rate	1985 Cases	Cumulative risk 1915	Cumulative risk 1940	Recent trend
CHINA									
Shanghai	A8C2	1.99	*37.8*	*467*	43.3	714	17.7	23.6	5.9
HONG KONG	A8P2C7	-0.45	*84.7*	*585*	66.2	726	33.5	38.3	*2.2*
INDIA									
Bombay	A3P2	1.73	41.1	232	51.3	542	21.6	30.3	10.3
JAPAN									
Miyagi	A7P3C3	1.44	27.8	118	61.2	361	16.3	43.0	26.4
Nagasaki	A3P2	1.28	*81.1*	*84*	53.1	67	19.4	28.8	*8.2*
Osaka	A4P3C3	2.36	26.9	407	48.8	1134	13.5	43.2	29.9
SINGAPORE									
Chinese	A4C4	-0.07	40.4	96	66.2	248	21.6	52.4	21.2
Indian	A2D	-1.52	46.3	4	69.8	15	28.0	54.7	*11.7*
Malay	A2D	-0.18	31.8	10	48.7	26	16.4	33.0	24.6

* : not enough cases for reliable estimation
− : incomplete or missing data
Best model: polynomial of the given degree in age (A), period (P) or cohort (C), or linear drift (D) model.
Goodness of fit: the normalised likelihood ratio chi-square for the best model (see Method).
Rate: world-standardised truncated rate per 100 000 per year (30-74 years) and number of **cases** are both estimated from the best-fitting model for the single years cited.
Cumulative risk per 1000 (30-74 years) is estimated from the best-fitting *age-cohort* model for cohorts of central birth year cited.
Recent trend: estimated mean percentage change per five-year period in the age-specific rates (30-74 years) over the period 1973-1987.
Italics denote recent trends not significant at 5 per cent level, or other figures which should be interpreted with caution (see Method).

FEMALES

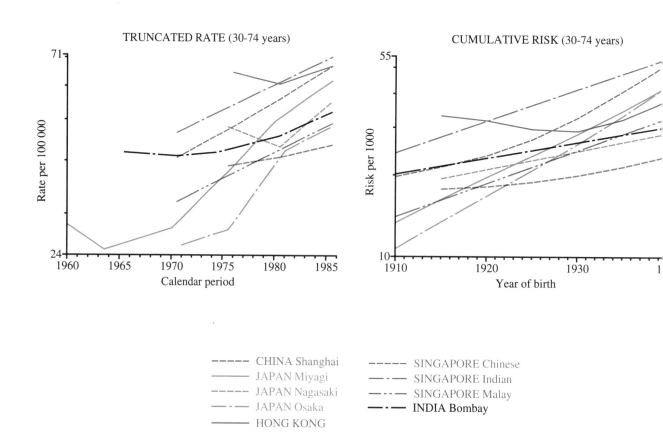

BREAST (ICD-9 174)

ASIA, INCIDENCE
Percentage change per five-year period, 1973-1987

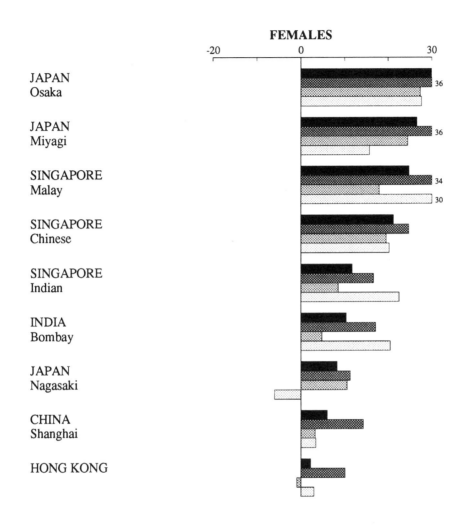

FEMALES

JAPAN
Osaka

JAPAN
Miyagi

SINGAPORE
Malay

SINGAPORE
Chinese

SINGAPORE
Indian

INDIA
Bombay

JAPAN
Nagasaki

CHINA
Shanghai

HONG KONG

30-74
30-44
45-64
65-74

OCEANIA, INCIDENCE

FEMALES	Best model	Goodness of fit	1970 Rate	Cases	1985 Rate	Cases	Cumulative risk 1915	1940	Recent trend
AUSTRALIA									
New South Wales	A6P2C2	3.37	*128.6*	*1441*	125.1	1603	52.6	73.3	6.1
South	A3	-1.08	*116.7*	*264*	116.7	403	58.7	58.7	*3.2*
HAWAII									
Caucasian	A7P3	0.58	177.1	66	204.3	115	86.0	132.4	7.0
Chinese	A3C2	0.68	109.4	10	142.4	22	62.8	82.3	*15.8*
Filipino	A3D	0.01	41.1	4	90.6	24	21.8	79.3	33.2
Hawaiian	A3D	-0.23	142.0	22	206.4	60	88.2	158.1	*8.1*
Japanese	A5P3C3	1.80	94.9	54	134.7	117	51.6	93.5	15.9
NEW ZEALAND									
Maori	A3D	0.83	105.3	23	139.7	54	56.4	88.9	*3.1*
Non-Maori	A7P4C2	2.04	111.7	649	128.0	897	60.0	74.2	*1.2*

* : not enough cases for reliable estimation
– : incomplete or missing data
Best model: polynomial of the given degree in age (A), period (P) or cohort (C), or linear drift (D) model.
Goodness of fit: the normalised likelihood ratio chi-square for the best model (see Method).
Rate: world-standardised truncated rate per 100 000 per year (30-74 years) and number of **cases** are both estimated from the best-fitting model for the single years cited.
Cumulative risk per 1000 (30-74 years) is estimated from the best-fitting *age-cohort* model for cohorts of central birth year cited.
Recent trend: estimated mean percentage change per five-year period in the age-specific rates (30-74 years) over the period 1973-1987.
Italics denote recent trends not significant at 5 per cent level, or other figures which should be interpreted with caution (see Method).

FEMALES

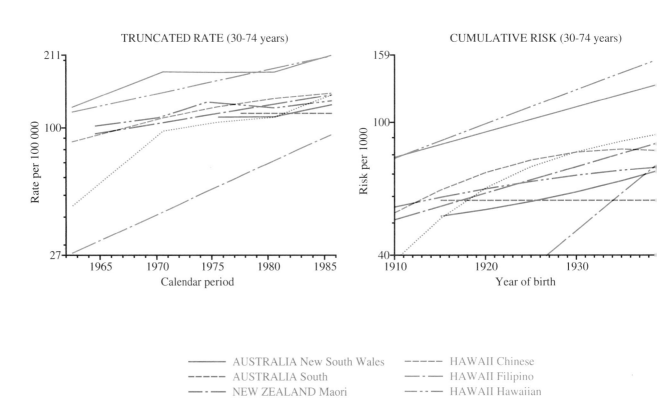

BREAST (ICD-9 174)

OCEANIA, INCIDENCE
Percentage change per five-year period, 1973-1987

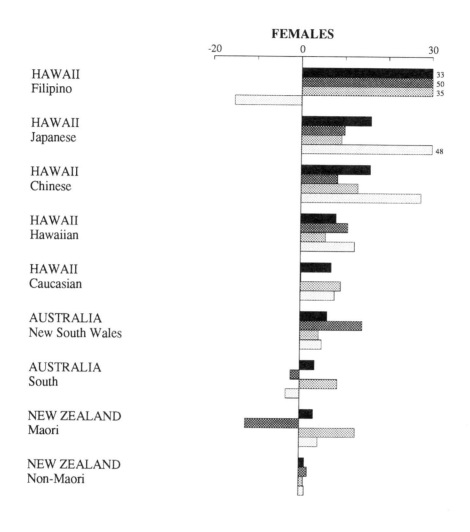

BREAST (ICD-9 174)

ASIA and OCEANIA, MORTALITY

FEMALES	Best model	Goodness of fit	1965 Rate	Deaths	1985 Rate	Deaths	Cumulative risk 1900	1940	Recent trend
AUSTRALIA	A3C4	1.71	38.3	999	40.7	1541	20.1	22.5	3.9
HONG KONG	A8C9	-0.38	18.7	108	17.8	167	9.8	9.1	-5.0
JAPAN	A5P4C6	3.02	8.1	1697	12.6	4239	3.5	7.7	8.8
MAURITIUS	A2D	0.68	8.2	7	15.0	21	3.7	12.3	15.8
NEW ZEALAND	A3D	0.83	46.7	269	53.8	407	24.4	32.2	4.9
SINGAPORE	A2P3	0.87	22.2	46	26.8	100	7.5	13.8	–

* : not enough deaths for reliable estimation
– : incomplete or missing data
Best model: polynomial of the given degree in age (A), period (P) or cohort (C), or linear drift (D) model.
Goodness of fit: the normalised likelihood ratio chi-square for the best model (see Method).
Rate: world-standardised truncated rate per 100 000 per year (30-74 years) and number of **deaths** are both estimated from the best-fitting model for the single years cited.
Cumulative risk per 1000 (30-74 years) is estimated from the best-fitting *age-cohort* model for cohorts of central birth year cited.
Recent trend: estimated mean percentage change per five-year period in the age-specific rates (30-74 years) over the period 1975-1988.
Italics denote recent trends not significant at 5 per cent level, or other figures which should be interpreted with caution (see Method).

FEMALES

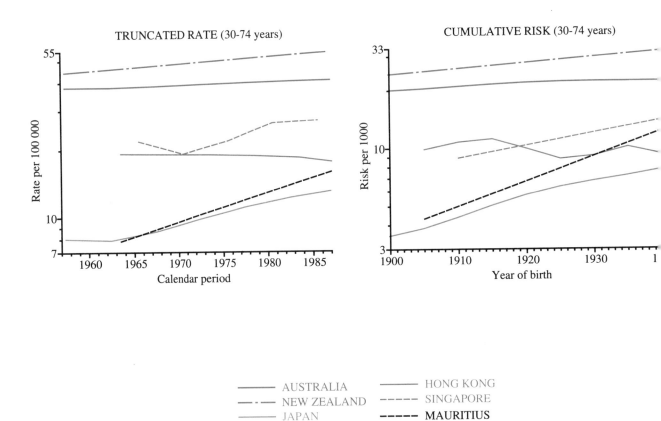

BREAST (ICD-9 174)

ASIA and OCEANIA, MORTALITY
Percentage change per five-year period, 1975-1988

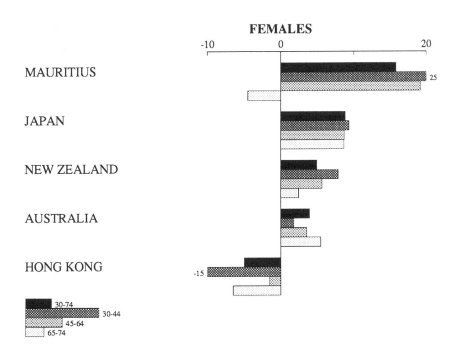

from page 411

Statistics (L. Raymond, personal communication). As a rule, trends in breast cancer incidence are more diverse when examined on a cohort basis: in addition to Switzerland, three populations show a deceleration of the rate of increase in risk — Sweden, Birmingham (UK) and Zaragoza (Spain) — and in South Thames (UK) there is even a decrease. The risk is increasing everywhere else except in Doubs (France), where an unexpected decrease in older women is seen. Strong period effects are seen in Saarland (FRG) and Scotland, where there has been a recent flattening of the increase in truncated rates. In most instances a complicated model is needed to describe the data, and the goodness of fit is often poor.

The trends in mortality are much simpler to interpret and still more diverse than the pattern of change in incidence. The truncated rate has increased everywhere, with the exception of the Netherlands, where cross-sectional mortality has barely changed, and Sweden and Norway, where there has actually been a small decline in more recent periods. The general increase in mortality has been especially steep in eastern Europe and in Spain and Greece. Again, the most interesting results come from the examination of the cumulative risks. In Norway, Sweden, and the Netherlands, there has been a very marked decrease in risk starting with the cohorts born 1915-1920. In Norway and Sweden, however, this decrease in

mortality appears to have stopped with cohorts born since 1935, as shown by the graph of cumulative risk and by the age-specific recent linear trends in younger women. Concomitantly, incidence has been increasing by more than 10% every five years among younger women in Norway, and there is no further decline in Sweden.

Mortality has also decreased cohort-wise in Switzerland, but less sharply than in Norway and Sweden; the trend parallels that for incidence in Geneva. In Denmark, Scotland, England and Wales and Finland, the risk of death has stopped increasing among recent birth cohorts, and the pattern of recent linear trends by age suggests that it may even be decreasing among successive birth cohorts in England and Wales: the estimated risk for the generation born in 1945 is lower than for the generation born in 1940 (data not shown). This trend is more marked for Scotland (3.0% versus 3.3%) where, in addition, a simple age-cohort model gives a good description of the data. The inflection seen in the curve for Germany and Belgium suggests that, after a deceleration around 1920, the risk is again increasing steeply for more recent birth cohorts. In several countries the recent linear trend in breast cancer mortality among younger women is negative, and it is possible that the decreasing risk already clearly seen in some countries will soon be observed; Czechoslovakia is perhaps the best example of this type of evolution.

425

continued page 431

BREAST (ICD-9 174)

AMERICAS (except USA), INCIDENCE

FEMALES	Best model	Goodness of fit	1970 Rate	1970 Cases	1985 Rate	1985 Cases	Cumulative risk 1915	Cumulative risk 1940	Recent trend
BRAZIL									
Sao Paulo	A3D	0.41	95.6	824	*149.1*	*1682*	43.1	*88.2*	–
CANADA									
Alberta	A8P5C9	0.83	118.2	354	135.7	636	69.7	73.1	3.8
British Columbia	A6P2C5	2.44	179.2	843	156.1	1150	87.1	64.1	2.9
Maritime Provinces	A8C8	0.13	124.1	391	134.0	500	65.4	66.7	4.1
Newfoundland	A3C4	3.01	92.8	77	109.1	123	50.9	67.7	*2.7*
Quebec	A6P3C4	2.57	117.6	1433	148.4	2419	70.0	86.0	4.4
COLOMBIA									
Cali	A3D	-1.47	59.4	57	70.7	139	31.8	42.2	*4.5*
CUBA	A3P2	7.52	58.3	788	66.6	1334	31.2	*40.1*	–
PUERTO RICO	A5P2	1.23	51.9	241	80.2	597	29.5	63.2	13.4

* : not enough cases for reliable estimation
– : incomplete or missing data
Best model: polynomial of the given degree in age (A), period (P) or cohort (C), or linear drift (D) model.
Goodness of fit: the normalised likelihood ratio chi-square for the best model (see Method).
Rate: world-standardised truncated rate per 100 000 per year (30-74 years) and number of **cases** are both estimated from the best-fitting model for the single years cited.
Cumulative risk per 1000 (30-74 years) is estimated from the best-fitting *age-cohort* model for cohorts of central birth year cited.
Recent trend: estimated mean percentage change per five-year period in the age-specific rates (30-74 years) over the period 1973-1987.
Italics denote recent trends not significant at 5 per cent level, or other figures which should be interpreted with caution (see Method).

FEMALES

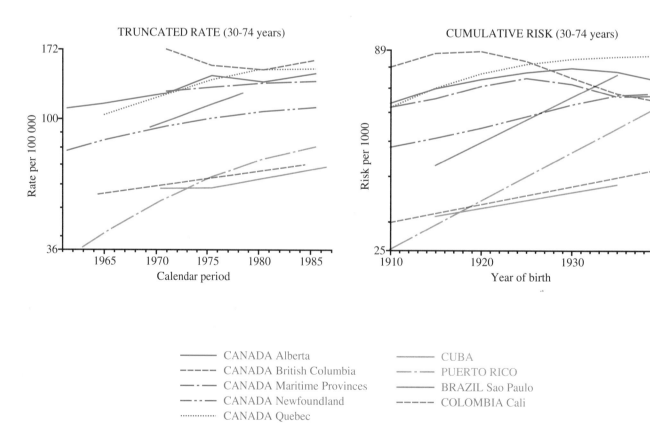

BREAST (ICD-9 174)

AMERICAS (except USA), INCIDENCE
Percentage change per five-year period, 1973-1987

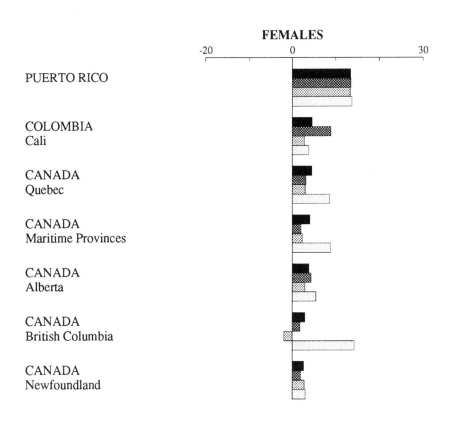

BREAST (ICD-9 174)

AMERICAS (USA), INCIDENCE

FEMALES	Best model	Goodness of fit	1970 Rate	1970 Cases	1985 Rate	1985 Cases	Cumulative risk 1915	Cumulative risk 1940	Recent trend
USA									
Bay Area, Black	A4D	-0.25	112.8	72	165.2	158	63.9	117.5	12.6
Bay Area, Chinese	A4	-0.36	97.8	18	*97.8*	*51*	47.1	*47.1*	–
Bay Area, White	A8P3C8	2.49	167.7	1123	216.1	1451	92.4	124.8	12.7
Connecticut	A8P5C9	0.23	152.8	1133	177.9	1556	82.2	97.9	7.5
Detroit, Black	A3P3C2	1.11	99.9	154	144.7	305	62.4	91.5	7.2
Detroit, White	A6P3C2	2.85	136.9	1121	188.5	1490	79.1	123.4	14.0
Iowa	A7P3C4	1.42	125.7	890	160.0	1183	73.1	96.2	8.4
New Orleans, Black	A3	0.58	*134.8*	*83*	134.8	106	66.7	66.7	*6.7*
New Orleans, White	A3P2	0.56	*176.2*	*321*	164.5	290	69.5	108.4	9.5
Seattle	A4P2C3	1.66	*223.6*	*1123*	192.0	1346	82.3	130.9	13.8

* : not enough cases for reliable estimation
– : incomplete or missing data
Best model: polynomial of the given degree in age (A), period (P) or cohort (C), or linear drift (D) model.
Goodness of fit: the normalised likelihood ratio chi-square for the best model (see Method).
Rate: world-standardised truncated rate per 100 000 per year (30-74 years) and number of **cases** are both estimated from the best-fitting model for the single years cited.
Cumulative risk per 1000 (30-74 years) is estimated from the best-fitting *age-cohort* model for cohorts of central birth year cited.
Recent trend: estimated mean percentage change per five-year period in the age-specific rates (30-74 years) over the period 1973-1987.
Italics denote recent trends not significant at 5 per cent level, or other figures which should be interpreted with caution (see Method).

FEMALES

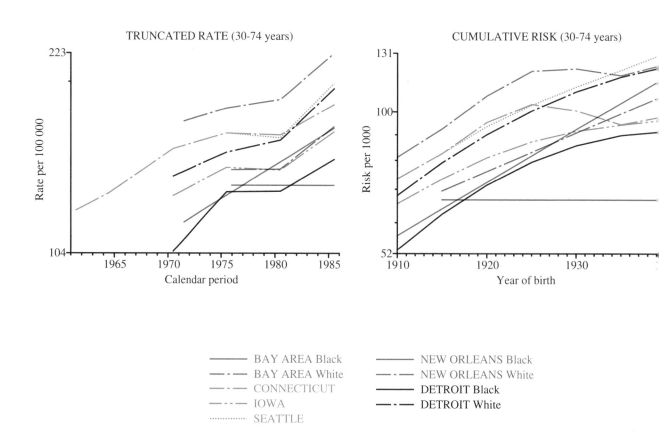

TRUNCATED RATE (30-74 years) — CUMULATIVE RISK (30-74 years)

——— BAY AREA Black ——— NEW ORLEANS Black
—·— BAY AREA White —··— NEW ORLEANS White
—·— CONNECTICUT ——— DETROIT Black
—··— IOWA —·— DETROIT White
·········· SEATTLE

428

BREAST (ICD-9 174)

AMERICAS (USA), INCIDENCE
Percentage change per five-year period, 1973-1987

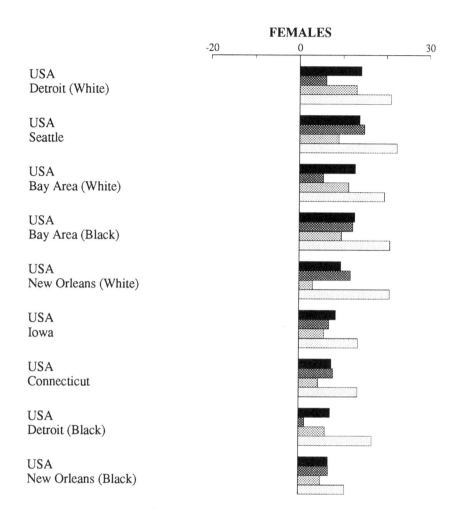

BREAST (ICD-9 174)

AMERICAS, MORTALITY

FEMALES	Best model	Goodness of fit	1965 Rate	1965 Deaths	1985 Rate	1985 Deaths	Cumulative risk 1900	Cumulative risk 1940	Recent trend
CANADA	A3P3C6	1.09	48.5	1917	47.6	2973	24.1	22.4	*1.3*
CHILE	A3P5C2	1.64	20.8	275	25.1	526	10.6	14.2	3.9
COSTA RICA	A3P2	0.74	*16.7*	*24*	22.2	66	*7.5*	15.9	17.1
PANAMA	A3D	2.40	14.0	20	15.6	45	7.2	9.0	–
PUERTO RICO	A3P3	1.54	14.0	59	25.8	156	*7.0*	19.8	14.7
URUGUAY	A3C2	-0.43	46.6	284	51.2	403	24.1	28.1	*3.7*
USA	A8P6C9	11.79	45.1	21107	46.1	28558	23.1	21.9	1.3
VENEZUELA	A3P2	0.80	17.2	171	*15.2*	*308*	8.5	11.2	–

* : not enough deaths for reliable estimation
– : incomplete or missing data
Best model: polynomial of the given degree in age (A), period (P) or cohort (C), or linear drift (D) model.
Goodness of fit: the normalised likelihood ratio chi-square for the best model (see Method).
Rate: world-standardised truncated rate per 100 000 per year (30-74 years) and number of **deaths** are both estimated from the best-fitting model for the single years cited.
Cumulative risk per 1000 (30-74 years) is estimated from the best-fitting *age-cohort* model for cohorts of central birth year cited.
Recent trend: estimated mean percentage change per five-year period in the age-specific rates (30-74 years) over the period 1975-1988.
Italics denote recent trends not significant at 5 per cent level, or other figures which should be interpreted with caution (see Method).

FEMALES

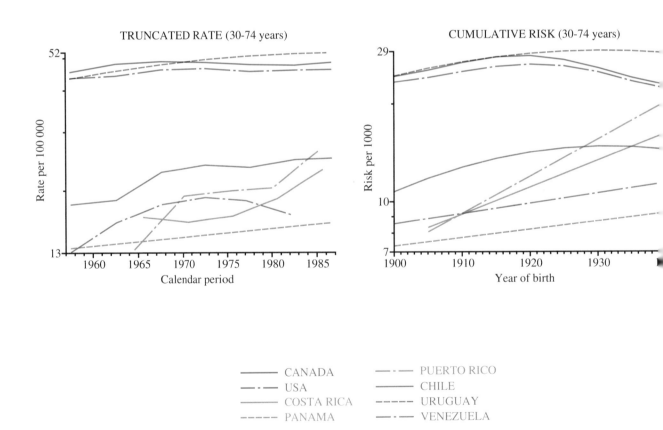

BREAST (ICD-9 174)

AMERICAS, MORTALITY
Percentage change per five-year period, 1975-1988

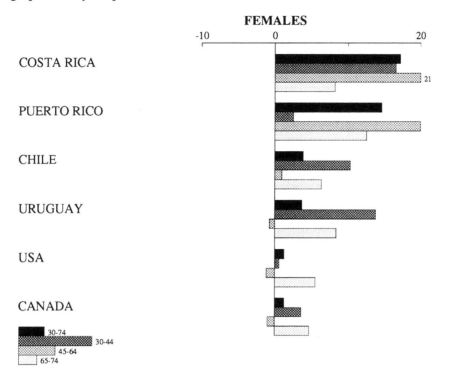

FEMALES

from page 425

Asia and Oceania

In Asia, the risk has been increasing rapidly in Japan and Singapore, more than doubling between the 1915 and 1940 birth cohorts, but the increase has been less marked in Bombay (India), Shanghai (China) and Hong Kong. The highest truncated rates (66 per 100 000) recorded in recent years in Asian populations (Hong Kong, Singapore) are of the same order of magnitude as the lowest rates recorded in Europe in 1970 (Spain). Mortality has decreased in Hong Kong but has been rising steadily in Singapore and Japan (9% every five years). Incidence rates for breast cancer in Hong Kong and among Chinese in Singapore were similar in 1985, whereas mortality in Hong Kong in 1985 was unexpectedly low compared to that in Singapore; this may be due to different patterns of change by period and birth cohort.

In Oceania, the results from the registry of Hawaii are especially interesting, since they show that the rates among Japanese and Filipinos are rapidly catching up with those recorded for other populations in the region. With a truncated rate of more than 200 per 100 000, Caucasians and Hawaiians in Hawaii have one of the highest risks of breast cancer in the world. The period effect observed among Caucasians is similar to that observed in other US populations: a steeper increase between 1980 and 1985 after a decelera-

tion in the previous period.

The incidence of breast cancer is increasing in New Zealand. An age-drift model describes the data for Maoris, whereas a poorly fitting age-period-cohort model is necessary in non-Maoris, showing a period effect similar to that observed in the Caucasian population of Hawaii. The recent trends are small, however, and not significant for either population. The Australian data are consistent with a steadily increasing risk. The mortality data in New Zealand and Australia are slightly divergent: whereas the cumulative risk of dying of breast cancer stopped increasing in Australia for generations born after 1925-30, the risk has been increasing steadily in New Zealand at 5% every five years.

Americas

In all US white populations, a period effect is needed to describe trends in the incidence of breast cancer; the main component of this effect in each case is a sharp increase in the truncated rate between 1980 and 1985. The truncated rate has also increased among black populations, but, except in Detroit, more steadily, without this characteristic period effect. In Canada, the slope of the curves is much less steep than in the USA, and the period effects are different in each of the five Canadian populations. British Columbia stands out as one of the few populations where the truncated rate decreased between 1970 and 1985. Another remarkable feature of the Canadian data is the downturn, or at least stabilisation, of the cumulative risk for the younger generations. This is particularly clear in Alberta and the Maritime Provinces. Only two of the ten US populations studied show a similar curvature: among whites in the Bay Area and in Connecticut, the risk has fallen for the generations born between 1925 and 1935, but it appears to increase for later birth cohorts.

The mortality data for Canada and the USA are remarkably similar, despite the disparities in incidence described above. The truncated rates have hardly changed over the period of the study, but the risk of death has shown a marked decrease for women born between 1920 and 1940. Unfortunately, the recent linear trend observed in younger women suggests that this decline may not continue beyond the 1940 generation.

In South America, incidence has increased in the four populations for which data were available. While women in São Paulo (Brazil) were already at relatively high risk in 1970, those in Cuba, Cali (Colombia) and Puerto Rico, especially, were at lower risk; Puerto Rico experienced the largest increase of all American populations, a 60% increase between 1970 and 1985. In Cali, the trend is well described by an age-drift model which suggests that the risk is increasing steadily at about 4% every five years.

The mortality data for Puerto Rico confirm the existence of a strong period effect and, together with the incidence data, they suggest that women in Puerto Rico, formerly at very low risk, may become a high-risk population in the near future. The high risk observed in Uruguay was very similar to that in North American populations, but it has remained almost constant, while the lower risk observed in other South American countries has steadily increased; the risk increased steeply in Costa Rica, but has reached a plateau in Chile.

Comment

The world-wide analysis presented here is not in complete agreement with the widely accepted notion of a large increase in incidence for breast cancer and a long-term stability of mortality[179]. This description of breast cancer trends derives from several publications on data from the USA which can in fact be interpreted differently. The analysis of incidence data reported here confirms the impressive and parallel increase in age-standar-

dised incidence in all USA registries between 1980 and 1985, following a plateau in the earlier periods. These characteristics have been noted by several authors[76,77,132,188], and various explanations have been given, among which the effect of screening has received most attention[165,185,267,277,302]. Despite the impressive increase in the use of mammography[188], however, the overall consensus is that screening does not account for all the increase[165,179,302], although it is probably difficult to quantify the effect of screening reliably from the available data. Mortality from breast cancer in the USA is stable only if it is analysed on a cross-sectional basis; it is in fact decreasing with year of birth, as has already been noted[28,279]. Furthermore, the change is correlated with trends in the pattern of childbearing[28,114,301]. These studies showed that the cohorts born during the period 1935-39 in the USA had the most favourable distribution of age at first birth. This observation is consistent with the trend in breast cancer mortality, and with the observed curvature of the risk by birth cohort in the San Francisco Bay Area and Connecticut. Mortality in Canada almost exactly parallels that of the USA, whereas the incidence data from Canada are substantially at variance with those of the USA, confirming the complexity of the relation between incidence and mortality for this cancer. The cancer registry of British Columbia has recorded a substantial increase in breast cancer incidence since 1987 (Band P., personal communication).

Breast cancer incidence trends have been analysed less extensively in other parts of the world, but all authors have noted that the trends are better described by birth cohort models[25,97,153,249,309]. It is thought that the impact of mammography has been less marked in European countries than in the USA[85,97,254]. In Asia, the increase in breast cancer has been ascribed to a shift towards a more westernised life-style. More specifically, changes in diet in Singapore have been considered as possibly relevant[155], while the change in age at first birth has been correlated with the increase of breast cancer incidence among Hindus in Bombay[309]. In developed countries, attempts to correlate aetiological factors and incidence changes have produced controversial results[49,140,245,246].

Our understanding of trends in breast cancer incidence and mortality is certainly incomplete. It is important to realise that the patterns of change are more diverse than is usually thought: incidence has reached a plateau, or is even decreasing in some countries[47], and mortality is decreasing in several countries in successive birth cohorts.

Chapter 18

CERVIX UTERI

Cervical cancer is the second most common cancer in females, representing 15% of all cancers. However, 80% of cervical cancers are diagnosed in developing countries, whereas the populations covered by this book are mainly in developed countries, where cervical cancer usually ranks lower, after cancers of the breast, colon and ovary, and is often less frequent than cancers of the uterine corpus and lung. The risk of cervical cancer varies by a factor of 20 between the populations which have been examined here. The cumulative risk (30-74 years) varies from 7% for the 1915 generation in Cali (Colombia) to 0.35% for the same generation in the non-Jewish population of Israel. Other high-risk populations are those in São Paulo (Brazil) and Hong Kong, Maoris in New Zealand, Indian populations and Singapore Chinese. Other low-risk populations are those in Spain, and Jews in Israel. As will be seen below, the risk in some countries is changing so rapidly that the rank order of the various populations for cervical cancer may change considerably in the near future.

There is growing evidence that cervical cancer disease is sexually transmitted; the human papilloma virus (HPV) has been convincingly identified as the most likely agent responsible for the disease[150,203]. The major risk factors for cervical cancer include age at first intercourse, multiple sexual partners, and low social class. It has been suggested that oral contraception may increase the risk[41] and that barrier contraceptives may be protective[40]. Screening for cervical cancer has been demonstrated to be effective[187], and the implementation of mass screening programmes is likely to be responsible for the decline observed in both mortality and incidence of invasive cancer in several countries[78,151,168].

Time trends in cervical cancer have been extensively studied, and the results may be summarised as a large overall decline in countries where well organised screening programmes are in operation, and a still unexplained increase in mortality in younger generations (born after 1930) in some countries.

Europe

Trends in the risk of cervical cancer in Europe may be described as a steep decline, except in Israel, County Vas (Hungary), Spain and the UK.

Among non-EC populations, the decline is particularly marked (14-30% every five years) in Geneva (Switzerland), Finland, Sweden and Slovenia, where well organised mass screening programmes are in operation[141,168]. The risk is also decreasing steeply in Cluj (Romania), where a screening programme is reported, but *in situ* lesions were reported as included in Volume V of *Cancer Incidence in Five Continents* for this population, and no information is provided for the data in Volume VI. The slight increase among younger women in Cluj is therefore difficult to interpret.

Among populations in the European Community, the decrease has been particularly steep in Saarland (FRG), but similar large declines are also seen in most populations where mass screening programmes are carried out. The data for Varese (Italy) show an upward turn in the cumulative risk curve, however, which suggests that the risk may have reached its minimum value. The UK populations are exceptional, with an overall increase of the standardised rate in 1983-87, and a large and similar increase (30% every five years) in the younger age groups in Birmingham and Scotland. The fit of the age-period-cohort model in South Thames is especially poor, and the fit of the best age-cohort model is therefore even worse; a detailed analysis of the data shows nevertheless that the increase in risk in the younger generation occurred later in South Thames than in Birmingham or Scotland. In South Thames, the risk first started to increase clearly for the generation born in 1945, and the description of the data obtained from the modelling approach is qualitatively correct. The lack of fit is mainly due to outlying data in the younger age group in 1975.

The mortality data for cervical cancer are not very informative, given the large number of deaths certified as 'uterus, not otherwise specified (NOS)'; the large differences between populations in certification of deaths to this rubric, and the decline over time in under-certification of deaths as due to cervical cancer, may bias the assessment of trends in mortality. Comparison of the information provided by incidence and mortality suggests that this bias is not as large as previously suspected, however, and it is probably reasonable to place some confidence in the mortality trends in those countries for which suitable long-term incidence data were not available. This is

continued page 447

CERVIX UTERI (ICD-9 180)

EUROPE (non-EC), INCIDENCE

FEMALES	Best model	Goodness of fit	1970 Rate	1970 Cases	1985 Rate	1985 Cases	Cumulative risk 1915	Cumulative risk 1940	Recent trend
FINLAND	A3P5C4	5.52	27.0	332	8.1	121	17.5	1.7	-29.3
HUNGARY									
County Vas	A2D	2.53	39.4	30	30.5	23	18.4	12.0	*0.3*
Szabolcs-Szatmar	A2D	-0.65	25.2	36	19.8	31	12.1	8.1	*-10.1*
ISRAEL									
All Jews	A3C6	0.43	9.7	48	8.9	62	4.7	3.5	*-6.5*
Non-Jews	A8C9	0.56	8.0	3	4.2	3	3.5	4.1	*21.2*
NORWAY	A3P2C6	3.98	40.6	390	27.0	285	18.0	11.1	-18.7
POLAND									
Warsaw City	A3P3	-1.62	45.6	181	33.1	165	22.2	13.1	-8.7
ROMANIA									
Cluj	A2C3	-0.12	*116.5*	*203*	35.4	69	59.0	9.3	-30.0
SWEDEN	A4P5C6	5.74	35.7	753	18.4	435	20.7	5.2	-16.8
SWITZERLAND									
Geneva	A2D	3.28	38.3	35	12.8	13	24.8	4.0	-28.0
YUGOSLAVIA									
Slovenia	A8P5C9	0.71	40.3	180	24.2	128	23.2	7.6	-13.9

* : not enough cases for reliable estimation
– : incomplete or missing data
Best model: polynomial of the given degree in age (A), period (P) or cohort (C), or linear drift (D) model.
Goodness of fit: the normalised likelihood ratio chi-square for the best model (see Method).
Rate: world-standardised truncated rate per 100 000 per year (30-74 years) and number of **cases** are both estimated from the best-fitting model for the single years cited.
Cumulative risk per 1000 (30-74 years) is estimated from the best-fitting *age-cohort* model for cohorts of central birth year cited.
Recent trend: estimated mean percentage change per five-year period in the age-specific rates (30-74 years) over the period 1973-1987.
Italics denote recent trends not significant at 5 per cent level, or other figures which should be interpreted with caution (see Method).

FEMALES

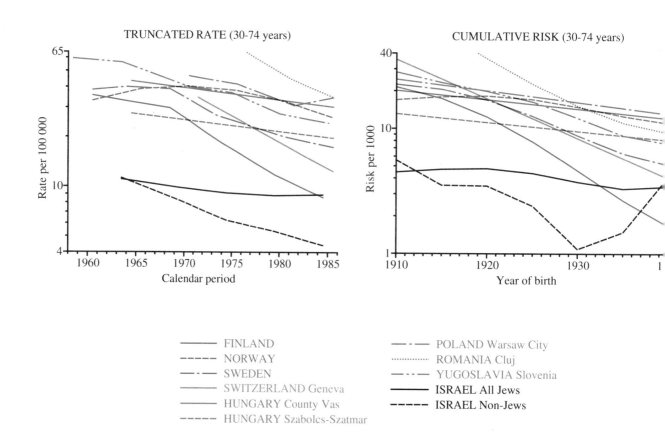

TRUNCATED RATE (30-74 years)

CUMULATIVE RISK (30-74 years)

——— FINLAND
------- NORWAY
—·— SWEDEN
——— SWITZERLAND Geneva
——— HUNGARY County Vas
------- HUNGARY Szabolcs-Szatmar

—·— POLAND Warsaw City
············ ROMANIA Cluj
—··— YUGOSLAVIA Slovenia
——— ISRAEL All Jews
------- ISRAEL Non-Jews

CERVIX UTERI (ICD-9 180)

EUROPE (non-EC), INCIDENCE
Percentage change per five-year period, 1973-1987

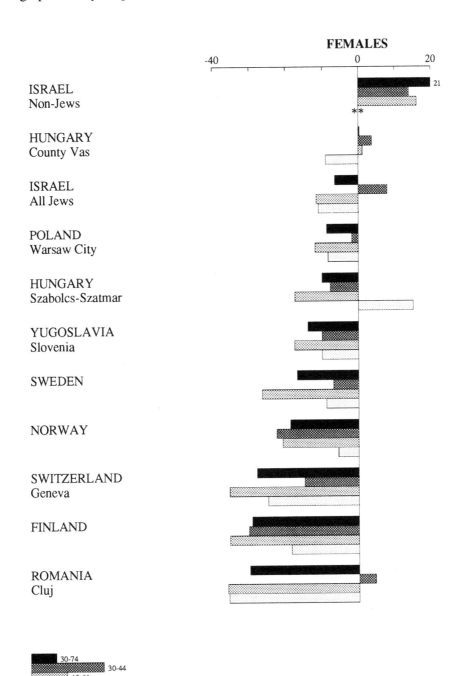

CERVIX UTERI (ICD-9 180)

EUROPE (EC), INCIDENCE

FEMALES	Best model	Goodness of fit	1970 Rate	1970 Cases	1985 Rate	1985 Cases	Cumulative risk 1915	Cumulative risk 1940	Recent trend
DENMARK	A4P5C7	6.67	61.7	758	33.7	463	28.7	11.4	-17.7
FRANCE									
Bas-Rhin	A4C5	-0.34	*95.9*	*328*	24.7	56	42.1	6.0	-24.6
Doubs	A5D	-0.18	*55.7*	*48*	20.1	23	29.7	5.5	-29.1
GERMANY (FRG)									
Hamburg	A8P4C9	0.99	74.3	423	*	*	41.1	*9.1*	–
Saarland	A7C3	0.23	75.6	239	21.7	72	75.2	5.8	-31.3
GERMANY (GDR)	A4P4C9	6.19	74.6	3598	43.6	1980	45.4	14.7	-16.4
ITALY									
Varese	A8C7	-0.90	*42.5*	*79*	14.9	34	35.5	5.0	-25.4
SPAIN									
Navarra	A2C2	0.33	*9.4*	*12*	16.9	20	3.5	14.3	33.0
Zaragoza	A2C2	0.21	10.1	20	11.9	29	5.7	6.1	*-2.4*
UK									
Birmingham	A3P3C8	2.07	28.5	379	27.7	377	14.4	9.8	*3.0*
Scotland	A3C9	1.51	26.3	371	27.0	369	15.1	10.1	*2.7*
South Thames	A4P5C6	14.76	28.5	695	21.7	393	14.0	5.5	3.9

* : not enough cases for reliable estimation
– : incomplete or missing data
Best model: polynomial of the given degree in age (A), period (P) or cohort (C), or linear drift (D) model.
Goodness of fit: the normalised likelihood ratio chi-square for the best model (see Method).
Rate: world-standardised truncated rate per 100 000 per year (30-74 years) and number of **cases** are both estimated from the best-fitting model for the single years cited.
Cumulative risk per 1000 (30-74 years) is estimated from the best-fitting *age-cohort* model for cohorts of central birth year cited.
Recent trend: estimated mean percentage change per five-year period in the age-specific rates (30-74 years) over the period 1973-1987.
Italics denote recent trends not significant at 5 per cent level, or other figures which should be interpreted with caution (see Method).

FEMALES

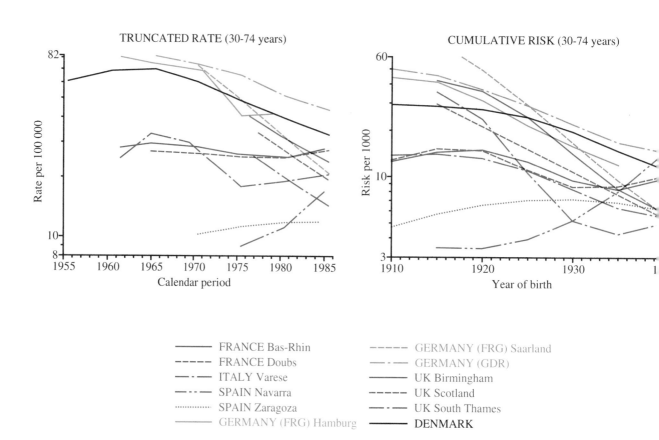

CERVIX UTERI (ICD-9 180)

EUROPE (EC), INCIDENCE
Percentage change per five-year period, 1973-1987

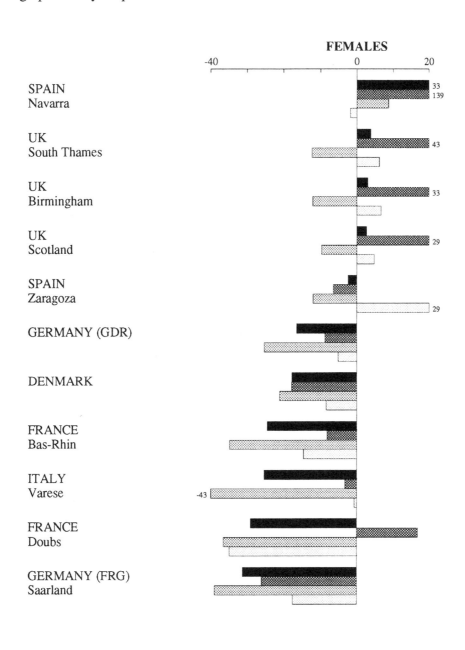

FEMALES

SPAIN
Navarra

UK
South Thames

UK
Birmingham

UK
Scotland

SPAIN
Zaragoza

GERMANY (GDR)

DENMARK

FRANCE
Bas-Rhin

ITALY
Varese

FRANCE
Doubs

GERMANY (FRG)
Saarland

30-74
30-44
45-64
65-74

CERVIX UTERI (ICD-9 180)

EUROPE (non-EC), MORTALITY

FEMALES	Best model	Goodness of fit	1965 Rate	1965 Deaths	1985 Rate	1985 Deaths	Cumulative risk 1900	Cumulative risk 1940	Recent trend
AUSTRIA	A8P6C9	-0.24	9.0	206	9.0	204	4.5	4.1	-12.1
CZECHOSLOVAKIA	A3P4C6	1.09	14.6	567	11.8	497	7.2	4.4	7.3
FINLAND	A3P3C6	-1.16	11.7	140	3.8	60	6.6	0.7	-24.0
HUNGARY	A3P4C7	2.46	11.4	329	15.7	508	4.7	9.3	6.5
NORWAY	A3P3C4	-1.48	12.9	130	9.4	109	7.0	3.4	-10.9
POLAND	A3P4C3	5.75	15.2	1132	17.7	1662	6.8	9.7	-3.4
ROMANIA	A5P3C8	4.17	21.1	977	*22.2*	*1334*	9.5	9.6	–
SWEDEN	A3P3C4	1.58	12.9	280	6.2	159	5.7	2.0	-17.0
SWITZERLAND	A3C2	0.37	13.1	211	7.0	131	8.6	2.4	-17.8
YUGOSLAVIA	A3P5C6	3.21	9.3	396	8.9	534	4.9	3.5	-12.1

* : not enough deaths for reliable estimation
– : incomplete or missing data
Best model: polynomial of the given degree in age (A), period (P) or cohort (C), or linear drift (D) model.
Goodness of fit: the normalised likelihood ratio chi-square for the best model (see Method).
Rate: world-standardised truncated rate per 100 000 per year (30-74 years) and number of **deaths** are both estimated from the best-fitting model for the single years cited.
Cumulative risk per 1000 (30-74 years) is estimated from the best-fitting *age-cohort* model for cohorts of central birth year cited.
Recent trend: estimated mean percentage change per five-year period in the age-specific rates (30-74 years) over the period 1975-1988.
Italics denote recent trends not significant at 5 per cent level, or other figures which should be interpreted with caution (see Method).

FEMALES

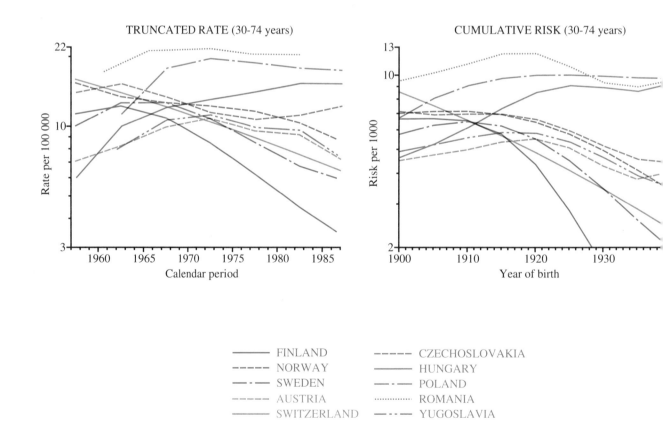

438

CERVIX UTERI (ICD-9 180)

EUROPE (non-EC), MORTALITY
Percentage change per five-year period, 1975-1988

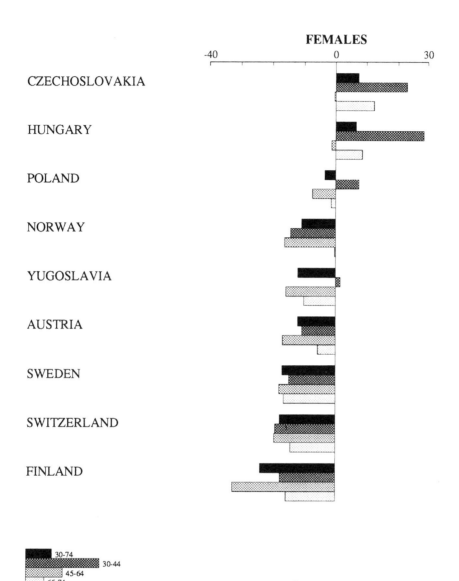

CERVIX UTERI (ICD-9 180)

EUROPE (EC), MORTALITY

FEMALES	Best model	Goodness of fit	1965 Rate	Deaths	1985 Rate	Deaths	Cumulative risk 1900	1940	Recent trend
BELGIUM	A3C4	3.96	8.5	238	5.1	151	5.0	1.7	-9.1
DENMARK	A3P6C7	2.60	26.1	325	12.6	184	11.9	3.7	-17.8
FRANCE	A3P2C6	2.49	6.1	806	4.2	628	3.1	1.5	-7.8
GERMANY (FRG)	A4P4C9	5.25	11.4	2049	7.2	1431	4.9	3.0	-19.2
GREECE	A3P2C3	1.55	1.1	23	2.7	78	*0.6*	2.5	*-4.1*
IRELAND	A2P4C4	2.80	6.9	46	5.8	45	3.0	2.6	*-1.4*
ITALY	A3P5C8	1.40	4.0	545	1.8	306	2.2	0.5	-15.8
NETHERLANDS	A3P2C9	2.16	12.5	363	5.6	217	7.2	1.5	-21.1
PORTUGAL	A5P5C3	1.88	18.9	426	4.3	119	14.4	1.8	-37.4
SPAIN	A3P6C6	0.60	1.6	132	2.8	296	0.5	2.8	22.6
UK ENGLAND & WALES	A7P3C9	8.21	14.4	2038	10.3	1491	7.4	3.6	-6.4
UK SCOTLAND	A3P2C8	-0.62	14.5	216	10.4	154	7.3	4.0	-7.1

* : not enough deaths for reliable estimation
– : incomplete or missing data
Best model: polynomial of the given degree in age (A), period (P) or cohort (C), or linear drift (D) model.
Goodness of fit: the normalised likelihood ratio chi-square for the best model (see Method).
Rate: world-standardised truncated rate per 100 000 per year (30-74 years) and number of **deaths** are both estimated from the best-fitting model for the single years cited.
Cumulative risk per 1000 (30-74 years) is estimated from the best-fitting *age-cohort* model for cohorts of central birth year cited.
Recent trend: estimated mean percentage change per five-year period in the age-specific rates (30-74 years) over the period 1975-1988.
Italics denote recent trends not significant at 5 per cent level, or other figures which should be interpreted with caution (see Method).

FEMALES

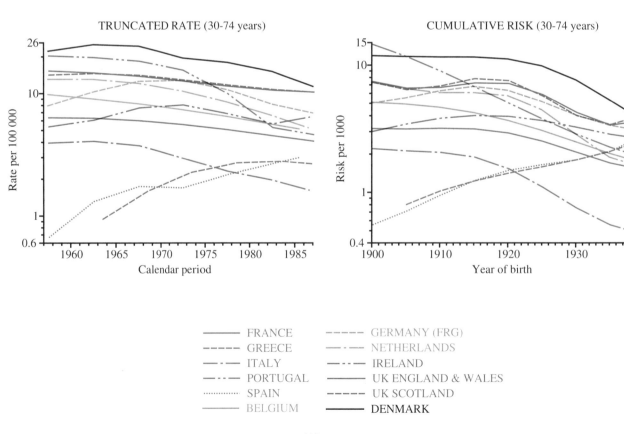

440

CERVIX UTERI (ICD-9 180)

EUROPE (EC), MORTALITY
Percentage change per five-year period, 1975-1988

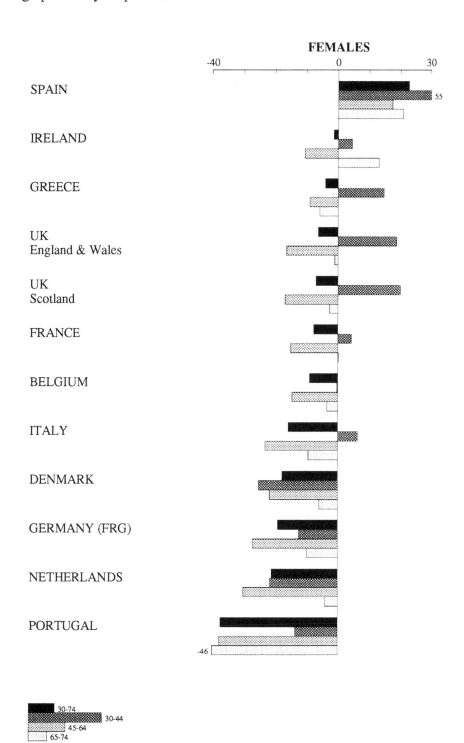

CERVIX UTERI (ICD-9 180)

ASIA, INCIDENCE

FEMALES	Best model	Goodness of fit	1970 Rate	1970 Cases	1985 Rate	1985 Cases	Cumulative risk 1915	Cumulative risk 1940	Recent trend
CHINA									
Shanghai	A4P2C4	0.33	*205.5*	*2462*	8.9	166	209.8	0.8	-58.5
HONG KONG	A3C4	2.44	*82.9*	*553*	42.4	468	41.3	13.0	-20.7
INDIA									
Bombay	A3C2	4.59	50.0	298	42.1	456	24.1	17.5	-6.8
JAPAN									
Miyagi	A5P4C3	2.97	31.3	130	14.1	86	17.8	4.4	-28.9
Nagasaki	A3D	0.08	*84.9*	*86*	26.9	34	49.5	7.5	-31.9
Osaka	A6P2C4	3.40	33.6	502	29.2	669	21.6	10.5	-13.5
SINGAPORE									
Chinese	A3C2	1.43	41.1	97	38.1	141	18.7	18.3	*-0.5*
Indian	A2P2	-0.64	42.4	4	34.0	7	28.3	13.6	-25.0
Malay	A2C3	1.15	23.6	7	19.7	10	9.0	9.2	*1.0*

* : not enough cases for reliable estimation
− : incomplete or missing data
Best model: polynomial of the given degree in age (A), period (P) or cohort (C), or linear drift (D) model.
Goodness of fit: the normalised likelihood ratio chi-square for the best model (see Method).
Rate: world-standardised truncated rate per 100 000 per year (30-74 years) and number of **cases** are both estimated from the best-fitting model for the single years cited.
Cumulative risk per 1000 (30-74 years) is estimated from the best-fitting *age-cohort* model for cohorts of central birth year cited.
Recent trend: estimated mean percentage change per five-year period in the age-specific rates (30-74 years) over the period 1973-1987.
Italics denote recent trends not significant at 5 per cent level, or other figures which should be interpreted with caution (see Method).

FEMALES

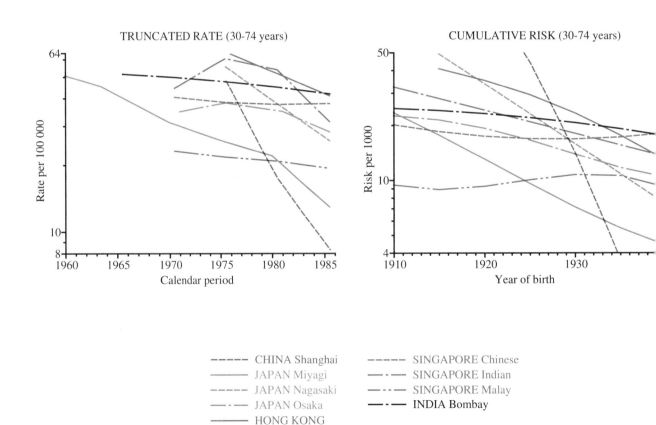

TRUNCATED RATE (30-74 years) — Rate per 100 000 — Calendar period

CUMULATIVE RISK (30-74 years) — Risk per 1000 — Year of birth

------ CHINA Shanghai
——— JAPAN Miyagi
------ JAPAN Nagasaki
—·— JAPAN Osaka
——— HONG KONG
------ SINGAPORE Chinese
—·— SINGAPORE Indian
—··— SINGAPORE Malay
—··— INDIA Bombay

CERVIX UTERI (ICD-9 180)

ASIA, INCIDENCE
Percentage change per five-year period, 1973-1987

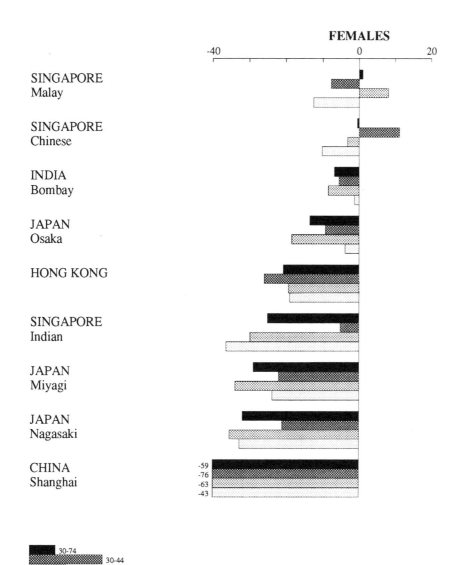

CERVIX UTERI (ICD-9 180)

OCEANIA, INCIDENCE

FEMALES	Best model	Goodness of fit	1970		1985		Cumulative risk		Recent trend
			Rate	Cases	Rate	Cases	1915	1940	
AUSTRALIA									
New South Wales	A8C7	0.96	*26.7*	*276*	20.9	261	13.5	8.3	-7.9
South	A1	0.80	*19.9*	*45*	19.9	68	9.5	9.5	*14.0*
HAWAII									
Caucasian	A1D	-0.44	23.7	10	16.4	10	11.8	6.4	*-5.7*
Chinese	A1D	-0.25	24.3	2	8.2	1	15.4	2.5	*-39.3*
Filipino	A1	-0.45	18.7	1	18.7	5	9.5	9.5	*27.7*
Hawaiian	A3C2	0.37	37.5	6	22.7	6	17.3	8.3	*-21.5*
Japanese	A1D	0.96	18.1	9	8.6	7	9.8	2.9	*-18.3*
NEW ZEALAND									
Maori	A2	1.25	66.2	17	66.2	29	29.6	29.6	*-7.0*
Non-Maori	A2P3C6	1.79	21.9	125	24.7	173	12.5	9.5	*2.8*

* : not enough cases for reliable estimation
– : incomplete or missing data
Best model: polynomial of the given degree in age (A), period (P) or cohort (C), or linear drift (D) model.
Goodness of fit: the normalised likelihood ratio chi-square for the best model (see Method).
Rate: world-standardised truncated rate per 100 000 per year (30-74 years) and number of **cases** are both estimated from the best-fitting model for the single years cited.
Cumulative risk per 1000 (30-74 years) is estimated from the best-fitting *age-cohort* model for cohorts of central birth year cited.
Recent trend: estimated mean percentage change per five-year period in the age-specific rates (30-74 years) over the period 1973-1987.
Italics denote recent trends not significant at 5 per cent level, or other figures which should be interpreted with caution (see Method).

FEMALES

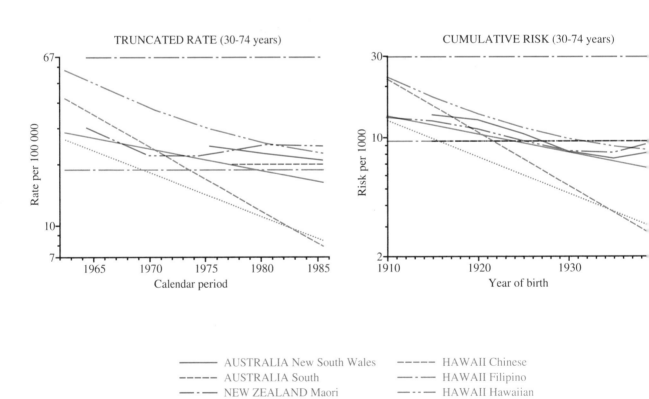

CERVIX UTERI (ICD-9 180)

OCEANIA, INCIDENCE
Percentage change per five-year period, 1973-1987

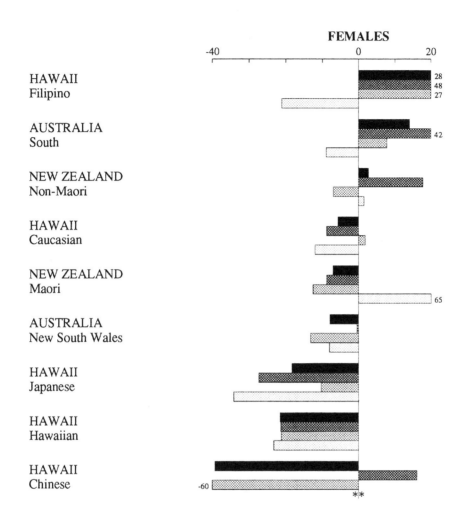

CERVIX UTERI (ICD-9 180)

ASIA and OCEANIA, MORTALITY

FEMALES	Best model	Goodness of fit	1965 Rate	1965 Deaths	1985 Rate	1985 Deaths	Cumulative risk 1900	Cumulative risk 1940	Recent trend
AUSTRALIA	A5P3C6	1.09	12.0	313	6.7	259	6.6	2.2	-9.0
HONG KONG	A3C5	-0.15	21.6	131	10.3	99	*13.6*	2.5	-17.1
JAPAN	A3P6C9	4.03	7.9	1614	3.9	1327	4.0	1.2	-12.8
MAURITIUS	A2D	1.51	19.9	18	10.6	15	*13.1*	3.7	*6.3*
NEW ZEALAND	A3C6	1.27	13.0	74	10.5	79	7.0	4.5	*-4.1*
SINGAPORE	A2C2	0.27	*20.0*	*42*	15.1	52	*8.8*	5.1	–

* : not enough deaths for reliable estimation
– : incomplete or missing data
Best model: polynomial of the given degree in age (A), period (P) or cohort (C), or linear drift (D) model.
Goodness of fit: the normalised likelihood ratio chi-square for the best model (see Method).
Rate: world-standardised truncated rate per 100 000 per year (30-74 years) and number of **deaths** are both estimated from the best-fitting model for the single years cited.
Cumulative risk per 1000 (30-74 years) is estimated from the best-fitting *age-cohort* model for cohorts of central birth year cited.
Recent trend: estimated mean percentage change per five-year period in the age-specific rates (30-74 years) over the period 1975-1988.
Italics denote recent trends not significant at 5 per cent level, or other figures which should be interpreted with caution (see Method).

FEMALES

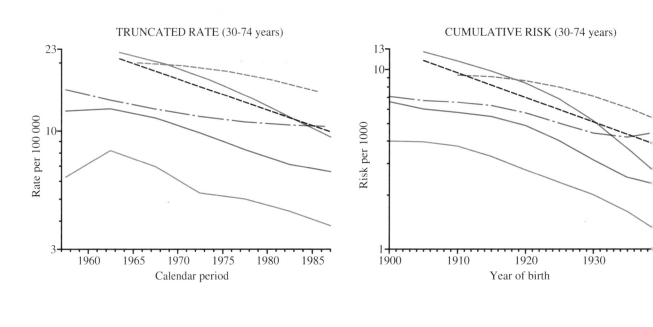

TRUNCATED RATE (30-74 years)

CUMULATIVE RISK (30-74 years)

——— AUSTRALIA ——— HONG KONG
—·— NEW ZEALAND ----- SINGAPORE
——— JAPAN ----- MAURITIUS

CERVIX UTERI (ICD-9 180)

ASIA and OCEANIA, MORTALITY
Percentage change per five-year period, 1975-1988

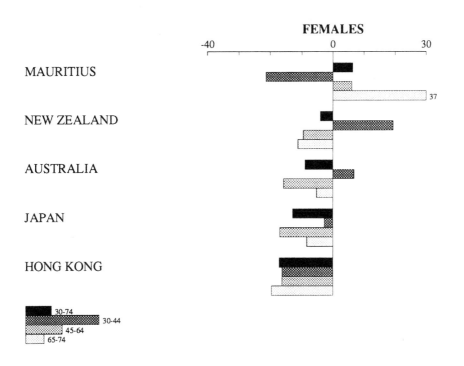

FEMALES

-40   0   30

MAURITIUS

37

NEW ZEALAND

AUSTRALIA

JAPAN

HONG KONG

30-74
30-44
45-64
65-74

from page 433

particularly relevant for the Netherlands, where relatively few deaths are certified as 'uterus, NOS' in any case[291]. It must also be noted that the true decrease in the risk of death from cervical cancer among younger women is probably larger than that observed, since in this age group deaths certified as 'uterus, NOS' are mainly deaths from cancer of the cervix uteri[137], and certification of death has improved. By contrast, an observed increase in mortality might be partly explained by a decrease in the number of deaths certified as due to cancer of the uterus, not otherwise specified.

Asia and Oceania

The decrease in the risk of cervical cancer (15-30% every five years) is seen for most Asian populations examined, except Chinese and Malays in Singapore. The rate of decline (7%) is somewhat lower in Bombay (India). In Shanghai (China), the recent rate of decline has been extremely rapid: more than 40% every five years in all age groups.

As in Europe, mortality data for Asian populations are remarkably consistent with the incidence data, and they confirm that the decrease in cervical cancer in Singapore is smaller than in other populations.

The most striking observation in Oceania is the absence of any substantial decline in the risk of cervical cancer in Australia and New Zealand. Among non-Maoris in New Zealand, the change in cumulative risk and the recent linear trends by age suggest an upward turn, similar to that observed in the UK, and in New South Wales (Australia), the decline has also stopped in young women. There is little suggestion that the very high lifetime risk (3%) observed among Maoris is declining; there has been a non-significant recent decrease in the rates of 7% every five years. In the population of South Australia, there is also little overall change, but the pattern of age-specific trends suggests an upward trend. In Hawaii, the risk of cervical cancer has decreased substantially among Chinese, Hawaiian and Japanese women, but not among Filipino women, for whom there has been a non-significant recent increase of 28% every five years.

The mortality data confirm the small rate of decline of cervical cancer in New Zealand and the increase in risk in younger generations. Although there is a similar pattern in Australia, it is certainly less marked. The data from Mauritius are consistent with a decline in the risk of death in successive birth cohorts.

447

continued page 453

CERVIX UTERI (ICD-9 180)

AMERICAS (except USA), INCIDENCE

FEMALES	Best model	Goodness of fit	1970 Rate	1970 Cases	1985 Rate	1985 Cases	Cumulative risk 1915	Cumulative risk 1940	Recent trend
BRAZIL									
Sao Paulo	A3P2	2.55	57.8	511	*27.2*	*316*	26.5	*42.3*	–
CANADA									
Alberta	A4P4C3	0.50	27.8	85	18.9	97	18.0	5.3	*3.3*
British Columbia	A8P3C8	0.49	43.3	199	14.7	108	34.6	4.5	-21.0
Maritime Provinces	A2P2C4	1.05	53.4	161	21.3	79	31.4	5.8	-18.8
Newfoundland	A2P3	-1.13	52.1	43	31.2	36	20.4	12.2	*-9.7*
Quebec	A4P4C6	8.97	34.9	429	19.5	327	30.2	4.2	-11.8
COLOMBIA									
Cali	A3P2C2	2.64	127.5	131	81.7	165	65.6	26.0	-12.4
CUBA	A5P2C2	1.09	41.3	568	38.8	786	17.7	*18.5*	–
PUERTO RICO	A7P5C8	2.28	55.4	258	26.3	196	30.4	6.7	-21.7

* : not enough cases for reliable estimation
– : incomplete or missing data
Best model: polynomial of the given degree in age (A), period (P) or cohort (C), or linear drift (D) model.
Goodness of fit: the normalised likelihood ratio chi-square for the best model (see Method).
Rate: world-standardised truncated rate per 100 000 per year (30-74 years) and number of **cases** are both estimated from the best-fitting model for the single years cited.
Cumulative risk per 1000 (30-74 years) is estimated from the best-fitting *age-cohort* model for cohorts of central birth year cited.
Recent trend: estimated mean percentage change per five-year period in the age-specific rates (30-74 years) over the period 1973-1987.
Italics denote recent trends not significant at 5 per cent level, or other figures which should be interpreted with caution (see Method).

FEMALES

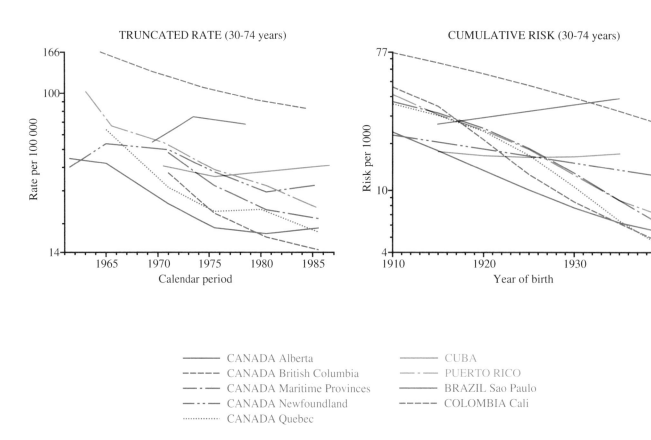

448

CERVIX UTERI (ICD-9 180)

AMERICAS (except USA), INCIDENCE
Percentage change per five-year period, 1973-1987

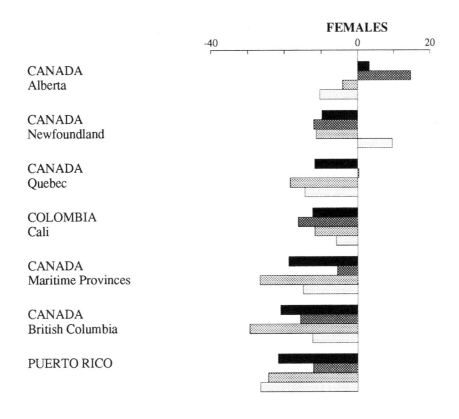

FEMALES

CANADA
Alberta

CANADA
Newfoundland

CANADA
Quebec

COLOMBIA
Cali

CANADA
Maritime Provinces

CANADA
British Columbia

PUERTO RICO

30-74
30-44
45-64
65-74

CERVIX UTERI (ICD-9 180)

AMERICAS (USA), INCIDENCE

FEMALES	Best model	Goodness of fit	1970 Rate	1970 Cases	1985 Rate	1985 Cases	Cumulative risk 1915	Cumulative risk 1940	Recent trend
USA									
Bay Area, Black	A3D	0.32	53.2	34	21.4	21	33.5	7.5	-25.3
Bay Area, Chinese	A1	0.33	26.9	4	*26.9*	*14*	14.4	*14.4*	–
Bay Area, White	A3C4	0.36	26.0	166	15.5	102	13.2	6.1	-15.1
Connecticut	A2P4C3	0.85	20.3	146	13.7	115	10.3	5.0	-7.6
Detroit, Black	A3D	0.00	66.1	102	28.2	60	38.2	9.4	-26.2
Detroit, White	A2D	0.22	28.1	223	15.4	117	15.1	5.5	-15.4
Iowa	A3P2	-0.67	34.4	221	16.5	113	18.6	5.8	-18.1
New Orleans, Black	A2D	-1.95	*61.8*	*37*	33.9	27	32.9	12.2	-17.5
New Orleans, White	A1D	-0.04	*22.8*	*38*	12.1	20	12.6	4.4	-19.7
Seattle	A1P2	0.45	*57.2*	*272*	14.7	105	15.1	5.4	-18.5

* : not enough cases for reliable estimation
– : incomplete or missing data
Best model: polynomial of the given degree in age (A), period (P) or cohort (C), or linear drift (D) model.
Goodness of fit: the normalised likelihood ratio chi-square for the best model (see Method).
Rate: world-standardised truncated rate per 100 000 per year (30-74 years) and number of **cases** are both estimated from the best-fitting model for the single years cited.
Cumulative risk per 1000 (30-74 years) is estimated from the best-fitting *age-cohort* model for cohorts of central birth year cited.
Recent trend: estimated mean percentage change per five-year period in the age-specific rates (30-74 years) over the period 1973-1987.
Italics denote recent trends not significant at 5 per cent level, or other figures which should be interpreted with caution (see Method).

FEMALES

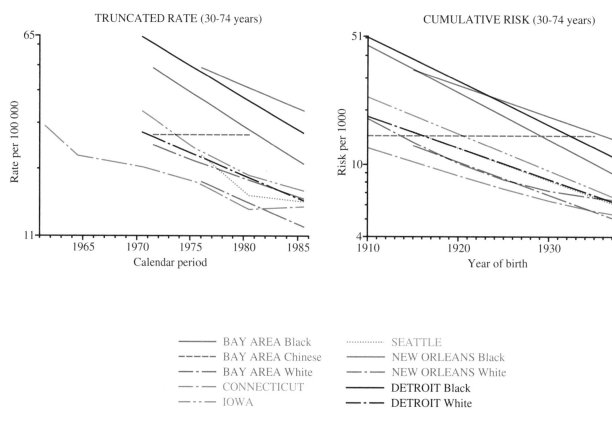

450

CERVIX UTERI (ICD-9 180)

AMERICAS (USA), INCIDENCE
Percentage change per five-year period, 1973-1987

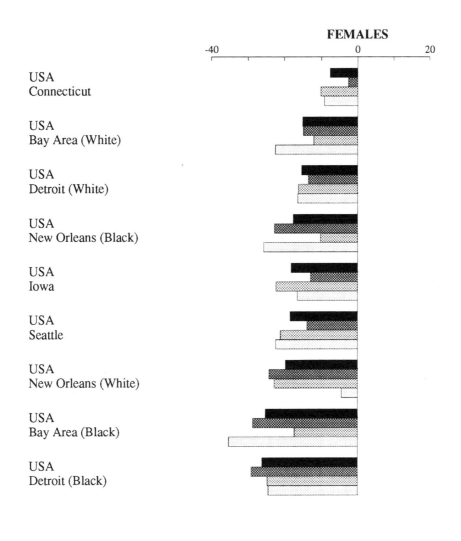

CERVIX UTERI (ICD-9 180)

AMERICAS, MORTALITY

FEMALES	Best model	Goodness of fit	1965 Rate	1965 Deaths	1985 Rate	1985 Deaths	Cumulative risk 1900	Cumulative risk 1940	Recent trend
CANADA	A4P5C4	0.05	14.0	555	5.2	327	9.9	1.6	-18.2
CHILE	A3P6C2	-0.58	25.1	346	28.1	602	11.6	15.9	-7.5
COSTA RICA	A3P2	1.24	*35.8*	*52*	22.2	66	*19.3*	8.5	*-3.3*
PANAMA	A3D	-1.52	22.3	34	19.8	59	12.0	9.5	–
PUERTO RICO	A2P3	0.46	14.7	62	6.6	39	*10.5*	1.7	*-9.0*
URUGUAY	A3P3C3	0.69	18.0	110	9.6	70	10.7	3.8	-11.0
USA	A5P6C7	3.55	14.5	6696	5.8	3506	11.3	1.8	-15.9
VENEZUELA	A3P2C2	2.46	25.9	272	*16.3*	*342*	12.6	9.0	–

* : not enough deaths for reliable estimation
– : incomplete or missing data
Best model: polynomial of the given degree in age (A), period (P) or cohort (C), or linear drift (D) model.
Goodness of fit: the normalised likelihood ratio chi-square for the best model (see Method).
Rate: world-standardised truncated rate per 100 000 per year (30-74 years) and number of **deaths** are both estimated from the best-fitting model for the single years cited.
Cumulative risk per 1000 (30-74 years) is estimated from the best-fitting *age-cohort* model for cohorts of central birth year cited.
Recent trend: estimated mean percentage change per five-year period in the age-specific rates (30-74 years) over the period 1975-1988.
Italics denote recent trends not significant at 5 per cent level, or other figures which should be interpreted with caution (see Method).

FEMALES

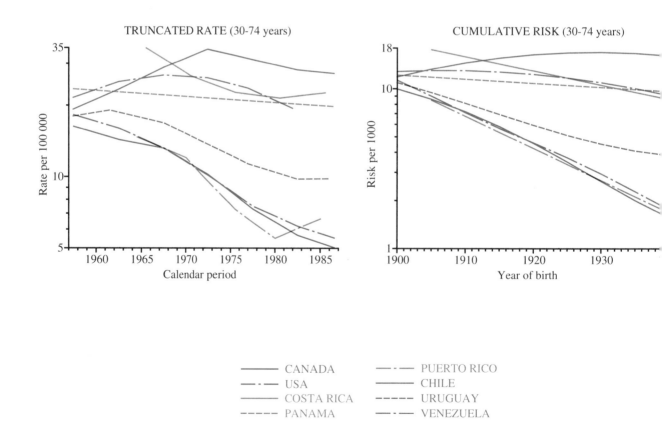

CERVIX UTERI (ICD-9 180)

AMERICAS, MORTALITY
Percentage change per five-year period, 1975-1988

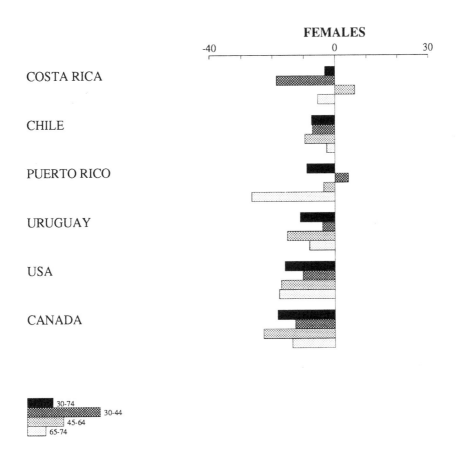

FEMALES

COSTA RICA

CHILE

PUERTO RICO

URUGUAY

USA

CANADA

■ 30-74
▨ 30-44
▨ 45-64
□ 65-74

from page 447

Americas

Among the Caribbean and South American populations examined there is a strong contrast between Cali (Colombia) and Puerto Rico on the one hand, and Cuba and São Paulo (Brazil) on the other. The decrease in incidence observed in Cali and Puerto Rico is consistent with the existence of mass screening programmes in these two populations. In Cuba, however, where a mass screening programme is also in operation, no decrease has been observed between 1975 and 1986, the only recent year for which data are available (no data were available around 1980).

In Canada, where there is a country-wide mass screening programme, the risk of cervical cancer has decreased steadily. The pattern of decrease varies between provinces, however. In particular, the data from Alberta show that the decrease stopped around 1975, and the incidence rate has even increased recently among younger age groups by a statistically significant 15% every five years. In Quebec, the risk has also stopped declining among young women, and in Newfoundland the rate of decline has been less pronounced.

In the USA, a rapid decline (15-25% every five years) is seen in every population, and it is exponential in five of the ten populations examined. In Seattle, and especially in Connecticut, there was no further decline during 1983-87, and in Iowa the rate of decrease has lessened. In the San Francisco Bay Area, the best-fitting model suggests that the risk for white females is no longer decreasing in young birth cohorts. The mortality data show a remarkably similar decline in the truncated rate in Canada, the USA and Puerto Rico up to 1980, but the significant period effect observed in Puerto Rico suggests that the rate has increased since then. The truncated rate and the cumulative risk have also declined recently in Chile and Uruguay, but to a lesser extent than in North America. Little change is seen in mortality for other South American countries.

453

Comment

The data described in this chapter support the concept that well organised screening programmes can prevent invasive cancer of the cervix[115,187]. Despite this optimistic note, it has been suggested that trends in cervical cancer may in the future come to be dominated by the increase in HPV infection[150]. Some authors have also considered that the change in distribution of histological types of cervical cancer among young women, with adenocarcinoma possibly becoming more frequent, reinforces the suspicion that oral contraceptives will play a role in incidence trends in the future[93,232,233]. Oral contraceptives may contribute to the increase in risk through an interaction with HPV infection[33,203].

The United Kingdom provides perhaps the clearest example of the increase in risk among young women, and the trend has been interpreted as evidence of lack of effectiveness of the screening programme in this country[21,205,222]. More recent analyses of these data[206,256,295] up to 1990 show that the situation is improving. It has been suggested that any future assessment of trends in cervical cancer should also take into account the change in sexual behaviour caused by the AIDS epidemic[207]. An increase in cervical cancer incidence in young women has also been reported in Switzerland[34], Belgium[69] and Slovakia[297], and an increase in incidence and/or mortality in the age-group 30-44 years is seen in several of the data sets analysed here. This emphasises the need for continuous monitoring of the incidence of cervical cancer, including its distribution by histological type, and of the known risk factors for this cancer.

The recent decline in the incidence of cervical cancer in Shanghai (China) seems remarkably rapid, at over 50% every five years, and by 1985 the truncated incidence (9 per 100 000) was less than a quarter of the levels in Hong Kong or among Chinese in Singapore, and of the same order of magnitude as in Finland and Israel. The incidence of cancer of the uterine corpus in Shanghai was also falling during this period, however, and the incidence of cervical cancer during 1983-87 in Qidong City (China) was similar to that in Shanghai[221]. Mortality from cervical cancer in Henan province (China) also fell by 50% between 1975 and 1985[169].

The declining trend in Bombay (India) has been attributed to an upward shift in age at marriage in the Hindu population[308].

The declining trend in New South Wales (Australia) has been analysed in detail by McCredie *et al.*[181], who did not observe any change in stage or histological type. This pattern is quite distinct from that seen in South Australia and among non-Maoris in New Zealand.

Trends in the incidence of cervical cancer have recently been reported for the whole of Canada[10]. This report showed a recent overall increase in the age group 30-39 years between 1981 and 1985, and a longer-term increase in the age group 20-29 years, while the analysis reported here shows an increase among young women in Alberta only.

The large decline in incidence seen here for the USA has been analysed previously by stage and histological type. Devesa *et al.*[78] noted an increase in adenocarcinoma and suggested that, while screening may be able to counterbalance the unfavourable trend in the prevalence of risk factors for squamous cell carcinoma, this may not be the case for adenocarcinoma, despite a smaller rate of increase for this histological type in the 1980s.

Chapter 19

CORPUS UTERI

Cancer of the uterine corpus, mainly carcinoma of the endometrium, was the fifth most frequent cancer among women around 1980, accounting for about 5% of all cancers in women. More than two-thirds of cases arise in developed countries, and it is relatively uncommon in developing countries. Incidence varies widely even in developed countries: the cumulative risk estimate (30-74 years) for the generation born in 1915 varied from about 0.1% in Zaragoza (Spain) and Osaka (Japan) to more than 3% among Caucasians in Hawaii or the San Francisco Bay Area (USA). The incidence of endometrial cancer is higher among more affluent populations, and increases with the adoption of a more westernised life-style. Since survival from endometrial cancer at five years is high (about 74%), it is not a major cause of mortality. The pattern of geographical variation and the main risk factors for endometrial cancer are broadly similar to those for cancers of the breast and ovary, and comparative epidemiology of these cancers and parallel analysis of their time trends should be rewarding. The known risk factors for cancer of the uterus are low parity, early menarche, late menopause, obesity and hormonal treatments. This last category is particularly important: it has been shown that unopposed oestrogen therapy used for alleviating the symptoms and harmful effects of the menopause increases the risk of endometrial cancer. Several case-control studies have shown that combined oral contraceptives have a protective effect, while sequential oral contraceptives may be a risk factor. The analyses reported here suggest that changes in the prevalence of these aetiological factors over time may be responsible for much of the observed change in incidence of cancer of the uterine corpus.

Europe

The patterns of change in risk for cancer of the uterine corpus in Europe appear complex on first examination. However, with the exception of Saarland (FRG), where there were problems of registration during the 1970s[299], it is possible to identify a group of populations with similar patterns of change in incidence by birth cohort. Finland, Sweden, and Denmark show an increase in lifetime risk (30-74 years) for older generations, a downward turn in risk for those born around 1925, and a clear decrease thereafter. The same is true in Germany (GDR) and in South Thames (UK), although the evidence for a peak in risk for cohorts born in the 1920s is less marked. It is likely that the decrease in risk in successive cohorts in Navarra (Spain), Bas-Rhin (France), and Varese (Italy) is of the same nature, although these trends are based on a shorter period of observation. Among eastern European populations, a similar pattern is seen for Slovenia, Warsaw City (Poland) and, although not statistically significant, for Szabolcs-Szatmar (Hungary). All these populations are characterised either by a recent decrease of the age-specific rate among young women or by a much smaller increase than for older women, and the trends are often well described by an age-cohort model.

Finally, in some populations, incidence is still increasing to some extent, such as among non-Jews in Israel and in County Vas (Hungary), Scotland and Birmingham (UK). In Zaragoza (Spain), the rate is small and the trend estimate is imprecise; despite the overall increase, it is worth noting that the rate has decreased among young women, as in Navarra (Spain).

The general pattern of mortality trends is consistent with an overall decrease. In Greece and Spain, where mortality rates have been very low by European standards, part of the observed increase may be attributable to improvement in death certification.

Asia and Oceania

The incidence of cancer of the uterine corpus in all nine Asian populations studied here is lower than in other parts of the world. Within Asia, incidence is highest in Hong Kong and among Chinese in Singapore, where it is clearly increasing in successive birth cohorts. The cohort increase in risk is especially marked in Japan, although clear period effects are also detected, and the recent trend is a 25-30% increase every five years (the data for Nagasaki are again inconsistent with those for Miyagi and Osaka). These observations are consistent with those for cancers of the breast and ovary, which share several risk factors linked to westernisation of life-style. The exponential increase in the risk of uterine cancer seen in Bom-

continued page 475

CORPUS UTERI (ICD-9 182)

EUROPE (non-EC), INCIDENCE

FEMALES	Best model	Goodness of fit	1970 Rate	1970 Cases	1985 Rate	1985 Cases	Cumulative risk 1915	Cumulative risk 1940	Recent trend
FINLAND	A8P5C9	-0.07	21.8	284	24.8	364	13.3	13.8	4.3
HUNGARY									
County Vas	A2D	-0.18	24.3	20	36.5	30	14.7	28.8	*9.0*
Szabolcs-Szatmar	A5	1.63	17.5	25	17.5	28	9.0	9.0	*-3.8*
ISRAEL									
All Jews	A4P3C2	-0.31	22.3	111	22.5	149	12.6	10.7	*2.8*
Non-Jews	A2D	0.98	5.0	1	5.9	4	3.0	4.0	*27.7*
NORWAY	A5P2	0.45	21.5	246	27.6	314	12.6	20.4	5.7
POLAND									
Warsaw City	A8P3C8	0.11	19.9	81	23.9	125	12.0	11.9	9.5
ROMANIA									
Cluj	A2	1.06	*11.8*	*20*	11.8	23	6.4	6.4	*-4.3*
SWEDEN	A7C7	2.83	27.0	669	28.1	725	15.0	11.5	*0.9*
SWITZERLAND									
Geneva	A2	1.58	32.7	32	32.7	36	19.0	19.0	*-6.0*
YUGOSLAVIA									
Slovenia	A4C4	-0.31	20.0	92	25.8	146	13.1	12.6	7.9

* : not enough cases for reliable estimation
− : incomplete or missing data
Best model: polynomial of the given degree in age (A), period (P) or cohort (C), or linear drift (D) model.
Goodness of fit: the normalised likelihood ratio chi-square for the best model (see Method).
Rate: world-standardised truncated rate per 100 000 per year (30-74 years) and number of **cases** are both estimated from the best-fitting model for the single years cited.
Cumulative risk per 1000 (30-74 years) is estimated from the best-fitting *age-cohort* model for cohorts of central birth year cited.
Recent trend: estimated mean percentage change per five-year period in the age-specific rates (30-74 years) over the period 1973-1987.
Italics denote recent trends not significant at 5 per cent level, or other figures which should be interpreted with caution (see Method).

FEMALES

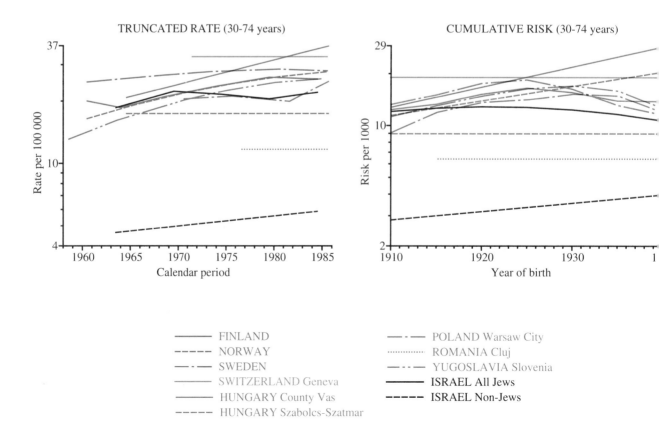

TRUNCATED RATE (30-74 years)

CUMULATIVE RISK (30-74 years)

———— FINLAND
------ NORWAY
—·—· SWEDEN
———— SWITZERLAND Geneva
———— HUNGARY County Vas
------ HUNGARY Szabolcs-Szatmar
—·— POLAND Warsaw City
············ ROMANIA Cluj
—··—·· YUGOSLAVIA Slovenia
———— ISRAEL All Jews
------ ISRAEL Non-Jews

CORPUS UTERI (ICD-9 182)

EUROPE (non-EC), INCIDENCE
Percentage change per five-year period, 1973-1987

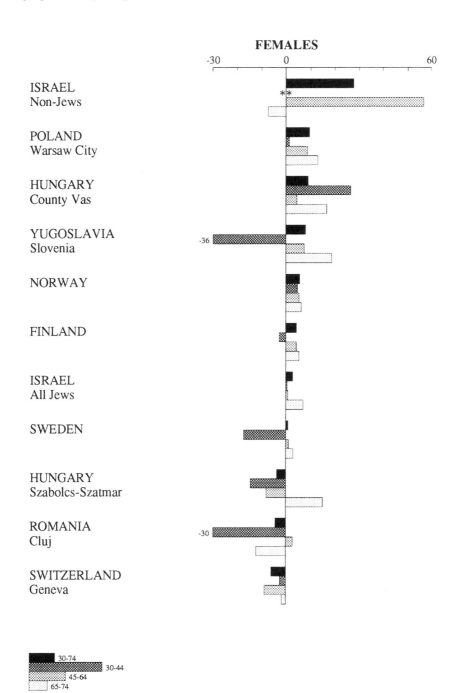

CORPUS UTERI (ICD-9 182)

EUROPE (EC), INCIDENCE

FEMALES	Best model	Goodness of fit	1970 Rate	1970 Cases	1985 Rate	1985 Cases	Cumulative risk 1915	Cumulative risk 1940	Recent trend
DENMARK	A4P2C9	2.53	26.9	390	34.0	523	17.5	16.9	9.7
FRANCE									
Bas-Rhin	A2P2C2	0.60	*117.1*	*298*	30.6	76	18.7	12.3	*1.5*
Doubs	A3D	-0.32	*36.6*	*30*	17.4	21	16.0	4.7	-21.6
GERMANY (FRG)									
Hamburg	A4D	0.08	18.7	133	*31.6*	*168*	13.5	*31.8*	–
Saarland	A4P2C4	1.04	53.6	191	27.8	109	30.3	3.1	-10.4
GERMANY (GDR)	A8C5	5.63	29.2	1716	30.8	1616	17.5	13.5	*0.4*
ITALY									
Varese	A2C3	1.46	*35.0*	*46*	29.2	72	14.7	15.3	*0.7*
SPAIN									
Navarra	A2C2	3.32	*26.8*	*31*	22.0	33	16.2	6.1	*-7.1*
Zaragoza	A4P2	2.45	8.5	18	16.7	42	7.2	21.4	*11.0*
UK									
Birmingham	A6D	4.54	19.3	291	21.1	321	11.1	12.9	*1.8*
Scotland	A5P2	0.66	14.8	239	16.0	247	8.4	9.0	4.8
South Thames	A8P5C5	1.65	17.3	512	18.2	380	10.6	8.0	*-1.4*

* : not enough cases for reliable estimation
– : incomplete or missing data
Best model: polynomial of the given degree in age (A), period (P) or cohort (C), or linear drift (D) model.
Goodness of fit: the normalised likelihood ratio chi-square for the best model (see Method).
Rate: world-standardised truncated rate per 100 000 per year (30-74 years) and number of **cases** are both estimated from the best-fitting model for the single years cited.
Cumulative risk per 1000 (30-74 years) is estimated from the best-fitting *age-cohort* model for cohorts of central birth year cited.
Recent trend: estimated mean percentage change per five-year period in the age-specific rates (30-74 years) over the period 1973-1987.
Italics denote recent trends not significant at 5 per cent level, or other figures which should be interpreted with caution (see Method).

FEMALES

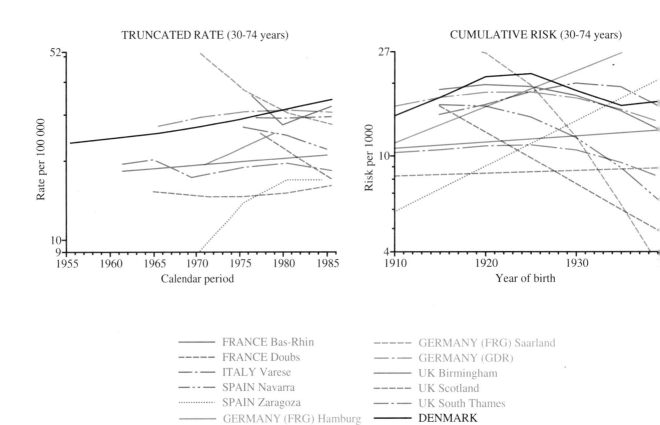

TRUNCATED RATE (30-74 years)   CUMULATIVE RISK (30-74 years)

———— FRANCE Bas-Rhin   ------ GERMANY (FRG) Saarland
------ FRANCE Doubs   —·— GERMANY (GDR)
—·— ITALY Varese   ———— UK Birmingham
—··— SPAIN Navarra   ------ UK Scotland
············ SPAIN Zaragoza   —·— UK South Thames
———— GERMANY (FRG) Hamburg   **———— DENMARK**

CORPUS UTERI (ICD-9 182)

EUROPE (EC), INCIDENCE
Percentage change per five-year period, 1973-1987

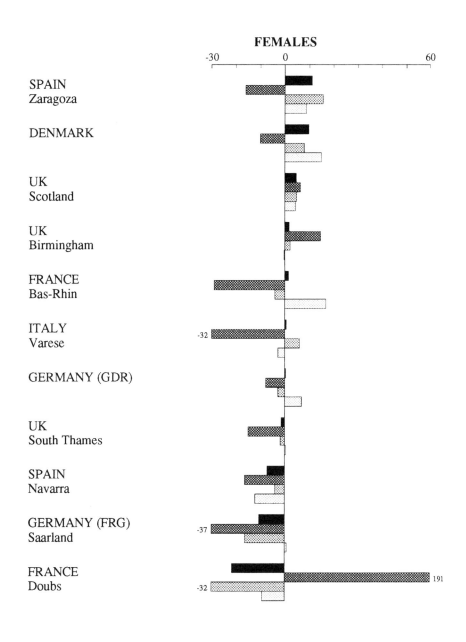

CORPUS UTERI (ICD-9 182)

EUROPE (non-EC), MORTALITY

FEMALES	Best model	Goodness of fit	1965 Rate	1965 Deaths	1985 Rate	1985 Deaths	Cumulative risk 1900	Cumulative risk 1940	Recent trend
AUSTRIA	A2D	-1.32	*1.1*	*31*	2.2	60	*0.8*	3.1	17.1
CZECHOSLOVAKIA	A2P4C9	2.64	4.8	202	6.6	300	3.9	6.2	-16.0
FINLAND	A2P4C2	3.16	4.7	59	3.8	64	4.0	0.8	-16.0
HUNGARY	A2P3C5	1.60	*72.2*	*2351*	7.6	271	*3.3*	3.7	12.2
NORWAY	A8C9	0.88	5.2	60	4.4	59	3.3	2.5	*-7.9*
POLAND	A3P2	0.33	2.9	223	*	*	2.7	*954.4*	–
ROMANIA	A3P2	6.72	*23.0*	*1094*	*33.7*	*2067*	*11.9*	*3.9*	–
SWEDEN	A8P6C9	-0.42	4.2	106	5.4	162	3.3	2.8	-18.8
SWITZERLAND	A2P4C6	-1.55	*0.1*	*2*	5.5	117	*3.0*	2.5	-13.7
YUGOSLAVIA	A4P5C4	3.45	10.2	437	2.9	175	5.7	1.5	-42.4

* : not enough deaths for reliable estimation
– : incomplete or missing data
Best model: polynomial of the given degree in age (A), period (P) or cohort (C), or linear drift (D) model.
Goodness of fit: the normalised likelihood ratio chi-square for the best model (see Method).
Rate: world-standardised truncated rate per 100 000 per year (30-74 years) and number of **deaths** are both estimated from the best-fitting model for the single years cited.
Cumulative risk per 1000 (30-74 years) is estimated from the best-fitting *age-cohort* model for cohorts of central birth year cited.
Recent trend: estimated mean percentage change per five-year period in the age-specific rates (30-74 years) over the period 1975-1988.
Italics denote recent trends not significant at 5 per cent level, or other figures which should be interpreted with caution (see Method).

FEMALES

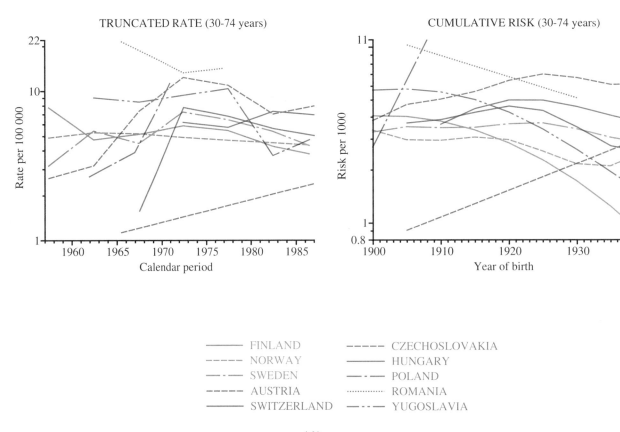

TRUNCATED RATE (30-74 years) CUMULATIVE RISK (30-74 years)

——— FINLAND	- - - - CZECHOSLOVAKIA
- - - - NORWAY	——— HUNGARY
—·— SWEDEN	—··— POLAND
- - - - AUSTRIA	············ ROMANIA
——— SWITZERLAND	—··—· YUGOSLAVIA

CORPUS UTERI (ICD-9 182)

EUROPE (non-EC), MORTALITY
Percentage change per five-year period, 1975-1988

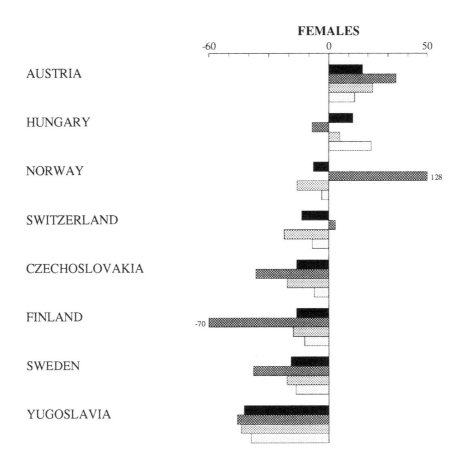

FEMALES

CORPUS UTERI (ICD-9 182)

EUROPE (EC), MORTALITY

FEMALES	Best model	Goodness of fit	1965 Rate	1965 Deaths	1985 Rate	1985 Deaths	Cumulative risk 1900	Cumulative risk 1940	Recent trend
BELGIUM	A2P6C6	0.34	7.6	227	2.6	82	3.5	0.7	-32.0
DENMARK	A8C9	-0.26	5.5	80	5.7	93	3.6	4.0	8.5
FRANCE	A5P3C2	0.26	1.3	196	1.6	260	0.9	0.8	*-1.6*
GERMANY (FRG)	A8P4C6	6.63	*13.5*	*2759*	2.5	574	*3.7*	0.3	-8.3
GREECE	A2C2	0.35	*0.1*	*2*	0.4	12	*0.1*	0.4	*12.3*
IRELAND	A2P5	3.12	2.1	15	3.9	32	1.7	6.5	-21.1
ITALY	A4P4C8	0.74	0.8	108	1.6	290	0.4	1.5	20.3
NETHERLANDS	A2P6C4	2.85	2.3	72	5.1	214	2.8	1.3	-9.0
PORTUGAL	–	–	–	–	–	–	–	–	–
SPAIN	A3P6C8	0.61	0.9	72	2.3	272	3.5	1.0	18.1
UK ENGLAND & WALES	A8P6C9	1.89	5.6	903	3.3	564	3.6	1.1	-10.0
UK SCOTLAND	A2P6C4	-0.01	3.2	55	3.1	53	2.1	2.7	-8.6

* : not enough deaths for reliable estimation
– : incomplete or missing data
Best model: polynomial of the given degree in age (A), period (P) or cohort (C), or linear drift (D) model.
Goodness of fit: the normalised likelihood ratio chi-square for the best model (see Method).
Rate: world-standardised truncated rate per 100 000 per year (30-74 years) and number of **deaths** are both estimated from the best-fitting model for the single years cited.
Cumulative risk per 1000 (30-74 years) is estimated from the best-fitting *age-cohort* model for cohorts of central birth year cited.
Recent trend: estimated mean percentage change per five-year period in the age-specific rates (30-74 years) over the period 1975-1988.
Italics denote recent trends not significant at 5 per cent level, or other figures which should be interpreted with caution (see Method).

FEMALES

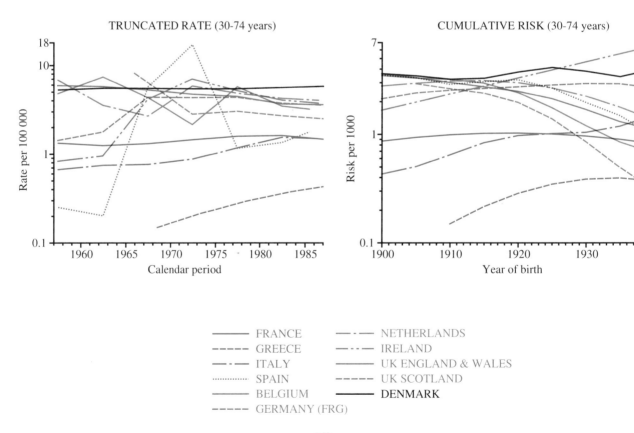

462

CORPUS UTERI (ICD-9 182)

EUROPE (EC), MORTALITY
Percentage change per five-year period, 1975-1988

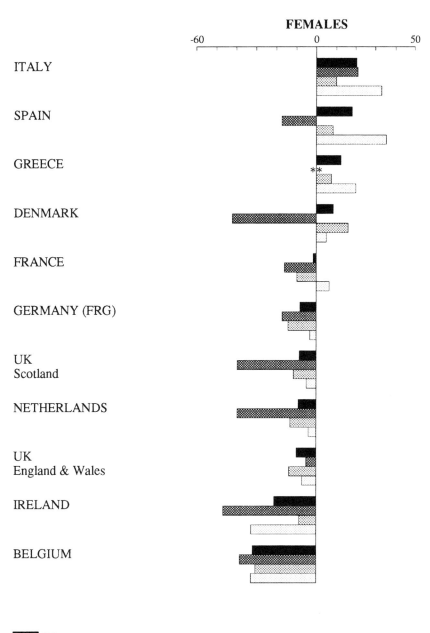

FEMALES

CORPUS UTERI (ICD-9 182)

ASIA, INCIDENCE

FEMALES	Best model	Goodness of fit	1970 Rate	1970 Cases	1985 Rate	1985 Cases	Cumulative risk 1915	Cumulative risk 1940	Recent trend
CHINA									
Shanghai	A8C7	0.21	*16.5*	*205*	5.9	107	3.9	2.2	-13.0
HONG KONG	A8C7	0.80	*11.2*	*84*	14.6	157	5.7	12.1	9.3
INDIA									
Bombay	A2D	0.68	3.1	15	4.7	44	2.1	4.1	19.6
JAPAN									
Miyagi	A2P3C2	1.58	2.6	10	7.3	43	1.9	8.2	24.5
Nagasaki	A2	-1.13	*6.4*	*6*	6.4	8	3.0	3.0	*2.3*
Osaka	A4P2	2.15	1.4	20	5.9	131	1.7	9.4	35.2
SINGAPORE									
Chinese	A2C2	0.76	9.6	22	13.0	46	5.0	11.1	25.1
Indian	A1C2	0.06	10.4	1	8.0	1	6.9	1.9	*-38.5*
Malay	A8C8	-0.70	4.1	1	4.7	2	2.0	5.1	*4.9*

* : not enough cases for reliable estimation
– : incomplete or missing data
Best model: polynomial of the given degree in age (A), period (P) or cohort (C), or linear drift (D) model.
Goodness of fit: the normalised likelihood ratio chi-square for the best model (see Method).
Rate: world-standardised truncated rate per 100 000 per year (30-74 years) and number of **cases** are both estimated from the best-fitting model for the single years cited.
Cumulative risk per 1000 (30-74 years) is estimated from the best-fitting *age-cohort* model for cohorts of central birth year cited.
Recent trend: estimated mean percentage change per five-year period in the age-specific rates (30-74 years) over the period 1973-1987.
Italics denote recent trends not significant at 5 per cent level, or other figures which should be interpreted with caution (see Method).

FEMALES

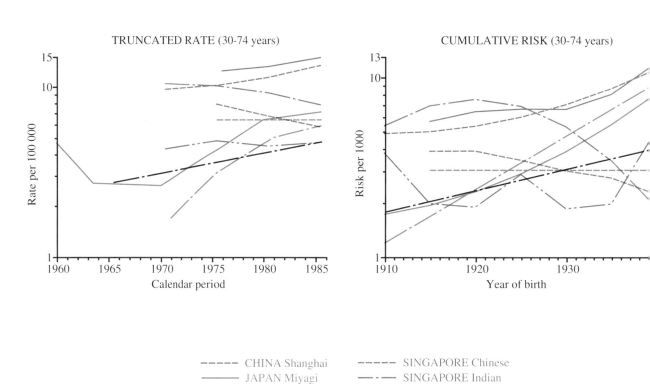

TRUNCATED RATE (30-74 years)   CUMULATIVE RISK (30-74 years)

----- CHINA Shanghai   ----- SINGAPORE Chinese
——— JAPAN Miyagi   —-— SINGAPORE Indian
----- JAPAN Nagasaki   —--— SINGAPORE Malay
—-— JAPAN Osaka   —--— INDIA Bombay
——— HONG KONG

CORPUS UTERI (ICD-9 182)

ASIA, INCIDENCE
Percentage change per five-year period, 1973-1987

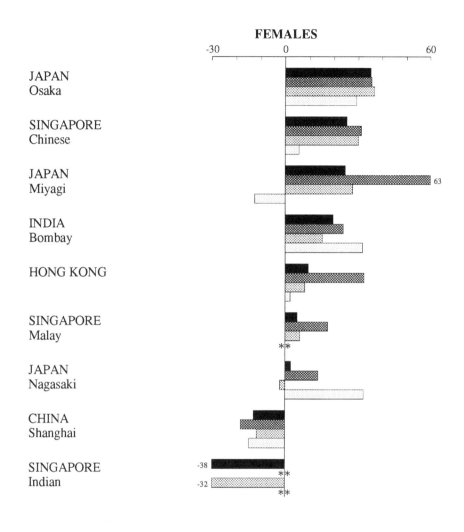

FEMALES

JAPAN
Osaka

SINGAPORE
Chinese

JAPAN
Miyagi   63

INDIA
Bombay

HONG KONG

SINGAPORE
Malay
**

JAPAN
Nagasaki

CHINA
Shanghai

SINGAPORE   -38
Indian   **
             -32
              **

30-74
30-44
45-64
65-74

CORPUS UTERI (ICD-9 182)

OCEANIA, INCIDENCE

FEMALES	Best model	Goodness of fit	1970 Rate	1970 Cases	1985 Rate	1985 Cases	Cumulative risk 1915	Cumulative risk 1940	Recent trend
AUSTRALIA									
New South Wales	A5D	1.35	*16.2*	*187*	18.5	253	9.6	12.0	4.3
South	A2P2	-0.65	*209.5*	*471*	23.2	83	14.8	11.2	*-4.4*
HAWAII									
Caucasian	A2P4C2	0.85	57.9	20	37.3	21	35.3	12.0	-27.8
Chinese	A2C2	0.07	47.1	4	38.5	6	28.2	9.7	-24.3
Filipino	A2	0.99	24.8	2	24.8	6	11.3	11.3	*-18.9*
Hawaiian	A2P2	-0.76	70.0	11	39.1	11	30.3	20.2	-27.5
Japanese	A4P2C5	-0.35	34.6	19	32.7	30	24.0	14.2	-14.5
NEW ZEALAND									
Maori	A2	0.93	39.4	8	39.4	14	21.0	21.0	*-1.2*
Non-Maori	A4D	0.26	22.9	139	20.7	150	12.2	10.3	-8.2

* : not enough cases for reliable estimation
– : incomplete or missing data
Best model: polynomial of the given degree in age (A), period (P) or cohort (C), or linear drift (D) model.
Goodness of fit: the normalised likelihood ratio chi-square for the best model (see Method).
Rate: world-standardised truncated rate per 100 000 per year (30-74 years) and number of **cases** are both estimated from the best-fitting model for the single years cited.
Cumulative risk per 1000 (30-74 years) is estimated from the best-fitting *age-cohort* model for cohorts of central birth year cited.
Recent trend: estimated mean percentage change per five-year period in the age-specific rates (30-74 years) over the period 1973-1987.
Italics denote recent trends not significant at 5 per cent level, or other figures which should be interpreted with caution (see Method).

FEMALES

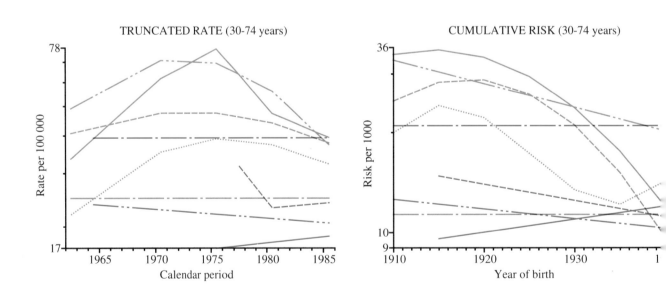

TRUNCATED RATE (30-74 years) — Rate per 100 000 — Calendar period

CUMULATIVE RISK (30-74 years) — Risk per 1000 — Year of birth

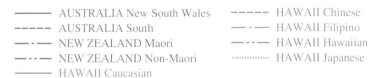

AUSTRALIA New South Wales
AUSTRALIA South
NEW ZEALAND Maori
NEW ZEALAND Non-Maori
HAWAII Caucasian
HAWAII Chinese
HAWAII Filipino
HAWAII Hawaiian
HAWAII Japanese

CORPUS UTERI (ICD-9 182)

OCEANIA, INCIDENCE
Percentage change per five-year period, 1973-1987

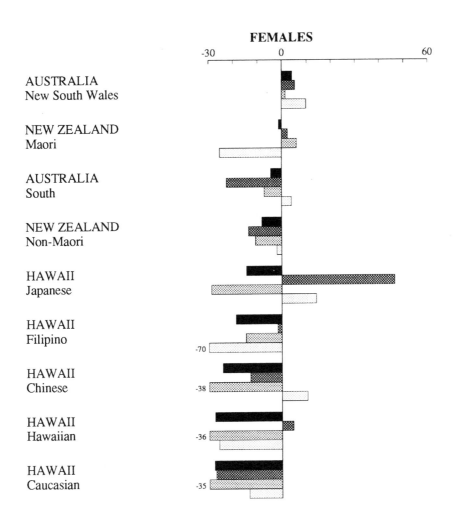

CORPUS UTERI (ICD-9 182)

ASIA and OCEANIA, MORTALITY

FEMALES	Best model	Goodness of fit	1965 Rate	1965 Deaths	1985 Rate	1985 Deaths	Cumulative risk 1900	Cumulative risk 1940	Recent trend
AUSTRALIA	A2P6C3	1.94	4.4	117	3.3	138	2.6	1.2	*-2.9*
HONG KONG	A2P3	-0.04	*1.5*	*8*	1.4	13	*2.9*	0.4	-20.7
JAPAN	A6P6C5	5.04	1.8	354	0.9	316	0.8	0.3	20.0
MAURITIUS	–	–	–	–	–	–	–	–	–
NEW ZEALAND	A2D	0.94	5.9	34	4.3	35	3.8	2.0	-16.7
SINGAPORE	A2	1.07	1.0	1	1.0	3	*0.5*	0.5	–

* : not enough deaths for reliable estimation
– : incomplete or missing data
Best model: polynomial of the given degree in age (A), period (P) or cohort (C), or linear drift (D) model.
Goodness of fit: the normalised likelihood ratio chi-square for the best model (see Method).
Rate: world-standardised truncated rate per 100 000 per year (30-74 years) and number of **deaths** are both estimated from the best-fitting model for the single years cited.
Cumulative risk per 1000 (30-74 years) is estimated from the best-fitting *age-cohort* model for cohorts of central birth year cited.
Recent trend: estimated mean percentage change per five-year period in the age-specific rates (30-74 years) over the period 1975-1988.
Italics denote recent trends not significant at 5 per cent level, or other figures which should be interpreted with caution (see Method).

FEMALES

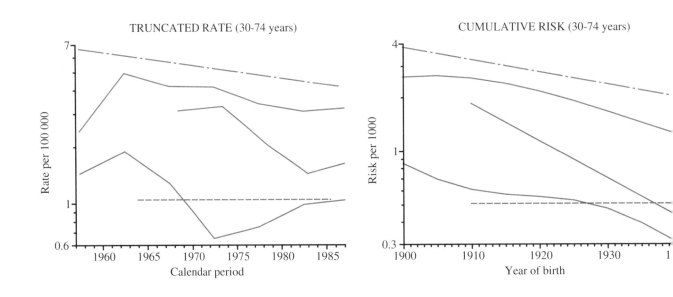

TRUNCATED RATE (30-74 years)

CUMULATIVE RISK (30-74 years)

——— AUSTRALIA   ——— HONG KONG
—·—· NEW ZEALAND   - - - - SINGAPORE
——— JAPAN

CORPUS UTERI (ICD-9 182)

ASIA and OCEANIA, MORTALITY
Percentage change per five-year period, 1975-1988

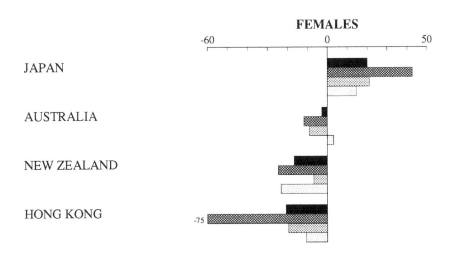

FEMALES

JAPAN

AUSTRALIA

NEW ZEALAND

HONG KONG

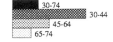

30-74
30-44
45-64
65-74

CORPUS UTERI (ICD-9 182)

AMERICAS (except USA), INCIDENCE

FEMALES	Best model	Goodness of fit	1970 Rate	1970 Cases	1985 Rate	1985 Cases	Cumulative risk 1915	Cumulative risk 1940	Recent trend
BRAZIL									
Sao Paulo	A2D	-0.69	17.8	121	*32.8*	*305*	11.2	*30.6*	–
CANADA									
Alberta	A5P5C7	-1.00	30.9	91	30.4	141	24.0	18.1	-9.2
British Columbia	A4P3C5	0.87	31.4	150	31.0	241	27.1	10.8	-12.7
Maritime Provinces	A6C2	1.45	26.4	85	28.7	113	17.3	12.8	*0.7*
Newfoundland	A3	-0.42	22.6	18	22.6	24	12.0	12.0	*1.7*
Quebec	A7P4C5	3.34	29.2	354	35.1	592	20.6	19.2	*2.7*
COLOMBIA									
Cali	A2P2C2	-0.85	10.4	9	12.3	21	6.9	4.2	*10.6*
CUBA	A2P2C3	4.85	22.3	291	10.7	213	8.5	*2.6*	–
PUERTO RICO	A3P4C3	1.08	12.3	56	18.0	137	8.1	15.4	12.8

* : not enough cases for reliable estimation
– : incomplete or missing data
Best model: polynomial of the given degree in age (A), period (P) or cohort (C), or linear drift (D) model.
Goodness of fit: the normalised likelihood ratio chi-square for the best model (see Method).
Rate: world-standardised truncated rate per 100 000 per year (30-74 years) and number of **cases** are both estimated from the best-fitting model for the single years cited.
Cumulative risk per 1000 (30-74 years) is estimated from the best-fitting *age-cohort* model for cohorts of central birth year cited.
Recent trend: estimated mean percentage change per five-year period in the age-specific rates (30-74 years) over the period 1973-1987.
Italics denote recent trends not significant at 5 per cent level, or other figures which should be interpreted with caution (see Method).

FEMALES

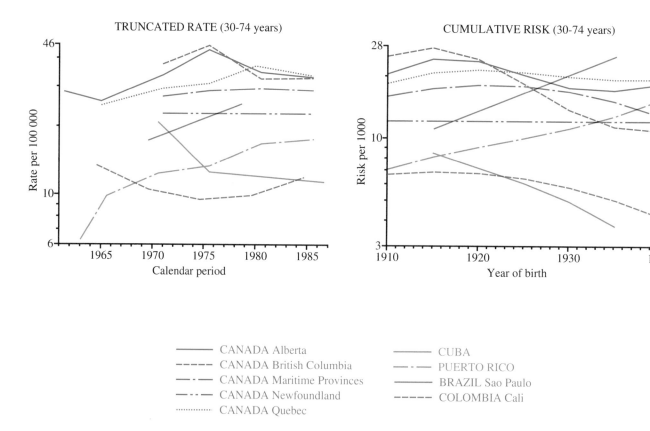

CORPUS UTERI (ICD-9 182)

AMERICAS (except USA), INCIDENCE
Percentage change per five-year period, 1973-1987

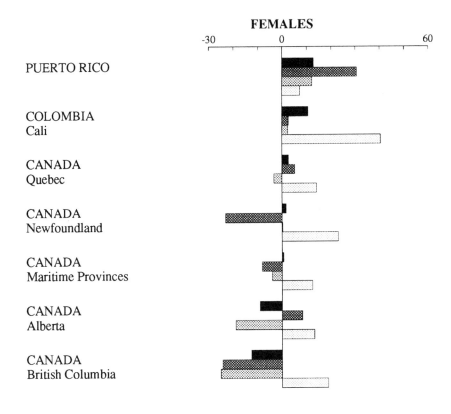

FEMALES

CORPUS UTERI (ICD-9 182)

AMERICAS (USA), INCIDENCE

FEMALES	Best model	Goodness of fit	1970 Rate	1970 Cases	1985 Rate	1985 Cases	Cumulative risk 1915	Cumulative risk 1940	Recent trend
USA									
Bay Area, Black	A3	1.24	22.3	13	22.3	22	13.2	13.2	*-4.2*
Bay Area, Chinese	A3	0.72	34.3	6	*34.3*	*17*	16.3	*16.3*	–
Bay Area, White	A8P3C7	1.46	46.6	322	44.6	315	43.9	13.3	-24.1
Connecticut	A6P2C6	2.92	40.5	306	36.9	337	25.2	18.0	-9.9
Detroit, Black	A5C2	0.53	21.2	31	20.6	45	14.0	8.5	*-3.5*
Detroit, White	A6P3C7	2.38	42.1	351	45.3	377	31.4	22.9	-8.1
Iowa	A5P3C5	2.65	32.9	240	39.0	301	26.5	20.8	-6.1
New Orleans, Black	A3	2.69	*20.9*	*13*	20.9	16	13.4	13.4	*-1.3*
New Orleans, White	A2C5	0.30	*37.5*	*83*	21.6	40	14.4	9.6	*-5.1*
Seattle	A4P2C5	1.02	*184.8*	*898*	46.8	340	55.6	11.1	-23.5

* : not enough cases for reliable estimation
– : incomplete or missing data
Best model: polynomial of the given degree in age (A), period (P) or cohort (C), or linear drift (D) model.
Goodness of fit: the normalised likelihood ratio chi-square for the best model (see Method).
Rate: world-standardised truncated rate per 100 000 per year (30-74 years) and number of **cases** are both estimated from the best-fitting model for the single years cited.
Cumulative risk per 1000 (30-74 years) is estimated from the best-fitting *age-cohort* model for cohorts of central birth year cited.
Recent trend: estimated mean percentage change per five-year period in the age-specific rates (30-74 years) over the period 1973-1987.
Italics denote recent trends not significant at 5 per cent level, or other figures which should be interpreted with caution (see Method).

FEMALES

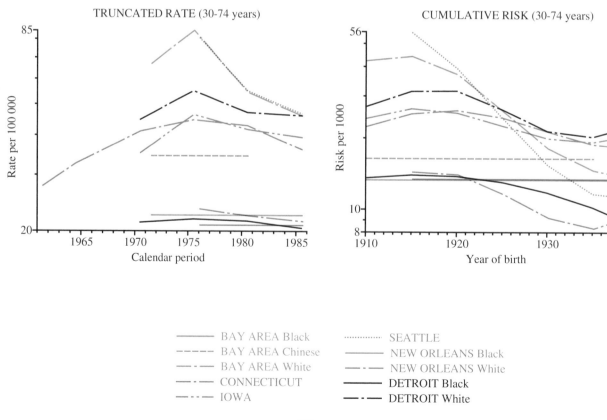

472

CORPUS UTERI (ICD-9 182)

AMERICAS (USA), INCIDENCE
Percentage change per five-year period, 1973-1987

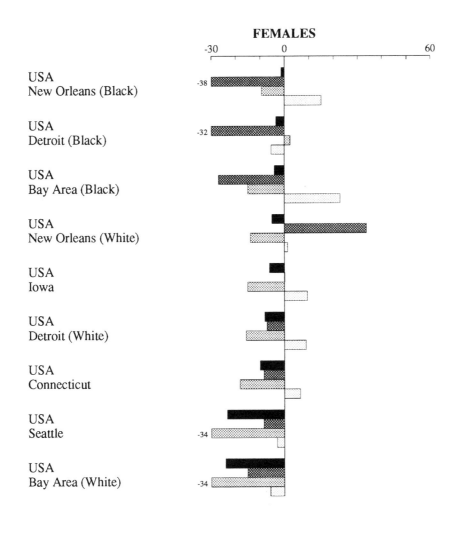

CORPUS UTERI (ICD-9 182)

AMERICAS, MORTALITY

FEMALES	Best model	Goodness of fit	1965 Rate	1965 Deaths	1985 Rate	1985 Deaths	Cumulative risk 1900	Cumulative risk 1940	Recent trend
CANADA	A3C2	-0.39	4.1	158	3.1	210	2.7	1.1	-7.2
CHILE	A2D	1.10	1.0	12	*2.8*	*58*	0.7	*5.4*	–
COSTA RICA	–	–	–	–	–	–	–	–	–
PANAMA	–	–	–	–	–	–	–	–	–
PUERTO RICO	–	–	–	–	–	–	–	–	–
URUGUAY	–	–	–	–	–	–	–	–	–
USA	A8P6C9	9.99	8.7	4198	4.3	2920	6.3	0.9	-28.2
VENEZUELA	A2D	2.14	1.5	14	*3.2*	*59*	0.9	*3.6*	–

* : not enough deaths for reliable estimation
– : incomplete or missing data
Best model: polynomial of the given degree in age (A), period (P) or cohort (C), or linear drift (D) model.
Goodness of fit: the normalised likelihood ratio chi-square for the best model (see Method).
Rate: world-standardised truncated rate per 100 000 per year (30-74 years) and number of **deaths** are both estimated from the best-fitting model for the single years cited.
Cumulative risk per 1000 (30-74 years) is estimated from the best-fitting *age-cohort* model for cohorts of central birth year cited.
Recent trend: estimated mean percentage change per five-year period in the age-specific rates (30-74 years) over the period 1975-1988.
Italics denote recent trends not significant at 5 per cent level, or other figures which should be interpreted with caution (see Method).

FEMALES

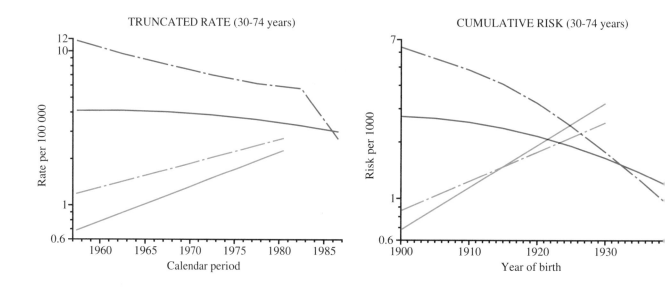

TRUNCATED RATE (30-74 years)

CUMULATIVE RISK (30-74 years)

——— CANADA
—·— USA
——— CHILE
—·— VENEZUELA

474

CORPUS UTERI (ICD-9 182)

AMERICAS, MORTALITY
Percentage change per five-year period, 1975-1988

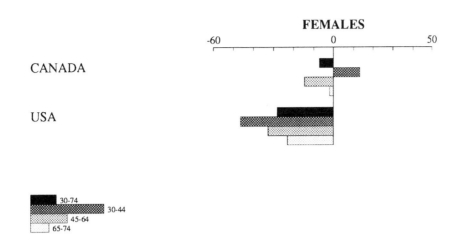

from page 455

bay (India) is even greater than that observed for breast cancer in this population. In contrast, the incidence of uterine cancer is decreasing in Shanghai (China), though less quickly than for cervix cancer, and among Indians in Singapore.

In the three Asian countries for which mortality data were available, mortality is quite low, with a truncated rate of about 1 per 100 000. Mortality is clearly declining in Hong Kong. In Japan, however, although the period effect is irregular, mortality has doubled since the mid-1970s, and there is a significant recent increase among 30-44 year-olds (42% every five years, three standard errors).

In Hawaii the pattern is extremely clear, and similar in all ethnic groups except Filipinos. The truncated rate increased up to 1975 and then declined. This pattern is similar to that observed in most North American white populations. A cohort effect similar to that observed in Europe may also be present, especially for Caucasians, for whom the decrease among young women is of the order of 30% every five years. The same may be true for the Chinese population.

Incidence rates for uterine cancer in Australia and the non-Maori population of New Zealand are in the European range, and about half the levels in Hawaii or North America. Incidence is increasing at a similar rate in New South Wales and in South Australia, where there is an irregular period effect. In contrast, the risk among non-Maoris in New Zealand has been declining steadily since the mid-1960s. There has been no

change among Maori women, who have retained a higher level of risk throughout the last 25 years. National mortality trends in both Australia and New Zealand show a steady decline, although the period effect in Australia suggests this rate of decline has slowed down in the decade up to 1988.

Americas

In North America, the pattern of change is extremely striking. It has two distinct components: a marked period effect with a peak in 1975, probably due to the use of unopposed oestrogen therapy for menopausal symptoms, and a cohort-wise decrease for women born since 1925. It is remarkable that the 1975 peak is absent among black and Chinese populations, while the cohort effect is present in all populations. Although it is not significant in the San Francisco Bay Area or New Orleans, it is clear that the cohort effect is the same among black populations, as can be seen from the recent linear trends by age. The white population of New Orleans is slightly atypical, in that the risk of uterine cancer is increasing again for women born since 1935. The data for 1945 (not shown) suggest that this trend is still continuing.

The data from South America confirm that the incidence of cancer of the uterine corpus was lower than in North America in the 1970s. The risk of this cancer has, however, changed differently in the four populations available: while in Cali (Colombia) the risk has decreased, as for ovarian cancer, in Puerto Rico the risk has increased, as for breast cancer. These observations are compatible with a smaller increase of breast cancer risk in Cali and a smaller decline in ovarian cancer risk in Puerto Rico. In São Paulo (Brazil), cancers of the breast, ovary, and uterine corpus cancers have been increasing at the same rate. In Cuba, the data are too sparse to permit any conclusion to be drawn, and even the best age-period-cohort model fits poorly.

The available mortality data show a steady decline in both Canada and the USA since the 1960s, but the rate of decline and its recent acceleration have been more marked in the USA, and the earlier two-fold difference in mortality between the countries had disappeared by 1985. Mortality from uterine cancer in Chile and Venezuela has risen steadily by three-fold from very low rates in the 1960s to reach about 3 per 100 000 in 1980, but more recent data were unavailable.

Comment

The change in cancer of the uterine corpus is particularly clear in the USA, where the overall decline has been previously noted[77,85]. These authors concluded that the observed 3% per year decline in mortality would in fact be only 1.5% if both hysterectomy and the lack of specificity of death certification were taken into account. They also suggest that the decline among women under 55 years of age may be partly explained by the use of combined oral contraceptives. The peak and decline of uterine cancer incidence in Connecticut (USA) around 1975, after correction of the population at risk for prior hysterectomy, was restricted to localised invasive carcinoma in women aged 45-64 and was closely related to trends in prescription of non-contraceptive oral oestrogens[177]. A recent and detailed analysis of the SEER data in relation to hormone prescription, including post-menopausal progestins, suggests that more recent formulations of post-menopausal treatment and oral contraceptives may be involved in the observed decline[230]. This hypothesis was also suggested from an earlier examination of the Connecticut data[126].

The protective effect of oral contraceptives has also been given as the explanation for the declining trend in England and Wales[294], and the cohort effect observed for both incidence and mortality in Sweden has also been ascribed to patterns of hormone prescription[231]. Further data on uterine cancer trend in the Pannonian region of central Europe (Austria, Czechoslovakia, Hungary and Yugoslavia) have been published by the Pannonian Tumor Epidemiology Study Group[218]. The incidence of uterine cancer is increasing in Burgenland county (Austria), on the Hungarian border adjacent to County Vas, where an increase has also been recorded; the data from Burgenland are consistent with the national increase in mortality in Austria shown here.

It may be that the similar patterns of decline seen for cancer of the uterus and cancer of the ovary are due to a protective effect of combined oral contraceptives; the data suggest that the effect is more marked for the uterus than for the ovary.

Chapter 20

OVARY

Ovarian cancer varies widely in frequency between geographical regions, and is generally more frequent in more affluent populations. Since survival is poor (25-35% at five years), it is an important cause of mortality among women in many developed countries. There is a six-fold geographical variation between the populations examined here, ranging from a cumulative risk of 1.7% to less than 0.3%. The high-risk countries are found in north-western Europe, especially Scandinavia, and in North America; Japanese populations and non-Jews in Israel are at low risk. The cumulative risk of dying from the disease between 30 and 74 years of age is highest in Denmark, where it was 1.7% for the generation born in 1915, and it is high (close to 1%) in several countries of Europe and North America. Except for countries where errors in death certification may be large, the geographical variation in mortality is generally consistent with that of incidence.

The aetiology of ovarian cancer is poorly understood, and only two protective factors have been consistently documented: parity and combined oral contraceptive use. The protection afforded by parity is of the order of 40% for two children, while the average effect of oral contraceptives is 50%, and may be as large as 80%, depending on duration of use. In addition, oral contraceptives further increase the protection given by parity[156].

There is some evidence that the survival of patients with ovarian cancer has improved in recent years[16], due to earlier stage at diagnosis and possibly to the introduction of combination chemotherapy with cisplatin.

Europe

In most European populations the frequency of ovarian cancer is either decreasing or stable. The main exceptions are County Vas (Hungary) and Navarra (Spain), where a large exponential increase is seen. For populations in which a decrease in risk of ovarian cancer is observed, this decrease is more evident on a cohort basis; Finland, Sweden, Slovenia, Denmark, and Saarland (FRG) are the best examples of this type of trend. In other countries there is often a suggestion of a recent decrease in the younger age groups, but the numbers are frequently too small to allow a

decline in risk to be clearly identified. In Birmingham (UK), the best age-cohort model may overemphasize the reduction in risk among the younger generations. The bar charts suggest that the age-specific rates among 30-44 year-old women are still increasing; this apparent contradiction, however, is almost entirely due to the large increase which occurred in the period 1983-87, as can be seen from the graph of truncated rates. This period effect is highly significant, as shown by the best model; it is hard to explain and needs further study.

The mortality data show the same pattern as incidence data, but the geographical differences are more marked. The reduction in mortality is seen in all Nordic countries, with the exception of Iceland (data not shown). This reduction is also seen in the Netherlands and Belgium, where no incidence data were available, and the decrease is especially large in the Netherlands. In France and Italy, where the risk of death was lower, the increase has stopped, as shown by the cumulative risk graph and the recent trend among 30-44 year-olds. The large increases seen in Yugoslavia, Poland, Spain and Portugal are outside the range observed for the rest of Europe, and greater than would be expected from the incidence data. The most likely explanation is under-certification of death in the 1960s; ovarian cancer is difficult to diagnose, and may have been incorrectly certified as other or unspecified abdominal malignancy. In Germany, the extremely bad fit is almost entirely due to outlying observations in the first period of observation (1965-66) for the age groups 45-49 and 50-54 years.

Asia and Oceania

The most striking changes in incidence arise in Japan and Hong Kong, where there has been an exponential increase of about 15-25% every five years. The data from Nagasaki (Japan) are inconsistent with the data from Miyagi and Osaka, as for other sites: the rates in the first two periods are clearly over-estimated. Among Singapore Chinese, the increase between the first two calendar periods and the last two periods is highly significant; the significance of the trend in cumulative risk among Indians in Singapore is slightly over-emphasised by the age-cohort model, given the

continued page 497

OVARY (ICD-9 183)

EUROPE (non-EC), INCIDENCE

FEMALES	Best model	Goodness of fit	1970 Rate	1970 Cases	1985 Rate	1985 Cases	Cumulative risk 1915	Cumulative risk 1940	Recent trend
FINLAND	A3P2C2	0.05	21.6	276	19.4	280	11.5	10.0	-5.0
HUNGARY									
County Vas	A7D	-1.41	17.5	14	24.0	19	10.4	17.6	22.9
Szabolcs-Szatmar	A3	-2.05	12.3	18	12.3	19	6.2	6.2	-9.2
ISRAEL									
All Jews	A3	0.32	24.7	122	24.7	164	13.1	13.1	-3.1
Non-Jews	A1	0.93	6.1	2	6.1	4	3.4	3.4	-27.0
NORWAY	A5P2C4	0.69	28.8	317	30.7	350	15.1	18.8	-0.1
POLAND									
Warsaw City	A3C3	-0.04	23.1	93	24.3	123	12.7	13.0	0.4
ROMANIA									
Cluj	A2	-0.49	14.7	25	14.7	29	7.6	7.6	8.6
SWEDEN	A5P2C2	2.92	31.9	768	30.7	773	17.0	16.2	-2.3
SWITZERLAND									
Geneva	A3	0.07	24.2	23	24.2	26	13.1	13.1	5.6
YUGOSLAVIA									
Slovenia	A3C2	-0.11	20.5	93	20.3	111	11.3	9.5	-3.8

* : not enough cases for reliable estimation
– : incomplete or missing data
Best model: polynomial of the given degree in age (A), period (P) or cohort (C), or linear drift (D) model.
Goodness of fit: the normalised likelihood ratio chi-square for the best model (see Method).
Rate: world-standardised truncated rate per 100 000 per year (30-74 years) and number of **cases** are both estimated from the best-fitting model for the single years cited.
Cumulative risk per 1000 (30-74 years) is estimated from the best-fitting *age-cohort* model for cohorts of central birth year cited.
Recent trend: estimated mean percentage change per five-year period in the age-specific rates (30-74 years) over the period 1973-1987.
Italics denote recent trends not significant at 5 per cent level, or other figures which should be interpreted with caution (see Method).

FEMALES

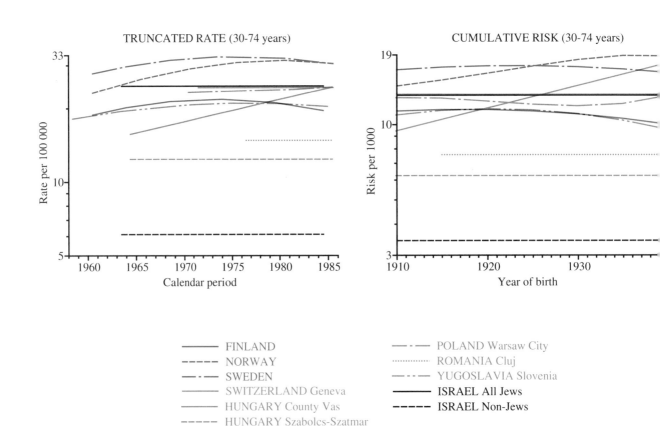

TRUNCATED RATE (30-74 years)   CUMULATIVE RISK (30-74 years)

——— FINLAND
----- NORWAY
—·— SWEDEN
——— SWITZERLAND Geneva
——— HUNGARY County Vas
----- HUNGARY Szabolcs-Szatmar
—·— POLAND Warsaw City
············ ROMANIA Cluj
—··— YUGOSLAVIA Slovenia
——— ISRAEL All Jews
----- ISRAEL Non-Jews

OVARY (ICD-9 183)

EUROPE (non-EC), INCIDENCE
Percentage change per five-year period, 1973-1987

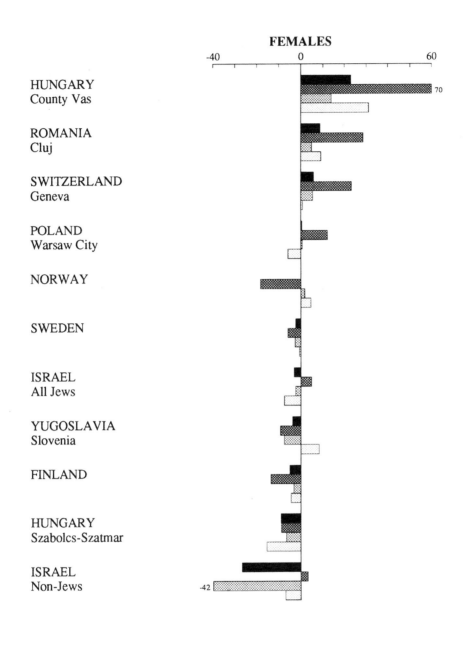

FEMALES

HUNGARY
County Vas

ROMANIA
Cluj

SWITZERLAND
Geneva

POLAND
Warsaw City

NORWAY

SWEDEN

ISRAEL
All Jews

YUGOSLAVIA
Slovenia

FINLAND

HUNGARY
Szabolcs-Szatmar

ISRAEL
Non-Jews

30-74
30-44
45-64
65-74

OVARY (ICD-9 183)

EUROPE (EC), INCIDENCE

FEMALES	Best model	Goodness of fit	1970 Rate	1970 Cases	1985 Rate	1985 Cases	Cumulative risk 1915	Cumulative risk 1940	Recent trend
DENMARK	A8P6C9	0.25	33.2	464	31.9	472	16.6	14.2	*1.0*
FRANCE									
Bas-Rhin	A2C2	0.33	*18.4*	*44*	26.4	64	12.6	16.6	13.1
Doubs	A2	0.56	*19.2*	*16*	19.2	22	10.1	10.1	*15.6*
GERMANY (FRG)									
Hamburg	A8P2	0.23	22.8	153	*16.1*	*83*	14.2	20.9	–
Saarland	A4C2	-1.38	19.2	67	19.0	69	11.4	8.6	*-1.2*
GERMANY (GDR)	A6C2	4.86	25.5	1485	25.5	1306	13.9	12.9	*0.1*
ITALY									
Varese	A3	-0.57	*21.6*	*38*	21.6	51	11.1	11.1	-2.5
SPAIN									
Navarra	A4D	0.84	*6.8*	*8*	17.8	24	5.3	26.3	37.5
Zaragoza	A2C2	2.41	7.8	15	12.1	30	5.2	8.1	*7.3*
UK									
Birmingham	A5P3C5	-0.64	24.0	343	27.9	412	13.0	12.6	10.8
Scotland	A4C2	-1.43	20.6	316	25.8	392	12.6	15.5	9.2
South Thames	A8C9	0.67	24.2	681	25.6	510	13.3	13.7	*2.3*

* : not enough cases for reliable estimation
– : incomplete or missing data
Best model: polynomial of the given degree in age (A), period (P) or cohort (C), or linear drift (D) model.
Goodness of fit: the normalised likelihood ratio chi-square for the best model (see Method).
Rate: world-standardised truncated rate per 100 000 per year (30-74 years) and number of **cases** are both estimated from the best-fitting model for the single years cited.
Cumulative risk per 1000 (30-74 years) is estimated from the best-fitting *age-cohort* model for cohorts of central birth year cited.
Recent trend: estimated mean percentage change per five-year period in the age-specific rates (30-74 years) over the period 1973-1987.
Italics denote recent trends not significant at 5 per cent level, or other figures which should be interpreted with caution (see Method).

FEMALES

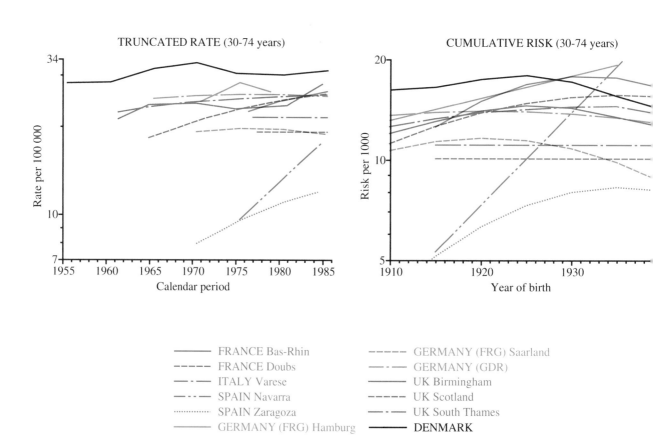

TRUNCATED RATE (30-74 years) — Rate per 100 000 — Calendar period

CUMULATIVE RISK (30-74 years) — Risk per 1000 — Year of birth

FRANCE Bas-Rhin
FRANCE Doubs
ITALY Varese
SPAIN Navarra
SPAIN Zaragoza
GERMANY (FRG) Hamburg
GERMANY (FRG) Saarland
GERMANY (GDR)
UK Birmingham
UK Scotland
UK South Thames
DENMARK

OVARY (ICD-9 183)

EUROPE (EC), INCIDENCE
Percentage change per five-year period, 1973-1987

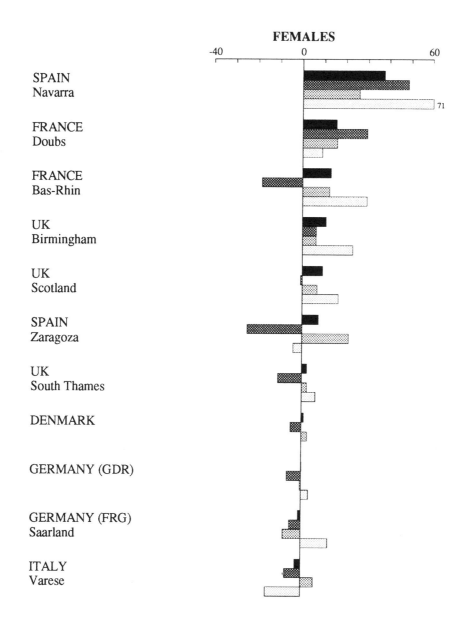

OVARY (ICD-9 183)

EUROPE (non-EC), MORTALITY

FEMALES	Best model	Goodness of fit	1965 Rate	Deaths	1985 Rate	Deaths	Cumulative risk 1900	1940	Recent trend
AUSTRIA	A5C2	1.11	*18.5*	*464*	16.8	414	*10.3*	7.3	-4.0
CZECHOSLOVAKIA	A8C2	0.72	14.3	579	17.3	741	7.4	10.3	3.9
FINLAND	A8P6C9	0.22	13.1	160	10.3	155	6.9	5.6	-9.9
HUNGARY	A8P3C8	0.82	*17.3*	*499*	15.1	507	*7.6*	8.2	*1.8*
NORWAY	A3C2	-1.42	17.7	192	17.4	213	9.6	8.6	*0.2*
POLAND	A5P3C2	2.99	7.8	585	13.7	1299	3.6	*11.0*	–
ROMANIA	–	–	–	–	–	–	–	–	–
SWEDEN	A8P6C9	-0.26	19.9	476	15.8	424	11.4	7.7	-9.3
SWITZERLAND	A3C2	0.18	17.0	284	14.5	288	9.9	6.2	-11.3
YUGOSLAVIA	A6P2C2	-0.36	5.7	244	9.2	554	2.8	6.6	7.5

∗ : not enough deaths for reliable estimation
– : incomplete or missing data
Best model: polynomial of the given degree in age (A), period (P) or cohort (C), or linear drift (D) model.
Goodness of fit: the normalised likelihood ratio chi-square for the best model (see Method).
Rate: world-standardised truncated rate per 100 000 per year (30-74 years) and number of **deaths** are both estimated from the best-fitting model for the single years cited.
Cumulative risk per 1000 (30-74 years) is estimated from the best-fitting *age-cohort* model for cohorts of central birth year cited.
Recent trend: estimated mean percentage change per five-year period in the age-specific rates (30-74 years) over the period 1975-1988.
Italics denote recent trends not significant at 5 per cent level, or other figures which should be interpreted with caution (see Method).

FEMALES

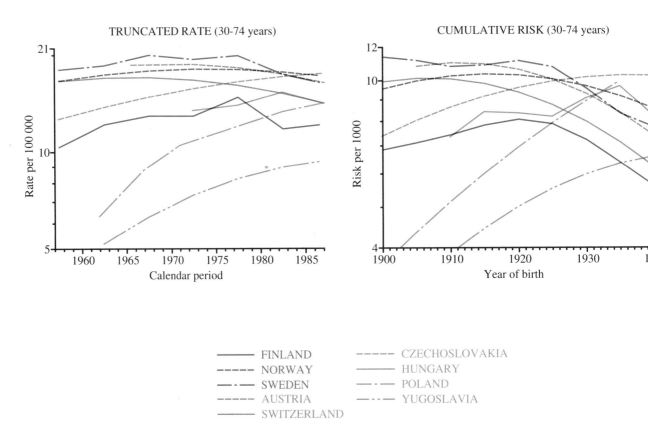

482

OVARY (ICD-9 183)

EUROPE (non-EC), MORTALITY
Percentage change per five-year period, 1975-1988

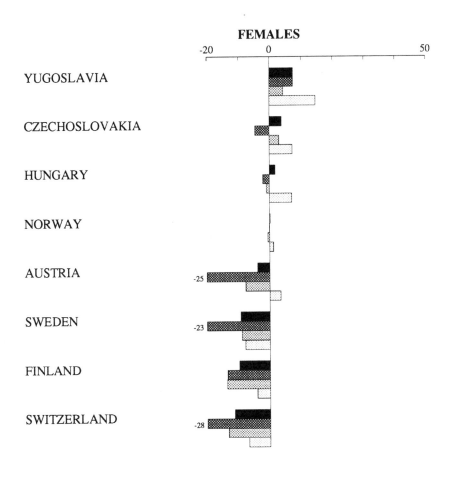

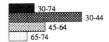

OVARY (ICD-9 183)

EUROPE (EC), MORTALITY

FEMALES	Best model	Goodness of fit	1965 Rate	1965 Deaths	1985 Rate	1985 Deaths	Cumulative risk 1900	Cumulative risk 1940	Recent trend
BELGIUM	A5P4C3	1.41	12.5	358	14.6	441	6.6	7.0	*1.1*
DENMARK	A3P2C2	-0.35	23.5	323	20.7	319	13.1	9.6	-5.2
FRANCE	A8P3C2	3.30	8.0	1124	11.5	1778	4.2	7.2	6.5
GERMANY (FRG)	A8C6	14.13	*15.8*	*3101*	15.8	3332	*8.2*	6.6	-0.9
GREECE	A8P4C9	0.03	*4.1*	*87*	5.7	164	*0.4*	6.2	16.7
IRELAND	A2C2	-0.18	11.6	81	16.1	129	5.7	9.8	*3.6*
ITALY	A8P3C2	4.09	6.8	957	9.5	1668	3.3	5.9	13.8
NETHERLANDS	A6P5C3	0.06	16.8	508	15.0	589	9.5	6.9	-8.3
PORTUGAL	–	–	–	–	–	–	–	–	–
SPAIN	A8P6C9	-0.04	1.7	134	6.2	658	0.6	7.6	35.2
UK ENGLAND & WALES	A6P4C6	2.93	17.8	2662	17.9	2743	9.7	8.2	*-1.3*
UK SCOTLAND	A3C2	-1.38	16.9	266	16.8	266	9.0	8.0	*0.2*

* : not enough deaths for reliable estimation
– : incomplete or missing data
Best model: polynomial of the given degree in age (A), period (P) or cohort (C), or linear drift (D) model.
Goodness of fit: the normalised likelihood ratio chi-square for the best model (see Method).
Rate: world-standardised truncated rate per 100 000 per year (30-74 years) and number of **deaths** are both estimated from the best-fitting model for the single years cited.
Cumulative risk per 1000 (30-74 years) is estimated from the best-fitting *age-cohort* model for cohorts of central birth year cited.
Recent trend: estimated mean percentage change per five-year period in the age-specific rates (30-74 years) over the period 1975-1988.
Italics denote recent trends not significant at 5 per cent level, or other figures which should be interpreted with caution (see Method).

FEMALES

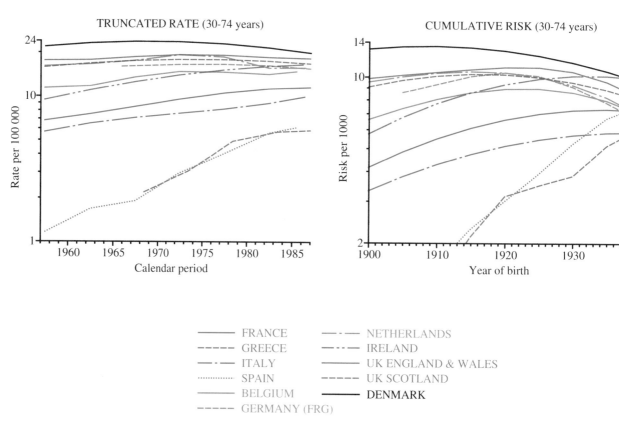

TRUNCATED RATE (30-74 years) — Rate per 100 000 — Calendar period
CUMULATIVE RISK (30-74 years) — Risk per 1000 — Year of birth

FRANCE — NETHERLANDS
GREECE — IRELAND
ITALY — UK ENGLAND & WALES
SPAIN — UK SCOTLAND
BELGIUM — DENMARK
GERMANY (FRG)

484

OVARY (ICD-9 183)

EUROPE (EC), MORTALITY
Percentage change per five-year period, 1975-1988

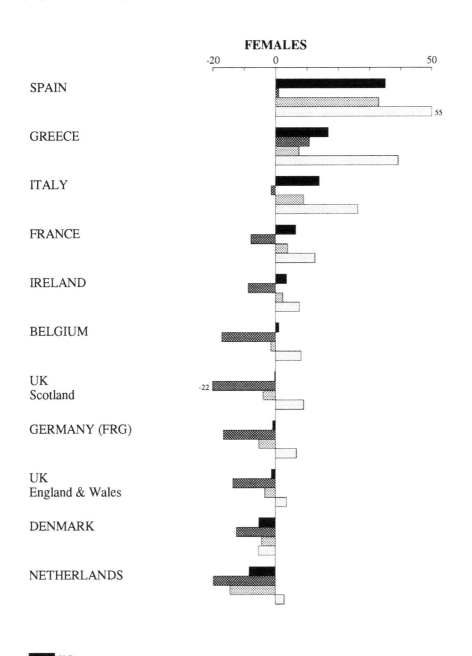

FEMALES

Legend:
- 30-74
- 30-44
- 45-64
- 65-74

OVARY (ICD-9 183)

ASIA, INCIDENCE

FEMALES	Best model	Goodness of fit	1970 Rate	1970 Cases	1985 Rate	1985 Cases	Cumulative risk 1915	Cumulative risk 1940	Recent trend
CHINA									
Shanghai	A2P2	-0.57	*3.8*	*46*	9.4	164	4.6	5.1	*2.1*
HONG KONG	A2D	-0.28	*9.2*	*61*	13.7	152	5.2	10.1	13.9
INDIA									
Bombay	A2P4	1.51	9.1	49	12.4	126	6.1	8.4	*-2.0*
JAPAN									
Miyagi	A8D	0.47	4.8	20	9.8	59	3.0	9.7	26.5
Nagasaki	A2D	-0.08	*17.7*	*18*	9.9	12	8.8	3.4	-18.1
Osaka	A4D	0.63	5.1	77	10.2	235	3.5	10.8	24.6
SINGAPORE									
Chinese	A2P3	-0.10	13.1	31	18.0	67	6.2	11.9	19.6
Indian	A2C2	1.33	14.7	1	14.3	3	5.0	10.2	*23.2*
Malay	A2	-0.40	17.6	5	17.6	9	8.3	8.3	*0.5*

* : not enough cases for reliable estimation
– : incomplete or missing data
Best model: polynomial of the given degree in age (A), period (P) or cohort (C), or linear drift (D) model.
Goodness of fit: the normalised likelihood ratio chi-square for the best model (see Method).
Rate: world-standardised truncated rate per 100 000 per year (30-74 years) and number of **cases** are both estimated from the best-fitting model for the single years cited.
Cumulative risk per 1000 (30-74 years) is estimated from the best-fitting *age-cohort* model for cohorts of central birth year cited.
Recent trend: estimated mean percentage change per five-year period in the age-specific rates (30-74 years) over the period 1973-1987.
Italics denote recent trends not significant at 5 per cent level, or other figures which should be interpreted with caution (see Method).

FEMALES

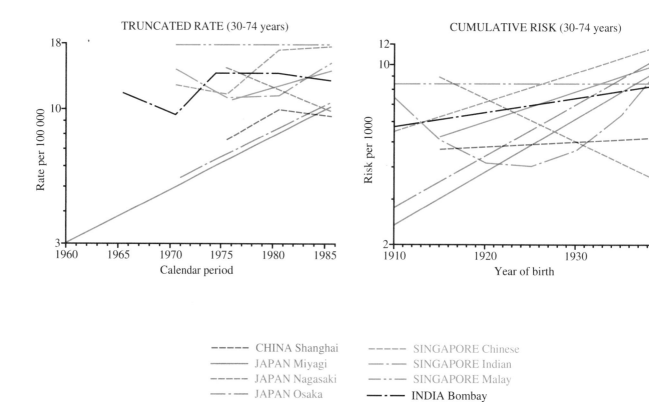

CHINA Shanghai   SINGAPORE Chinese
JAPAN Miyagi   SINGAPORE Indian
JAPAN Nagasaki   SINGAPORE Malay
JAPAN Osaka   INDIA Bombay
HONG KONG

OVARY (ICD-9 183)

ASIA, INCIDENCE
Percentage change per five-year period, 1973-1987

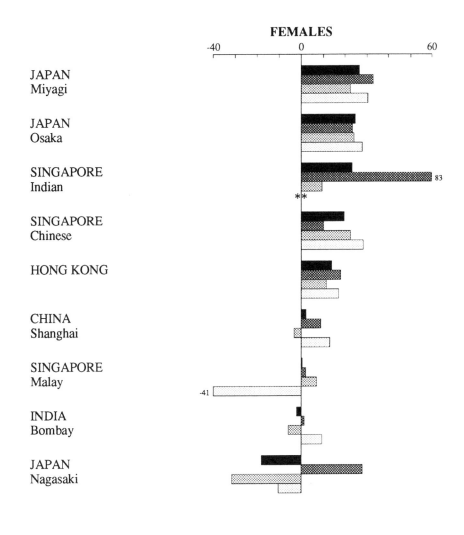

OVARY (ICD-9 183)

OCEANIA, INCIDENCE

FEMALES	Best model	Goodness of fit	1970 Rate	1970 Cases	1985 Rate	1985 Cases	Cumulative risk 1915	Cumulative risk 1940	Recent trend
AUSTRALIA									
New South Wales	A2	1.61	*18.3*	*207*	18.3	243	9.7	9.7	*-1.3*
South	A2	-0.26	*17.2*	*37*	17.2	61	9.6	9.6	*-1.8*
HAWAII									
Caucasian	A2P2	1.50	22.7	8	25.8	15	13.4	11.8	*19.1*
Chinese	A2	0.88	18.1	1	18.1	2	9.2	9.2	*22.9*
Filipino	A2	0.88	15.1	1	15.1	4	7.8	7.8	*40.4*
Hawaiian	A2	-0.75	24.2	4	24.2	7	12.4	12.4	*-10.1*
Japanese	A2	-0.47	15.0	8	15.0	13	7.3	7.3	*2.0*
NEW ZEALAND									
Maori	A1	0.22	20.7	4	20.7	7	11.2	11.2	*-6.7*
Non-Maori	A5C4	-0.70	23.9	141	20.5	149	13.1	8.2	*-4.6*

* : not enough cases for reliable estimation
− : incomplete or missing data
Best model: polynomial of the given degree in age (A), period (P) or cohort (C), or linear drift (D) model.
Goodness of fit: the normalised likelihood ratio chi-square for the best model (see Method).
Rate: world-standardised truncated rate per 100 000 per year (30-74 years) and number of **cases** are both estimated from the best-fitting model for the single years cited.
Cumulative risk per 1000 (30-74 years) is estimated from the best-fitting *age-cohort* model for cohorts of central birth year cited.
Recent trend: estimated mean percentage change per five-year period in the age-specific rates (30-74 years) over the period 1973-1987.
Italics denote recent trends not significant at 5 per cent level, or other figures which should be interpreted with caution (see Method).

FEMALES

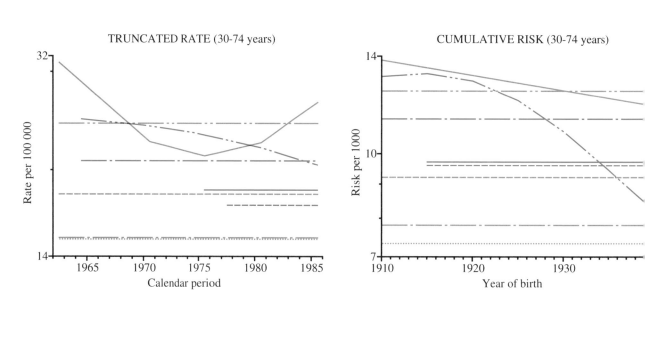

OVARY (ICD-9 183)

OCEANIA, INCIDENCE
Percentage change per five-year period, 1973-1987

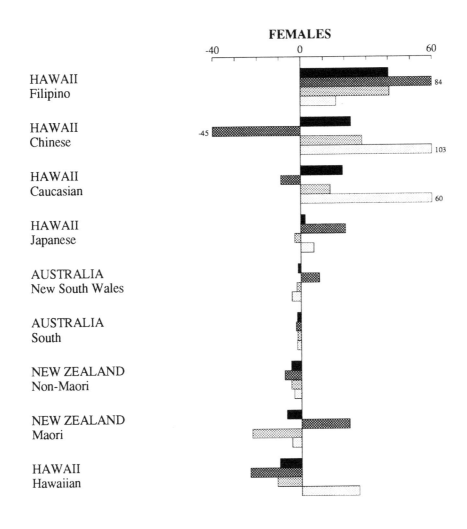

OVARY (ICD-9 183)

ASIA and OCEANIA, MORTALITY

FEMALES	Best model	Goodness of fit	1965 Rate	Deaths	1985 Rate	Deaths	Cumulative risk 1900	1940	Recent trend
AUSTRALIA	A4C5	0.05	13.3	347	11.6	452	7.4	4.6	-5.6
HONG KONG	A2C2	-1.53	*6.3*	*37*	6.4	61	*3.0*	2.8	*-2.7*
JAPAN	A8P6C3	5.33	3.6	744	6.3	2135	1.4	4.5	10.6
MAURITIUS	A2	0.12	*2.9*	*2*	2.9	4	*1.5*	1.5	*-2.4*
NEW ZEALAND	A3C4	-0.15	16.3	94	14.6	114	8.8	6.0	*-5.9*
SINGAPORE	A2D	0.91	5.0	10	7.4	26	*1.9*	4.3	–

* : not enough deaths for reliable estimation
– : incomplete or missing data
Best model: polynomial of the given degree in age (A), period (P) or cohort (C), or linear drift (D) model.
Goodness of fit: the normalised likelihood ratio chi-square for the best model (see Method).
Rate: world-standardised truncated rate per 100 000 per year (30-74 years) and number of **deaths** are both estimated from the best-fitting model for the single years cited.
Cumulative risk per 1000 (30-74 years) is estimated from the best-fitting *age-cohort* model for cohorts of central birth year cited.
Recent trend: estimated mean percentage change per five-year period in the age-specific rates (30-74 years) over the period 1975-1988.
Italics denote recent trends not significant at 5 per cent level, or other figures which should be interpreted with caution (see Method).

FEMALES

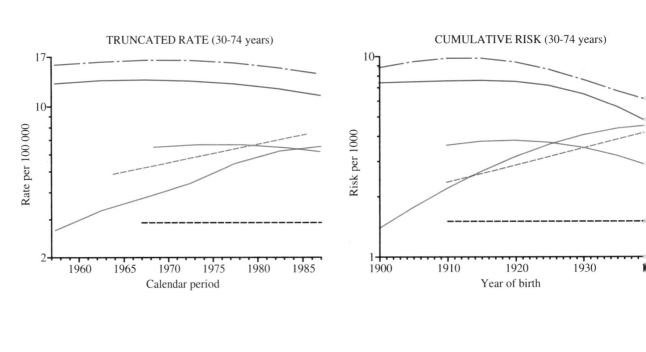

OVARY (ICD-9 183)

ASIA and OCEANIA, MORTALITY
Percentage change per five-year period, 1975-1988

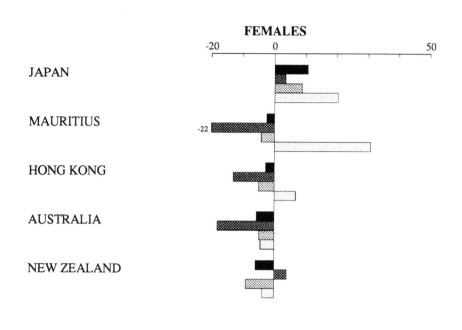

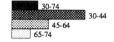

OVARY (ICD-9 183)

AMERICAS (except USA), INCIDENCE

FEMALES	Best model	Goodness of fit	1970 Rate	1970 Cases	1985 Rate	1985 Cases	Cumulative risk 1915	Cumulative risk 1940	Recent trend
BRAZIL									
Sao Paulo	A2D	0.98	13.2	114	*24.7*	*283*	6.4	*18.0*	–
CANADA									
Alberta	A2D	-0.02	20.5	61	23.9	111	11.4	14.6	7.8
British Columbia	A2P2C3	0.36	31.4	148	24.4	178	13.4	11.0	*1.9*
Maritime Provinces	A2	-0.68	21.1	67	21.1	79	11.3	11.3	*1.2*
Newfoundland	A2	0.39	18.8	15	18.8	21	9.7	9.7	*-5.7*
Quebec	A2P4C2	0.78	19.7	239	24.0	392	10.7	14.7	6.9
COLOMBIA									
Cali	A2C3	0.78	18.8	19	15.0	28	11.4	5.1	-12.5
CUBA	A2P2	1.51	8.9	121	10.5	209	4.8	*6.8*	–
PUERTO RICO	A4C5	-0.34	10.7	49	10.3	77	5.6	5.0	*-5.2*

* : not enough cases for reliable estimation
– : incomplete or missing data
Best model: polynomial of the given degree in age (A), period (P) or cohort (C), or linear drift (D) model.
Goodness of fit: the normalised likelihood ratio chi-square for the best model (see Method).
Rate: world-standardised truncated rate per 100 000 per year (30-74 years) and number of **cases** are both estimated from the best-fitting model for the single years cited.
Cumulative risk per 1000 (30-74 years) is estimated from the best-fitting *age-cohort* model for cohorts of central birth year cited.
Recent trend: estimated mean percentage change per five-year period in the age-specific rates (30-74 years) over the period 1973-1987.
Italics denote recent trends not significant at 5 per cent level, or other figures which should be interpreted with caution (see Method).

FEMALES

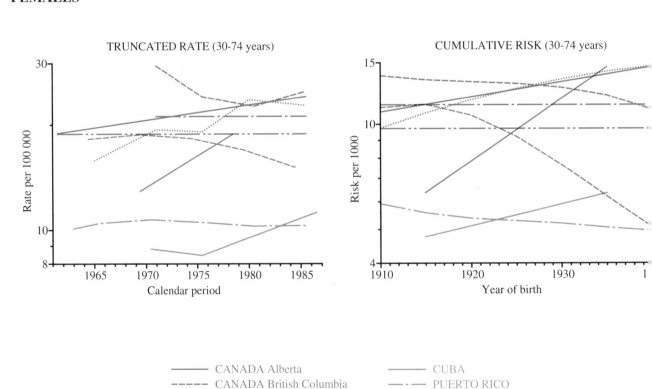

492

OVARY (ICD-9 183)

AMERICAS (except USA), INCIDENCE
Percentage change per five-year period, 1973-1987

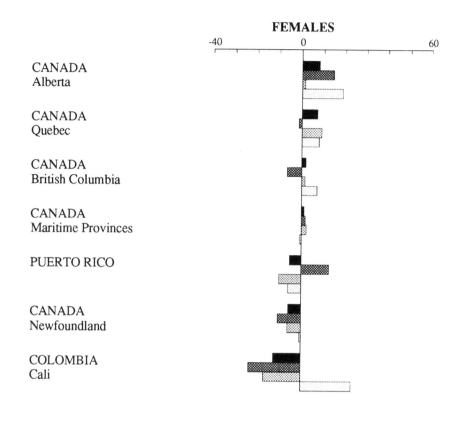

OVARY (ICD-9 183)

AMERICAS (USA), INCIDENCE

FEMALES	Best model	Goodness of fit	1970 Rate	1970 Cases	1985 Rate	1985 Cases	Cumulative risk 1915	Cumulative risk 1940	Recent trend
USA									
Bay Area, Black	A1C3	1.55	16.4	10	15.7	15	11.8	5.7	*-3.8*
Bay Area, Chinese	A4	0.20	16.9	3	*16.9*	*8*	8.4	*8.4*	–
Bay Area, White	A2C2	2.11	29.1	196	26.8	181	15.8	12.5	*-4.7*
Connecticut	A5C4	2.17	25.4	189	24.2	213	14.2	10.8	*1.9*
Detroit, Black	A3	-0.83	18.3	27	18.3	39	10.0	10.0	*-3.0*
Detroit, White	A3C2	0.58	25.1	206	26.6	213	14.3	13.8	*2.7*
Iowa	A8C8	0.18	26.5	188	24.5	181	14.6	9.3	*-1.1*
New Orleans, Black	A8D	0.92	*6.8*	*4*	15.7	11	4.8	19.2	32.2
New Orleans, White	A3P2	0.07	*7.6*	*14*	19.4	34	11.1	10.4	*-0.9*
Seattle	A2C2	0.67	*25.0*	*126*	25.0	176	14.5	11.8	*-0.8*

* : not enough cases for reliable estimation
– : incomplete or missing data
Best model: polynomial of the given degree in age (A), period (P) or cohort (C), or linear drift (D) model.
Goodness of fit: the normalised likelihood ratio chi-square for the best model (see Method).
Rate: world-standardised truncated rate per 100 000 per year (30-74 years) and number of **cases** are both estimated from the best-fitting model for the single years cited.
Cumulative risk per 1000 (30-74 years) is estimated from the best-fitting *age-cohort* model for cohorts of central birth year cited.
Recent trend: estimated mean percentage change per five-year period in the age-specific rates (30-74 years) over the period 1973-1987.
Italics denote recent trends not significant at 5 per cent level, or other figures which should be interpreted with caution (see Method).

FEMALES

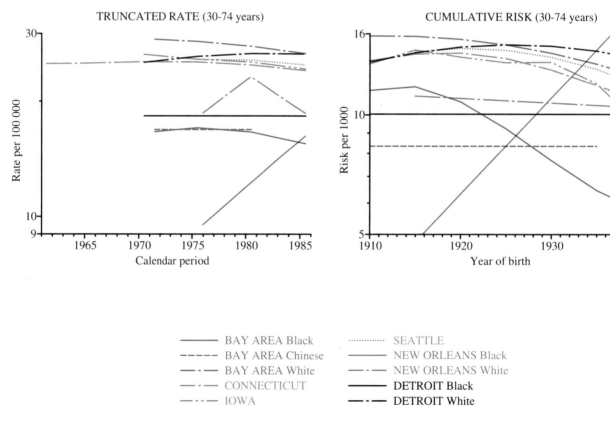

494

OVARY (ICD-9 183)

AMERICAS (USA), INCIDENCE
Percentage change per five-year period, 1973-1987

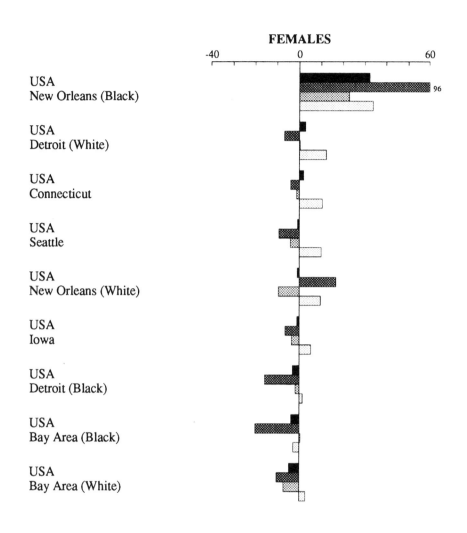

OVARY (ICD-9 183)

AMERICAS, MORTALITY

FEMALES	Best model	Goodness of fit	1965 Rate	1965 Deaths	1985 Rate	1985 Deaths	Cumulative risk 1900	Cumulative risk 1940	Recent trend
CANADA	A5C2	1.39	15.4	604	12.9	820	8.9	5.4	-6.4
CHILE	A2C2	0.87	4.7	62	*8.6*	*178*	2.3	*6.6*	–
COSTA RICA	–	–	–	–	–	–	–	–	–
PANAMA	–	–	–	–	–	–	–	–	–
PUERTO RICO	–	–	–	–	–	–	–	–	–
URUGUAY	–	–	–	–	–	–	–	–	–
USA	A7P4C9	3.82	15.5	7302	12.5	8036	8.8	4.5	-5.4
VENEZUELA	A2P2C2	-2.09	4.7	47	*5.4*	*103*	1.9	*5.7*	–

* : not enough deaths for reliable estimation
– : incomplete or missing data
Best model: polynomial of the given degree in age (A), period (P) or cohort (C), or linear drift (D) model.
Goodness of fit: the normalised likelihood ratio chi-square for the best model (see Method).
Rate: world-standardised truncated rate per 100 000 per year (30-74 years) and number of **deaths** are both estimated from the best-fitting model for the single years cited.
Cumulative risk per 1000 (30-74 years) is estimated from the best-fitting *age-cohort* model for cohorts of central birth year cited.
Recent trend: estimated mean percentage change per five-year period in the age-specific rates (30-74 years) over the period 1975-1988.
Italics denote recent trends not significant at 5 per cent level, or other figures which should be interpreted with caution (see Method).

FEMALES

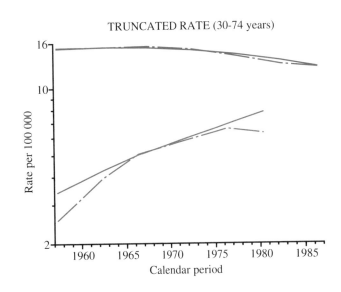

TRUNCATED RATE (30-74 years)

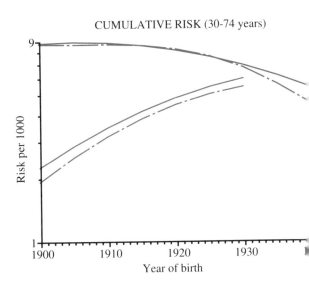

CUMULATIVE RISK (30-74 years)

——— CANADA
—·—· USA
——— CHILE
—··— VENEZUELA

OVARY (ICD-9 183)

AMERICAS, MORTALITY
Percentage change per five-year period, 1975-1988

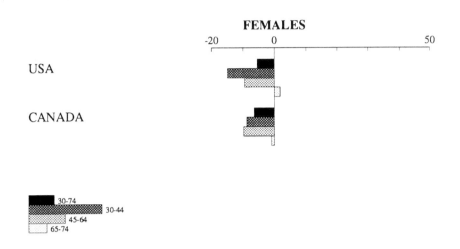

FEMALES

from page 477

number of cases on which it is based, and it should be interpreted with caution. The mortality data for Japan and Singapore are consistent with the incidence data, whereas those in Hong Kong are not, and incidence in Hong Kong may have been under-estimated for the period 1974-82, since about 10% of cases in 1983-87 were reported from death certificates, excluded from earlier data (see Chapter 2). There is a suggestion of a deceleration of the rate of increase in younger Japanese cohorts. In Mauritius, the number of cases is too small to evaluate reliably the large increase seen in the linear trend histogram.

In Australia and New Zealand, the risk of ovarian cancer is decreasing, but the decline is significant only for non-Maoris in New Zealand, where a spectacular cohort decline may be seen for females born since 1920. In Hawaii, the small number of cases complicates interpretation of the apparent increase. The period effect among Caucasians is caused by the high rate observed in the first period, while the cohort effect and the age-specific linear trends suggest the beginning of a decline in risk for the younger generations.

The mortality data in Australia and New Zealand show a clear decrease in the risk of death from ovarian cancer; this decrease is particularly evident when evaluated on a cohort basis, since in these two countries age-cohort models fit the mortality data perfectly.

Americas

In Alberta and Quebec (Canada), the risk of ovarian cancer is increasing. In Alberta, the increase is exponential, while in Quebec there is some suggestion that the rate of increase is slowing down for more recent generations; in British Columbia and in the Maritime Provinces, the cohort effect is more pronounced, and there is a notable reduction in risk for cohorts born since the 1930s.

In South America, the contrast between São Paulo (Brazil) and Cali (Colombia) is worth noting. The large and significant rate of decline in Cali is particularly impressive. The rate of increase in São Paulo up to 1978 is also striking.

In the USA, the cohort-wise decrease in the risk of ovarian cancer is seen in all populations, except among black females in New Orleans, where perhaps the disease may have been under-diagnosed or incompletely registered in earlier periods.

Finally, the risk of dying from ovarian cancer has decreased similarly in successive birth cohorts in Canada and the USA, while it has risen in Venezuela and Chile. The lifetime risk (30-74 years) is now similar in all four countries, at around 0.5%.

Comment

The pattern of change in ovarian cancer incidence and mortality has been discussed by seve-

497

ral authors. Doll[83] ascribed some of the early increase in mortality to better diagnosis, but considered that reduced parity and prolonged use of steroid contraceptives play a more important role in explaining the pattern of change in mortality. Detailed examination of these hypotheses, based on both incidence and mortality data, has been carried out for the UK, Sweden and Denmark[1,99,296]. Quantification of the use of oral contraceptives is difficult[186], and despite increasingly widespread birth control with oral contraceptives in Colombia[180], it is impossible to ascribe the large decrease in ovarian cancer observed in Cali to oral contraceptives with any certainty. More detailed studies of the correlation between the decline in ovarian cancer incidence and the use of steroid contraceptives should be encouraged.

Chapter 21

PROSTATE

Cancer of the prostate ranks as the fifth most common cancer in men, with an estimated 235 000 new cases a year around 1980, or over 7% of all cancers in males. It is much more common in developed than developing countries, and the global range in incidence is at least 70-fold. Adenocarcinoma accounts for over 90% of cases. Incidence is generally low until 50 years of age in most populations, then increases rapidly with age. Survival at five years is typically 40% to 50%.

Latent carcinoma of the prostate is common, and is frequently discovered on microscopic examination after prostatectomy for benign prostatic hypertrophy, or at autopsy. Small non-invasive carcinomas are common over 45 years of age, and where they are registered alongside cases diagnosed clinically, the incidence will be affected by the frequency of prostatectomy or autopsy. Among the 48 registries from which data are analysed here, 41 include prostate cancers diagnosed incidentally at biopsy, while Varese (Italy), Miyagi (Japan), Cali (Colombia), Quebec (Canada) and Cuba reported not doing so. Prostate cancers diagnosed incidentally at autopsy are included by 39 of the registries: only two, Singapore and Cali (Colombia) reported not doing so. Cases diagnosed incidentally at biopsy or autopsy are likely to have less influence on these analyses (30-74 years) than if all age groups had been included.

Europe

There is a 7-fold range of incidence in Europe, from about 10 per 100 000 among non-Jews in Israel to over 70 among men in Sweden. Incidence is increasing rapidly in most populations. Mortality is also increasing, although less rapidly. Incidence rates of 50 per 100 000 or more are seen in the Nordic countries and in Geneva (Switzerland). These rates are continuing to increase at 10-20% every five years, and the risk up to age 74 for the 1940 birth cohort in these countries is between 4% and 9%. Incidence in Szabolcs-Szatmar and County Vas (Hungary), Varese (Italy) and Navarra (Spain) is lower, but is increasing even more rapidly, at over 20% every five years, and only slightly less quickly in Bas-Rhin (France) and in the UK. Cumulative risk up to age 74 for the 1940 birth cohort in Varese is estimated at 9%.

The exception to this general increase is the significant and steady decline in Warsaw City (Poland), which is significant both in the 65-74 years age group (14% every five years) and for men aged 75 and over (10%, data not shown). This decline is not reflected in national mortality statistics, which show a significant recent increase of 8% every five years, and Warsaw City may represent a local departure from the national pattern of incidence in Poland.

In the southern countries of Italy, Spain and Portugal, the available incidence data from Varese (Italy), where cases diagnosed at incidental biopsy are excluded, and from Navarra (Spain) suggest that prostate cancer is increasing more rapidly than anywhere else in Europe, at more than 25% every five years, yet mortality in Italy is stable, and in Spain and Portugal it is actually falling steadily. This is in contrast to all other European countries except Romania, where mortality has also fallen significantly since the mid-1960s. The increase in truncated incidence (30-74 years) in Cluj (Romania) is not significant, however, and there has been a significant fall in incidence at ages 75 and over (22% every five years, data not shown).

Asia

Prostate cancer is much less common in the Asian populations studied here than in Europe, with a range of 2 to 10 per 100 000. It is increasing even more rapidly, however, especially in Japan, where the truncated rates have more than doubled in the last 20 years to around 10 per 100 000, and are still increasing at over 30% every five years (more than 5% on an annual basis). Similar increases are seen at age 75 years and over (data not shown). The truncated rate in Nagasaki (Japan) is about 12 per 100 000, but it is not increasing, and incidence at age 75 and over is also stable. Prostate cancer is four times more frequent among Japanese men in Hawaii than in Japan, but rates are increasing much more slowly (8% every five years). Men in Shanghai (China) have a particularly low truncated rate of prostate cancer, around 2 per 100 000, and there is no evidence of it increasing substantially. Incidence in Hong Kong and among Chinese in Singapore is about four times higher than in Shanghai, but

continued page 519

PROSTATE (ICD-9 185)

EUROPE (non-EC), INCIDENCE

MALES	Best model	Goodness of fit	1970 Rate	1970 Cases	1985 Rate	1985 Cases	Cumulative risk 1915	Cumulative risk 1940	Recent trend
FINLAND	A3P5C2	0.66	34.0	346	48.7	588	40.0	66.6	15.9
HUNGARY									
County Vas	A2P2	0.45	25.6	22	32.6	26	21.3	21.0	27.5
Szabolcs-Szatmar	A2D	0.24	12.8	18	22.4	31	16.4	41.5	22.2
ISRAEL									
All Jews	A4D	-0.13	19.6	69	27.2	124	20.1	34.5	7.9
Non-Jews	A3D	-0.52	6.4	1	10.8	4	7.0	16.6	*21.5*
NORWAY	A2P2	0.39	47.7	562	63.6	872	48.7	87.0	5.7
POLAND									
Warsaw City	A2D	-0.59	21.7	58	17.1	62	13.5	9.1	-10.3
ROMANIA									
Cluj	*	..	..	..	..	..	..	..	..
SWEDEN	A8P5C9	-1.15	58.4	1559	74.7	2256	54.4	61.1	7.9
SWITZERLAND									
Geneva	A2D	0.58	41.1	33	59.2	53	44.5	80.3	10.4
YUGOSLAVIA									
Slovenia	A8P5	0.85	23.1	89	23.2	95	20.7	29.9	*3.0*

* : not enough cases for reliable estimation
– : incomplete or missing data
Best model: polynomial of the given degree in age (A), period (P) or cohort (C), or linear drift (D) model.
Goodness of fit: the normalised likelihood ratio chi-square for the best model (see Method).
Rate: world-standardised truncated rate per 100 000 per year (30-74 years) and number of **cases** are both estimated from the best-fitting model for the single years cited.
Cumulative risk per 1000 (30-74 years) is estimated from the best-fitting *age-cohort* model for cohorts of central birth year cited.
Recent trend: estimated mean percentage change per five-year period in the age-specific rates (30-74 years) over the period 1973-1987.
Italics denote recent trends not significant at 5 per cent level, or other figures which should be interpreted with caution (see Method).

MALES

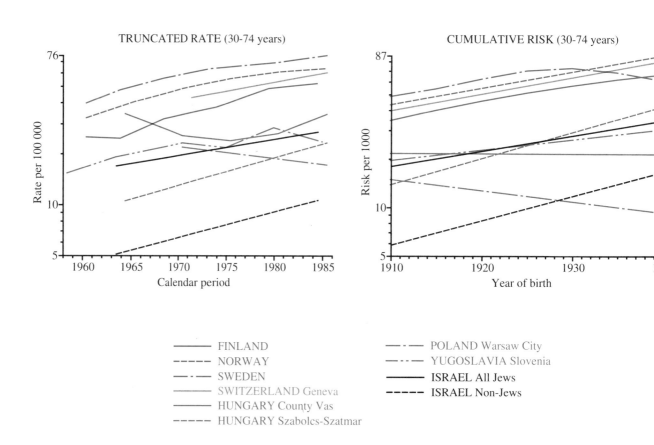

——— FINLAND	—·— POLAND Warsaw City	
----- NORWAY	—··— YUGOSLAVIA Slovenia	
—·— SWEDEN	——— ISRAEL All Jews	
——— SWITZERLAND Geneva	----- ISRAEL Non-Jews	
——— HUNGARY County Vas		
----- HUNGARY Szabolcs-Szatmar		

PROSTATE (ICD-9 185)

EUROPE (non-EC), INCIDENCE

Percentage change per five-year period, 1973-1987

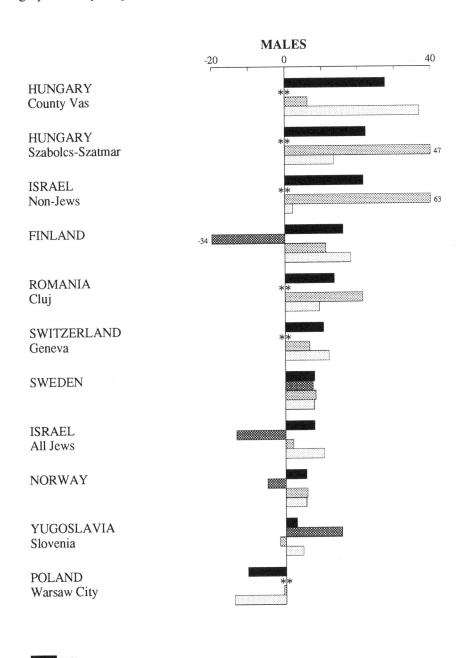

PROSTATE (ICD-9 185)

EUROPE (EC), INCIDENCE

MALES	Best model	Goodness of fit	1970 Rate	1970 Cases	1985 Rate	1985 Cases	Cumulative risk 1915	Cumulative risk 1940	Recent trend
DENMARK	A2C4	-0.50	31.7	456	43.3	695	31.8	40.3	12.8
FRANCE									
Bas-Rhin	A2D	-0.49	*28.7*	*78*	46.8	92	34.1	75.6	19.9
Doubs	A2	-0.99	*38.3*	*14*	38.3	42	29.4	29.4	*2.7*
GERMANY (FRG)									
Hamburg	A2P3C5	-1.05	31.5	191	*32.5*	*136*	50.3	*43.9*	–
Saarland	A2P3	-1.45	28.3	86	42.6	119	33.9	50.8	*-4.1*
GERMANY (GDR)	A8P4C4	0.63	22.6	1203	33.2	1181	28.1	50.3	9.2
ITALY									
Varese	A5D	-0.84	*17.3*	*13*	36.8	77	26.7	91.0	26.9
SPAIN									
Navarra	A2C2	-2.18	*11.8*	*14*	36.4	56	31.5	13.2	38.4
Zaragoza	A2	-1.06	19.6	38	19.6	50	15.2	15.2	*3.4*
UK									
Birmingham	A4P5	-2.15	23.4	316	32.9	529	22.9	32.7	14.1
Scotland	A2C3	0.83	22.5	318	37.5	571	28.7	29.3	19.3
South Thames	A4P5C8	-0.56	22.2	597	32.4	699	24.1	34.7	12.3

* : not enough cases for reliable estimation
– : incomplete or missing data
Best model: polynomial of the given degree in age (A), period (P) or cohort (C), or linear drift (D) model.
Goodness of fit: the normalised likelihood ratio chi-square for the best model (see Method).
Rate: world-standardised truncated rate per 100 000 per year (30-74 years) and number of **cases** are both estimated from the best-fitting model for the single years cited.
Cumulative risk per 1000 (30-74 years) is estimated from the best-fitting *age-cohort* model for cohorts of central birth year cited.
Recent trend: estimated mean percentage change per five-year period in the age-specific rates (30-74 years) over the period 1973-1987.
Italics denote recent trends not significant at 5 per cent level, or other figures which should be interpreted with caution (see Method).

MALES

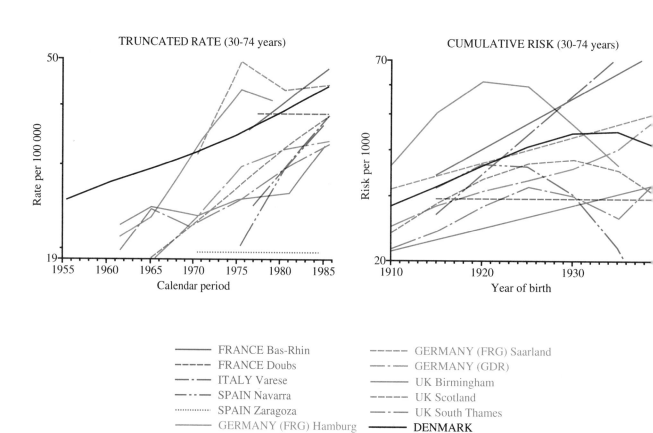

TRUNCATED RATE (30-74 years)

CUMULATIVE RISK (30-74 years)

——— FRANCE Bas-Rhin
------ FRANCE Doubs
—·— ITALY Varese
—··— SPAIN Navarra
············ SPAIN Zaragoza
——— GERMANY (FRG) Hamburg
------ GERMANY (FRG) Saarland
—·— GERMANY (GDR)
——— UK Birmingham
------ UK Scotland
—··— UK South Thames
——— DENMARK

PROSTATE (ICD-9 185)

EUROPE (EC), INCIDENCE
Percentage change per five-year period, 1973-1987

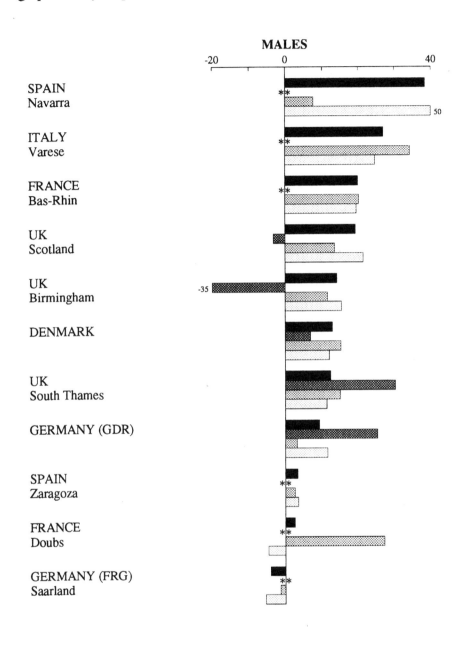

PROSTATE (ICD-9 185)

EUROPE (non-EC), MORTALITY

MALES	Best model	Goodness of fit	1965 Rate	1965 Deaths	1985 Rate	1985 Deaths	Cumulative risk 1900	Cumulative risk 1940	Recent trend
AUSTRIA	A3D	2.13	15.5	323	16.6	329	12.5	14.3	*2.0*
CZECHOSLOVAKIA	A2P3C5	2.03	11.8	408	16.7	643	10.0	19.3	7.9
FINLAND	A2P2	0.40	14.4	125	17.1	208	11.9	15.3	8.3
HUNGARY	A6P3	2.07	15.6	406	17.9	527	12.4	19.3	*0.9*
NORWAY	A2C2	1.92	17.3	189	22.2	309	14.3	30.0	4.8
POLAND	A8P5C9	0.59	9.1	506	11.9	910	8.2	12.3	8.5
ROMANIA	A3P2	1.51	11.2	435	*9.2*	*473*	8.7	6.3	–
SWEDEN	A8P6	-0.07	19.8	482	21.6	674	16.4	19.5	*0.6*
SWITZERLAND	A2D	1.33	18.7	271	20.6	386	15.2	18.5	7.2
YUGOSLAVIA	A4P4	2.88	8.2	274	11.1	503	7.0	12.9	*-2.0*

* : not enough deaths for reliable estimation
– : incomplete or missing data
Best model: polynomial of the given degree in age (A), period (P) or cohort (C), or linear drift (D) model.
Goodness of fit: the normalised likelihood ratio chi-square for the best model (see Method).
Rate: world-standardised truncated rate per 100 000 per year (30-74 years) and number of **deaths** are both estimated from the best-fitting model for the single years cited.
Cumulative risk per 1000 (30-74 years) is estimated from the best-fitting *age-cohort* model for cohorts of central birth year cited.
Recent trend: estimated mean percentage change per five-year period in the age-specific rates (30-74 years) over the period 1975-1988.
Italics denote recent trends not significant at 5 per cent level, or other figures which should be interpreted with caution (see Method).

MALES

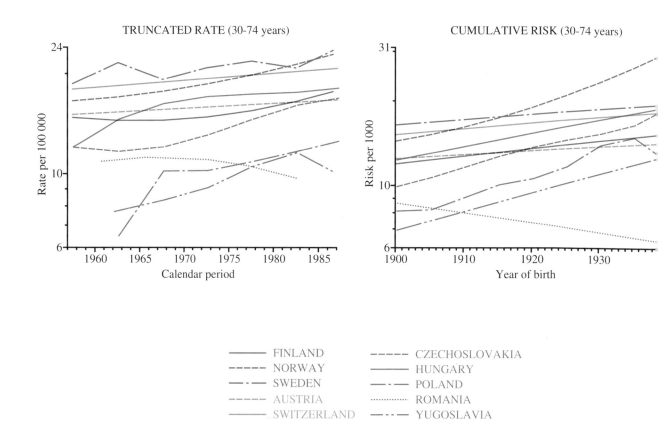

PROSTATE (ICD-9 185)

EUROPE (non-EC), MORTALITY
Percentage change per five-year period, 1975-1988

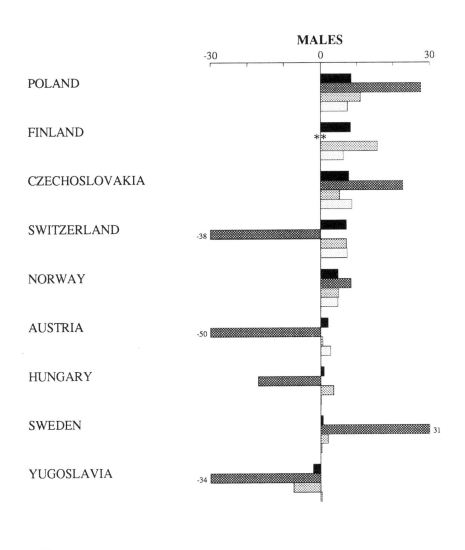

MALES

PROSTATE (ICD-9 185)

EUROPE (EC), MORTALITY

MALES	Best model	Goodness of fit	1965 Rate	1965 Deaths	1985 Rate	1985 Deaths	Cumulative risk 1900	Cumulative risk 1940	Recent trend
BELGIUM	A8D	2.42	16.9	468	18.6	531	13.8	16.6	-2.2
DENMARK	A2P4C2	-0.07	16.0	215	20.5	335	12.7	29.9	12.7
FRANCE	A4P4	3.29	16.3	2036	16.7	2458	12.7	13.6	4.5
GERMANY (FRG)	A4P5C9	8.63	14.6	2308	16.7	2743	12.5	15.8	*-0.3*
GREECE	A4C4	2.19	6.0	111	8.6	258	*5.2*	9.8	*5.8*
IRELAND	A2C2	0.41	14.1	112	16.2	147	11.8	10.5	*0.0*
ITALY	A3P3C4	2.46	12.5	1508	12.6	2096	9.9	7.7	*1.0*
NETHERLANDS	A3D	0.21	14.1	411	16.3	612	11.7	15.7	5.2
PORTUGAL	A3P3	1.45	14.4	256	14.2	393	10.8	13.0	-4.3
SPAIN	A3P5C3	3.82	12.5	865	12.8	1289	10.4	12.2	-4.4
UK ENGLAND & WALES	A8P3C7	0.38	12.3	1596	15.2	2414	8.6	12.9	13.4
UK SCOTLAND	A8P6	0.77	10.7	140	13.0	191	7.4	7.9	13.5

∗ : not enough deaths for reliable estimation
− : incomplete or missing data
Best model: polynomial of the given degree in age (A), period (P) or cohort (C), or linear drift (D) model.
Goodness of fit: the normalised likelihood ratio chi-square for the best model (see Method).
Rate: world-standardised truncated rate per 100 000 per year (30-74 years) and number of **deaths** are both estimated from the best-fitting model for the single years cited.
Cumulative risk per 1000 (30-74 years) is estimated from the best-fitting *age-cohort* model for cohorts of central birth year cited.
Recent trend: estimated mean percentage change per five-year period in the age-specific rates (30-74 years) over the period 1975-1988.
Italics denote recent trends not significant at 5 per cent level, or other figures which should be interpreted with caution (see Method).

MALES

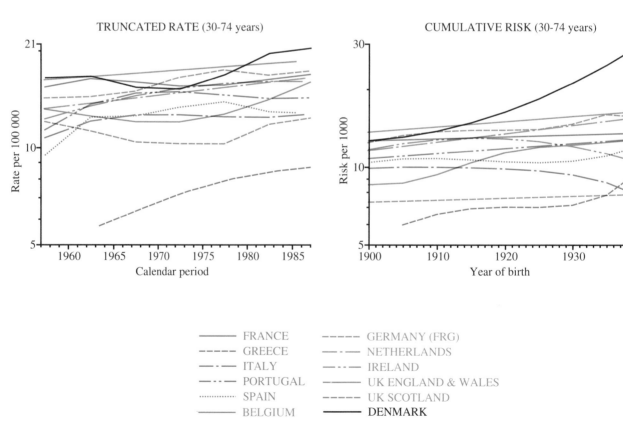

506

PROSTATE (ICD-9 185)

EUROPE (EC), MORTALITY
Percentage change per five-year period, 1975-1988

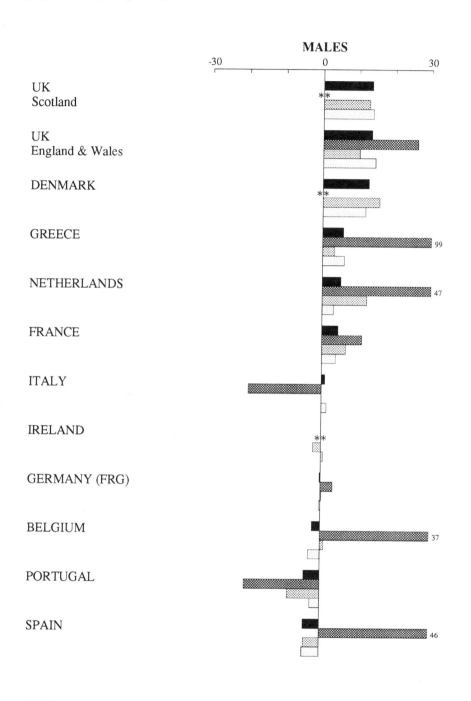

MALES

PROSTATE (ICD-9 185)

ASIA, INCIDENCE

MALES	Best model	Goodness of fit	1970 Rate	1970 Cases	1985 Rate	1985 Cases	Cumulative risk 1915	Cumulative risk 1940	Recent trend
CHINA									
Shanghai	A3P2	-0.08	*0.3*	*2*	2.5	42	1.9	2.4	*4.3*
HONG KONG	A2D	-0.28	*6.7*	*18*	8.8	98	6.6	10.2	*6.5*
INDIA									
Bombay	A2P2	0.03	7.7	38	9.2	77	6.4	7.4	17.3
JAPAN									
Miyagi	A1P3	-0.80	3.9	13	10.1	52	7.5	17.4	30.2
Nagasaki	A3	0.40	*11.8*	*9*	11.8	12	9.1	9.1	*-10.7*
Osaka	A2D	-0.38	3.0	33	8.0	135	6.2	31.9	38.0
SINGAPORE									
Chinese	A2D	0.81	5.3	9	9.4	26	6.5	16.5	22.0
Indian	A2	-1.04	11.7	2	11.7	4	8.7	8.7	*28.5*
Malay	A2D	-3.08	5.6	1	12.2	5	8.7	31.7	*34.6*

* : not enough cases for reliable estimation
− : incomplete or missing data
Best model: polynomial of the given degree in age (A), period (P) or cohort (C), or linear drift (D) model.
Goodness of fit: the normalised likelihood ratio chi-square for the best model (see Method).
Rate: world-standardised truncated rate per 100 000 per year (30-74 years) and number of **cases** are both estimated from the best-fitting model for the single years cited.
Cumulative risk per 1000 (30-74 years) is estimated from the best-fitting *age-cohort* model for cohorts of central birth year cited.
Recent trend: estimated mean percentage change per five-year period in the age-specific rates (30-74 years) over the period 1973-1987.
Italics denote recent trends not significant at 5 per cent level, or other figures which should be interpreted with caution (see Method).

MALES

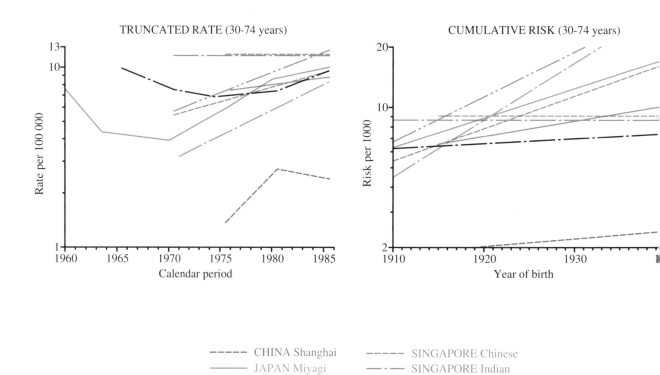

TRUNCATED RATE (30-74 years)

CUMULATIVE RISK (30-74 years)

------- CHINA Shanghai
——— JAPAN Miyagi
------- JAPAN Nagasaki
—·— JAPAN Osaka
——— HONG KONG

------- SINGAPORE Chinese
—·— SINGAPORE Indian
—··— SINGAPORE Malay
——·— INDIA Bombay

PROSTATE (ICD-9 185)

ASIA, INCIDENCE
Percentage change per five-year period, 1973-1987

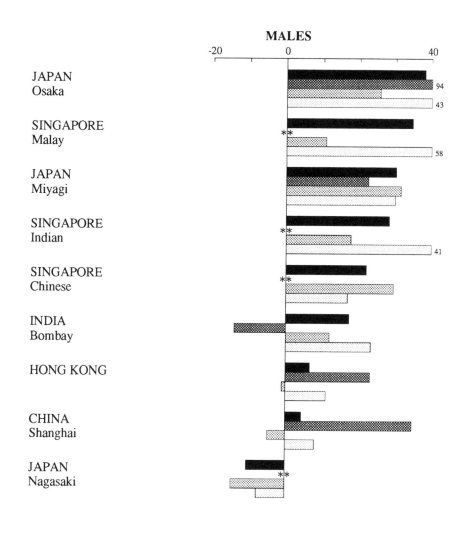

PROSTATE (ICD-9 185)

OCEANIA, INCIDENCE

MALES	Best model	Goodness of fit	1970 Rate	1970 Cases	1985 Rate	1985 Cases	Cumulative risk 1915	Cumulative risk 1940	Recent trend
AUSTRALIA									
New South Wales	A4D	0.30	*30.8*	*319*	55.0	770	40.0	101.6	21.0
South	A4C3	0.23	*84.5*	*46*	58.4	221	44.1	15.3	*3.0*
HAWAII									
Caucasian	A2D	0.24	76.2	22	102.8	64	73.0	117.4	*8.7*
Chinese	A2C2	-3.19	26.3	3	40.3	8	34.0	5.2	*14.9*
Filipino	A2D	0.22	24.2	7	46.3	20	34.0	97.3	*1.0*
Hawaiian	A2P3	-2.14	29.5	3	66.8	14	46.9	75.2	*17.4*
Japanese	A2C2	-1.34	30.7	13	44.3	43	36.0	21.4	*7.6*
NEW ZEALAND									
Maori	A4P3	-2.77	32.6	5	59.6	14	40.2	55.6	*11.6*
Non-Maori	A2P3C3	-0.40	34.9	196	46.7	352	34.4	31.8	6.5

* : not enough cases for reliable estimation
– : incomplete or missing data
Best model: polynomial of the given degree in age (A), period (P) or cohort (C), or linear drift (D) model.
Goodness of fit: the normalised likelihood ratio chi-square for the best model (see Method).
Rate: world-standardised truncated rate per 100 000 per year (30-74 years) and number of **cases** are both estimated from the best-fitting model for the single years cited.
Cumulative risk per 1000 (30-74 years) is estimated from the best-fitting *age-cohort* model for cohorts of central birth year cited.
Recent trend: estimated mean percentage change per five-year period in the age-specific rates (30-74 years) over the period 1973-1987.
Italics denote recent trends not significant at 5 per cent level, or other figures which should be interpreted with caution (see Method).

MALES

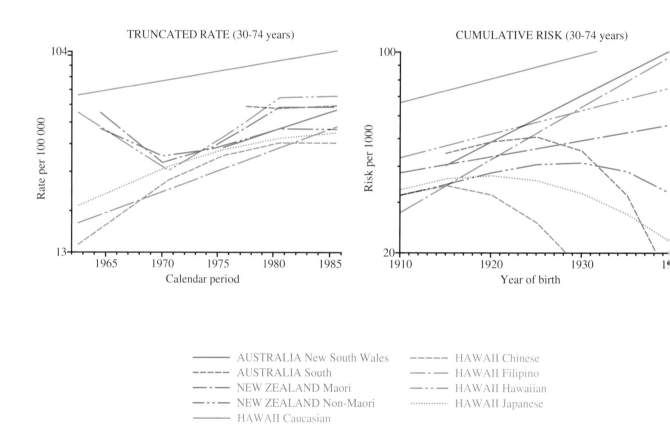

PROSTATE (ICD-9 185)

OCEANIA, INCIDENCE
Percentage change per five-year period, 1973-1987

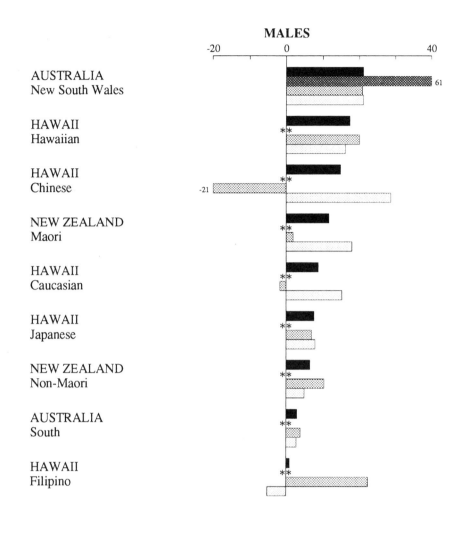

PROSTATE (ICD-9 185)

ASIA and OCEANIA, MORTALITY

MALES	Best model	Goodness of fit	1965 Rate	1965 Deaths	1985 Rate	1985 Deaths	Cumulative risk 1900	Cumulative risk 1940	Recent trend
AUSTRALIA	A2	2.88	16.2	379	16.2	627	12.9	12.9	5.0
HONG KONG	A2	0.07	2.9	6	2.9	19	*2.3*	2.3	*-1.3*
JAPAN	A4P3C2	3.71	2.3	399	3.3	930	2.0	2.5	10.1
MAURITIUS	A1	-1.72	3.7	1	3.7	2	*2.8*	2.8	*14.7*
NEW ZEALAND	A8D	1.13	14.9	77	18.3	143	12.3	18.3	10.5
SINGAPORE	A2D	-1.69	*1.5*	2	2.9	6	*0.8*	2.9	–

*   : not enough deaths for reliable estimation
– : incomplete or missing data
Best model: polynomial of the given degree in age (A), period (P) or cohort (C), or linear drift (D) model.
Goodness of fit: the normalised likelihood ratio chi-square for the best model (see Method).
Rate: world-standardised truncated rate per 100 000 per year (30-74 years) and number of **deaths** are both estimated from the best-fitting model for the single years cited.
Cumulative risk per 1000 (30-74 years) is estimated from the best-fitting *age-cohort* model for cohorts of central birth year cited.
Recent trend: estimated mean percentage change per five-year period in the age-specific rates (30-74 years) over the period 1975-1988.
Italics denote recent trends not significant at 5 per cent level, or other figures which should be interpreted with caution (see Method).

MALES

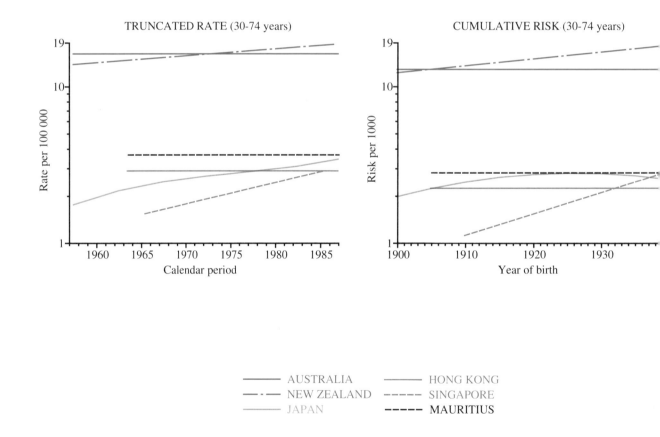

PROSTATE (ICD-9 185)

ASIA and OCEANIA, MORTALITY
Percentage change per five-year period, 1975-1988

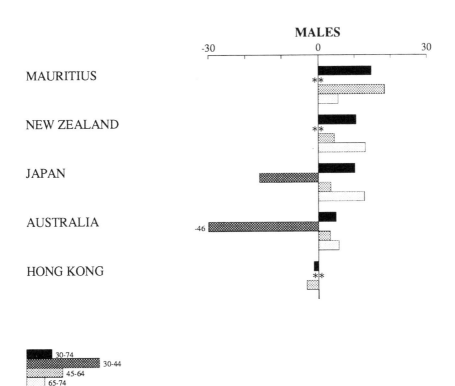

PROSTATE (ICD-9 185)

AMERICAS (except USA), INCIDENCE

MALES	Best model	Goodness of fit	1970 Rate	1970 Cases	1985 Rate	1985 Cases	Cumulative risk 1915	Cumulative risk 1940	Recent trend
BRAZIL									
Sao Paulo	A3D	0.38	15.6	56	*45.4*	*212*	17.8	*101.4*	–
CANADA									
Alberta	A4D	0.02	44.2	132	82.1	360	57.8	154.3	22.2
British Columbia	A4P2C3	-0.49	55.9	263	94.1	720	63.9	122.4	29.7
Maritime Provinces	A4P3	-1.21	38.8	127	64.0	256	46.1	96.7	18.0
Newfoundland	A2C5	-0.20	28.1	23	51.6	62	35.7	3.7	14.8
Quebec	A8P4C9	0.56	38.5	397	71.1	1039	50.5	70.3	23.7
COLOMBIA									
Cali	A5P3	-0.71	25.5	11	36.8	36	27.9	39.6	*10.4*
CUBA	A4P2	5.60	20.7	288	27.5	611	21.7	*32.4*	–
PUERTO RICO	A8C9	0.32	29.9	136	48.9	365	32.2	136.9	16.6

* : not enough cases for reliable estimation
– : incomplete or missing data
Best model: polynomial of the given degree in age (A), period (P) or cohort (C), or linear drift (D) model.
Goodness of fit: the normalised likelihood ratio chi-square for the best model (see Method).
Rate: world-standardised truncated rate per 100 000 per year (30-74 years) and number of **cases** are both estimated from the best-fitting model for the single years cited.
Cumulative risk per 1000 (30-74 years) is estimated from the best-fitting *age-cohort* model for cohorts of central birth year cited.
Recent trend: estimated mean percentage change per five-year period in the age-specific rates (30-74 years) over the period 1973-1987.
Italics denote recent trends not significant at 5 per cent level, or other figures which should be interpreted with caution (see Method).

MALES

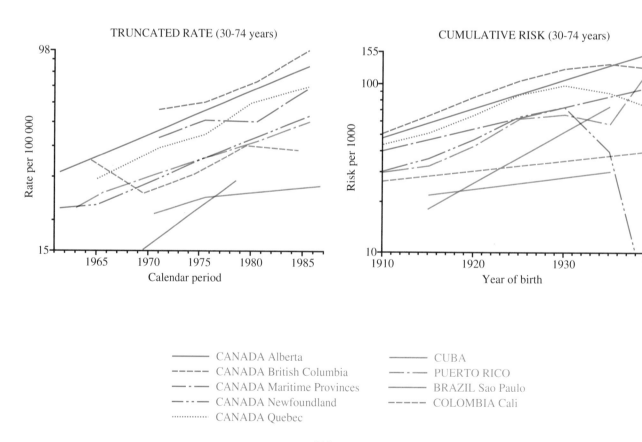

TRUNCATED RATE (30-74 years)

CUMULATIVE RISK (30-74 years)

——— CANADA Alberta
－－－－ CANADA British Columbia
—·— CANADA Maritime Provinces
—··— CANADA Newfoundland
············ CANADA Quebec

——— CUBA
—·—· PUERTO RICO
——— BRAZIL Sao Paulo
－－－－ COLOMBIA Cali

514

PROSTATE (ICD-9 185)

AMERICAS (except USA), INCIDENCE
Percentage change per five-year period, 1973-1987

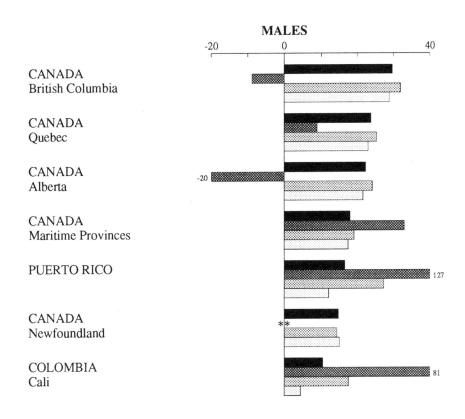

PROSTATE (ICD-9 185)

AMERICAS (USA), INCIDENCE

MALES	Best model	Goodness of fit	1970 Rate	Cases	1985 Rate	Cases	Cumulative risk 1915	1940	Recent trend
USA									
Bay Area, Black	A2P3	1.10	93.7	45	151.6	123	107.1	153.5	*3.1*
Bay Area, Chinese	*	..	..	..	..	..	..	..	..
Bay Area, White	A2P2	0.08	66.5	389	88.5	582	61.3	104.2	12.6
Connecticut	A2P3	1.13	53.2	345	73.5	631	52.8	86.4	9.2
Detroit, Black	A2P3	-0.71	114.8	147	158.2	292	103.4	180.4	13.5
Detroit, White	A3C2	-1.69	52.3	374	92.6	698	62.7	*223.0*	23.8
Iowa	A2C3	0.67	56.1	409	88.1	685	61.6	102.3	18.9
New Orleans, Black	A2	0.99	*114.2*	*61*	114.2	69	79.5	79.5	*-1.8*
New Orleans, White	A2D	1.10	*46.2*	*66*	79.6	128	52.9	125.8	19.9
Seattle	A2P2	1.02	*93.2*	*461*	129.4	919	84.9	*231.6*	25.1

* : not enough cases for reliable estimation
– : incomplete or missing data
Best model: polynomial of the given degree in age (A), period (P) or cohort (C), or linear drift (D) model.
Goodness of fit: the normalised likelihood ratio chi-square for the best model (see Method).
Rate: world-standardised truncated rate per 100 000 per year (30-74 years) and number of **cases** are both estimated from the best-fitting model for the single years cited.
Cumulative risk per 1000 (30-74 years) is estimated from the best-fitting *age-cohort* model for cohorts of central birth year cited.
Recent trend: estimated mean percentage change per five-year period in the age-specific rates (30-74 years) over the period 1973-1987.
Italics denote recent trends not significant at 5 per cent level, or other figures which should be interpreted with caution (see Method).

MALES

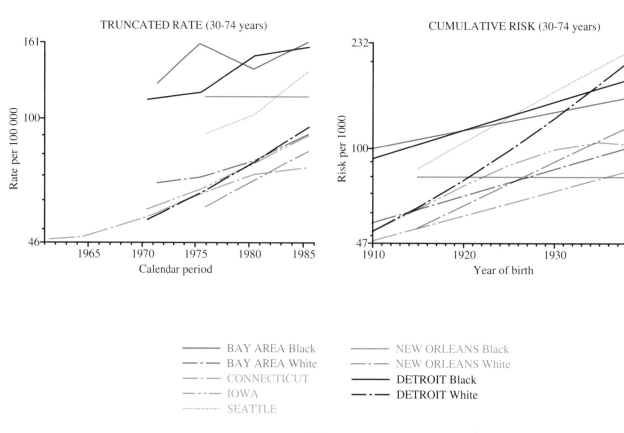

516

PROSTATE (ICD-9 185)

AMERICAS (USA), INCIDENCE
Percentage change per five-year period, 1973-1987

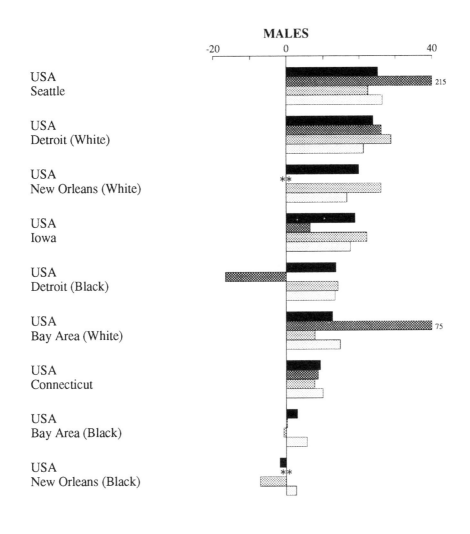

MALES

PROSTATE (ICD-9 185)

AMERICAS, MORTALITY

MALES	Best model	Goodness of fit	1965 Rate	1965 Deaths	1985 Rate	1985 Deaths	Cumulative risk 1900	Cumulative risk 1940	Recent trend
CANADA	A4P5C4	1.81	14.7	555	16.2	987	11.7	15.1	8.4
CHILE	A8P6C9	-0.38	10.1	108	11.0	184	8.6	4.7	6.6
COSTA RICA	A2P2	0.56	*11.9*	*16*	12.8	38	*8.2*	12.1	16.0
PANAMA	A3D	-0.72	10.5	13	12.6	35	8.4	12.2	–
PUERTO RICO	A2P3	1.34	12.1	48	16.6	61	*10.1*	16.1	*5.8*
URUGUAY	A2	1.11	19.6	113	19.6	151	15.2	15.2	*2.7*
USA	A5P4C8	1.90	17.0	7391	17.5	10661	13.5	11.8	2.3
VENEZUELA	A2P4C3	0.86	14.0	97	*19.5*	*219*	10.8	7.8	–

* : not enough deaths for reliable estimation
– : incomplete or missing data
Best model: polynomial of the given degree in age (A), period (P) or cohort (C), or linear drift (D) model.
Goodness of fit: the normalised likelihood ratio chi-square for the best model (see Method).
Rate: world-standardised truncated rate per 100 000 per year (30-74 years) and number of **deaths** are both estimated from the best-fitting model for the single years cited.
Cumulative risk per 1000 (30-74 years) is estimated from the best-fitting *age-cohort* model for cohorts of central birth year cited.
Recent trend: estimated mean percentage change per five-year period in the age-specific rates (30-74 years) over the period 1975-1988.
Italics denote recent trends not significant at 5 per cent level, or other figures which should be interpreted with caution (see Method).

MALES

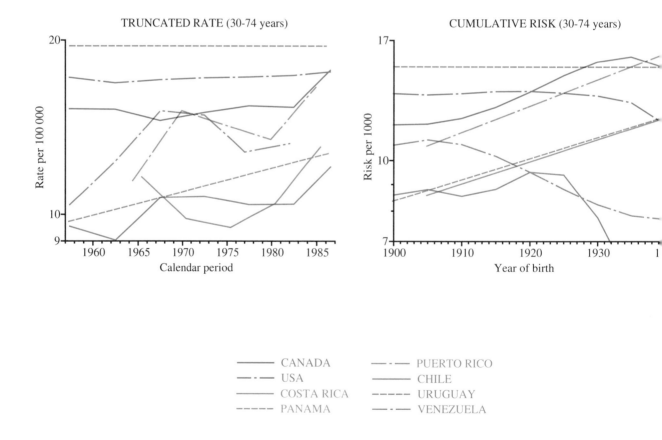

PROSTATE (ICD-9 185)

AMERICAS, MORTALITY
Percentage change per five-year period, 1975-1988

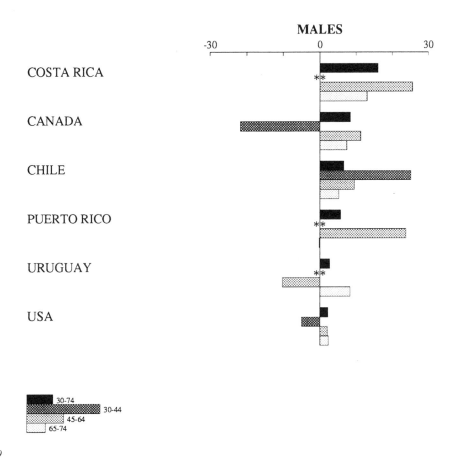

from page 499

while recent increases in Hong Kong are small (6% every five years), Chinese men in Singapore have experienced a rapid increase in the rate of prostate cancer, in common with Indians and Malays.

Incidence in the five ethnic groups in Hawaii, especially the Caucasians, is more similar to that in Europe or among North American whites than to incidence in Asian populations, but except for Hawaiians, these incidence rates are increasing only slowly.

Incidence among non-Maoris (and Maoris) in New Zealand and in both Australian populations resembles that in other Caucasian populations, and in New South Wales it is increasing rapidly (21% every five years). Mortality in New Zealand has been increasing at 10% every five years, a similar trend to that seen for incidence (6% for non-Maoris, 12% for Maoris), but the rate of increase in mortality in Australia (5%) is much smaller than the rise in incidence in New South Wales. This suggests either that the incidence trend in New South Wales, which covers a third of the national population, is not typical of Australia

as a whole, or perhaps that an increasing number of cases diagnosed at incidental biopsy have been registered in New South Wales.

Americas

The incidence of prostate cancer in North American populations is higher than anywhere else in the world, particularly among blacks (truncated rates of 110-150 per 100 000), for whom lifetime risks were already around 10% for the 1915 birth cohort, and may reach 15% or more for the 1940 birth cohort if current trends continue. Incidence in Seattle is also very high, however, although 88% of the population is white; the recent rate of increase (25% every five years) is the highest of the US populations examined, and more similar to that in the adjacent Canadian province of British Columbia (30%), where the incidence is also the highest among the Canadian populations examined. The rates of increase in incidence among black populations are generally lower than for whites. With this exception, the increasing trends for other American and Canadian populations are substantial, around 15-25% every five years. Mortality is increasing much more slowly, at around 2% every five years in the USA, and more recently at 8% in Canada. This suggests both that incidence may be increasing partly as a result of incidental diagnosis of latent carcinomas, and, perhaps, that treatment of invasive carcinoma of the prostate and survival are also improving.

Mortality from prostate cancer in Uruguayan males is even higher than in the USA and Canada, but stable, and there is little evidence of an increase elsewhere in South America: mortality in Venezuela has been unstable, and recent data are lacking; the recent increase in Chile is explained by the higher rate recorded in the period 1985-87, especially among the elderly, while the cohort effect is caused by the very low rate recorded in younger men in the period 1980-84. In São Paulo (Brazil), incidence appeared to be increasing up to 1978, but there is little change in Cali (Colombia).

In Central America, mortality is increasing steadily in Panama and Puerto Rico, where incidence is also rising quite rapidly (17% every five years). Incidence is lower in Cuba, but also appears to be increasing at a similar rate.

Comment

Restriction of the analyses reported here to the age range 30-74 years should in principle enable a clearer description of the trends in risk, since large increases have been observed at older ages due to more widespread use of minimally invasive diagnostic techniques[50,77], including transrectal ultrasonography, serum biomarkers and needle biopsy. A strong correlation between the increase in localised prostatic carcinoma and the increase in transurethral resection of the prostate for benign prostatic hypertrophy has been documented in the USA[241]. Improvements in diagnostic techniques have also led to increases in diagnosis in younger age groups, as seen in these analyses, where the trends are mostly better described by age-period models. There is a systematic difference between the trends in incidence and mortality, but the modest improvements in survival observed in some countries are difficult to assess, due to the more frequent diagnosis of relatively benign lesions[27,239,241].

The problem of examining trends in survival and mortality in very elderly patients is further complicated by the difficulty of adjusting for competing risks of death, given that many elderly males with localised prostate cancer will die of other causes even if they are not treated[48]. Taking this difficulty into consideration, most investigators have concluded that while improvement in diagnostic practice is the main explanation for the observed increase in prostate cancer incidence, a real increase in risk cannot be excluded on the basis of the available data[6,50,182,199,241,262]. There is some interesting evidence on this point. There has been an increase in latent invasive carcinoma of the prostate discovered at autopsy in Japan[307], and the frequency among Japanese men aged 50 or more during the period 1982-86 (34%) was similar to that in US white men, in sharp contrast to the difference in the incidence of clinical carcinoma between the two countries. The increase in latent carcinoma in Japan was interpreted as being due to a change in risk factors, and as presaging a large increase in incidence for men in Japan, who are currently at low risk.

The incidence of prostate cancer in Kingston and St Andrew (Jamaica), where it is the commonest cancer in men, has been stable or slightly decreasing over the 30-year period 1958-87[42], in contrast to the patterns reported here for Cuba and Puerto Rico.

Chapter 22

TESTIS

Cancer of the testis accounts for less than 1% of all male cancers. There are several morphological types, with distinct age-incidence and clinical behaviour. Seminoma comprises half or more of all testicular cancer, especially in the age range 15-50 years. Teratoma and other germ cell tumours account for a further 40%, and lymphoma and sarcoma the remainder, although lymphoma of the testis is rare before the age of 50. The age-incidence pattern of testicular cancer is unusual. In whites, peak incidence occurs at ages 20-34 years, at which age it is the commonest malignancy in males, while this peak is much less marked in blacks. Overall incidence is also much higher in whites. Cryptorchidism is associated with an increased risk of testicular cancer, and there is evidence that cryptorchidism has been increasing in some countries. There are marked socio-economic and racial differences, and genetic factors may also influence risk. Five-year survival has increased to 85%, and 90% or more in stage I or II tumours, since the introduction of cis-platin in the late 1970s.

Trends in testicular cancer have been examined for the age groups 15-29, 30-44 and 45-64 years. The unusual age pattern of the disease enables risk to be examined for more recent birth cohorts than for most other cancers, since the incidence peak for 20-34 year-olds has already been recorded for the 1950 birth cohort. Truncated rates per 100 000 (15-64 years) are tabulated for the same reference years as for other sites (1970 and 1985). Cumulative risks (15-64 years) are tabulated for the 1925 and 1950 birth cohorts for incidence (instead of 1915 and 1940) and for the 1910 and 1950 cohorts for mortality (1900, 1940). The graphs of cumulative risk by year of birth have also been extended to include 1950. The risk (15-64 years) for the 1950 birth cohort is 1-7 per 1000 in the populations at highest risk.

Europe

The incidence of testicular cancer is increasing almost everywhere, most rapidly in Hungary and Slovenia, where the rates have doubled since 1970, and are still rising at 35% or more every five years. Incidence in Hungary and Slovenia was well within the European range in the 1960s, and the increase since then is unlikely to be due solely to better registration. The rates of increase are almost as great in France, Germany and Italy, where cumulative risks (15-64 years) for the 1950 birth cohort are 3-5 per 1000. The exception is Spain, where the cumulative risk is very low by European standards — less than 1 per 1000 for the 1950 cohort — and shows no sign of increasing, either in Navarra or Zaragoza. The risk in five other populations in Spain and Portugal around 1985 was also low[221]. Most data are well fitted by linear drift or cohort effects, and the cumulative risk ranges up to 7 per 1000 for the 1950 birth cohort in Denmark, Germany and Switzerland. Unusually, there is a 4-fold range of incidence among the Nordic countries, and the differentials have persisted since the 1960s. Incidence is lowest in Finland, but it is increasing significantly among 15-29 year-olds (17% every five years). Both Norway and Denmark show a clear dip in the upward trend in risk for successive birth cohorts for men born around the time of the second world war, 1935-45, with a further acceleration in the increase for later cohorts.

Mortality from testicular cancer in Europe has fallen substantially in most countries since about 1970, and is now in the range 0.2 to 1 per 100 000 (15-64 years). Where it has not fallen, the rate of increase in mortality has decelerated sharply. The fall in mortality was seen after 1970 in Norway, the Netherlands, Belgium and Italy, and after 1975 in the UK and the other Nordic countries, where the decline has been most marked. Mortality has stopped increasing in eastern Europe, and may now be declining in Poland and Czechoslovakia. Overall mortality in Spain is low, reflecting incidence, and it has also declined, after reaching a peak around 1980; but there is a small increase in mortality among men aged 15-29 years, whereas incidence at this age is declining in both Navarra and Zaragoza.

Asia and Oceania

The risk of testicular cancer in Asian populations is a third or less of that in European or North American populations, and it has changed very little, except in Japan. In Osaka and Miyagi prefectures, truncated rates (15-64 years) have more than doubled since 1970, and are increasing at more than 20% every five years, and twice as

continued page 541

TESTIS (ICD-9 186)

EUROPE (non-EC), INCIDENCE

MALES	Best model	Goodness of fit	1970 Rate	1970 Cases	1985 Rate	1985 Cases	Cumulative risk 1925	Cumulative risk 1950	Recent trend
FINLAND	A3C2	0.39	1.5	23	2.9	50	0.6	1.5	*9.6*
HUNGARY									
County Vas	A3D	-0.35	2.2	1	8.4	7	0.8	7.7	53.8
Szabolcs-Szatmar	A3C2	0.28	1.7	3	3.5	7	0.7	1.6	52.3
ISRAEL									
All Jews	A3D	-1.46	2.4	18	3.4	36	1.0	1.8	*10.2*
Non-Jews	A0C2	-1.09	*0.9*	*0*	1.4	2	0.5	1.2	*6.2*
NORWAY	A4C6	-0.08	6.1	71	10.2	139	2.9	4.1	21.4
POLAND									
Warsaw City	A5D	2.04	2.3	9	4.4	24	0.8	2.2	22.1
ROMANIA									
Cluj	A0C4	1.40	*1.2*	*2*	2.0	5	0.7	2.6	*11.0*
SWEDEN	A4C2	0.88	3.8	98	5.9	161	1.6	2.9	14.3
SWITZERLAND									
Geneva	A2D	2.67	6.9	7	10.2	13	2.8	5.2	*11.5*
YUGOSLAVIA									
Slovenia	A3C4	0.81	2.4	13	5.3	36	0.8	2.9	35.3

* : not enough cases for reliable estimation
– : incomplete or missing data
Best model: polynomial of the given degree in age (A), period (P) or cohort (C), or linear drift (D) model.
Goodness of fit: the normalised likelihood ratio chi-square for the best model (see Method).
Rate: world-standardised truncated rate per 100 000 per year (15-64 years) and number of **cases** are both estimated from the best-fitting model for the single years cited.
Cumulative risk per 1000 (15-64 years) is estimated from the best-fitting *age-cohort* model for cohorts of central birth year cited.
Recent trend: estimated mean percentage change per five-year period in the age-specific rates (15-64 years) over the period 1973-1987.
Italics denote recent trends not significant at 5 per cent level, or other figures which should be interpreted with caution (see Method).

MALES

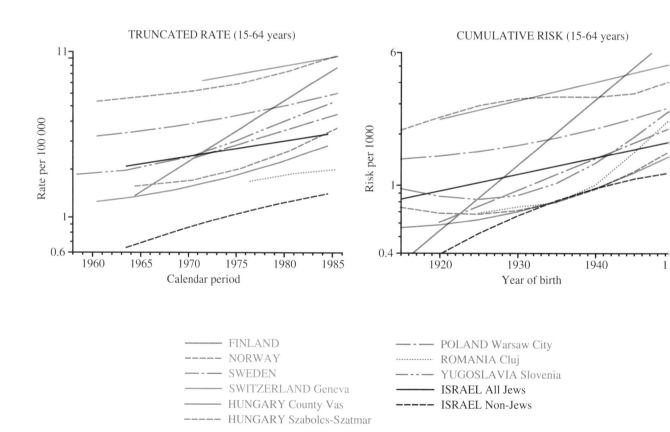

TRUNCATED RATE (15-64 years) CUMULATIVE RISK (15-64 years)

FINLAND	POLAND Warsaw City
NORWAY	ROMANIA Cluj
SWEDEN	YUGOSLAVIA Slovenia
SWITZERLAND Geneva	ISRAEL All Jews
HUNGARY County Vas	ISRAEL Non-Jews
HUNGARY Szabolcs-Szatmar	

TESTIS (ICD-9 186)

EUROPE (non-EC), INCIDENCE
Percentage change per five-year period, 1973-1987

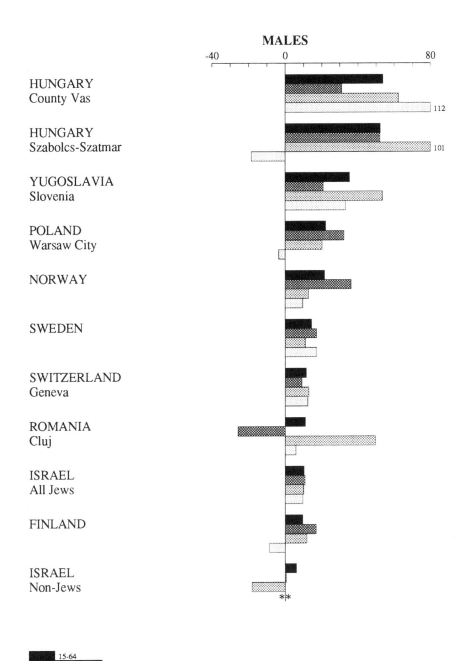

MALES

TESTIS (ICD-9 186)

EUROPE (EC), INCIDENCE

MALES	Best model	Goodness of fit	1970 Rate	1970 Cases	1985 Rate	1985 Cases	Cumulative risk 1925	Cumulative risk 1950	Recent trend
DENMARK	A6C8	-0.40	8.4	131	13.4	234	3.8	6.6	12.6
FRANCE									
Bas-Rhin	A3D	0.51	*3.7*	*10*	8.6	28	1.2	4.8	32.5
Doubs	A2	0.05	*5.2*	*8*	5.2	8	2.5	2.5	*11.8*
GERMANY (FRG)									
Hamburg	A3D	-0.63	6.5	36	*11.8*	*64*	2.3	6.4	–
Saarland	A3D	0.51	4.1	14	9.4	34	1.3	5.1	33.3
GERMANY (GDR)	A5C8	0.91	4.7	232	10.6	590	1.2	5.3	33.2
ITALY									
Varese	A2D	-0.26	*2.9*	*6*	6.1	16	1.0	3.5	28.2
SPAIN									
Navarra	A2	-1.23	*1.7*	*2*	1.7	2	0.8	0.8	*6.2*
Zaragoza	A3	0.94	1.8	4	1.8	4	0.9	0.9	*-8.9*
UK									
Birmingham	A5D	-1.70	3.8	60	5.2	90	1.5	2.7	10.3
Scotland	A3D	0.26	4.7	69	7.6	127	1.8	4.0	15.0
South Thames	A4P2C4	-0.44	4.5	116	5.3	113	1.9	2.8	*2.2*

* : not enough cases for reliable estimation
– : incomplete or missing data
Best model: polynomial of the given degree in age (A), period (P) or cohort (C), or linear drift (D) model.
Goodness of fit: the normalised likelihood ratio chi-square for the best model (see Method).
Rate: world-standardised truncated rate per 100 000 per year (15-64 years) and number of **cases** are both estimated from the best-fitting model for the single years cited.
Cumulative risk per 1000 (15-64 years) is estimated from the best-fitting *age-cohort* model for cohorts of central birth year cited.
Recent trend: estimated mean percentage change per five-year period in the age-specific rates (15-64 years) over the period 1973-1987.
Italics denote recent trends not significant at 5 per cent level, or other figures which should be interpreted with caution (see Method).

MALES

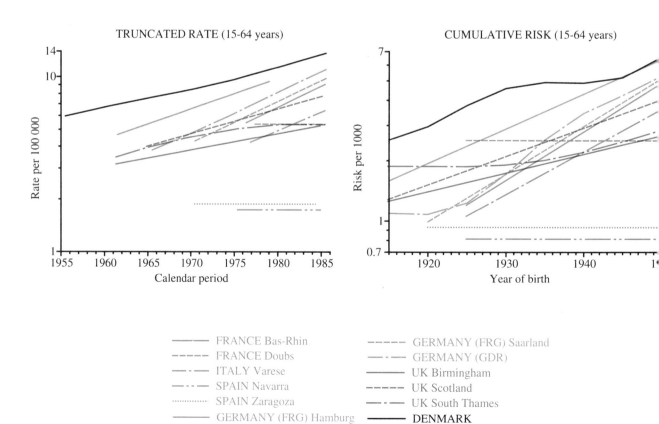

TRUNCATED RATE (15-64 years) — CUMULATIVE RISK (15-64 years)

FRANCE Bas-Rhin — GERMANY (FRG) Saarland
FRANCE Doubs — GERMANY (GDR)
ITALY Varese — UK Birmingham
SPAIN Navarra — UK Scotland
SPAIN Zaragoza — UK South Thames
GERMANY (FRG) Hamburg — DENMARK

TESTIS (ICD-9 186)

EUROPE (EC), INCIDENCE
Percentage change per five-year period, 1973-1987

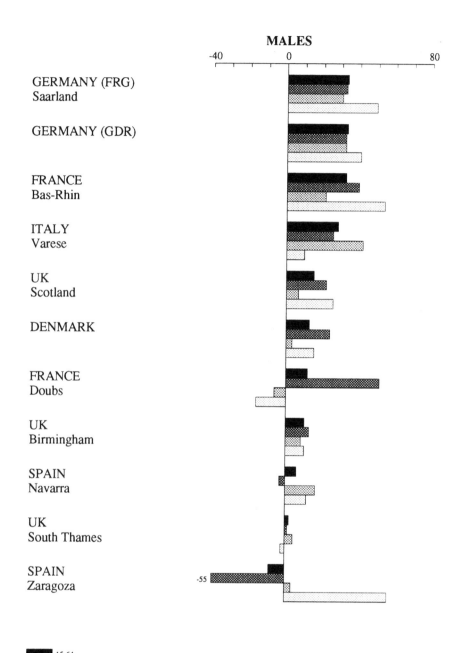

TESTIS (ICD-9 186)

EUROPE (non-EC), MORTALITY

MALES	Best model	Goodness of fit	1965 Rate	1965 Deaths	1985 Rate	1985 Deaths	Cumulative risk 1910	Cumulative risk 1950	Recent trend
AUSTRIA	A4P2C3	0.30	1.5	32	1.1	26	0.6	0.7	-31.3
CZECHOSLOVAKIA	A4P2C4	1.06	0.9	38	1.6	83	0.3	1.1	*-2.6*
FINLAND	A4P3	0.31	0.5	6	0.4	7	0.3	0.3	-32.5
HUNGARY	A4C4	-0.49	*1.2*	*35*	1.7	58	*0.4*	0.8	*5.1*
NORWAY	A4P5	1.17	1.9	21	0.5	7	1.6	0.5	-52.3
POLAND	A4P3C4	-0.79	0.4	41	1.1	138	0.2	0.7	–
ROMANIA	A3D	0.96	*0.4*	*24*	*0.7*	*53*	*0.1*	0.5	–
SWEDEN	A4P5	0.41	1.1	26	0.5	13	0.8	0.4	-41.1
SWITZERLAND	A4P3C3	0.71	1.6	30	1.2	27	0.7	0.8	-31.8
YUGOSLAVIA	A4P2	-0.04	0.5	29	0.6	50	0.2	0.4	*-5.5*

* : not enough deaths for reliable estimation
– : incomplete or missing data
Best model: polynomial of the given degree in age (A), period (P) or cohort (C), or linear drift (D) model.
Goodness of fit: the normalised likelihood ratio chi-square for the best model (see Method).
Rate: world-standardised truncated rate per 100 000 per year (15-64 years) and number of **deaths** are both estimated from the best-fitting model for the single years cited.
Cumulative risk per 1000 (15-64 years) is estimated from the best-fitting *age-cohort* model for cohorts of central birth year cited.
Recent trend: estimated mean percentage change per five-year period in the age-specific rates (15-64 years) over the period 1975-1988.
Italics denote recent trends not significant at 5 per cent level, or other figures which should be interpreted with caution (see Method).

MALES

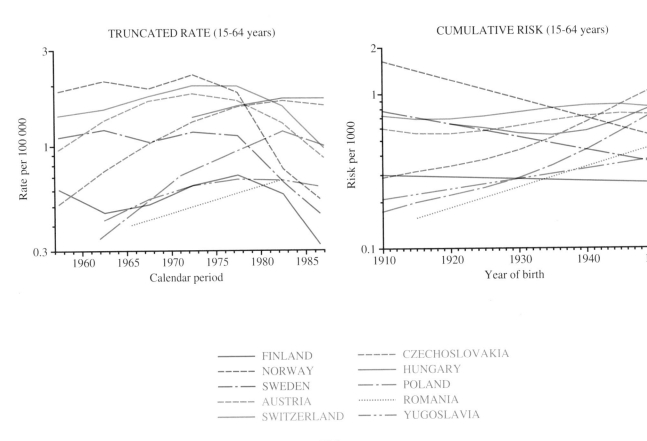

TRUNCATED RATE (15-64 years)

CUMULATIVE RISK (15-64 years)

———— FINLAND   - - - - - CZECHOSLOVAKIA
- - - - - NORWAY   ———— HUNGARY
—·—· SWEDEN   —··— POLAND
- - - - - AUSTRIA   ·········· ROMANIA
———— SWITZERLAND   —···— YUGOSLAVIA

TESTIS (ICD-9 186)

EUROPE (non-EC), MORTALITY
Percentage change per five-year period, 1975-1988

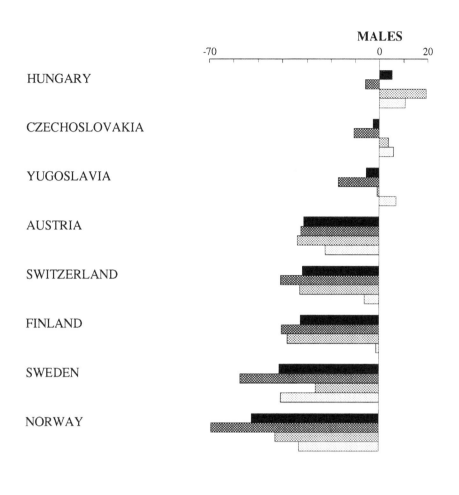

TESTIS (ICD-9 186)

EUROPE (EC), MORTALITY

MALES	Best model	Goodness of fit	1965		1985		Cumulative risk		Recent trend
			Rate	Deaths	Rate	Deaths	1910	1950	
BELGIUM	A4P4	1.80	0.7	20	0.2	7	0.4	0.2	-35.7
DENMARK	A4P5C2	2.66	2.7	39	0.9	16	1.7	0.8	-33.6
FRANCE	A9P6C9	-0.42	0.9	132	0.8	148	0.4	0.4	-18.7
GERMANY (FRG)	A4P5C9	4.87	1.5	281	1.1	227	0.8	0.7	-26.9
GREECE	A3P2	2.03	*0.3*	*9*	0.4	12	*0.3*	0.2	*-20.4*
IRELAND	A4P2	-0.33	0.9	7	0.8	8	0.4	0.5	*-21.1*
ITALY	A5P3C4	2.06	1.0	170	0.5	98	0.7	0.3	-30.3
NETHERLANDS	A4P2C6	1.48	1.9	69	0.6	30	1.1	0.3	-32.4
PORTUGAL	–	–	–	–	–	–	–	–	–
SPAIN	A3P2C2	0.73	0.2	20	0.3	34	0.1	0.2	-17.9
UK ENGLAND & WALES	A4P5	1.61	1.2	184	0.7	108	0.7	0.5	-32.4
UK SCOTLAND	A4P2C3	1.70	1.7	24	1.0	16	0.6	0.7	-32.6

* : not enough deaths for reliable estimation
– : incomplete or missing data
Best model: polynomial of the given degree in age (A), period (P) or cohort (C), or linear drift (D) model.
Goodness of fit: the normalised likelihood ratio chi-square for the best model (see Method).
Rate: world-standardised truncated rate per 100 000 per year (15-64 years) and number of **deaths** are both estimated from the best-fitting model for the single years cited.
Cumulative risk per 1000 (15-64 years) is estimated from the best-fitting *age-cohort* model for cohorts of central birth year cited.
Recent trend: estimated mean percentage change per five-year period in the age-specific rates (15-64 years) over the period 1975-1988.
Italics denote recent trends not significant at 5 per cent level, or other figures which should be interpreted with caution (see Method).

MALES

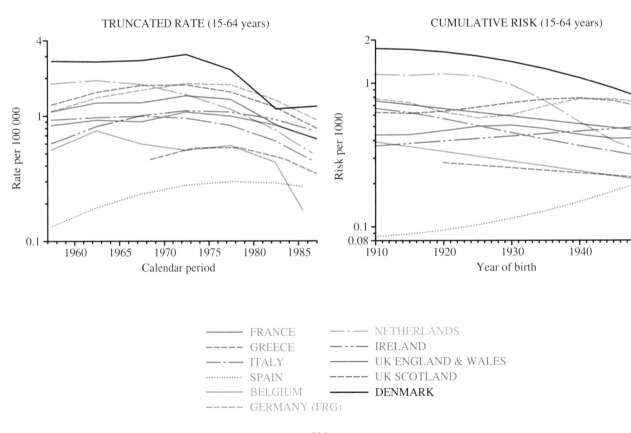

TESTIS (ICD-9 186)

EUROPE (EC), MORTALITY
Percentage change per five-year period, 1975-1988

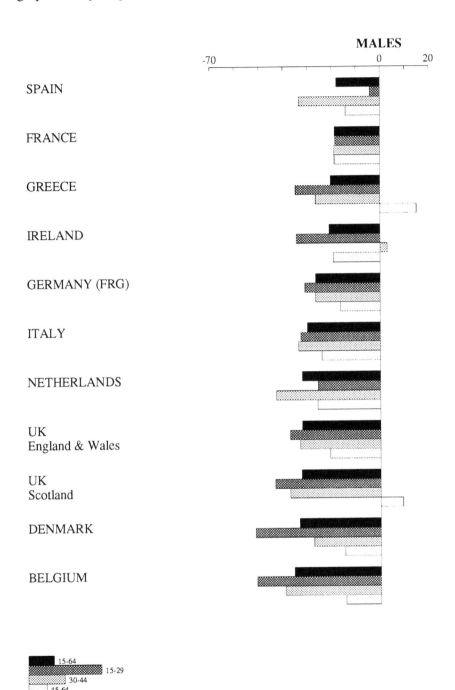

MALES

TESTIS (ICD-9 186)

ASIA, INCIDENCE

MALES	Best model	Goodness of fit	1970 Rate	1970 Cases	1985 Rate	1985 Cases	Cumulative risk 1925	Cumulative risk 1950	Recent trend
CHINA									
Shanghai	A9C8	-0.25	*1.1*	20	0.8	21	0.6	0.8	*0.6*
HONG KONG	A3D	-0.95	*1.9*	*21*	1.2	24	1.2	0.6	-16.0
INDIA									
Bombay	A3P3	0.73	0.8	18	1.2	40	0.4	0.7	*1.8*
JAPAN									
Miyagi	A3D	0.48	0.8	4	1.7	12	0.3	1.1	22.3
Nagasaki	A0	0.35	*1.5*	*2*	1.5	2	0.7	0.7	*50.1*
Osaka	A9C9	-0.31	0.8	22	1.9	58	0.2	1.3	37.2
SINGAPORE									
Chinese	A2	0.96	1.2	5	1.2	8	0.6	0.6	*8.0*
Indian	*	..	..	..	..	..	..	..	..
Malay	A0C2	0.68	*0.7*	*0*	1.4	1	0.5	1.4	-22.7

* : not enough cases for reliable estimation
− : incomplete or missing data
Best model: polynomial of the given degree in age (A), period (P) or cohort (C), or linear drift (D) model.
Goodness of fit: the normalised likelihood ratio chi-square for the best model (see Method).
Rate: world-standardised truncated rate per 100 000 per year (15-64 years) and number of **cases** are both estimated from the best-fitting model for the single years cited.
Cumulative risk per 1000 (15-64 years) is estimated from the best-fitting *age-cohort* model for cohorts of central birth year cited.
Recent trend: estimated mean percentage change per five-year period in the age-specific rates (15-64 years) over the period 1973-1987.
Italics denote recent trends not significant at 5 per cent level, or other figures which should be interpreted with caution (see Method).

MALES

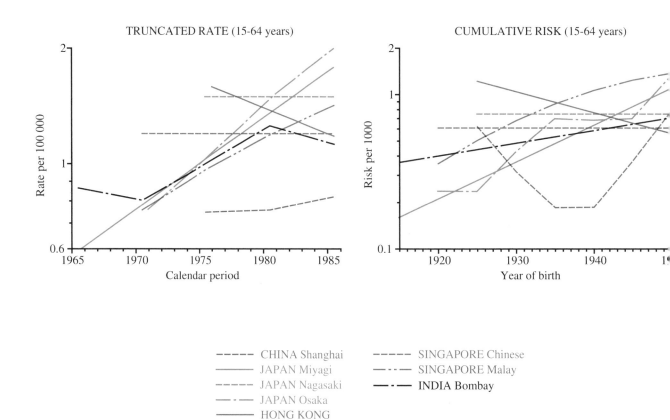

TESTIS (ICD-9 186)

ASIA, INCIDENCE
Percentage change per five-year period, 1973-1987

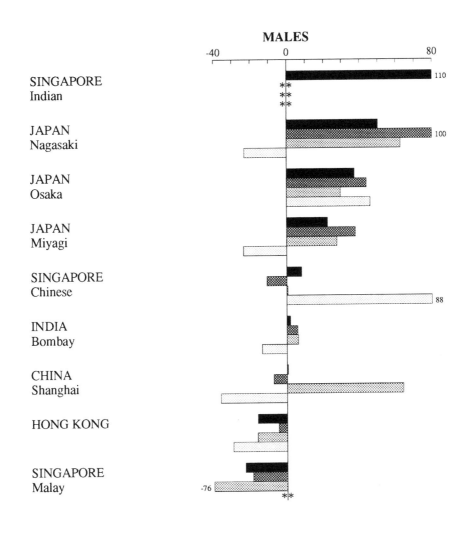

MALES

SINGAPORE Indian	** ** ** 110
JAPAN Nagasaki	100
JAPAN Osaka	
JAPAN Miyagi	
SINGAPORE Chinese	88
INDIA Bombay	
CHINA Shanghai	
HONG KONG	
SINGAPORE Malay	-76 **

15-64
15-29
30-44
45-64

TESTIS (ICD-9 186)

OCEANIA, INCIDENCE

MALES	Best model	Goodness of fit	1970		1985		Cumulative risk		Recent trend
			Rate	Cases	Rate	Cases	1925	1950	
AUSTRALIA									
New South Wales	A4D	0.45	*3.9*	*59*	5.6	106	1.6	2.8	12.2
South	A3	-0.86	*5.1*	*19*	5.1	24	2.4	2.4	*4.4*
HAWAII									
Caucasian	A3D	0.25	5.4	5	8.2	11	2.2	4.4	*12.2*
Chinese	A0D	-1.59	*1.7*	*0*	*6.4*	*0*	1.1	9.6	261.6
Filipino	*	..	..	..	..	..	..	..	..
Hawaiian	A4	-0.64	4.7	1	4.7	2	2.2	2.2	*13.2*
Japanese	A2C2	0.31	*1.2*	*0*	3.8	2	0.5	1.4	69.4
NEW ZEALAND									
Maori	A3D	-0.21	6.3	3	10.5	10	2.2	5.2	*13.2*
Non-Maori	A4D	-0.18	5.7	43	8.4	84	2.2	4.2	7.2

* : not enough cases for reliable estimation
− : incomplete or missing data
Best model: polynomial of the given degree in age (A), period (P) or cohort (C), or linear drift (D) model.
Goodness of fit: the normalised likelihood ratio chi-square for the best model (see Method).
Rate: world-standardised truncated rate per 100 000 per year (15-64 years) and number of **cases** are both estimated from the best-fitting model for the single years cited.
Cumulative risk per 1000 (15-64 years) is estimated from the best-fitting *age-cohort* model for cohorts of central birth year cited.
Recent trend: estimated mean percentage change per five-year period in the age-specific rates (15-64 years) over the period 1973-1987.
Italics denote recent trends not significant at 5 per cent level, or other figures which should be interpreted with caution (see Method).

MALES

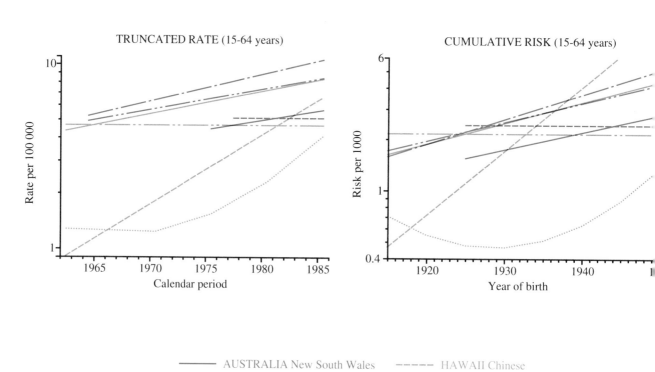

TESTIS (ICD-9 186)

OCEANIA, INCIDENCE
Percentage change per five-year period, 1973-1987

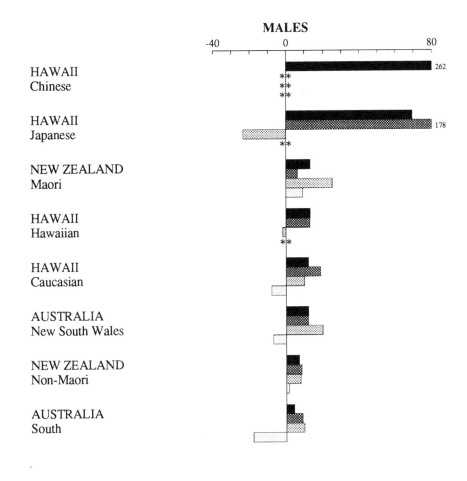

TESTIS (ICD-9 186)

ASIA and OCEANIA, MORTALITY

MALES	Best model	Goodness of fit	1965		1985		Cumulative risk		Recent trend
			Rate	Deaths	Rate	Deaths	1910	1950	
AUSTRALIA	A4P2C3	1.63	1.2	42	0.5	29	0.7	0.4	-34.4
HONG KONG	A3P2	0.15	*0.1*	*0*	0.1	2	*0.6*	0.1	-57.3
JAPAN	A4P2C8	1.76	0.3	107	0.3	123	0.2	0.2	-18.3
MAURITIUS	A0	-1.96	*0.1*	*0*	*0.1*	*0*	*0.1*	0.1	*
NEW ZEALAND	A3P2C2	0.44	2.0	15	1.0	10	0.8	0.6	-28.1
SINGAPORE	A0	0.27	0.4	1	0.4	3	*0.2*	0.2	*-4.5*

* : not enough deaths for reliable estimation
– : incomplete or missing data
Best model: polynomial of the given degree in age (A), period (P) or cohort (C), or linear drift (D) model.
Goodness of fit: the normalised likelihood ratio chi-square for the best model (see Method).
Rate: world-standardised truncated rate per 100 000 per year (15-64 years) and number of **deaths** are both estimated from the best-fitting model for the single years cited.
Cumulative risk per 1000 (15-64 years) is estimated from the best-fitting *age-cohort* model for cohorts of central birth year cited.
Recent trend: estimated mean percentage change per five-year period in the age-specific rates (15-64 years) over the period 1975-1988.
Italics denote recent trends not significant at 5 per cent level, or other figures which should be interpreted with caution (see Method).

MALES

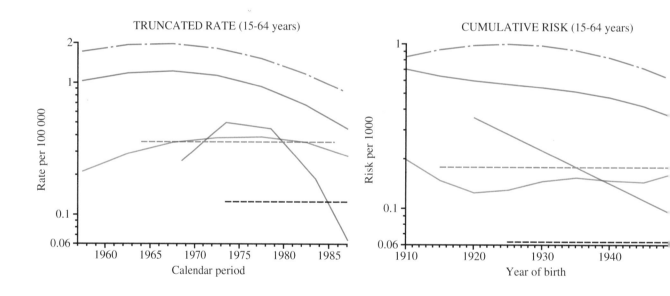

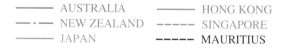

534

TESTIS (ICD-9 186)

ASIA and OCEANIA, MORTALITY
Percentage change per five-year period, 1975-1988

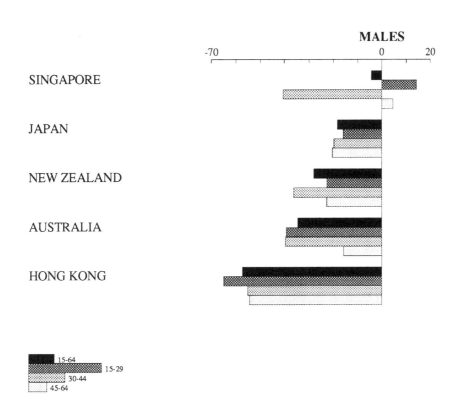

TESTIS (ICD-9 186)

AMERICAS (except USA), INCIDENCE

MALES	Best model	Goodness of fit	1970 Rate	1970 Cases	1985 Rate	1985 Cases	Cumulative risk 1925	Cumulative risk 1950	Recent trend
BRAZIL									
Sao Paulo	A2C2	1.17	1.5	28	*5.5*	*135*	0.6	1.5	–
CANADA									
Alberta	A5C2	0.49	4.7	22	6.1	55	2.1	2.9	*3.3*
British Columbia	A4C5	0.55	4.5	29	6.0	61	2.4	2.5	15.8
Maritime Provinces	A3C2	1.10	3.0	13	4.7	25	1.3	2.2	17.8
Newfoundland	A3	-0.63	3.1	4	3.1	6	1.5	1.5	*5.0*
Quebec	A5C3	2.15	1.8	34	3.5	81	0.8	1.4	28.1
COLOMBIA									
Cali	A0	0.97	1.9	3	1.9	7	0.9	0.9	*17.5*
CUBA	A2D	-0.33	0.3	6	0.7	24	0.1	0.6	–
PUERTO RICO	A3C2	1.31	0.6	4	1.7	15	0.2	0.9	61.1

* : not enough cases for reliable estimation
– : incomplete or missing data
Best model: polynomial of the given degree in age (A), period (P) or cohort (C), or linear drift (D) model.
Goodness of fit: the normalised likelihood ratio chi-square for the best model (see Method).
Rate: world-standardised truncated rate per 100 000 per year (15-64 years) and number of **cases** are both estimated from the best-fitting model for the single years cited.
Cumulative risk per 1000 (15-64 years) is estimated from the best-fitting *age-cohort* model for cohorts of central birth year cited.
Recent trend: estimated mean percentage change per five-year period in the age-specific rates (15-64 years) over the period 1973-1987.
Italics denote recent trends not significant at 5 per cent level, or other figures which should be interpreted with caution (see Method).

MALES

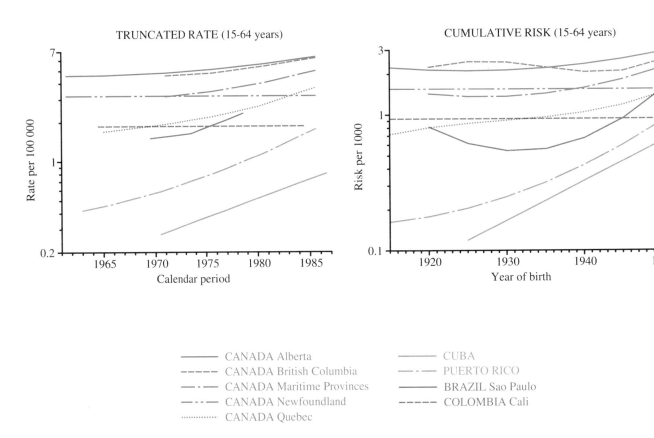

TRUNCATED RATE (15-64 years) — Rate per 100 000 — Calendar period

CUMULATIVE RISK (15-64 years) — Risk per 1000 — Year of birth

——— CANADA Alberta
------ CANADA British Columbia
—·— CANADA Maritime Provinces
—··— CANADA Newfoundland
············ CANADA Quebec

——— CUBA
—·— PUERTO RICO
——— BRAZIL Sao Paulo
------ COLOMBIA Cali

TESTIS (ICD-9 186)

AMERICAS (except USA), INCIDENCE
Percentage change per five-year period, 1973-1987

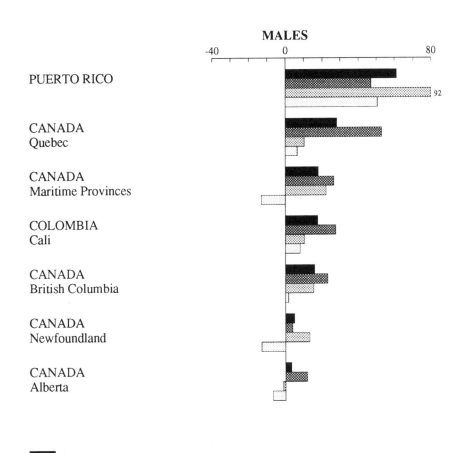

TESTIS (ICD-9 186)

AMERICAS (USA), INCIDENCE

MALES	Best model	Goodness of fit	1970 Rate	Cases	1985 Rate	Cases	Cumulative risk 1925	1950	Recent trend
USA									
Bay Area, Black	A2	0.04	1.6	1	1.6	2	0.8	0.8	-22.6
Bay Area, Chinese	A2	-0.54	*3.1*	*0*	*3.1*	2	1.4	1.4	–
Bay Area, White	A4C2	0.72	6.5	53	8.0	81	3.0	3.4	14.8
Connecticut	A4D	-1.06	4.3	36	7.1	76	1.6	3.7	13.6
Detroit, Black	A3	0.87	1.2	2	1.2	3	0.6	0.6	*12.5*
Detroit, White	A7C3	-0.08	4.5	44	7.7	78	1.6	3.9	22.5
Iowa	A3D	0.88	5.0	38	6.8	65	2.0	3.4	11.8
New Orleans, Black	A2	0.41	*1.5*	*0*	1.5	1	0.7	0.7	*2.9*
New Orleans, White	A4	-1.85	*5.7*	*11*	5.7	15	2.6	2.6	*-2.1*
Seattle	A6D	0.88	*5.4*	*30*	8.5	95	2.1	4.4	16.9

* : not enough cases for reliable estimation
– : incomplete or missing data
Best model: polynomial of the given degree in age (A), period (P) or cohort (C), or linear drift (D) model.
Goodness of fit: the normalised likelihood ratio chi-square for the best model (see Method).
Rate: world-standardised truncated rate per 100 000 per year (15-64 years) and number of **cases** are both estimated from the best-fitting model for the single years cited.
Cumulative risk per 1000 (15-64 years) is estimated from the best-fitting *age-cohort* model for cohorts of central birth year cited.
Recent trend: estimated mean percentage change per five-year period in the age-specific rates (15-64 years) over the period 1973-1987.
Italics denote recent trends not significant at 5 per cent level, or other figures which should be interpreted with caution (see Method).

MALES

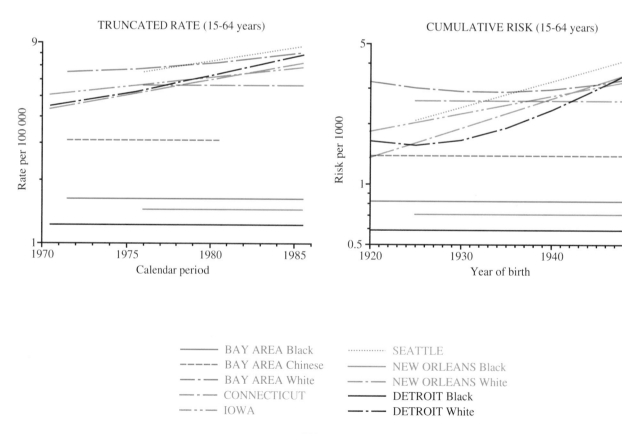

TESTIS (ICD-9 186)

AMERICAS (USA), INCIDENCE
Percentage change per five-year period, 1973-1987

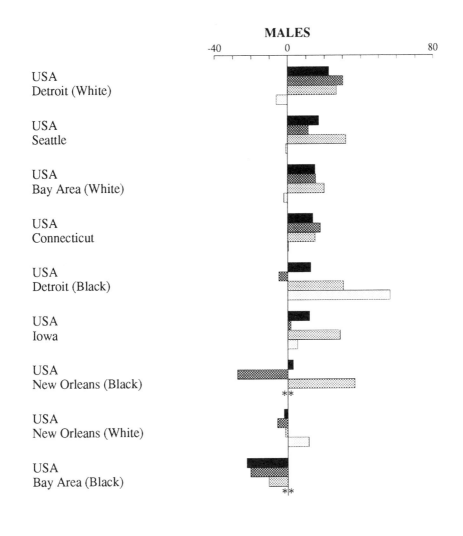

TESTIS (ICD-9 186)

AMERICAS, MORTALITY

MALES	Best model	Goodness of fit	1965 Rate	Deaths	1985 Rate	Deaths	Cumulative risk 1910	1950	Recent trend
CANADA	A4P4	1.10	1.0	57	0.4	39	0.7	0.3	-30.0
CHILE	A3C2	0.43	1.4	33	*3.6*	*145*	0.5	*1.8*	–
COSTA RICA	–	–	–	–	–	–	–	–	–
PANAMA	–	–	–	–	–	–	–	–	–
PUERTO RICO	–	–	–	–	–	–	–	–	–
URUGUAY	–	–	–	–	–	–	–	–	–
USA	A6P5C9	1.72	1.1	588	0.4	344	0.9	0.3	-32.1
VENEZUELA	A3D	2.14	0.2	5	*0.3*	*11*	0.1	*0.1*	–

* : not enough deaths for reliable estimation
– : incomplete or missing data
Best model: polynomial of the given degree in age (A), period (P) or cohort (C), or linear drift (D) model.
Goodness of fit: the normalised likelihood ratio chi-square for the best model (see Method).
Rate: world-standardised truncated rate per 100 000 per year (15-64 years) and number of **deaths** are both estimated from the best-fitting model for the single years cited.
Cumulative risk per 1000 (15-64 years) is estimated from the best-fitting *age-cohort* model for cohorts of central birth year cited.
Recent trend: estimated mean percentage change per five-year period in the age-specific rates (15-64 years) over the period 1975-1988.
Italics denote recent trends not significant at 5 per cent level, or other figures which should be interpreted with caution (see Method).

MALES

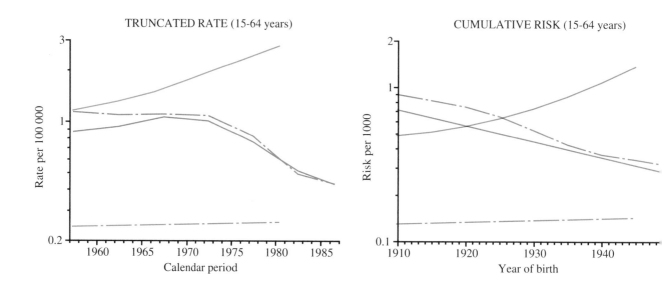

TRUNCATED RATE (15-64 years)

CUMULATIVE RISK (15-64 years)

—————— CANADA
— · — USA
—————— CHILE
— · — VENEZUELA

540

TESTIS (ICD-9 186)

AMERICAS, MORTALITY
Percentage change per five-year period, 1975-1988

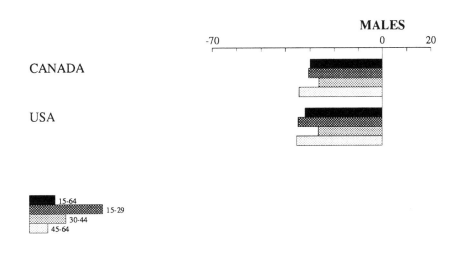

MALES

from page 521

rapidly again among 15-29 year-olds. The rapid increases in the truncated rates for both Chinese in Hawaii and Malays in Singapore are based on very few cases, and are not reliable. The significance of these overall trends is due to a very irregular distribution of the few cases that were observed over the calendar period under examination.

Testicular cancer risk in Australian men is lower than in other Caucasian populations, and it has increased more slowly: cumulative risk (15-64 years) is still less than 3 per 1000 for the 1950 birth cohort. Incidence has increased for younger men and declined among 55-64 year-olds. Incidence among both Maoris and non-Maoris in New Zealand is higher than in Australia, at 8-10 per 100 000, and it has been increasing as rapidly, most recently at 8-10% every five years. Mortality has fallen sharply since 1970 in both Australia and New Zealand (particularly for men aged 15-44) and since 1975 in Hong Kong. The decline in mortality in Japan is slightly less marked, but it is still falling at 15-20% every five years in all age groups.

Americas

Testicular cancer risk in white or predominantly white populations is lower in North America than in Europe, and is increasing less rapidly. The low risk in blacks and Chinese (1-3 per 100 000) has not changed significantly. The most rapid increase has occurred in Puerto Rico, where risk was an order of magnitude lower than in North America in the 1960s, but is now only about 50% less, and is still increasing very quickly, at 61% every five years. Incidence in Quebec (Canada) has also been rising sharply, at 28% every five years, but the cumulative risk (15-64 years) for the 1950 birth cohort is still 1.4 per 1000, not more than half the risk in the other Canadian provinces studied. Men born in 1930-40 in British Columbia have a lower risk than earlier or later birth cohorts, and the inflection in the trend in cumulative risk is more marked than in Norway and Denmark.

Mortality in both Canada and the USA has fallen substantially and steadily since 1970 at all ages, and is still declining at around 30% every five years.

Comment

The patterns of mortality for cancer of the testis are often fitted by period effects as well as cohort effects. This reflects the dramatic improvement in survival at all ages brought about by cisplatin treatment after the 1970s, providing a sharp period effect on mortality, superimposed on the underlying increase in incidence in successive birth cohorts born since 1920.

The incidence trend for Finland reported here,

using data for the period 1955-87 and showing a clear increase in successive birth cohorts, extends a previous report covering the period 1972-83[119], during which no significant change in the incidence of either seminoma or non-seminoma tumours was observed. Interestingly, there was no change in the stage distribution either, but survival improved markedly for both tumour types following the addition of cisplatin to chemotherapy regimes. This suggests that improvement in survival is not due to earlier diagnosis. The steady increase in incidence in Geneva (Switzerland) is echoed by a combined analysis from the six population-based registries in Switzerland[251], which showed a significant overall rise during the period 1970-85 in both seminoma and non-seminoma tumours. Data from the canton of Vaud (Switzerland), where incidence is high (world-standardised rate 8.4 per 100 000), were included in this analysis, though separate reports from Vaud covering the period 1974-87 gave conflicting results[162-164]. Reports from Slovakia[237] and the former Czechoslovakia as a whole[80] give comparable increases of around 35% every five years in age-standardised rates, consistent with the trends in Hungary, Poland and Slovenia.

Mortality from testicular cancer in Ireland increased substantially in the period 1961-84[282], more than doubling in the age groups of peak incidence, 15-24 and 25-34 years, while mortality in England and Wales fell slightly during the period up to 1984[213]; small increases in mortality occurred in both countries among older men (75 years and over). A small overall increase in mortality occurred in France between 1952 and 1985[128], but, as in Ireland and England and Wales, the trends have clearly been downward since the late 1970s. A report on mortality from testicular cancer in Spain[7] up to 1983 also noted the recent slight decline in overall mortality, with the same unexpected increase in mortality among younger males (25-34 years) noted here; this was attributed to increased exposure to various risk factors in recent birth cohorts, but with little evidence of increase in the low incidence rates of testicular cancer in Spain, the increase in mortality in younger males is difficult to explain.

In New Zealand, incidence has been increasing by about 3% a year since 1948, the increase affecting all age groups similarly, and under-ascertainment in the early part of the period was ruled out as an explanation[226]. Although the increase in the USA has principally affected younger men (15-44 years), improvements in diagnosis were excluded as an explanation[193], and the increase in adolescents (15-19 years) in Connecticut was particularly large, almost 20% every five years during the 45 years up to 1979[293]. The 50% decline in mortality in Ontario (Canada) between 1964 and 1982 was attributed largely to cisplatin[178].

The increases in incidence around the world are too large, consistent and long-standing to be due to improvements in diagnosis or registration. Undescended testis and mumps orchitis are associated with the risk of testicular cancer, but it is unclear whether the increase in maldescent could account for such large trends in testicular cancer[192]. The exceptions to this widespread increase are provided by black and Chinese populations, and apparently by men in Spain; rapid increases in the incidence of other cancers have occurred in Zaragoza and Navarra, and it seems unlikely that any such trend has been missed for cancer of the testis, since incidence elsewhere in Spain and Portugal is also low, as is mortality in Spain.

The transient dip in the cohort risk trends seen for males born around 1935-45 in Denmark, Norway and British Columbia (Canada) is intriguing.

The dramatic impact of cisplatin in improving the prognosis of testicular cancer is widely acknowledged. Mortality has declined in most countries since the 1970s, often by more than 50%, and despite continuing increases in incidence in many of these countries. While the trends in mortality underline a major therapeutic advance, therefore, they camouflage the underlying trends in incidence, which now constitute an important preventive challenge to public health.

Chapter 23

BLADDER

Cancer of the urinary bladder accounted for about 3.5% of all malignancies in the world in 1980, with some 219 000 new cases a year, ranking eleventh in frequency on a global scale. It is three times more common in males than in females, accounting for 5.2% of all cancers among men, and ranking eighth. Geographical variation in incidence is greater than ten-fold, and until recently recorded incidence was highest in white male populations in developed countries, and lowest among Indian, Chinese and Japanese populations. Bladder cancers are mostly transitional cell carcinomas (90-95%) in developed countries, although 10-15% are squamous cell carcinomas in some populations, and this can exceed 50% where schistosomiasis is common[264]. Tobacco smoking is a cause of bladder cancer, with attributable risks of 40% or more in males and 30% in females in developed countries, and a number of organic chemicals used in industry are known to be carcinogenic to the bladder.

When reporting their data, most cancer registries exclude bladder papillomas specified as benign, and those unspecified as to whether benign or malignant. The data for 20 of the 60 populations, however, explicitly included among malignant neoplasms of the bladder those which were registered as 'benign' and/or unspecified papilloma (ICD-9 223.3 and 236.7 respectively) in one or more calendar periods. For nine of these populations, practice appears to have changed during the 1980s (Table 23.1). Since 'benign' papillomas of the bladder may comprise a substantial proportion of all bladder neoplasms[264], this clearly complicates both the interpretation of trends for the minority of registries which appear to have changed their practice, and the comparison of risks and trends between registries which include 'benign' and unspecified bladder papillomas in their data and the remainder which do not[196].

The tendency for pathologists to classify as malignant some papillomas which would previously have been classified as benign further complicates the issue, since these papillomas would be included among malignant tumours, even by registries which do not register papillomas classified by the pathologist as benign or of unspecified behaviour. With these variations in registration practice around the world, it is

perhaps surprising that geographical variation in recorded incidence is not greater than it is.

Trends in incidence and mortality from bladder cancer vary widely around the world. Recent incidence trends range from declines of 30% or more every five years to rates of increase of a similar magnitude, while mortality trends have a narrower range. Opposite trends are seen for males and females in some countries.

Europe

Incidence has been increasing in almost all populations, particularly in males: truncated rates are mostly between 15 and 40 per 100 000, increasing at 5-20% every five years. In Denmark, where truncated incidence rates (30-74 years) are among the highest in the world, at 45 per 100 000 in males and 12 per 100 000 in females, the recent trend has been a further rise of 8-9% every five years, although there are signs of a deceleration for cohorts born since 1930. Benign and unspecified papillomas comprise up to 50% of the Danish data, but registration practice has not changed, and this seems unlikely to account for the increase. In Varese (Italy), where benign and unspecified papillomas are also included, incidence in males is even higher (57 per 100 000), and increasing steadily. In Norway, cumulative risks up to age 75 for the 1940 birth cohort may exceed 5% (56 per 1000) for males, and 2% for females. Incidence in the GDR is less than half that in Denmark, but has been increasing more rapidly, at around 15% every five years.

The sharp peak in incidence among males in Geneva (Switzerland) around 1975 is due to the inclusion of non-invasive bladder papillomas for the period 1973-77 but not in earlier or later periods; incidence has declined since that time in both sexes, in contrast to the trends in other countries. A similar peak in 1975 among males in County Vas (Hungary) may have the same explanation; the underlying trend is similar to that in Szabolcs-Szatmar (Hungary), as can be seen from the period curves. The data for Zaragoza (Spain) also show irregularity, and the recent linear trend values given for County Vas and Zaragoza should therefore be ignored. The rate of increase in incidence in both sexes in

Saarland (FRG) seems very high, and warrants investigation; benign papillomas are not included.

Mortality rates for males in northern Europe show a gradual increase, peak and decline, with the peak occurring variously between 1970 and 1985. The decline is evident first in Austria and Finland, and later in most countries of northern and western Europe. Evidence of the peak is less clear for the southern countries of Greece, Italy and Spain, and the increase continues unchecked in Hungary, Poland and Romania, although there are signs of deceleration in Czechoslovakia. Among males in Europe, there is now a geographical gradient in bladder cancer mortality trends: upward in the east, a plateau in the south and downward in the north and west of the continent.

The trends in bladder cancer mortality for successive birth cohorts suggest a decline for males born since 1920 in almost all European countries. France and Spain are the exceptions, and the cumulative risks (30-74 years) for males born in 1940 seem set to exceed not only those of previous birth cohorts but also those of males in other countries. Mortality patterns among females in Europe are more homogeneous, and there is a slight but general decline since the 1970s in most countries. Females born since about 1925 are likely to have a lower risk of bladder cancer mortality than previous birth cohorts. France and Spain provide a different contrast here, since bladder cancer mortality among females is already among the lowest in the European Community, and falling for successive birth cohorts, in line with other countries.

Asia and Oceania

Incidence has increased steadily since the mid-1960s in the Japanese prefectures of Osaka and Miyagi, particularly in males, and lifetime risks for the 1940 birth cohort are around 2%. The recent upward trends are about 25% (4 standard errors) every five years for Japanese males in both prefectures, and 10% or more in Japanese females. The very high rates among Chinese in Hong Kong have declined steadily, but in both sexes bladder cancer incidence is still much higher than elsewhere in Asia, and more than twice as high as among Chinese in Shanghai (China) or Singapore. Chinese in Hawaii also have high bladder cancer risks, comparable with those of Caucasian populations elsewhere. Incidence among Caucasian males in Hawaii is particularly high (47 per 100 000), and still increasing steadily, whereas it is declining among females.

Truncated mortality rates have declined slowly but steadily in Australia and New Zealand since the 1960s, from around 8 per 100 000 in males and 2.5 in females to around 6 and 2, respectively, in the 1980s. Mortality has fallen more sharply in Japan and Hong Kong.

Americas

In the Americas, the most striking changes have occurred in Canada. In British Columbia, truncated incidence rates (30-74 years) have fallen from around 32 per 100 000 in males and 9 in females, among the highest in the Americas in the 1970s, to around 20 and 6, respectively, in the middle of the range for the continent. In other Canadian provinces, such as Alberta and the Maritime Provinces, the underlying trend is upward, and in Quebec, incidence has been increasing at 15% every five years in males and 25% in females, even though papillomas of unspecified behaviour were apparently excluded from the data after 1978. Cumulative risks for those born around 1940 in several Canadian provinces look set to reach 5% in males and 1% or more in females.

In the USA, incidence is similar to that in Canada, with cumulative risks in the range 2-5% in males and up to 1% in females. Risks are about twice as high in whites as in blacks, although the difference (ratio of rates) is more marked among males. The trends suggest that these racial differences are diminishing among males, since the rates of increase are somewhat higher among blacks. The risk is lowest among Chinese in the San Francisco Bay Area, and is stable. Rates are increasing in most populations at about 5-15% every five years, although there is little evidence of any change among black females in Detroit, New Orleans or the Bay Area. Incidence is increasing in Puerto Rican males (10% every five years) but truncated rates in both sexes are still much lower than in neighbouring countries (15 and 5 per 100 000). A slight increase in recorded incidence in Puerto Rican females since the mid-1970s is reflected by a sharper increase in mortality, which has almost doubled since 1980.

Bladder cancer mortality in Canada, the USA and Venezuela has declined steadily since the 1960s, by almost 50% in females and by about 25% in males, to around 0.8 and 2.5 per 100 000 respectively, and recent rates of further decline are around 7-15% every five years. For females in North America, the rates of decline are most rapid for the age group 30-44 years, at around 12% (five standard errors) every five years in the USA and 16% (two standard errors) in Canada.

544

continued page 566

Table 23.1: Inclusion of papillomas of bladder in data for *Cancer Incidence in Five Continents*

Population		Volume IV	Volume V	Volume VI
Period (approx.)		1975	1980	1985

Europe (except European Community)

Hungary	County Vas	Benign and unspecified	-	-
Israel	All Jews	Benign and unspecified	Benign and unspecified	Benign and unspecified
	Non-Jews	Benign and unspecified	Benign and unspecified	Benign and unspecified
Norway		If Bergkvist grading of cellular atypia > 1		
Romania	County Cluj	-	Unspecified	-
Sweden		Benign and unspecified	Benign and unspecified	Benign and unspecified
Switzerland	Geneva	Benign and unspecified	-	-

Europe (European Community)

Denmark		Benign and unspecified	Benign and unspecified	Benign and unspecified
France	Doubs	Benign and unspecified	-	Benign and unspecified
Italy	Varese	Benign and unspecified	Benign and unspecified	Benign and unspecified
UK	Birmingham	Benign and unspecified	Benign and unspecified	Benign and unspecified
	S Thames	Benign and unspecified	Benign and unspecified	Benign and unspecified

Asia

India	Bombay	-	Unspecified	-
Singapore	Chinese	Unspecified	Unspecified	-
	Indian	Unspecified	Unspecified	-
	Malay	Unspecified	Unspecified	-

Americas (except USA)

Brazil	São Paulo	Unspecified	-	..
Canada	Alberta	-	Benign and unspecified	-
	Quebec	Unspecified	-	-
Colombia	Cali	-	Unspecified	Unspecified

.. Data not included in this volume

- Benign and unspecified papillomas of bladder not included with data for this period

EUROPE (non-EC), INCIDENCE

MALES	Best model	Goodness of fit	1970		1985		Cumulative risk		Recent trend
			Rate	Cases	Rate	Cases	1915	1940	
FINLAND	A4P3	2.20	15.6	159	22.6	269	14.5	28.4	13.6
HUNGARY									
County Vas	A1P4	-0.11	6.5	5	13.8	10	12.3	45.9	*1.6*
Szabolcs-Szatmar	A2D	-0.05	8.0	11	18.2	25	9.9	38.2	56.6
ISRAEL									
All Jews	A8P4C9	-0.73	28.6	134	38.3	226	21.1	47.0	*2.2*
Non-Jews	A2P2	2.73	17.5	5	15.8	8	11.3	16.0	*-4.1*
NORWAY	A3P4C2	1.80	17.3	192	34.6	428	21.4	56.0	15.1
POLAND									
Warsaw City	A2	-1.09	17.5	48	17.5	66	11.8	11.8	*8.0*
ROMANIA									
Cluj	A2D	1.97	*11.3*	*17*	21.1	38	11.9	33.1	23.4
SWEDEN	A4P2C4	-0.71	23.0	573	30.3	817	18.6	28.0	9.0
SWITZERLAND									
Geneva	A5P3	1.71	10.3	8	26.1	24	23.8	13.2	-29.8
YUGOSLAVIA									
Slovenia	A2D	2.98	11.9	45	18.8	79	11.6	24.5	15.9

FEMALES	Best model	Goodness of fit	1970		1985		Cumulative risk		Recent trend
			Rate	Cases	Rate	Cases	1915	1940	
FINLAND	A4P2	0.54	3.4	47	4.0	64	2.6	4.6	*-0.6*
HUNGARY									
County Vas	A1D	0.22	1.6	1	3.3	3	1.7	5.5	*29.0*
Szabolcs-Szatmar	A1D	0.42	0.9	1	2.4	4	1.3	7.3	71.2
ISRAEL									
All Jews	A4P4	-0.13	6.3	26	8.9	53	5.2	9.2	*1.6*
Non-Jews	A1P3	-0.57	4.3	1	1.9	1	1.3	1.1	*-5.2*
NORWAY	A2P2C2	0.01	5.2	67	9.1	122	5.0	19.7	11.6
POLAND									
Warsaw City	A2	-0.09	3.9	17	3.9	20	2.6	2.6	*-2.2*
ROMANIA									
Cluj	A1C2	-1.31	*1.5*	*2*	5.2	11	3.2	7.0	45.0
SWEDEN	A4P2	-0.71	7.0	189	8.2	241	5.0	7.2	4.5
SWITZERLAND									
Geneva	A2C2	-0.39	8.1	8	6.7	7	6.0	0.9	*-18.2*
YUGOSLAVIA									
Slovenia	A2D	-0.69	2.3	11	3.2	19	2.0	3.6	*15.9*

* : not enough cases for reliable estimation
− : incomplete or missing data
Best model: polynomial of the given degree in age (A), period (P) or cohort (C), or linear drift (D) model.
Goodness of fit: the normalised likelihood ratio chi-square for the best model (see Method).
Rate: world-standardised truncated rate per 100 000 per year (30-74 years) and number of **cases** are both estimated from the best-fitting model for the single years cited.
Cumulative risk per 1000 (30-74 years) is estimated from the best-fitting *age-cohort* model for cohorts of central birth year cited.
Recent trend: estimated mean percentage change per five-year period in the age-specific rates (30-74 years) over the period 1973-1987.
Italics denote recent trends not significant at 5 per cent level, or other figures which should be interpreted with caution (see Method).

BLADDER (ICD-9 188)

EUROPE (non-EC), INCIDENCE

MALES

TRUNCATED RATE (30-74 years)

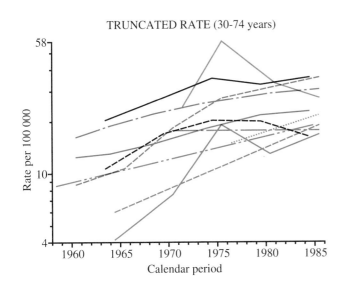

CUMULATIVE RISK (30-74 years)

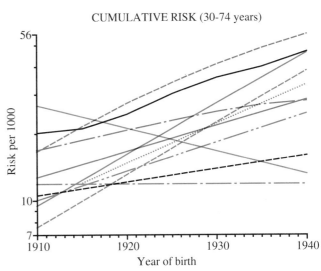

FEMALES

TRUNCATED RATE (30-74 years)

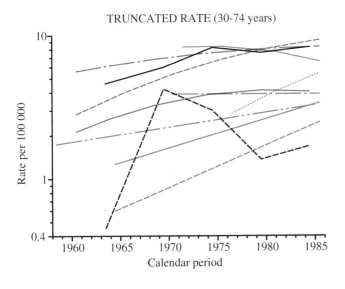

CUMULATIVE RISK (30-74 years)

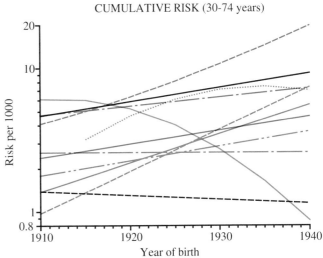

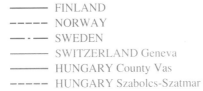

——— FINLAND	—·—· POLAND Warsaw City
- - - - NORWAY	········· ROMANIA Cluj
—·—· SWEDEN	—··—·· YUGOSLAVIA Slovenia
——— SWITZERLAND Geneva	——— ISRAEL All Jews
——— HUNGARY County Vas	- - - - ISRAEL Non-Jews
- - - - HUNGARY Szabolcs-Szatmar	

BLADDER (ICD-9 188)

EUROPE (EC), INCIDENCE

MALES	Best model	Goodness of fit	1970 Rate	Cases	1985 Rate	Cases	Cumulative risk 1915	1940	Recent trend
DENMARK	A3P4C2	0.61	37.6	513	48.0	711	30.8	40.1	8.0
FRANCE									
Bas-Rhin	A2D	0.07	*30.9*	*73*	44.4	88	24.9	45.1	14.0
Doubs	A4C2	0.54	*44.1*	*22*	39.2	43	21.1	64.1	*9.6*
GERMANY (FRG)									
Hamburg	A2	0.85	24.0	139	*24.0*	*87*	16.6	*16.6*	–
Saarland	A2P2	0.44	16.2	47	43.1	121	25.6	100.0	23.0
GERMANY (GDR)	A2P3C5	5.11	16.4	808	27.9	1013	16.2	41.9	22.9
ITALY									
Varese	A2D	0.43	*41.6*	*53*	56.9	116	31.5	52.5	11.0
SPAIN									
Navarra	A4D	-0.43	*25.0*	*30*	44.0	62	23.6	59.5	20.8
Zaragoza	A2P3	0.05	14.0	26	44.8	108	19.9	65.4	19.1
UK									
Birmingham	A2P5	2.32	31.4	424	33.3	500	20.7	32.9	*2.4*
Scotland	A2P4C2	0.45	29.6	405	40.5	569	23.8	38.2	12.9
South Thames	A2P5C5	2.87	35.9	914	35.4	699	22.4	21.0	*1.6*

FEMALES	Best model	Goodness of fit	1970 Rate	Cases	1985 Rate	Cases	Cumulative risk 1915	1940	Recent trend
DENMARK	A2P2C6	1.00	9.2	140	12.5	203	6.8	10.9	8.2
FRANCE									
Bas-Rhin	A1	0.87	*6.8*	*22*	6.8	17	4.3	4.3	*-3.4*
Doubs	A1	0.20	*5.1*	*3*	5.1	6	3.3	3.3	*12.8*
GERMANY (FRG)									
Hamburg	A2	0.59	5.4	47	*5.4*	*32*	3.8	*3.8*	–
Saarland	A2C2	0.30	3.1	12	8.8	36	5.0	13.1	37.2
GERMANY (GDR)	A2D	2.68	2.7	201	4.9	290	2.9	7.7	23.8
ITALY									
Varese	A1D	-1.02	*4.0*	*5*	8.8	23	4.8	17.8	29.1
SPAIN									
Navarra	A1	0.99	*3.6*	*5*	3.6	5	2.3	2.3	*8.6*
Zaragoza	A1P3	0.49	2.0	4	6.3	17	2.3	7.0	32.1
UK									
Birmingham	A2P4	1.93	7.3	116	9.7	163	5.7	11.9	7.1
Scotland	A3P3C2	1.38	7.4	128	13.3	226	7.5	14.3	15.5
South Thames	A2P3	4.40	7.7	251	9.1	211	5.4	8.1	6.7

* : not enough cases for reliable estimation
– : incomplete or missing data
Best model: polynomial of the given degree in age (A), period (P) or cohort (C), or linear drift (D) model.
Goodness of fit: the normalised likelihood ratio chi-square for the best model (see Method).
Rate: world-standardised truncated rate per 100 000 per year (30-74 years) and number of **cases** are both estimated from the best-fitting model for the single years cited.
Cumulative risk per 1000 (30-74 years) is estimated from the best-fitting *age-cohort* model for cohorts of central birth year cited.
Recent trend: estimated mean percentage change per five-year period in the age-specific rates (30-74 years) over the period 1973-1987.
Italics denote recent trends not significant at 5 per cent level, or other figures which should be interpreted with caution (see Method).

BLADDER (ICD-9 188)

EUROPE (EC), INCIDENCE

MALES

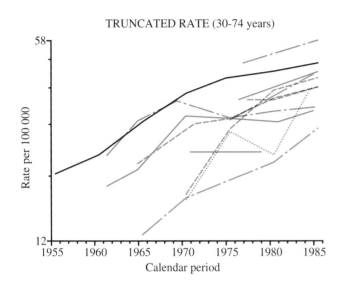

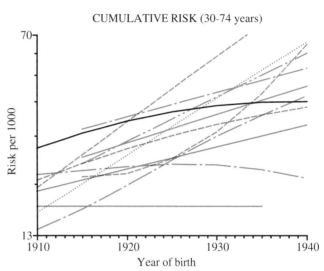

FEMALES

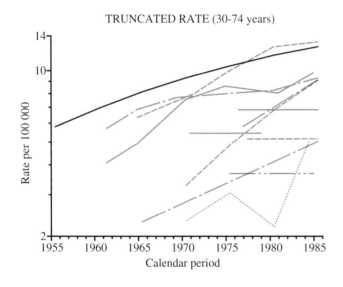

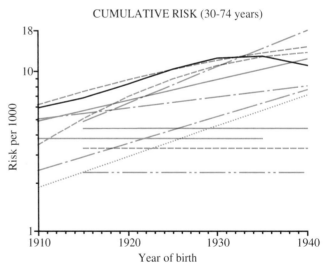

—— FRANCE Bas-Rhin	— — — GERMANY (FRG) Saarland
— — — FRANCE Doubs	—·— GERMANY (GDR)
—·—·— ITALY Varese	—— UK Birmingham
—··—··— SPAIN Navarra	— — — UK Scotland
·········· SPAIN Zaragoza	—·—·— UK South Thames
—— GERMANY (FRG) Hamburg	—— DENMARK

BLADDER (ICD-9 188)

EUROPE (non-EC), INCIDENCE
Percentage change per five-year period, 1973-1987

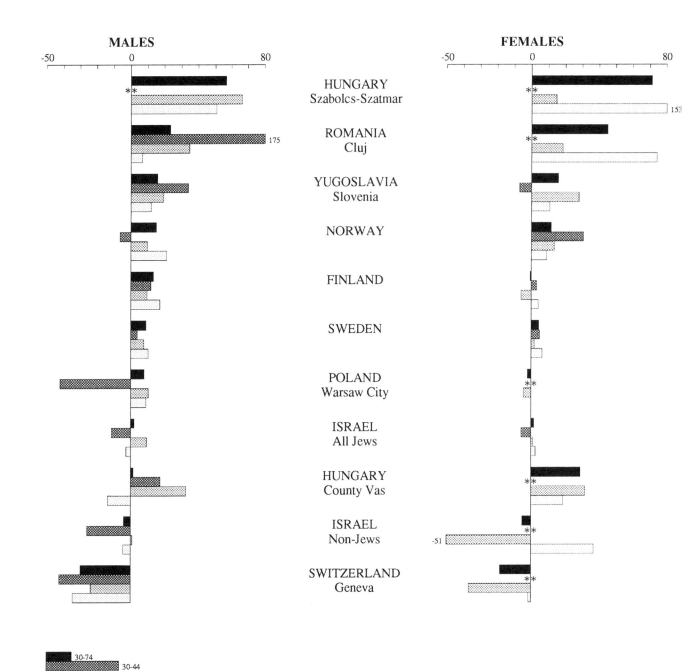

MALES

-50   0   80

FEMALES

-50   0   80

HUNGARY
Szabolcs-Szatmar

ROMANIA
Cluj

YUGOSLAVIA
Slovenia

NORWAY

FINLAND

SWEDEN

POLAND
Warsaw City

ISRAEL
All Jews

HUNGARY
County Vas

ISRAEL
Non-Jews

SWITZERLAND
Geneva

30-74
30-44
45-64
65-74

BLADDER (ICD-9 188)

EUROPE (EC), INCIDENCE
Percentage change per five-year period, 1973-1987

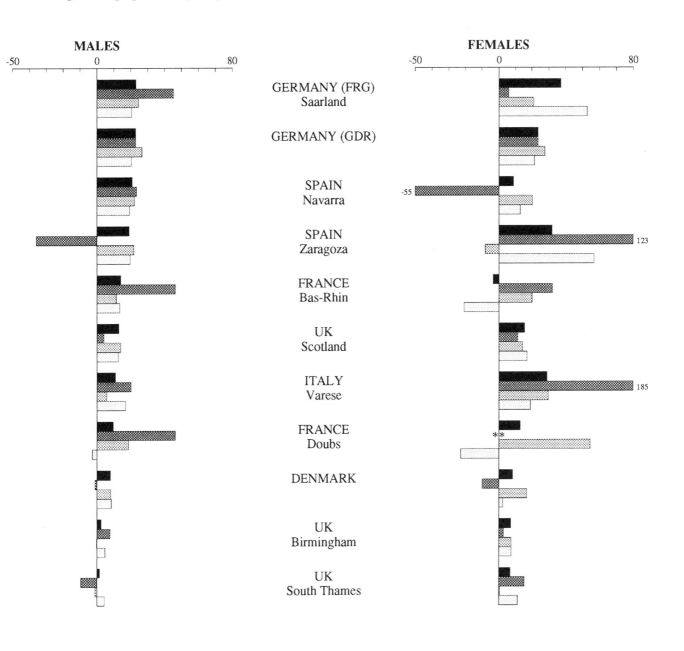

BLADDER (ICD-9 188)

EUROPE (non-EC), MORTALITY

MALES	Best model	Goodness of fit	1965 Rate	Deaths	1985 Rate	Deaths	Cumulative risk 1900	1940	Recent trend
AUSTRIA	A4D	0.89	*12.5*	*257*	8.7	167	*8.8*	4.3	-7.8
CZECHOSLOVAKIA	A2P4C7	0.95	11.0	386	11.8	440	7.9	7.8	6.2
FINLAND	A2P2C2	0.04	7.5	67	5.8	69	5.3	2.3	-11.4
HUNGARY	A2D	-0.04	*8.6*	*224*	10.6	303	*6.3*	9.6	*3.8*
NORWAY	A2P2C2	0.62	7.3	77	7.9	104	5.4	3.9	*-7.3*
POLAND	A5D	4.45	7.8	454	12.2	936	5.7	*13.6*	–
ROMANIA	A2D	0.16	*6.7*	*268*	*7.9*	*413*	*4.6*	6.3	–
SWEDEN	A4P4C4	0.27	6.2	147	5.7	165	4.8	4.1	-6.8
SWITZERLAND	A2P5C2	0.82	7.6	109	9.3	166	5.9	6.3	*-0.4*
YUGOSLAVIA	A3D	1.80	5.6	197	7.3	347	4.0	6.7	9.7

FEMALES	Best model	Goodness of fit	1965 Rate	Deaths	1985 Rate	Deaths	Cumulative risk 1900	1940	Recent trend
AUSTRIA	A3C2	0.32	*2.3*	*66*	2.5	72	*1.7*	1.1	*-0.9*
CZECHOSLOVAKIA	A4P4C2	0.56	2.3	100	2.2	107	1.5	1.1	13.0
FINLAND	A2P2	0.47	1.6	20	1.0	16	1.0	0.6	-23.6
HUNGARY	A2P3	0.86	*14.4*	*475*	2.1	80	*1.0*	2.1	18.4
NORWAY	A2D	1.53	2.7	32	2.2	33	1.9	1.3	*-4.0*
POLAND	A2P2C2	0.97	1.5	116	1.6	164	1.0	*0.8*	–
ROMANIA	A2D	0.84	*1.4*	*70*	*2.1*	*134*	*1.0*	2.1	–
SWEDEN	A2C2	-0.02	2.1	54	1.8	57	1.5	0.7	-11.7
SWITZERLAND	A3P3	0.94	2.1	38	2.4	51	1.6	1.7	*-6.4*
YUGOSLAVIA	A2P4C4	2.42	1.7	75	1.7	102	1.3	0.3	*5.1*

* : not enough deaths for reliable estimation
– : incomplete or missing data
Best model: polynomial of the given degree in age (A), period (P) or cohort (C), or linear drift (D) model.
Goodness of fit: the normalised likelihood ratio chi-square for the best model (see Method).
Rate: world-standardised truncated rate per 100 000 per year (30-74 years) and number of **deaths** are both estimated from the best-fitting model for the single years cited.
Cumulative risk per 1000 (30-74 years) is estimated from the best-fitting *age-cohort* model for cohorts of central birth year cited.
Recent trend: estimated mean percentage change per five-year period in the age-specific rates (30-74 years) over the period 1975-1988.
Italics denote recent trends not significant at 5 per cent level, or other figures which should be interpreted with caution (see Method).

BLADDER (ICD-9 188)

EUROPE (non-EC), MORTALITY

MALES

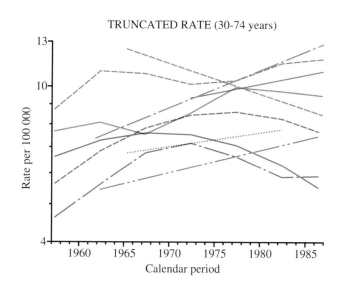

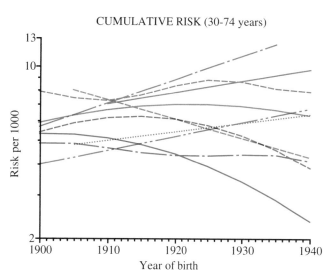

FEMALES

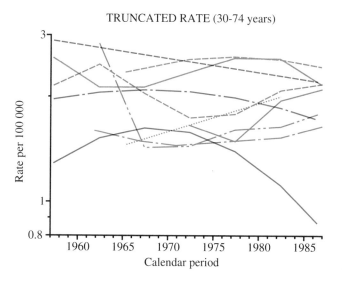

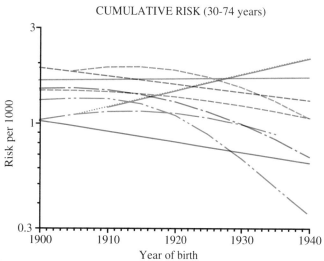

—— FINLAND	----- CZECHOSLOVAKIA
----- NORWAY	—— HUNGARY
—·—· SWEDEN	—·—· POLAND
----- AUSTRIA	········· ROMANIA
—— SWITZERLAND	—··—·· YUGOSLAVIA

BLADDER (ICD-9 188)

EUROPE (EC), MORTALITY

MALES	Best model	Goodness of fit	1965 Rate	1965 Deaths	1985 Rate	1985 Deaths	Cumulative risk 1900	Cumulative risk 1940	Recent trend
BELGIUM	A2P6C2	0.75	11.2	303	11.5	320	7.8	6.7	-9.2
DENMARK	A2C3	-0.13	12.1	158	14.4	222	8.5	5.9	*2.1*
FRANCE	A7P4C6	2.14	8.3	1039	10.4	1476	6.2	9.9	2.6
GERMANY (FRG)	A2P3C2	6.54	*11.8*	*1858*	10.0	1604	*8.3*	4.8	-5.7
GREECE	A4P4C2	-0.12	*15.3*	*289*	10.0	288	*5.4*	6.7	*3.2*
IRELAND	A2C2	1.71	6.2	46	6.3	54	4.5	2.4	*-0.9*
ITALY	A4P4C6	3.51	10.0	1219	14.0	2253	7.4	8.3	5.1
NETHERLANDS	A2P2C2	0.89	9.3	264	10.1	368	6.8	5.2	*-3.3*
PORTUGAL	–	–	–	–	–	–	–	–	–
SPAIN	A2P5C2	1.74	7.2	500	11.4	1129	6.0	11.7	*-1.5*
UK ENGLAND & WALES	A2P4C2	1.12	12.3	1603	10.7	1644	8.7	4.8	-4.6
UK SCOTLAND	A2P2C2	0.43	12.1	159	11.4	166	8.5	5.3	*-4.5*

FEMALES	Best model	Goodness of fit	1965 Rate	1965 Deaths	1985 Rate	1985 Deaths	Cumulative risk 1900	Cumulative risk 1940	Recent trend
BELGIUM	A5C2	0.31	2.7	89	2.5	87	1.9	1.4	*-0.9*
DENMARK	A2C4	-0.17	3.7	54	4.0	69	2.4	2.3	*-6.3*
FRANCE	A2P2C2	1.37	1.9	315	1.7	290	1.3	0.8	-5.5
GERMANY (FRG)	A2C4	2.33	*2.4*	*549*	2.3	564	*1.7*	1.1	-4.8
GREECE	A2P3	-0.07	*3.3*	*74*	1.9	64	*1.3*	1.3	*4.3*
IRELAND	A2	-0.85	2.4	18	2.4	21	1.6	1.6	*-5.8*
ITALY	A2P3C2	0.63	1.8	271	1.8	373	1.4	0.8	-5.6
NETHERLANDS	A2D	1.09	2.4	78	2.1	91	1.7	1.3	*4.6*
PORTUGAL	–	–	–	–	–	–	–	–	–
SPAIN	A2P5C4	-0.48	1.3	109	1.5	187	1.0	0.5	*-4.8*
UK ENGLAND & WALES	A2C5	0.53	3.2	540	3.3	597	2.1	1.5	*-0.9*
UK SCOTLAND	A2C2	0.96	4.0	68	4.3	77	2.7	2.4	*-3.9*

* : not enough deaths for reliable estimation
– : incomplete or missing data
Best model: polynomial of the given degree in age (A), period (P) or cohort (C), or linear drift (D) model.
Goodness of fit: the normalised likelihood ratio chi-square for the best model (see Method).
Rate: world-standardised truncated rate per 100 000 per year (30-74 years) and number of **deaths** are both estimated from the best-fitting model for the single years cited.
Cumulative risk per 1000 (30-74 years) is estimated from the best-fitting *age-cohort* model for cohorts of central birth year cited.
Recent trend: estimated mean percentage change per five-year period in the age-specific rates (30-74 years) over the period 1975-1988.
Italics denote recent trends not significant at 5 per cent level, or other figures which should be interpreted with caution (see Method).

BLADDER (ICD-9 188)

EUROPE (EC), MORTALITY

MALES

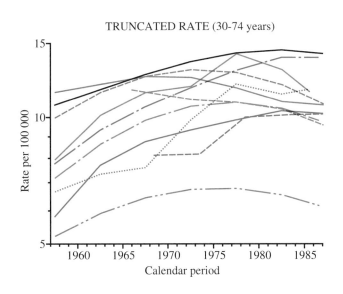

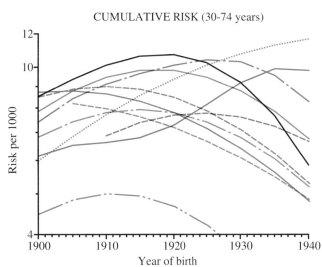

FEMALES

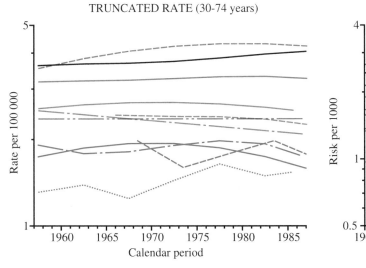

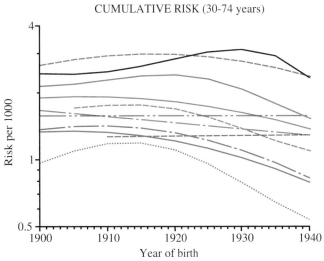

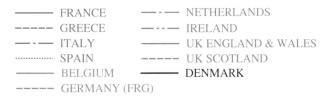

BLADDER (ICD-9 188)

EUROPE (non-EC), MORTALITY
Percentage change per five-year period, 1975-1988

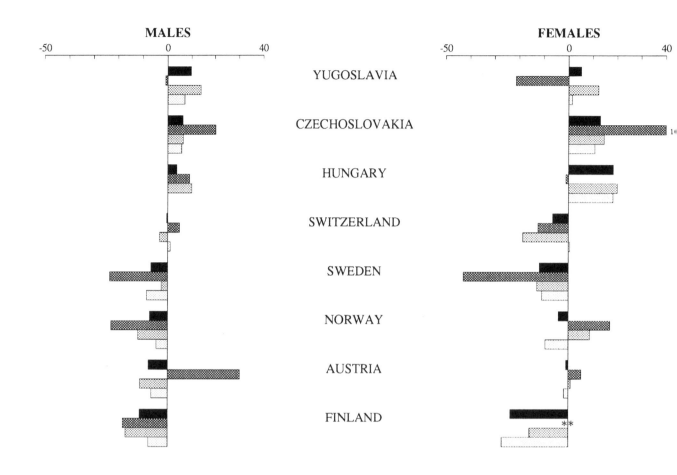

MALES | FEMALES

-50　0　40

YUGOSLAVIA
CZECHOSLOVAKIA
HUNGARY
SWITZERLAND
SWEDEN
NORWAY
AUSTRIA
FINLAND

30-74
30-44
45-64
65-74

BLADDER (ICD-9 188)

EUROPE (EC), MORTALITY
Percentage change per five-year period, 1975-1988

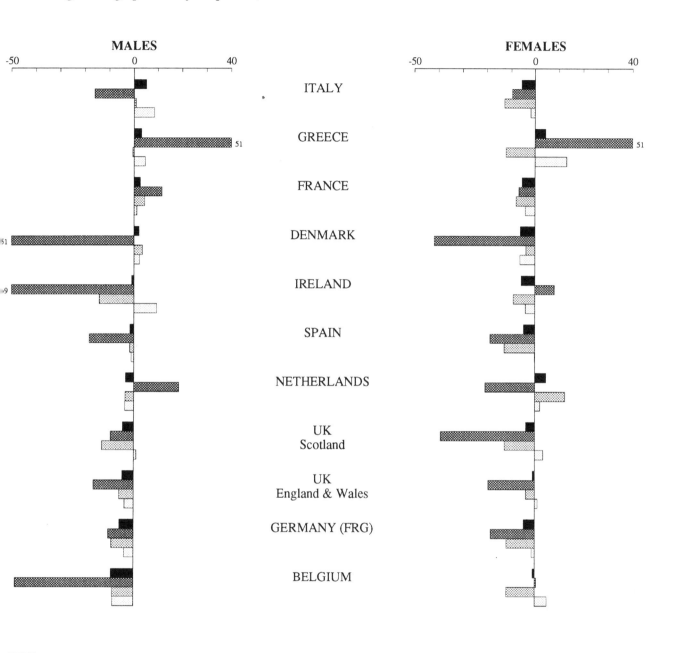

557

BLADDER (ICD-9 188)

ASIA, INCIDENCE

MALES	Best model	Goodness of fit	1970 Rate	1970 Cases	1985 Rate	1985 Cases	Cumulative risk 1915	Cumulative risk 1940	Recent trend
CHINA									
Shanghai	A1C2	1.21	*14.4*	*139*	11.2	191	8.6	4.5	-10.4
HONG KONG	A5C2	-1.06	*29.6*	*140*	26.7	303	19.2	11.4	-7.8
INDIA									
Bombay	A2D	1.28	4.6	30	6.2	66	3.6	6.0	10.3
JAPAN									
Miyagi	A4P4	-0.06	6.8	22	14.3	75	7.6	17.0	25.7
Nagasaki	A1D	0.39	*12.4*	*10*	20.0	21	11.3	24.9	*16.1*
Osaka	A2P3	0.10	9.3	110	13.5	245	7.9	20.2	23.8
SINGAPORE									
Chinese	A2	1.02	12.4	24	12.4	36	8.4	8.4	*0.1*
Indian	A1	-0.61	6.9	1	6.9	2	4.7	4.7	*-0.1*
Malay	A2	-0.27	8.2	2	8.2	4	5.4	5.4	*28.2*

FEMALES	Best model	Goodness of fit	1970 Rate	1970 Cases	1985 Rate	1985 Cases	Cumulative risk 1915	Cumulative risk 1940	Recent trend
CHINA									
Shanghai	A3	-1.44	*3.2*	*35*	3.2	58	2.1	2.1	*-0.6*
HONG KONG	A3D	0.80	*12.9*	*61*	7.6	90	6.1	2.5	-17.3
INDIA									
Bombay	A1	-0.31	1.6	7	1.6	13	1.0	1.0	*6.2*
JAPAN									
Miyagi	A1P2	2.13	2.6	10	3.7	24	2.2	3.0	17.7
Nagasaki	A1	-0.76	*3.2*	*3*	3.2	4	2.3	2.3	*-3.7*
Osaka	A2C2	1.45	2.3	31	3.2	70	1.9	7.6	9.5
SINGAPORE									
Chinese	A3C3	-0.13	3.5	7	3.9	13	2.4	6.7	*18.5*
Indian	A4	-3.63	*0.4*	*0*	*0.4*	*0*	0.3	0.3	*-5.9*
Malay	A2	-2.04	*2.1*	*0*	*2.1*	*0*	1.4	1.4	*36.5*

* : not enough cases for reliable estimation
– : incomplete or missing data
Best model: polynomial of the given degree in age (A), period (P) or cohort (C), or linear drift (D) model.
Goodness of fit: the normalised likelihood ratio chi-square for the best model (see Method).
Rate: world-standardised truncated rate per 100 000 per year (30-74 years) and number of **cases** are both estimated from the best-fitting model for the single years cited.
Cumulative risk per 1000 (30-74 years) is estimated from the best-fitting *age-cohort* model for cohorts of central birth year cited.
Recent trend: estimated mean percentage change per five-year period in the age-specific rates (30-74 years) over the period 1973-1987.
Italics denote recent trends not significant at 5 per cent level, or other figures which should be interpreted with caution (see Method).

BLADDER (ICD-9 188)

ASIA, INCIDENCE

MALES

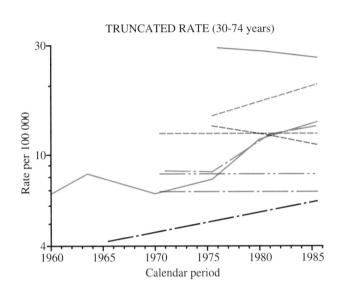

TRUNCATED RATE (30-74 years)

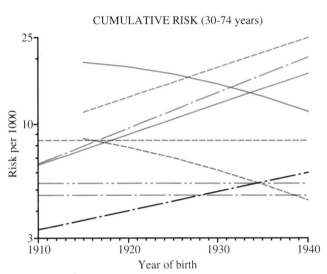

CUMULATIVE RISK (30-74 years)

FEMALES

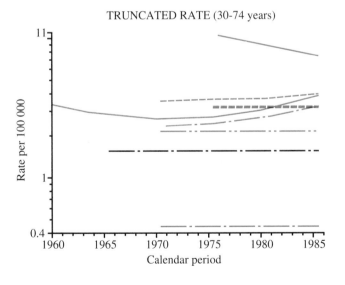

TRUNCATED RATE (30-74 years)

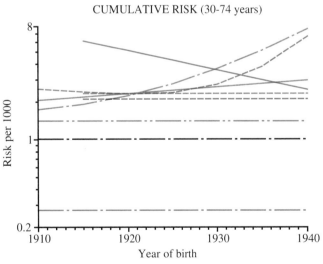

CUMULATIVE RISK (30-74 years)

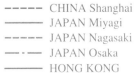

------ CHINA Shanghai
——— JAPAN Miyagi
------ JAPAN Nagasaki
—·—· JAPAN Osaka
——— HONG KONG

------ SINGAPORE Chinese
—·—· SINGAPORE Indian
—··—· SINGAPORE Malay
—··— INDIA Bombay

BLADDER (ICD-9 188)

OCEANIA, INCIDENCE

MALES	Best model	Goodness of fit	1970 Rate	1970 Cases	1985 Rate	1985 Cases	Cumulative risk 1915	Cumulative risk 1940	Recent trend
AUSTRALIA									
New South Wales	A3P2	-0.69	*18.7*	*193*	28.9	390	18.3	22.4	4.1
South	A2C3	-0.59	*88.1*	*125*	20.3	73	32.3	2.2	-36.5
HAWAII									
Caucasian	A3D	-0.37	36.9	12	46.8	29	27.7	40.8	*10.2*
Chinese	A1C2	-1.34	17.4	2	23.3	4	12.3	48.0	*3.8*
Filipino	A1	0.99	6.5	1	6.5	2	4.1	4.1	*38.5*
Hawaiian	A2	-0.04	16.1	2	16.1	3	10.2	10.2	*-1.3*
Japanese	A1C3	1.08	16.5	8	14.6	13	11.2	3.7	*-2.2*
NEW ZEALAND									
Maori	A2P2	0.26	5.5	1	8.1	2	4.6	12.0	*-13.9*
Non-Maori	A2P3	0.76	18.8	106	22.0	158	14.6	16.7	*-1.2*

FEMALES	Best model	Goodness of fit	1970 Rate	1970 Cases	1985 Rate	1985 Cases	Cumulative risk 1915	Cumulative risk 1940	Recent trend
AUSTRALIA									
New South Wales	A4P2	0.46	*4.1*	*51*	9.4	136	5.4	8.5	9.1
South	A8	2.13	*4.8*	*10*	4.8	17	2.7	2.7	-27.1
HAWAII									
Caucasian	A1C3	0.94	10.1	3	8.4	5	6.8	3.0	*12.9*
Chinese	*	..	..	..	..	..	..	..	..
Filipino	A2	-2.04	*5.6*	*0*	5.6	1	3.7	3.7	*50.0*
Hawaiian	A1	0.37	7.9	1	7.9	2	5.4	5.4	*-29.9*
Japanese	A1	-0.44	4.5	2	4.5	4	3.0	3.0	*-1.9*
NEW ZEALAND									
Maori	A1	-1.90	*6.4*	*0*	6.4	1	4.7	4.7	*36.9*
Non-Maori	A2P2	1.37	5.0	31	5.7	44	3.7	5.5	*-4.7*

* : not enough cases for reliable estimation
– : incomplete or missing data
Best model: polynomial of the given degree in age (A), period (P) or cohort (C), or linear drift (D) model.
Goodness of fit: the normalised likelihood ratio chi-square for the best model (see Method).
Rate: world-standardised truncated rate per 100 000 per year (30-74 years) and number of **cases** are both estimated from the best-fitting model for the single years cited.
Cumulative risk per 1000 (30-74 years) is estimated from the best-fitting *age-cohort* model for cohorts of central birth year cited.
Recent trend: estimated mean percentage change per five-year period in the age-specific rates (30-74 years) over the period 1973-1987.
Italics denote recent trends not significant at 5 per cent level, or other figures which should be interpreted with caution (see Method).

BLADDER (ICD-9 188)

OCEANIA, INCIDENCE

MALES

TRUNCATED RATE (30-74 years)

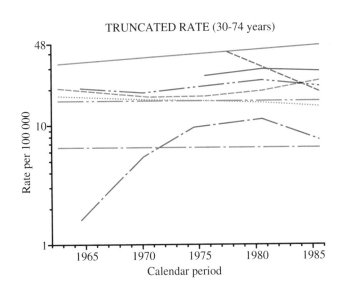

CUMULATIVE RISK (30-74 years)

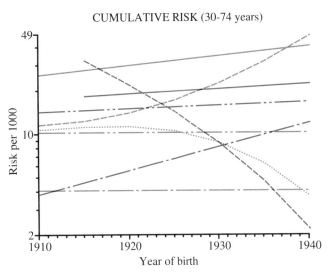

FEMALES

TRUNCATED RATE (30-74 years)

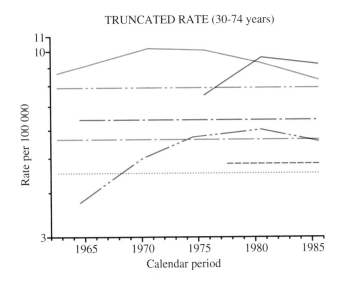

CUMULATIVE RISK (30-74 years)

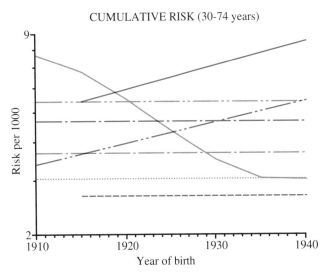

――――― AUSTRALIA New South Wales
― ― ― ― AUSTRALIA South
―・―・― NEW ZEALAND Maori
―・・―・・ NEW ZEALAND Non-Maori
――――― HAWAII Caucasian

――――― HAWAII Chinese
―・―・― HAWAII Filipino
―・・―・・ HAWAII Hawaiian
················· HAWAII Japanese

BLADDER (ICD-9 188)

ASIA, INCIDENCE
Percentage change per five-year period, 1973-1987

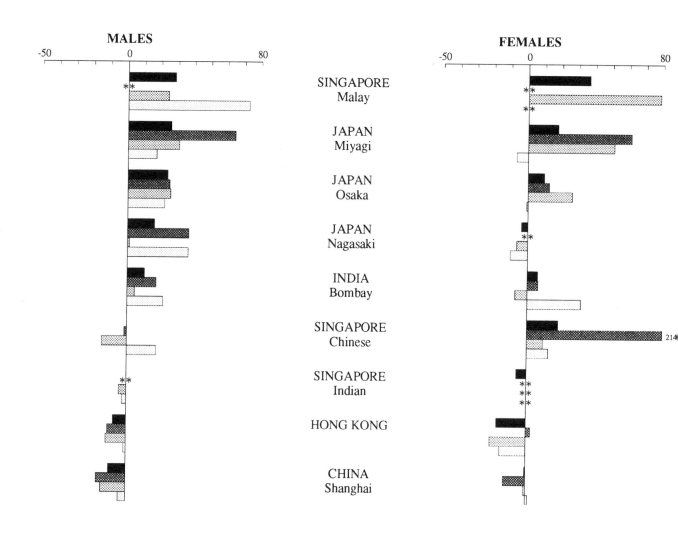

MALES

FEMALES

SINGAPORE
Malay

JAPAN
Miyagi

JAPAN
Osaka

JAPAN
Nagasaki

INDIA
Bombay

SINGAPORE
Chinese

SINGAPORE
Indian

HONG KONG

CHINA
Shanghai

30-74
30-44
45-64
65-74

BLADDER (ICD-9 188)

OCEANIA, INCIDENCE
Percentage change per five-year period, 1973-1987

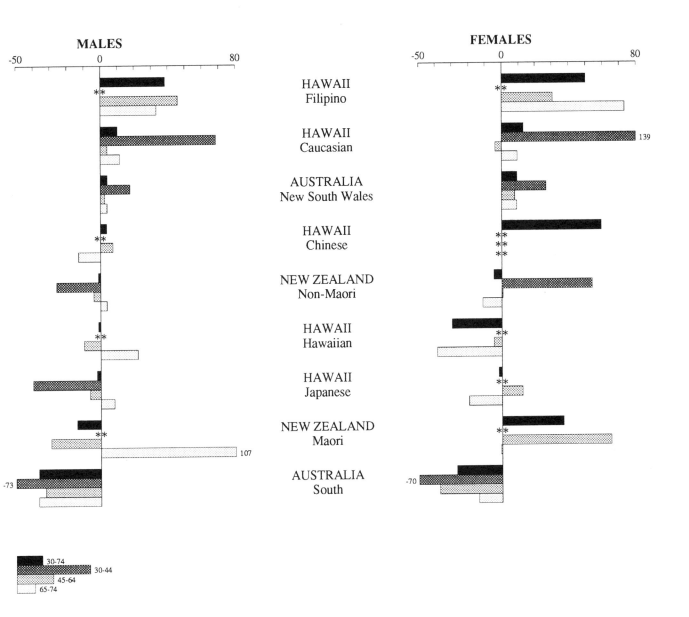

BLADDER (ICD-9 188)

ASIA and OCEANIA, MORTALITY

MALES	Best model	Goodness of fit	1965 Rate	1965 Deaths	1985 Rate	1985 Deaths	Cumulative risk 1900	Cumulative risk 1940	Recent trend
AUSTRALIA	A2C2	1.24	7.5	178	6.6	249	5.4	3.4	*-1.8*
HONG KONG	A3P3C2	1.62	*2.2*	*7*	6.2	48	*4.5*	2.4	-17.2
JAPAN	A3P2C3	0.43	3.4	596	3.0	870	2.5	1.8	-9.0
MAURITIUS	A2	-0.28	*5.4*	*3*	5.4	6	*3.4*	3.4	*-23.3*
NEW ZEALAND	A2C2	1.51	7.7	40	6.5	50	5.5	3.0	*-10.2*
SINGAPORE	A2	0.46	3.7	5	3.7	8	*2.0*	2.0	—

FEMALES	Best model	Goodness of fit	1965 Rate	1965 Deaths	1985 Rate	1985 Deaths	Cumulative risk 1900	Cumulative risk 1940	Recent trend
AUSTRALIA	A2D	1.66	2.3	62	2.0	86	1.6	1.3	-8.1
HONG KONG	A2C2	0.63	*3.5*	*17*	1.9	13	*2.6*	0.1	-35.0
JAPAN	A4P3C3	0.59	1.8	344	0.9	321	1.3	0.3	-17.7
MAURITIUS	A2	0.22	*1.7*	*1*	1.7	2	*1.1*	1.1	*-23.6*
NEW ZEALAND	A2	-1.45	2.2	13	2.2	19	1.6	1.6	*-11.1*
SINGAPORE	A1	-0.82	1.3	1	1.3	3	*0.7*	0.7	—

* : not enough deaths for reliable estimation
− : incomplete or missing data
Best model: polynomial of the given degree in age (A), period (P) or cohort (C), or linear drift (D) model.
Goodness of fit: the normalised likelihood ratio chi-square for the best model (see Method).
Rate: world-standardised truncated rate per 100 000 per year (30-74 years) and number of **deaths** are both estimated from the best-fitting model for the single years cited.
Cumulative risk per 1000 (30-74 years) is estimated from the best-fitting *age-cohort* model for cohorts of central birth year cited.
Recent trend: estimated mean percentage change per five-year period in the age-specific rates (30-74 years) over the period 1975-1988.
Italics denote recent trends not significant at 5 per cent level, or other figures which should be interpreted with caution (see Method).

BLADDER (ICD-9 188)

ASIA and OCEANIA, MORTALITY

MALES

TRUNCATED RATE (30-74 years)

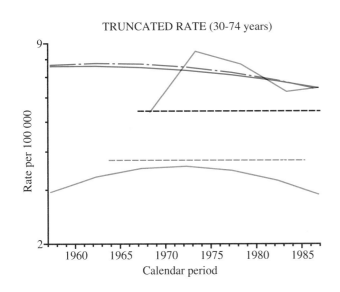

CUMULATIVE RISK (30-74 years)

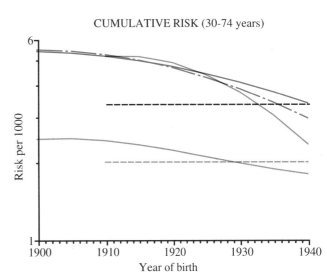

FEMALES

TRUNCATED RATE (30-74 years)

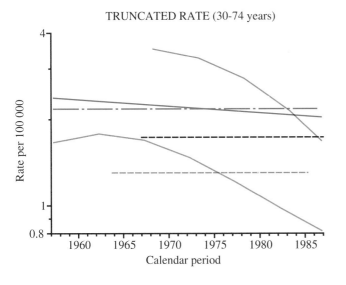

CUMULATIVE RISK (30-74 years)

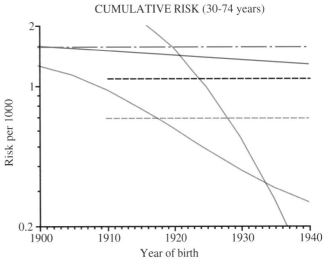

—————— AUSTRALIA ⁣ —————— HONG KONG
—·—·— NEW ZEALAND ⁣ – – – – SINGAPORE
—————— JAPAN ⁣ ▬ ▬ ▬ MAURITIUS

BLADDER (ICD-9 188)

ASIA and OCEANIA, MORTALITY
Percentage change per five-year period, 1975-1988

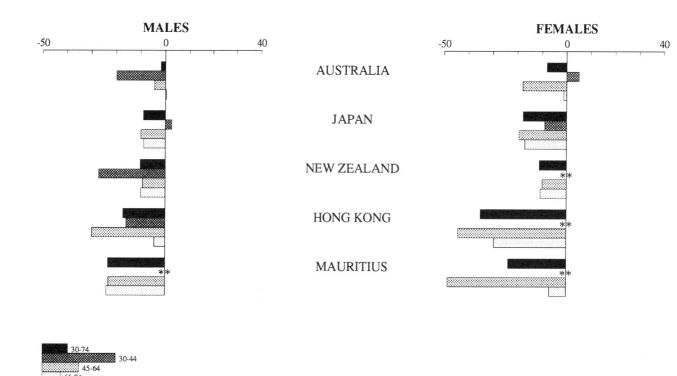

from page 544

Comment

The inclusion in a registry's data of papillomas not classified as malignant will obviously affect the recorded incidence rate, but provided there is no change in practice, it should have little effect on trends, unless there is a substantial change in diagnostic intensity. In Denmark (up to 50% papillomas), incidence is high, while in Sweden (5%), South Thames (UK; 2%) and Israel (1%), incidence is correspondingly lower, but the trends are broadly similar. None of these registries has changed its practice with respect to bladder papillomas since 1973. A change in practice may either attenuate or inflate a trend. In Singapore, papillomas of unspecified histology were included in the data up to 1982, and there was a significant rate of increase in world-standardised incidence of 2.3% per year among Chinese males between 1968 and 1982[152,154]; such papillomas were no longer included in the data for 1983-87, and the trend for the period 1968-1987 is not significant. Even a

reversal of practice may not be obvious, however; in Cluj (Romania), papillomas of unspecified histology were included for the period 1978-82 only, but there has been a steady increase in incidence up to 1987, while in Bombay (India), where the same change in practice occurred, there was a slight decline in recorded incidence between 1978-82 and 1983-87, but the overall trend is still upward.

Incidence in Czechoslovakia increased by 2.3% a year in males and 3.8% in females during the period 1968-85[80]; in Slovakia (formerly the eastern part of Czechoslovakia), incidence was similar to that in the western part (Bohemia and Moravia) and also rose slightly faster among females than males — by 24% and 20%, respectively, between the two quinquennia ending in 1988[237]. Mortality is still increasing in both sexes, but a decline in females born since 1920 seems imminent. In Vaud (Switzerland), the increase in the same period in females was similar (22%), but only 2.6% in males, a sex difference in trends seen for other tobacco-related cancers in Vaud[164]. The trend in Vaud is the converse of

566

that seen in Geneva. In Saarland (FRG), the lifetime probability at birth (similar to a cross-sectional cumulative risk: see Chapter 3) of developing bladder cancer increased from 1% to 2.5% in males and from 0.3% to 0.8% in females between 1970-72 and 1980-85[37], confirming the rapid increase in risk reported here: rates in the 1970s were low by European standards, and under-ascertainment at that time may explain part of the increase.

In France, the steady increase in mortality between 1952 and 1985 was attributed largely to tobacco, consumption of which increased from 4.7 to 6.3 grams per day for adults aged 15 or over in the 25 years up to 1976, a much larger increase than that recorded in the first half of the century[128]. In Northern Ireland (UK), no significant trend in bladder cancer mortality was observed in males or females aged 30-74 during the period 1979-88[224]; mortality rates are similar to those in other parts of the UK, and there are few deaths from bladder cancer. Previous analyses of bladder cancer mortality in England and Wales[213] showed a decline for males born after 1900, and a slight peak among females in the 1920 birth cohort, followed by a clear decline in mortality for subsequent cohorts; these observations are confirmed by the analyses reported here, incorporating data up to 1988. The timing of the cohort-related decline in each sex resembles that for lung cancer mortality, although the changes are less marked.

Previous analyses of incidence and mortality data from the USA[77] showed incidence in whites to have increased by about 2% and 1% a year in males and females, respectively, in the 35 years up to 1984, and mortality to have declined, but more slowly. *In situ* carcinomas represented 1% of the data in 1969-71 and 7% in the 1980s, but this change could not account for the sex differential in the incidence trends. In males, incidence increased most at age 65 and over, and while mortality increased substantially at ages 85 and over, it fell considerably in the age range 45-64 years. The incidence and mortality trends were attributed to cohort-specific changes in smoking habits and occupational exposures, with a possible effect due to opportunistic screening for benign prostatic hypertrophy in males, and divergence of the trends was attributed to the effects of improved treatment. The analyses of US data reported here demonstrate remarkable similarity in risks and trends, particularly among males, but also clear racial differences, with blacks showing the highest rates of increase among males and the least evidence of change among females.

BLADDER (ICD-9 188)

AMERICAS (except USA), INCIDENCE

MALES	Best model	Goodness of fit	1970 Rate	1970 Cases	1985 Rate	1985 Cases	Cumulative risk 1915	Cumulative risk 1940	Recent trend
BRAZIL									
Sao Paulo	A2	-0.90	19.2	96	*19.2*	*118*	10.1	*10.1*	–
CANADA									
Alberta	A3P2	-1.37	24.7	75	31.8	142	19.6	34.6	6.9
British Columbia	A2P3	-0.54	32.1	150	20.7	151	17.5	6.9	-15.9
Maritime Provinces	A3D	-0.06	24.1	77	35.1	130	20.3	37.6	12.2
Newfoundland	A2P5	2.39	26.8	23	34.9	40	20.3	38.0	*-2.6*
Quebec	A4P4	0.92	27.2	291	44.2	644	24.8	51.2	14.7
COLOMBIA									
Cali	A2	0.79	14.6	7	14.6	16	10.1	10.1	*-13.9*
CUBA	A2P2	2.66	12.6	183	14.8	314	10.6	*12.7*	–
PUERTO RICO	A3P3	-0.60	12.4	56	12.9	91	9.1	9.0	*-4.8*

FEMALES	Best model	Goodness of fit	1970 Rate	1970 Cases	1985 Rate	1985 Cases	Cumulative risk 1915	Cumulative risk 1940	Recent trend
BRAZIL									
Sao Paulo	A7P2C6	0.07	3.1	12	*	*	1.7	*3.3*	–
CANADA									
Alberta	A2D	0.43	6.0	17	8.9	42	4.8	9.4	*7.3*
British Columbia	A8P3C8	0.64	8.8	42	5.8	47	4.9	1.7	-19.8
Maritime Provinces	A2	0.88	7.7	25	7.7	31	4.9	4.9	15.1
Newfoundland	A1D	1.07	4.5	3	7.5	9	4.5	10.6	*10.3*
Quebec	A2P4	-0.12	6.9	83	13.1	224	6.2	16.8	25.4
COLOMBIA									
Cali	A4P2	0.93	4.3	2	5.8	8	3.2	3.4	*20.9*
CUBA	A1	0.80	3.6	43	3.6	75	2.5	*2.5*	–
PUERTO RICO	A2C3	0.65	5.2	23	4.3	33	3.1	2.1	*-4.8*

* : not enough cases for reliable estimation
– : incomplete or missing data
Best model: polynomial of the given degree in age (A), period (P) or cohort (C), or linear drift (D) model.
Goodness of fit: the normalised likelihood ratio chi-square for the best model (see Method).
Rate: world-standardised truncated rate per 100 000 per year (30-74 years) and number of **cases** are both estimated from the best-fitting model for the single years cited.
Cumulative risk per 1000 (30-74 years) is estimated from the best-fitting *age-cohort* model for cohorts of central birth year cited.
Recent trend: estimated mean percentage change per five-year period in the age-specific rates (30-74 years) over the period 1973-1987.
Italics denote recent trends not significant at 5 per cent level, or other figures which should be interpreted with caution (see Method).

BLADDER (ICD-9 188)

AMERICAS (except USA), INCIDENCE

MALES

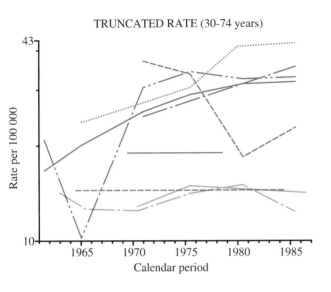

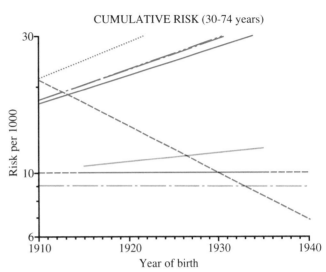

FEMALES

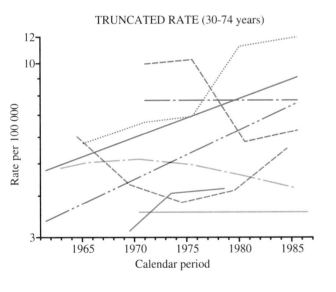

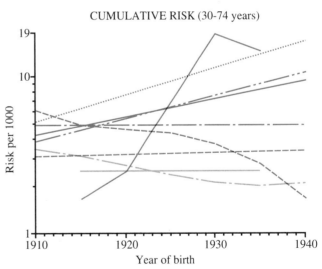

—— CANADA Alberta	—— CUBA
- - - - CANADA British Columbia	- · - · PUERTO RICO
- · - · CANADA Maritime Provinces	—— BRAZIL Sao Paulo
- · · - CANADA Newfoundland	- - - - - COLOMBIA Cali
· · · · · · CANADA Quebec	

BLADDER (ICD-9 188)

AMERICAS (USA), INCIDENCE

MALES	Best model	Goodness of fit	1970 Rate	1970 Cases	1985 Rate	1985 Cases	Cumulative risk 1915	Cumulative risk 1940	Recent trend
USA									
Bay Area, Black	A2D	0.45	16.3	8	24.8	20	14.2	28.5	*12.4*
Bay Area, Chinese	A1	-0.56	16.6	3	*16.6*	*8*	11.5	*11.5*	–
Bay Area, White	A3D	-0.83	33.1	195	40.1	255	24.8	34.0	7.6
Connecticut	A2C3	3.23	36.9	242	45.0	366	27.4	33.9	6.4
Detroit, Black	A2D	0.62	15.4	20	22.1	39	13.0	23.6	14.1
Detroit, White	A8D	1.39	34.4	252	48.5	353	28.0	49.1	13.2
Iowa	A3D	1.05	29.3	201	40.6	292	24.1	41.0	9.9
New Orleans, Black	A1	0.38	*18.5*	*9*	18.5	11	12.5	12.5	*14.5*
New Orleans, White	A2	-0.79	*42.3*	*61*	42.3	66	27.1	27.1	*8.4*
Seattle	A2D	-0.14	*33.7*	*164*	42.6	290	25.8	37.8	8.6

FEMALES	Best model	Goodness of fit	1970 Rate	1970 Cases	1985 Rate	1985 Cases	Cumulative risk 1915	Cumulative risk 1940	Recent trend
USA									
Bay Area, Black	A3C3	-0.82	8.6	4	6.5	6	4.7	0.1	*0.7*
Bay Area, Chinese	A1	-0.42	*3.0*	*0*	*3.0*	*1*	2.3	*2.3*	–
Bay Area, White	A5P3	1.12	9.5	68	11.5	86	7.1	10.7	*2.5*
Connecticut	A2C3	0.78	10.1	77	13.0	123	7.5	8.8	8.9
Detroit, Black	A2D	-0.24	5.8	8	8.7	19	4.9	9.4	*3.2*
Detroit, White	A2D	0.94	8.8	73	13.0	112	7.1	13.7	17.1
Iowa	A2C2	0.06	7.2	58	9.2	76	5.0	11.0	*4.5*
New Orleans, Black	A1	0.81	*7.2*	*4*	7.2	5	4.8	4.8	*-3.1*
New Orleans, White	A5D	0.00	*9.0*	*17*	13.9	26	7.2	14.8	*15.7*
Seattle	A2	0.65	*11.1*	*64*	11.1	84	7.1	7.1	*4.4*

* : not enough cases for reliable estimation
– : incomplete or missing data
Best model: polynomial of the given degree in age (A), period (P) or cohort (C), or linear drift (D) model.
Goodness of fit: the normalised likelihood ratio chi-square for the best model (see Method).
Rate: world-standardised truncated rate per 100 000 per year (30-74 years) and number of **cases** are both estimated from the best-fitting model for the single years cited.
Cumulative risk per 1000 (30-74 years) is estimated from the best-fitting *age-cohort* model for cohorts of central birth year cited.
Recent trend: estimated mean percentage change per five-year period in the age-specific rates (30-74 years) over the period 1973-1987.
Italics denote recent trends not significant at 5 per cent level, or other figures which should be interpreted with caution (see Method).

BLADDER (ICD-9 188)

AMERICAS (USA), INCIDENCE

MALES

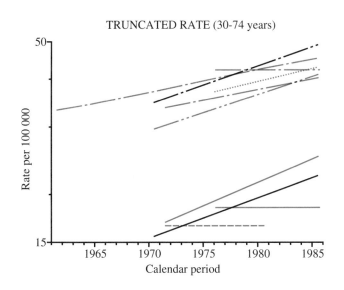

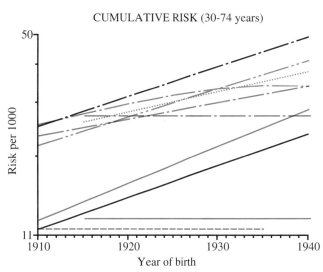

FEMALES

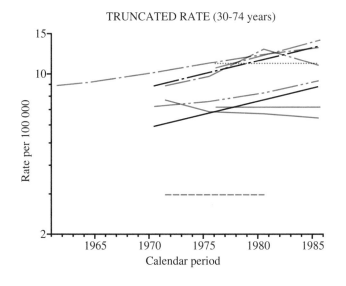

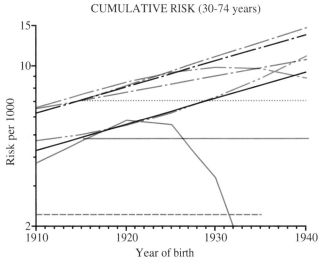

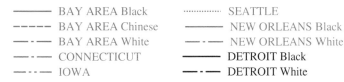

—— BAY AREA Black	·········· SEATTLE	
- - - BAY AREA Chinese	—— NEW ORLEANS Black	
—·— BAY AREA White	—·—·— NEW ORLEANS White	
—··— CONNECTICUT	—— DETROIT Black	
—···— IOWA	—··— DETROIT White	

BLADDER (ICD-9 188)

AMERICAS (except USA), INCIDENCE
Percentage change per five-year period, 1973-1987

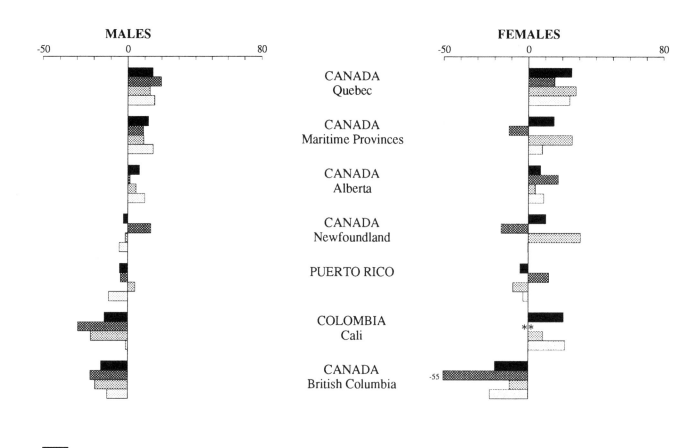

BLADDER (ICD-9 188)

AMERICAS (USA), INCIDENCE
Percentage change per five-year period, 1973-1987

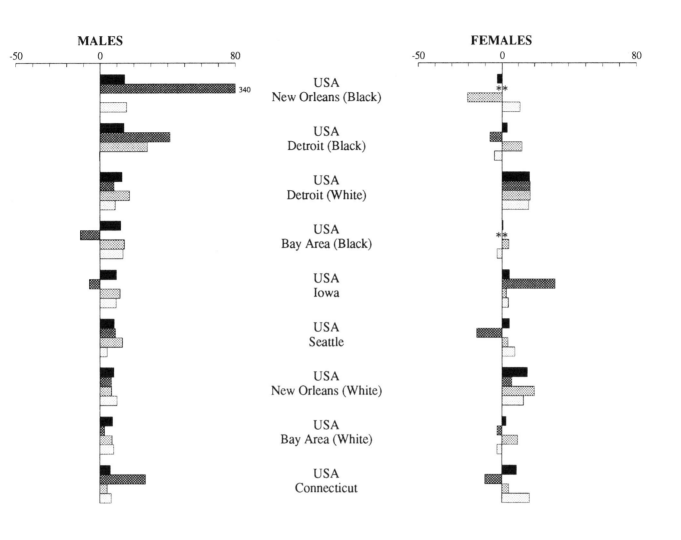

BLADDER (ICD-9 188)

AMERICAS, MORTALITY

MALES	Best model	Goodness of fit	1965 Rate	1965 Deaths	1985 Rate	1985 Deaths	Cumulative risk 1900	Cumulative risk 1940	Recent trend
CANADA	A2C4	-0.49	8.2	309	6.2	370	5.9	2.7	-7.4
CHILE	A5P4C4	9.09	6.9	81	3.6	61	3.7	*1.2*	–
COSTA RICA	A1	-1.13	3.0	4	3.0	9	*2.3*	*2.3*	–
PANAMA	–	–	–	–	–	–	–	–	–
PUERTO RICO	A1	0.33	3.2	12	3.2	12	*2.3*	*2.3*	–
URUGUAY	A4	0.29	*10.8*	*63*	10.8	82	*7.6*	*7.6*	–
USA	A5P4C6	-0.24	8.3	3561	5.5	3260	6.1	2.3	-14.7
VENEZUELA	A2P2	1.64	4.8	36	*2.3*	*33*	2.8	*1.5*	–

FEMALES	Best model	Goodness of fit	1965 Rate	1965 Deaths	1985 Rate	1985 Deaths	Cumulative risk 1900	Cumulative risk 1940	Recent trend
CANADA	A2D	0.71	2.5	98	1.7	115	1.7	0.8	-13.6
CHILE	A1P4C2	6.21	3.8	49	1.5	30	1.9	*0.4*	–
COSTA RICA	A1	-0.37	*0.7*	*0*	0.7	1	*0.5*	*0.5*	–
PANAMA	–	–	–	–	–	–	–	–	–
PUERTO RICO	A1P2	-0.14	1.0	4	1.6	7	*0.7*	*1.7*	–
URUGUAY	A1	-0.81	*1.7*	*10*	1.7	15	*1.2*	*1.2*	–
USA	A3P5C3	0.10	2.6	1318	1.7	1221	1.8	0.6	-12.5
VENEZUELA	A2C2	1.21	1.8	15	*1.3*	*20*	1.2	*0.4*	–

* : not enough deaths for reliable estimation
– : incomplete or missing data
Best model: polynomial of the given degree in age (A), period (P) or cohort (C), or linear drift (D) model.
Goodness of fit: the normalised likelihood ratio chi-square for the best model (see Method).
Rate: world-standardised truncated rate per 100 000 per year (30-74 years) and number of **deaths** are both estimated from the best-fitting model for the single years cited.
Cumulative risk per 1000 (30-74 years) is estimated from the best-fitting *age-cohort* model for cohorts of central birth year cited.
Recent trend: estimated mean percentage change per five-year period in the age-specific rates (30-74 years) over the period 1975-1988.
Italics denote recent trends not significant at 5 per cent level, or other figures which should be interpreted with caution (see Method).

BLADDER (ICD-9 188)

AMERICAS, MORTALITY

MALES

TRUNCATED RATE (30-74 years)

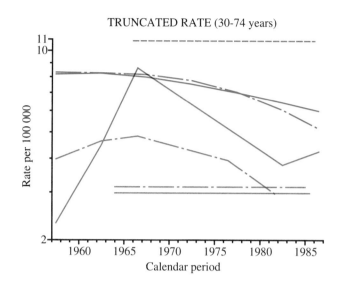

CUMULATIVE RISK (30-74 years)

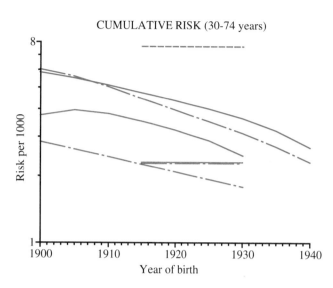

FEMALES

TRUNCATED RATE (30-74 years)

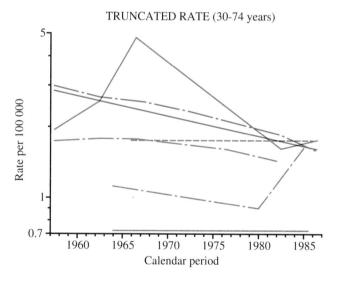

CUMULATIVE RISK (30-74 years)

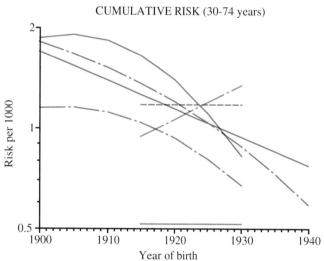

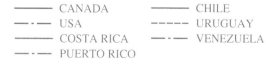

CANADA	CHILE
USA	URUGUAY
COSTA RICA	VENEZUELA
PUERTO RICO	

BLADDER (ICD-9 188)

AMERICAS, MORTALITY
Percentage change per five-year period, 1975-1988

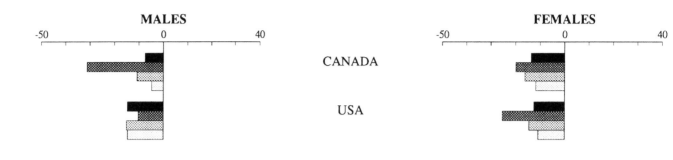

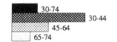

Chapter 24

KIDNEY AND OTHER URINARY ORGANS

Cancers of the kidney, renal pelvis and ureter account for about 1.5% of all cancers, and an estimated 100 000 new cases occur in the world each year. Clear cell adenocarcinomas of the kidney account for more than three quarters of the cases in adults, and transitional cell carcinomas of the renal pelvis for most of the remainder. Cancer of the ureter is rare. World-wide, there is at least a ten-fold range in incidence, which is highest in Europe and lowest in Asia and South America. Survival at five years is of the order of 40% to 50%. Tobacco smoking is a well established causal agent, associated with a 2-fold or greater increase in risk, and a third or more of cases are attributable to this exposure. Industrial exposure to airborne aromatic hydrocarbons from coke production and abuse of analgesics containing phenacetin are also known risk factors, but the percentage of cases attributable to these exposures is much smaller than for tobacco.

Europe

An increase in incidence and mortality from carcinoma of the kidney is occurring in all parts of Europe. Incidence in males is roughly twice that in females, as elsewhere, but in general the rates of increase in incidence are similar in the two sexes. Males in Bas-Rhin (France) have the highest truncated rate (30-74 years) in Europe (30 per 100 000) and this has been increasing steadily at 31% every five years. Males in the Nordic countries also have high rates (around 20 per 100 000), but these rates are increasing less rapidly than in Bas-Rhin, and showing signs of deceleration, in that smaller rates of increase, or even a decline, are observed in younger males. Incidence in the UK is lower (11 and 7 per 100 000), but still increasing steadily at 10% or more every five years. Mortality in these countries is increasing rather more slowly, but given the patterns of increase by age, it is likely to slow down still further or begin to decline within the next ten years.

The incidence of kidney cancer in Hungary, Poland, Slovenia and Romania has been moderate on a European scale, but it is generally increasing more rapidly than in other parts of Europe, and this is also true of mortality in Czechoslovakia, Hungary and Yugoslavia.

Asia and Oceania

Incidence rates in Asia and Oceania are highest among Japanese and Caucasian populations, but the male-to-female ratio is smaller and the levels of incidence are generally lower than in Europe. The most notable increases are occurring among both sexes in Miyagi and Osaka (Japan), where incidence has been rising by up to 40% every five years (4 or more standard errors) and the cumulative risk (30-74 years) for Japanese males born around 1940 approaches 2%. The rates of increase are smaller in Nagasaki City and among Japanese males in Hawaii, but the populations covered by these registries are much smaller than in the prefectural registries of Osaka and Miyagi, and the trends are correspondingly less precise. Mortality in Japan is increasing rapidly, especially in males, but the age-specific trends suggest a deceleration and eventual decline in the cross-sectional rates, with the peak mortality risk occurring in cohorts born around 1930-40.

Substantial increases in incidence are seen in both sexes in Caucasian populations of Australia and New Zealand. In Australia, the rate of increase in mortality is similar in females and males (6-8% every five years), and in both sexes the rate of increase is decelerating. The age-specific patterns, well fitted by simple age-cohort models, suggest that lifetime risk is likely to decline for males born after 1925, while for females the cohort at peak risk cannot yet be identified. The rate of increase in New Zealand males is 7% every five years, and although the recent trend over the last 15 years is not significant, the data are well fitted by an age-drift model, and this figure is a good estimate of the continuing rate of increase.

The extremely rapid rate of increase in incidence among Hawaii Chinese males (more than doubling every five years) is statistically significant (2.7 standard errors), but it is based on very few cases occurring each year, and is thus imprecise — the 95% confidence interval for the recent linear trend of 132% every five years is from 26% to 326% (see Chapter 3). The data for Caucasian males in Hawaii are not well fitted even by the best model, which is an age-drift model suggesting a steady increase in risk, averaged over the entire data set. Whilst there has been a steady overall increase in the truncated rate over the entire period 1960-87, the rate has been falling more

577

continued page 598

KIDNEY (ICD-9 189)

EUROPE (non-EC), INCIDENCE

MALES	Best model	Goodness of fit	1970 Rate	1970 Cases	1985 Rate	1985 Cases	Cumulative risk 1915	Cumulative risk 1940	Recent trend
FINLAND	A8P5C9	0.71	12.7	129	20.2	238	10.0	17.9	17.2
HUNGARY									
County Vas	A2D	2.05	8.0	6	12.1	8	5.9	11.9	*11.8*
Szabolcs-Szatmar	A4D	-0.38	4.1	5	7.1	9	3.1	7.8	*13.5*
ISRAEL									
All Jews	A2P3	-0.80	13.4	61	13.1	73	7.8	9.1	*-0.9*
Non-Jews	A1D	0.34	*2.4*	*0*	6.5	3	3.2	16.9	25.7
NORWAY	A2D	-0.05	12.8	139	19.6	228	10.0	20.2	16.1
POLAND									
Warsaw City	A2P3C3	-0.12	11.3	31	15.4	61	8.0	14.1	*3.6*
ROMANIA									
Cluj	A2P2	-0.40	*23.7*	*37*	6.0	10	2.2	23.9	59.3
SWEDEN	A2P2C5	0.08	19.3	468	21.5	554	12.6	14.2	2.7
SWITZERLAND									
Geneva	A2	-1.04	18.4	14	18.4	17	11.2	11.2	*7.2*
YUGOSLAVIA									
Slovenia	A2C3	0.67	6.6	24	11.1	48	5.4	10.3	33.2

FEMALES	Best model	Goodness of fit	1970 Rate	1970 Cases	1985 Rate	1985 Cases	Cumulative risk 1915	Cumulative risk 1940	Recent trend
FINLAND	A2C5	-0.91	7.0	94	11.1	173	5.8	9.2	17.3
HUNGARY									
County Vas	A2D	0.62	4.8	4	9.5	8	4.0	12.5	44.6
Szabolcs-Szatmar	A4D	-1.36	2.6	3	3.9	6	1.7	3.4	*29.6*
ISRAEL									
All Jews	A2	-0.61	7.1	32	7.1	46	4.3	4.3	*3.6*
Non-Jews	A1	-0.52	*2.1*	*0*	2.1	1	1.2	1.2	24.0
NORWAY	A2D	1.50	7.3	89	9.1	119	5.1	7.3	*2.1*
POLAND									
Warsaw City	A2P3	0.79	5.6	23	6.9	36	4.0	5.7	*7.1*
ROMANIA									
Cluj	A1	1.05	*2.9*	*5*	2.9	6	1.8	1.8	*11.8*
SWEDEN	A4P3C2	1.84	11.9	313	11.9	337	7.4	7.6	*0.3*
SWITZERLAND									
Geneva	A1	0.51	6.4	6	6.4	7	4.1	4.1	*14.7*
YUGOSLAVIA									
Slovenia	A2D	0.62	3.4	16	4.8	27	2.4	4.3	*13.6*

* : not enough cases for reliable estimation
− : incomplete or missing data
Best model: polynomial of the given degree in age (A), period (P) or cohort (C), or linear drift (D) model.
Goodness of fit: the normalised likelihood ratio chi-square for the best model (see Method).
Rate: world-standardised truncated rate per 100 000 per year (30-74 years) and number of **cases** are both estimated from the best-fitting model for the single years cited.
Cumulative risk per 1000 (30-74 years) is estimated from the best-fitting *age-cohort* model for cohorts of central birth year cited.
Recent trend: estimated mean percentage change per five-year period in the age-specific rates (30-74 years) over the period 1973-1987.
Italics denote recent trends not significant at 5 per cent level, or other figures which should be interpreted with caution (see Method).

KIDNEY (ICD-9 189)

EUROPE (non-EC), INCIDENCE

MALES

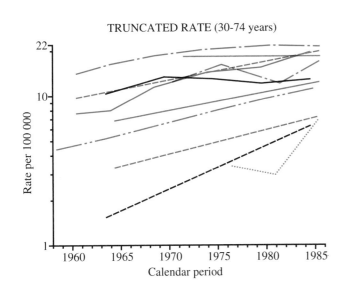
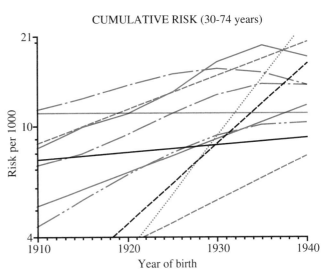

FEMALES

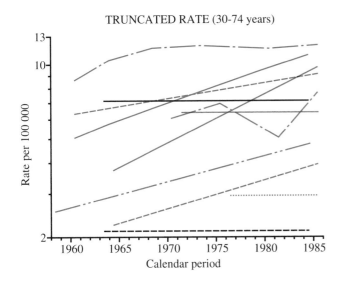
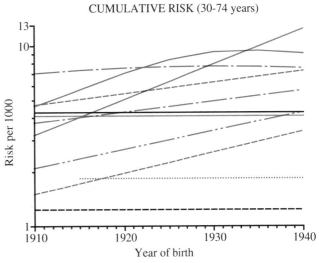

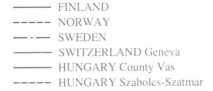

——— FINLAND	—·— POLAND Warsaw City
– – – NORWAY	········· ROMANIA Cluj
—·—· SWEDEN	—··—·· YUGOSLAVIA Slovenia
——— SWITZERLAND Geneva	——— ISRAEL All Jews
——— HUNGARY County Vas	– – – ISRAEL Non-Jews
– – – HUNGARY Szabolcs-Szatmar	

KIDNEY (ICD-9 189)

EUROPE (EC), INCIDENCE

MALES	Best model	Goodness of fit	1970 Rate	1970 Cases	1985 Rate	1985 Cases	Cumulative risk 1915	Cumulative risk 1940	Recent trend
DENMARK	A2P4C4	-0.76	16.7	222	19.0	273	11.7	14.9	*4.0*
FRANCE									
Bas-Rhin	A2D	-0.80	*14.3*	*32*	30.2	60	14.0	47.8	30.7
Doubs	A1	1.81	*13.3*	*8*	13.3	14	8.4	8.4	*-2.2*
GERMANY (FRG)									
Hamburg	A8	0.86	15.1	79	*15.1*	*59*	8.9	*8.9*	–
Saarland	A8C8	0.71	12.4	34	20.8	57	8.8	24.3	13.5
GERMANY (GDR)	A3D	3.63	11.4	485	22.2	825	9.6	28.5	25.0
ITALY									
Varese	A2C2	0.96	*10.7*	*17*	22.1	45	11.8	16.6	20.5
SPAIN									
Navarra	A2C2	0.22	*10.1*	*12*	11.8	15	4.5	20.7	*12.7*
Zaragoza	A2D	1.01	7.0	13	6.6	15	4.0	3.6	*-8.0*
UK									
Birmingham	A2D	1.67	8.2	110	11.7	169	5.9	10.6	12.5
Scotland	A8C9	-0.28	9.5	128	13.9	189	6.9	12.2	11.3
South Thames	A2C4	-1.23	8.4	207	10.7	198	5.8	8.0	10.4

FEMALES	Best model	Goodness of fit	1970 Rate	1970 Cases	1985 Rate	1985 Cases	Cumulative risk 1915	Cumulative risk 1940	Recent trend
DENMARK	A8P6C9	-0.66	11.6	173	14.8	238	7.1	7.9	12.3
FRANCE									
Bas-Rhin	A2D	0.21	*7.0*	*20*	10.4	25	4.9	9.5	*13.9*
Doubs	A1	-0.48	*5.9*	*4*	5.9	7	3.6	3.6	*34.8*
GERMANY (FRG)									
Hamburg	A2	-1.25	6.9	50	*6.9*	*37*	4.0	*4.0*	–
Saarland	A2D	1.14	6.4	23	10.8	40	4.9	11.8	25.4
GERMANY (GDR)	A5P4	0.76	6.8	440	10.9	582	4.9	12.2	22.5
ITALY									
Varese	A1D	1.42	*2.8*	*4*	7.5	19	3.3	16.9	36.7
SPAIN									
Navarra	A1D	0.37	*1.3*	*1*	6.8	10	2.9	45.4	75.9
Zaragoza	A2	-0.97	3.1	6	3.1	7	1.7	1.7	*-4.8*
UK									
Birmingham	A4P2	0.82	3.3	50	5.5	88	2.6	5.0	20.3
Scotland	A2D	0.46	4.7	79	7.2	118	3.6	7.5	11.4
South Thames	A2D	0.25	3.5	107	4.7	100	2.4	3.9	11.0

* : not enough cases for reliable estimation
– : incomplete or missing data
Best model: polynomial of the given degree in age (A), period (P) or cohort (C), or linear drift (D) model.
Goodness of fit: the normalised likelihood ratio chi-square for the best model (see Method).
Rate: world-standardised truncated rate per 100 000 per year (30-74 years) and number of **cases** are both estimated from the best-fitting model for the single years cited.
Cumulative risk per 1000 (30-74 years) is estimated from the best-fitting *age-cohort* model for cohorts of central birth year cited.
Recent trend: estimated mean percentage change per five-year period in the age-specific rates (30-74 years) over the period 1973-1987.
Italics denote recent trends not significant at 5 per cent level, or other figures which should be interpreted with caution (see Method).

580

KIDNEY (ICD-9 189)

EUROPE (EC), INCIDENCE

MALES

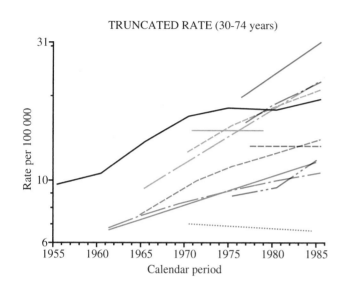

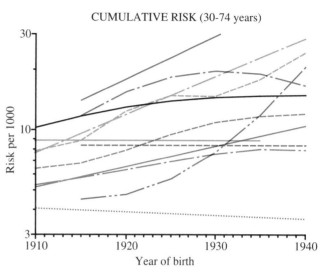

FEMALES

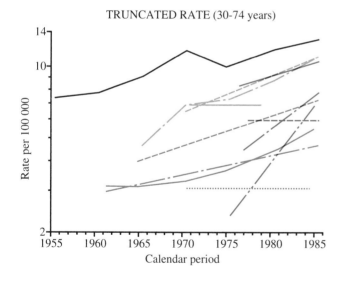

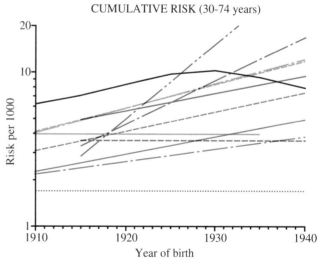

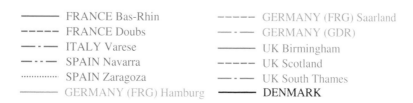

—— FRANCE Bas-Rhin	----- GERMANY (FRG) Saarland
----- FRANCE Doubs	–·– GERMANY (GDR)
–·– ITALY Varese	—— UK Birmingham
–··– SPAIN Navarra	----- UK Scotland
·········· SPAIN Zaragoza	–··– UK South Thames
—— GERMANY (FRG) Hamburg	—— DENMARK

KIDNEY (ICD-9 189)

EUROPE (non-EC), INCIDENCE
Percentage change per five-year period, 1973-1987

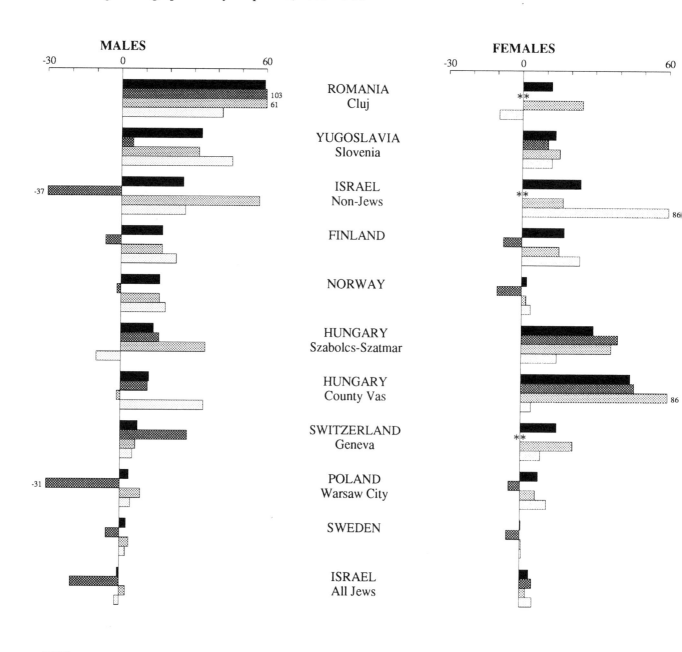

KIDNEY (ICD-9 189)

EUROPE (EC), INCIDENCE
Percentage change per five-year period, 1973-1987

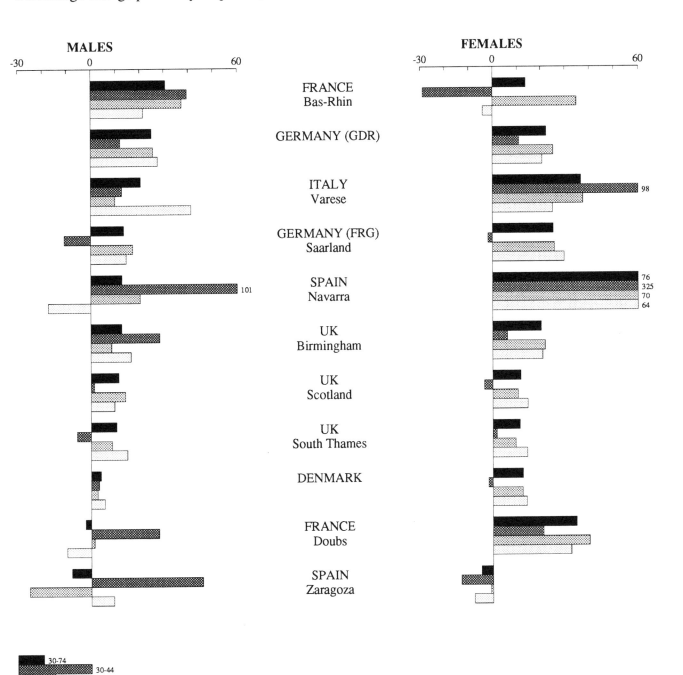

KIDNEY (ICD-9 189)

EUROPE (non-EC), MORTALITY

MALES	Best model	Goodness of fit	1965 Rate	1965 Deaths	1985 Rate	1985 Deaths	Cumulative risk 1900	Cumulative risk 1940	Recent trend
AUSTRIA	A5D	0.01	*8.7*	*172*	10.2	189	*5.5*	7.5	*2.1*
CZECHOSLOVAKIA	A8P6C9	1.15	8.3	293	16.6	599	5.7	17.1	12.0
FINLAND	A3C4	-1.57	6.5	61	10.2	119	3.7	7.1	*2.0*
HUNGARY	A3D	1.26	*5.5*	*142*	9.9	275	*3.4*	11.1	15.2
NORWAY	A2D	-1.36	7.0	72	9.2	110	4.4	7.5	*4.3*
POLAND	A2D	-1.23	3.3	197	*8.9*	*690*	1.8	*13.5*	–
ROMANIA	–	–	–	–	–	–	–	–	–
SWEDEN	A2P2C4	0.75	9.7	224	10.6	281	6.0	6.8	-7.3
SWITZERLAND	A2C2	-1.27	7.5	107	8.6	149	4.8	5.3	*0.6*
YUGOSLAVIA	A2C3	2.23	2.3	83	4.3	215	1.3	3.7	20.0

FEMALES	Best model	Goodness of fit	1965 Rate	1965 Deaths	1985 Rate	1985 Deaths	Cumulative risk 1900	Cumulative risk 1940	Recent trend
AUSTRIA	A3C3	0.40	*4.7*	*127*	5.4	143	*2.8*	3.2	*4.1*
CZECHOSLOVAKIA	A8D	2.30	3.8	164	6.5	293	2.3	6.7	14.6
FINLAND	A2D	0.26	3.5	43	5.4	84	2.2	5.2	*7.7*
HUNGARY	A2P3	-0.13	*0.7*	*23*	4.1	147	*1.9*	4.2	8.6
NORWAY	A8C9	0.23	4.2	49	4.0	55	2.9	1.8	*-7.5*
POLAND	A4C2	1.51	1.9	141	*3.2*	*324*	1.1	*2.3*	–
ROMANIA	–	–	–	–	–	–	–	–	–
SWEDEN	A2P2	0.66	5.8	147	6.3	185	3.6	4.8	*-2.0*
SWITZERLAND	A2C2	0.35	4.0	69	4.5	94	2.5	2.6	*-0.2*
YUGOSLAVIA	A2C2	0.77	1.4	60	2.5	148	0.8	1.8	9.9

* : not enough deaths for reliable estimation
– : incomplete or missing data
Best model: polynomial of the given degree in age (A), period (P) or cohort (C), or linear drift (D) model.
Goodness of fit: the normalised likelihood ratio chi-square for the best model (see Method).
Rate: world-standardised truncated rate per 100 000 per year (30-74 years) and number of **deaths** are both estimated from the best-fitting model for the single years cited.
Cumulative risk per 1000 (30-74 years) is estimated from the best-fitting *age-cohort* model for cohorts of central birth year cited.
Recent trend: estimated mean percentage change per five-year period in the age-specific rates (30-74 years) over the period 1975-1988.
Italics denote recent trends not significant at 5 per cent level, or other figures which should be interpreted with caution (see Method).

KIDNEY (ICD-9 189)

EUROPE (non-EC), MORTALITY

MALES

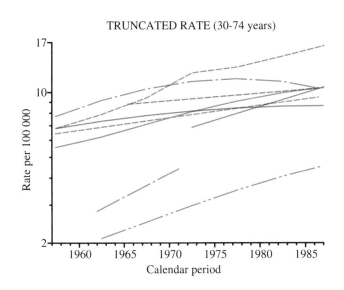

TRUNCATED RATE (30-74 years)

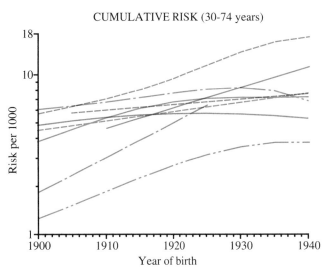

CUMULATIVE RISK (30-74 years)

FEMALES

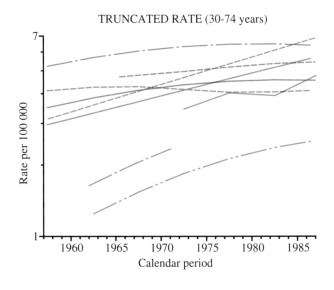

TRUNCATED RATE (30-74 years)

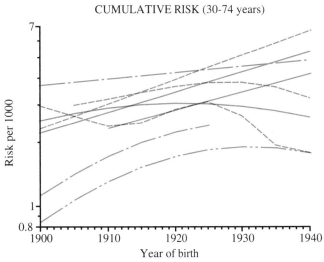

CUMULATIVE RISK (30-74 years)

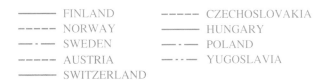

FINLAND   CZECHOSLOVAKIA
NORWAY   HUNGARY
SWEDEN   POLAND
AUSTRIA   YUGOSLAVIA
SWITZERLAND

KIDNEY (ICD-9 189)

EUROPE (EC), MORTALITY

MALES	Best model	Goodness of fit	1965 Rate	Deaths	1985 Rate	Deaths	Cumulative risk 1900	1940	Recent trend
BELGIUM	A2C5	0.92	5.8	151	7.8	211	3.8	6.5	*1.7*
DENMARK	A3C3	-0.40	8.7	111	10.3	149	5.3	6.3	*3.2*
FRANCE	A4C8	0.98	4.9	605	7.6	1055	3.2	6.4	11.6
GERMANY (FRG)	A3P3C2	10.17	*9.1*	*1371*	11.4	1800	*4.7*	7.4	7.4
GREECE	A2D	-1.07	*2.4*	*44*	4.2	116	*1.5*	4.8	20.3
IRELAND	A2C2	0.67	3.9	27	6.4	50	2.2	4.9	*2.2*
ITALY	A3P3C6	3.75	3.6	437	7.4	1146	2.2	6.7	22.0
NETHERLANDS	A2C4	1.20	6.9	191	9.5	334	4.3	6.1	8.1
PORTUGAL	–	–	–	–	–	–	–	–	–
SPAIN	A2D	0.48	2.4	168	4.0	388	1.6	4.3	11.9
UK ENGLAND & WALES	A8P6C9	-0.07	5.4	699	6.6	942	3.1	4.5	8.3
UK SCOTLAND	A2C2	-0.40	7.4	97	8.0	110	4.5	4.7	*3.4*

FEMALES	Best model	Goodness of fit	1965 Rate	Deaths	1985 Rate	Deaths	Cumulative risk 1900	1940	Recent trend
BELGIUM	A3C2	-0.17	3.1	97	4.4	138	1.9	3.2	*4.1*
DENMARK	A2C4	0.73	5.9	84	7.2	117	3.6	4.4	*-0.1*
FRANCE	A3P2C2	1.55	2.7	414	3.0	484	1.7	1.8	*-2.5*
GERMANY (FRG)	A2P3C3	4.73	*4.3*	*905*	4.8	1079	*2.4*	2.7	3.4
GREECE	A2D	1.86	*1.0*	*22*	1.6	51	*0.7*	1.7	*10.1*
IRELAND	A2C2	-1.25	2.0	14	3.0	25	1.1	2.1	*10.0*
ITALY	A4P2C2	-0.93	1.7	249	2.7	507	1.1	2.3	17.1
NETHERLANDS	A2C4	1.96	3.7	115	4.8	195	2.3	3.8	9.9
PORTUGAL	–	–	–	–	–	–	–	–	–
SPAIN	A2P2	0.50	1.4	117	1.5	166	0.8	1.2	*-3.4*
UK ENGLAND & WALES	A2D	2.61	2.3	361	3.1	492	1.4	2.4	12.1
UK SCOTLAND	A2D	1.10	3.4	56	4.2	70	2.0	3.2	10.1

* : not enough deaths for reliable estimation
– : incomplete or missing data
Best model: polynomial of the given degree in age (A), period (P) or cohort (C), or linear drift (D) model.
Goodness of fit: the normalised likelihood ratio chi-square for the best model (see Method).
Rate: world-standardised truncated rate per 100 000 per year (30-74 years) and number of **deaths** are both estimated from the best-fitting model for the single years cited.
Cumulative risk per 1000 (30-74 years) is estimated from the best-fitting *age-cohort* model for cohorts of central birth year cited.
Recent trend: estimated mean percentage change per five-year period in the age-specific rates (30-74 years) over the period 1975-1988.
Italics denote recent trends not significant at 5 per cent level, or other figures which should be interpreted with caution (see Method).

KIDNEY (ICD-9 189)

EUROPE (EC), MORTALITY

MALES

TRUNCATED RATE (30-74 years)

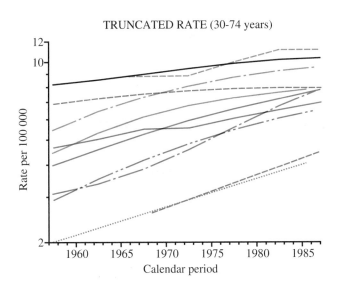

CUMULATIVE RISK (30-74 years)

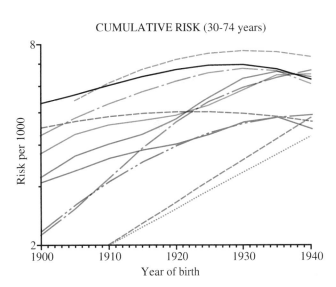

FEMALES

TRUNCATED RATE (30-74 years)

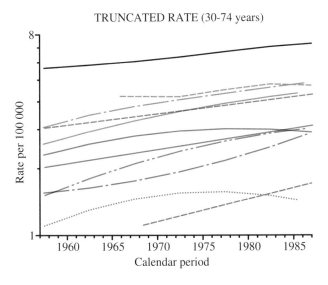

CUMULATIVE RISK (30-74 years)

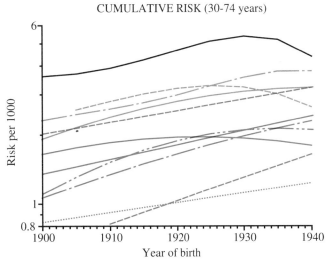

—— FRANCE	—·—·— NETHERLANDS
— — — GREECE	—··—··— IRELAND
—·—·— ITALY	—— UK ENGLAND & WALES
············ SPAIN	— — — UK SCOTLAND
—— BELGIUM	—— DENMARK
— — — GERMANY (FRG)	

KIDNEY (ICD-9 189)

EUROPE (non-EC), MORTALITY
Percentage change per five-year period, 1975-1988

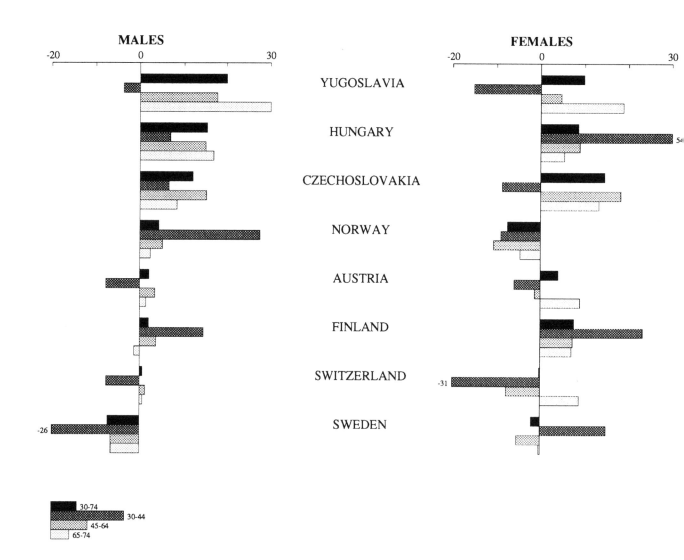

KIDNEY (ICD-9 189)

EUROPE (EC), MORTALITY
Percentage change per five-year period, 1975-1988

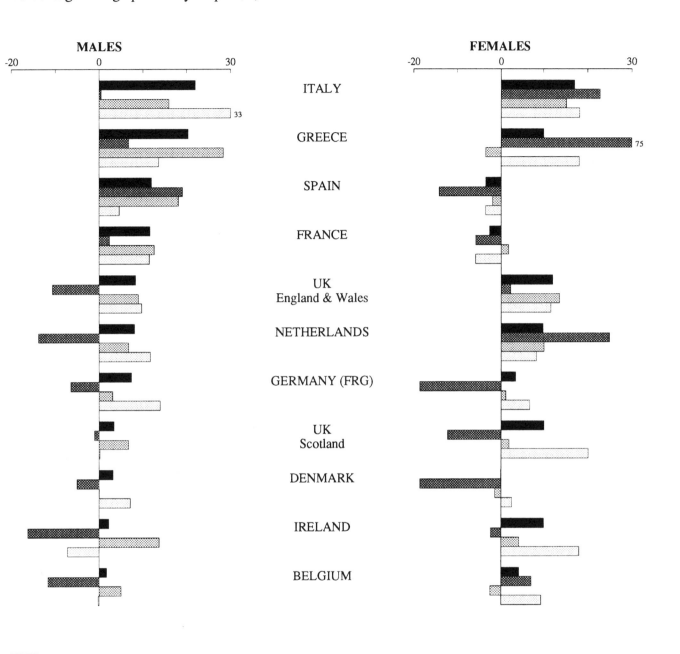

ASIA, INCIDENCE

MALES	Best model	Goodness of fit	1970 Rate	1970 Cases	1985 Rate	1985 Cases	Cumulative risk 1915	Cumulative risk 1940	Recent trend
CHINA									
Shanghai	A2D	1.45	*2.3*	*23*	3.6	62	1.9	4.0	15.1
HONG KONG	A8P2	-1.47	*16.1*	*89*	5.6	63	2.6	4.6	*9.4*
INDIA									
Bombay	A3	0.21	2.2	16	2.2	26	1.3	1.3	*9.7*
JAPAN									
Miyagi	A2D	1.54	3.5	12	9.3	49	4.2	21.2	43.4
Nagasaki	A1P2	0.57	*63.9*	*52*	9.8	10	5.6	9.8	*10.9*
Osaka	A2D	0.95	3.0	36	7.8	144	3.9	18.7	40.6
SINGAPORE									
Chinese	A2	-1.31	6.1	12	6.1	18	3.8	3.8	*11.9*
Indian	A1	0.34	4.7	1	4.7	1	3.1	3.1	*-12.5*
Malay	A1C4	0.52	*1.8*	*0*	4.8	2	3.0	0.9	*22.7*

FEMALES	Best model	Goodness of fit	1970 Rate	1970 Cases	1985 Rate	1985 Cases	Cumulative risk 1915	Cumulative risk 1940	Recent trend
CHINA									
Shanghai	A2D	-0.05	*1.3*	*14*	2.4	42	1.1	3.0	20.7
HONG KONG	A2D	0.05	*2.4*	*14*	3.9	43	1.7	3.8	15.7
INDIA									
Bombay	A2	-1.01	1.2	6	1.2	11	0.7	0.7	*-9.6*
JAPAN									
Miyagi	A1D	1.59	1.8	7	3.9	24	1.9	6.6	41.3
Nagasaki	A3	-0.20	*3.0*	*3*	3.0	4	2.0	2.0	*19.6*
Osaka	A3C2	0.29	1.4	19	3.0	66	1.6	3.9	25.4
SINGAPORE									
Chinese	A3	1.31	3.2	7	3.2	11	1.9	1.9	*10.7*
Indian	A0	-0.19	*1.7*	*0*	*1.7*	*0*	0.8	0.8	*75.9*
Malay	A1	-0.35	*1.9*	*0*	*1.9*	*0*	1.0	1.0	*21.6*

* : not enough cases for reliable estimation
− : incomplete or missing data
Best model: polynomial of the given degree in age (A), period (P) or cohort (C), or linear drift (D) model.
Goodness of fit: the normalised likelihood ratio chi-square for the best model (see Method).
Rate: world-standardised truncated rate per 100 000 per year (30-74 years) and number of **cases** are both estimated from the best-fitting model for the single years cited.
Cumulative risk per 1000 (30-74 years) is estimated from the best-fitting *age-cohort* model for cohorts of central birth year cited.
Recent trend: estimated mean percentage change per five-year period in the age-specific rates (30-74 years) over the period 1973-1987.
Italics denote recent trends not significant at 5 per cent level, or other figures which should be interpreted with caution (see Method).

KIDNEY (ICD-9 189)

ASIA, INCIDENCE

MALES

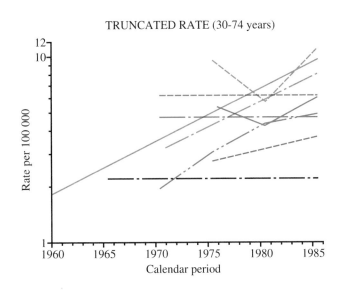

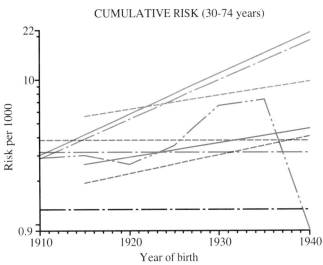

FEMALES

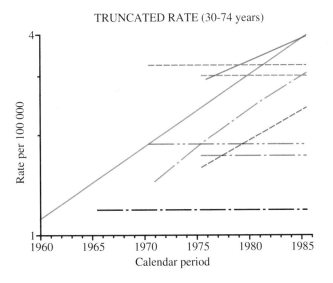

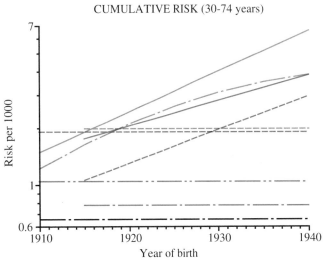

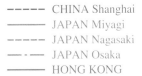

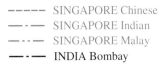

----- CHINA Shanghai
——— JAPAN Miyagi
----- JAPAN Nagasaki
—·—· JAPAN Osaka
——— HONG KONG

----- SINGAPORE Chinese
—·—· SINGAPORE Indian
—··—·· SINGAPORE Malay
—··—·· INDIA Bombay

KIDNEY (ICD-9 189)

OCEANIA, INCIDENCE

MALES	Best model	Goodness of fit	1970		1985		Cumulative risk		Recent trend
			Rate	Cases	Rate	Cases	1915	1940	
AUSTRALIA									
New South Wales	A2D	-0.40	*9.9*	*102*	15.0	198	7.7	15.3	14.9
South	A2	-0.38	*15.0*	*28*	15.0	52	9.1	9.1	*7.5*
HAWAII									
Caucasian	A1D	3.12	13.0	4	17.8	11	10.4	17.4	*-1.9*
Chinese	A1P2	0.23	*5.8*	*0*	16.3	2	6.2	10.8	132.2
Filipino	A1	-0.79	7.5	1	7.5	2	4.5	4.5	*1.9*
Hawaiian	A8	0.78	9.4	1	9.4	2	4.7	4.7	*10.8*
Japanese	A3D	-0.46	8.5	4	13.7	11	6.6	14.7	*15.0*
NEW ZEALAND									
Maori	A8	0.38	10.9	2	10.9	3	5.3	5.3	*1.1*
Non-Maori	A3P3	-0.63	10.5	59	14.8	102	8.0	10.6	11.2

FEMALES	Best model	Goodness of fit	1970		1985		Cumulative risk		Recent trend
			Rate	Cases	Rate	Cases	1915	1940	
AUSTRALIA									
New South Wales	A2C2	-2.75	*4.8*	*55*	10.4	148	5.0	11.5	26.9
South	A2P2	0.05	*0.1*	*0*	9.2	33	3.8	11.2	26.1
HAWAII									
Caucasian	A8C9	-0.30	6.3	2	10.1	6	8.7	4.9	45.3
Chinese	*	..	..	..	..	..	..	..	..
Filipino	A1	-0.64	*5.3*	*0*	5.3	1	3.3	3.3	*39.7*
Hawaiian	A1	-0.75	*4.9*	*0*	4.9	1	3.1	3.1	*-18.7*
Japanese	A2	-0.97	3.2	1	3.2	3	2.0	2.0	*10.9*
NEW ZEALAND									
Maori	A1	1.30	8.1	1	8.1	2	4.9	4.9	*-15.6*
Non-Maori	A2P3	-0.21	5.8	35	6.5	48	3.9	2.0	*9.1*

* : not enough cases for reliable estimation
− : incomplete or missing data
Best model: polynomial of the given degree in age (A), period (P) or cohort (C), or linear drift (D) model.
Goodness of fit: the normalised likelihood ratio chi-square for the best model (see Method).
Rate: world-standardised truncated rate per 100 000 per year (30-74 years) and number of **cases** are both estimated from the best-fitting model for the single years cited.
Cumulative risk per 1000 (30-74 years) is estimated from the best-fitting *age-cohort* model for cohorts of central birth year cited.
Recent trend: estimated mean percentage change per five-year period in the age-specific rates (30-74 years) over the period 1973-1987.
Italics denote recent trends not significant at 5 per cent level, or other figures which should be interpreted with caution (see Method).

KIDNEY (ICD-9 189)

OCEANIA, INCIDENCE

MALES

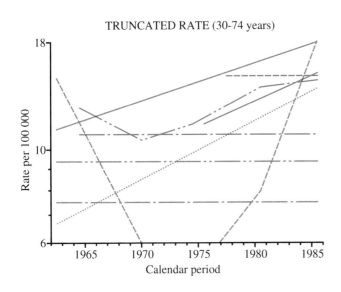

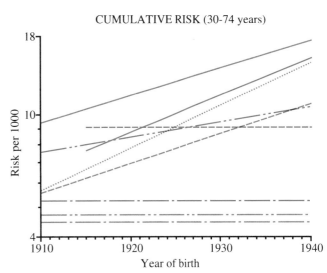

FEMALES

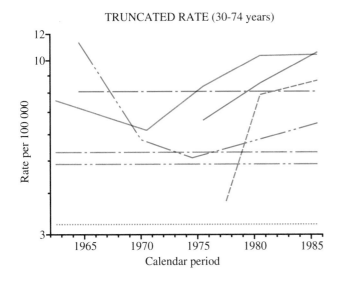

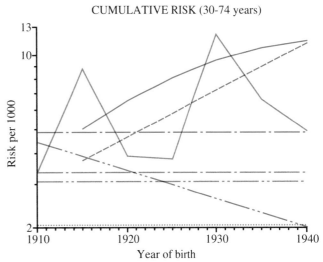

——— AUSTRALIA New South Wales	– – – – HAWAII Chinese
– – – – AUSTRALIA South	– · – · – HAWAII Filipino
– · – · – NEW ZEALAND Maori	– ·· – ·· – HAWAII Hawaiian
– ·· – ·· – NEW ZEALAND Non-Maori	············· HAWAII Japanese
——— HAWAII Caucasian	

ASIA, INCIDENCE
Percentage change per five-year period, 1973-1987

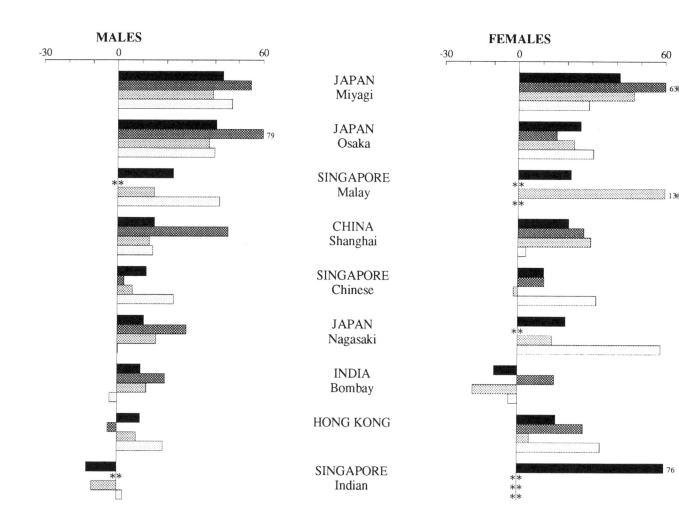

MALES

FEMALES

JAPAN
Miyagi

JAPAN
Osaka

SINGAPORE
Malay

CHINA
Shanghai

SINGAPORE
Chinese

JAPAN
Nagasaki

INDIA
Bombay

HONG KONG

SINGAPORE
Indian

30-74
30-44
45-64
65-74

KIDNEY (ICD-9 189)

OCEANIA, INCIDENCE
Percentage change per five-year period, 1973-1987

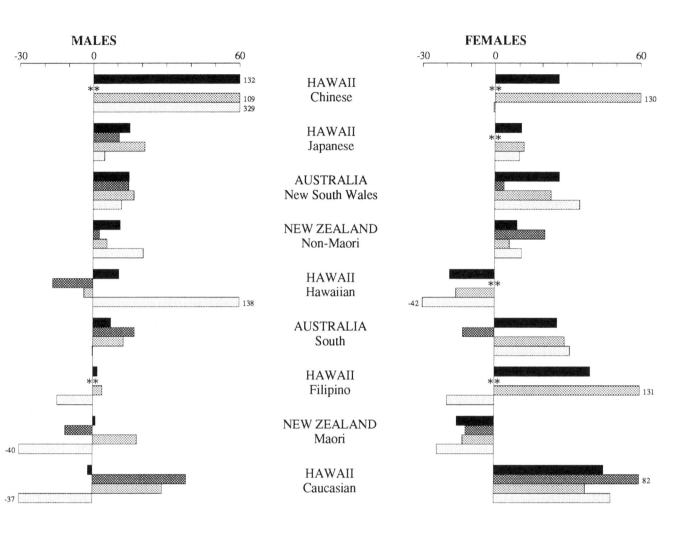

KIDNEY (ICD-9 189)

ASIA and OCEANIA, MORTALITY

MALES	Best model	Goodness of fit	1965 Rate	1965 Deaths	1985 Rate	1985 Deaths	Cumulative risk 1900	Cumulative risk 1940	Recent trend
AUSTRALIA	A2C3	0.84	5.9	143	6.7	247	3.6	3.7	6.8
HONG KONG	A2C2	-0.14	*1.4*	*6*	2.8	24	*0.8*	2.0	*-5.1*
JAPAN	A8P6C9	0.12	1.5	275	3.8	1102	1.0	3.4	20.9
MAURITIUS	*	..	..	..	..	..	..	..	..
NEW ZEALAND	A2D	0.83	6.7	36	7.6	55	4.1	5.2	*6.6*
SINGAPORE	A1D	1.51	1.8	3	3.1	8	*0.9*	2.6	–

FEMALES	Best model	Goodness of fit	1965 Rate	1965 Deaths	1985 Rate	1985 Deaths	Cumulative risk 1900	Cumulative risk 1940	Recent trend
AUSTRALIA	A2C2	-0.30	2.7	71	3.9	157	1.7	3.0	8.1
HONG KONG	A1	0.10	*1.4*	*6*	1.4	11	*0.9*	0.9	*-0.7*
JAPAN	A4C3	1.22	0.8	159	1.3	451	0.5	0.9	11.4
MAURITIUS	A1	-0.43	*0.7*	*0*	*0.7*	*0*	*0.4*	0.4	*14.6*
NEW ZEALAND	A2	1.33	3.1	18	3.1	25	2.0	2.0	*5.5*
SINGAPORE	A7	0.12	1.2	2	1.2	3	*0.6*	0.6	–

* : not enough deaths for reliable estimation
– : incomplete or missing data
Best model: polynomial of the given degree in age (A), period (P) or cohort (C), or linear drift (D) model.
Goodness of fit: the normalised likelihood ratio chi-square for the best model (see Method).
Rate: world-standardised truncated rate per 100 000 per year (30-74 years) and number of **deaths** are both estimated from the best-fitting model for the single years cited.
Cumulative risk per 1000 (30-74 years) is estimated from the best-fitting *age-cohort* model for cohorts of central birth year cited.
Recent trend: estimated mean percentage change per five-year period in the age-specific rates (30-74 years) over the period 1975-1988.
Italics denote recent trends not significant at 5 per cent level, or other figures which should be interpreted with caution (see Method).

KIDNEY (ICD-9 189)

ASIA and OCEANIA, MORTALITY

MALES

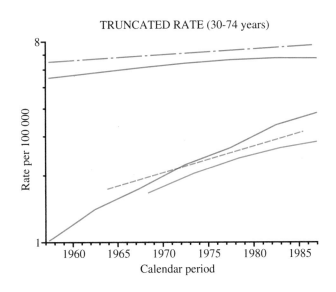

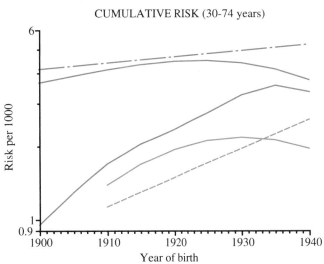

FEMALES

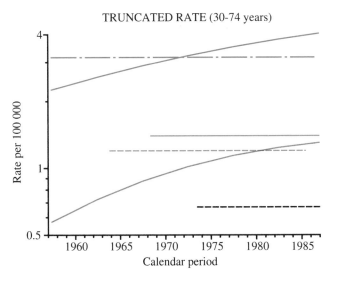

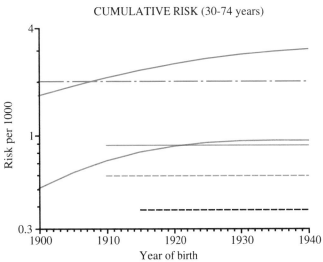

AUSTRALIA   HONG KONG
NEW ZEALAND   SINGAPORE
JAPAN   MAURITIUS

KIDNEY (ICD-9 189)

ASIA and OCEANIA, MORTALITY
Percentage change per five-year period, 1975-1988

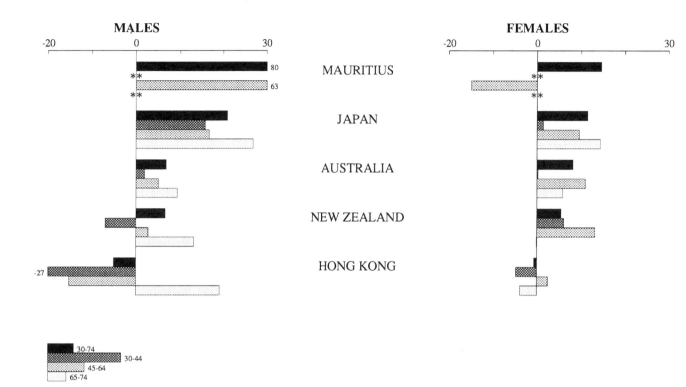

from page 577

recently by 2% (not significant) every five years, as shown in the table and histogram; the recent decrease needs to be re-evaluated in the future.

Americas

Incidence and mortality from cancer of the kidney are twice as high in North America as in Central and South America, and similar to the levels seen in western Europe. Cumulative risks for the 1940 birth cohort are about 1% in males and 0.7% in females. Chinese in the San Francisco Bay Area (USA) are a striking exception; while incidence is about twice as high as in Chinese populations in Shanghai (China) and Singapore, it is about half the levels seen in other North American populations, and shows little sign of change. Increasing trends in incidence are observed in almost all North American populations, including that of Puerto Rico, but incidence is changing very little, if at all, among those populations of Central and South America for which data have been examined.

There is little racial or geographical variation in incidence or in the rate with which it is changing in the USA, and still less geographical variation in incidence rates or trends across Canada. There is little evidence of (non-linear) cohort effects in these data. The large recent increase in incidence observed among black males in New Orleans is derived from a poorly-fitting age-drift model, based on only three periods of observation, and it should not be given too much weight.

Overall mortality is still increasing steadily in both the USA and Canada. In the USA, however, mortality below the age of 45 years is now decreasing slightly in both sexes at about 3% every five years, and overall mortality appears likely to start declining by the end of the century, but there is no evidence of any deceleration in the rate of increase in mortality observed in Canada. In this respect, the slightly more favourable outlook in the USA than in Canada for mortality from cancer of the kidney resembles the situation observed for cancers of the bladder and pancreas. Mortality from renal cancer does appear to be increasing among males in Chile and Venezuela, although more recent data would be necessary to confirm this observation.

598

Comment

There are few published reports on trends in the incidence of cancers of the kidney and other urinary organs. Incidence rates in Vaud (Switzerland) are similar to those in Geneva, but the recent rate of increase between the two quinquennia ending in 1988 is slightly higher at 14% and 20% in males and females, respectively[164], although these rates of change appear unstable[162]. Larger recent rates of increase for the same period have been reported from Slovakia[237], at 23% and 30% every five years among males and females, respectively. There was little or no change in incidence among Chinese males in Singapore in the 15 years up to 1982[154], and there has been no significant increase since then.

Incidence in the USA more than doubled between 1947 and 1984, the rate of increase slowing down since 1970[77]. Connecticut data were included in those analyses, and the series from Connecticut analysed here, dating from 1960, continues to reflect these trends, with a larger rate of increase among males than females. The age-specific mortality trends in the USA up to 1984, increasing in the elderly and stable in younger persons[77], have become more marked: mortality is now declining by 3-4% every five years among younger persons (30-44 years) and continues to increase significantly at 3-5% every five years among the elderly (65-74 years).

The increases in incidence may be partly due to better diagnosis in the 1950s and 1960s, and partly to true increases associated with tobacco smoking. Survival has also improved, which probably accounts for the disparity between trends in incidence and mortality in many countries. The geographical variation in speed and direction of trends in the incidence of kidney cancer is likely to reflect trends in exposure to tobacco.

Mortality trends reported here complement previous reports from France up to 1985[128], England and Wales up to 1980, Europe up to 1989[148] and the USA up to 1984[77]. The sharp peak in mortality seen for the 1930-40 birth cohorts in England and Wales[213] has become less marked with the inclusion of mortality data up to 1988 in the analyses. The underlying trend is still upward, with recent linear trends of about 8% every five years, although these are less than the rates of increase in incidence in Birmingham and South Thames (UK).

Overall, there is a similarity between the European patterns of mortality from cancer of the kidney and those for cancer of the pancreas in both sexes, both in the range of mortality rates and in the variation in time trends across the continent. This can perhaps best be summarised as a deceleration in the rate of increase or even a small decline in mortality in the north and west of the continent, and a rapid increase in mortality in the east and the south. The evidence for an actual inversion of the rankings, with the highest rates being observed (or expected soon) in the south and east of Europe, rather than in the north and west as hitherto[269], is less clear for cancer of the kidney than for cancers of the pancreas, bladder and lung.

In contrast with the situation in Europe, trends in cancer of the kidney in Asia and Oceania do not resemble those for cancers of the bladder. Mortality from cancer of the kidney is increasing rapidly among Japanese and, less rapidly, in Australia and New Zealand, while mortality from cancer of the bladder is stable or declining.

KIDNEY (ICD-9 189)

AMERICAS (except USA), INCIDENCE

MALES	Best model	Goodness of fit	1970		1985		Cumulative risk		Recent trend
			Rate	Cases	Rate	Cases	1915	1940	
BRAZIL									
Sao Paulo	A5C2	-0.35	2.8	23	6.2	39	2.5	1.6	–
CANADA									
Alberta	A3P4C3	1.00	13.4	41	17.4	78	9.5	16.0	22.3
British Columbia	A2D	0.48	12.9	60	15.6	110	8.6	11.8	9.4
Maritime Provinces	A2P2	0.02	11.9	37	18.7	67	8.7	22.9	27.9
Newfoundland	A2D	-0.66	9.1	7	18.4	20	8.5	27.3	13.7
Quebec	A2P4	1.66	10.9	119	21.2	307	9.3	28.4	32.6
COLOMBIA									
Cali	A1	0.03	3.9	2	3.9	5	2.5	2.5	-6.8
CUBA	A2D	-0.10	2.8	42	3.9	78	2.1	3.6	–
PUERTO RICO	A4D	0.38	3.0	13	7.3	48	2.9	12.7	37.9

FEMALES	Best model	Goodness of fit	1970		1985		Cumulative risk		Recent trend
			Rate	Cases	Rate	Cases	1915	1940	
BRAZIL									
Sao Paulo	A1	1.69	2.7	19	2.7	26	1.3	1.3	–
CANADA									
Alberta	A2P2	0.85	6.3	18	10.3	48	4.9	9.2	24.6
British Columbia	A2D	-0.48	5.5	26	7.5	58	3.9	6.4	12.9
Maritime Provinces	A2D	0.86	6.4	20	9.2	35	4.4	8.0	18.2
Newfoundland	A8C9	-1.13	5.9	4	8.9	9	2.8	7.2	21.0
Quebec	A2P2	-0.30	5.3	64	10.1	170	4.6	12.5	33.3
COLOMBIA									
Cali	A2C2	3.19	1.7	1	4.1	7	1.8	3.8	12.1
CUBA	A2	0.95	1.9	25	1.9	38	1.1	1.1	–
PUERTO RICO	A1D	0.23	2.0	9	3.0	23	1.6	3.2	21.9

* : not enough cases for reliable estimation
– : incomplete or missing data
Best model: polynomial of the given degree in age (A), period (P) or cohort (C), or linear drift (D) model.
Goodness of fit: the normalised likelihood ratio chi-square for the best model (see Method).
Rate: world-standardised truncated rate per 100 000 per year (30-74 years) and number of **cases** are both estimated from the best-fitting model for the single years cited.
Cumulative risk per 1000 (30-74 years) is estimated from the best-fitting *age-cohort* model for cohorts of central birth year cited.
Recent trend: estimated mean percentage change per five-year period in the age-specific rates (30-74 years) over the period 1973-1987.
Italics denote recent trends not significant at 5 per cent level, or other figures which should be interpreted with caution (see Method).

KIDNEY (ICD-9 189)

AMERICAS (except USA), INCIDENCE

MALES

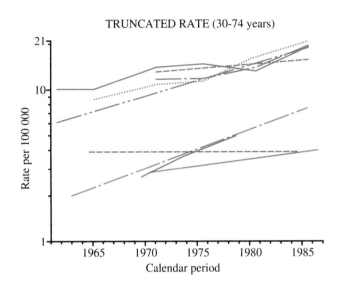

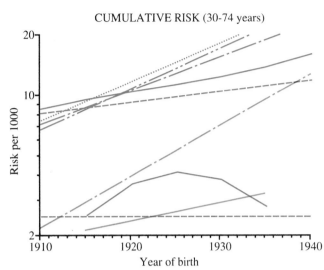

FEMALES

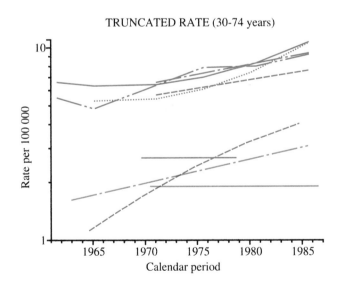

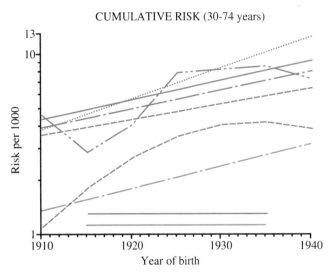

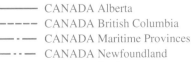

CANADA Alberta
CANADA British Columbia
CANADA Maritime Provinces
CANADA Newfoundland
CANADA Quebec
CUBA
PUERTO RICO
BRAZIL Sao Paulo
COLOMBIA Cali

KIDNEY (ICD-9 189)

AMERICAS (USA), INCIDENCE

MALES	Best model	Goodness of fit	1970 Rate	Cases	1985 Rate	Cases	Cumulative risk 1915	1940	Recent trend
USA									
Bay Area, Black	A2	0.18	16.4	9	16.4	13	9.7	9.7	*16.2*
Bay Area, Chinese	A1	0.25	7.8	1	*7.8*	*4*	4.7	*4.7*	–
Bay Area, White	A2D	0.42	14.5	86	17.0	106	9.6	12.4	2.4
Connecticut	A2C2	0.50	15.9	104	19.7	156	11.3	13.4	7.1
Detroit, Black	A4C2	-0.21	11.8	16	20.8	36	10.4	17.6	19.5
Detroit, White	A2P2	-0.13	15.4	114	23.2	166	11.2	24.9	20.7
Iowa	A3D	-1.03	14.2	95	19.7	136	10.6	18.1	9.9
New Orleans, Black	A1D	2.93	*6.0*	*3*	24.9	15	10.0	102.3	63.9
New Orleans, White	A2	1.06	*21.5*	*31*	21.5	33	12.8	12.8	*12.5*
Seattle	A2D	1.15	*15.6*	*74*	20.9	139	11.2	18.0	10.9

FEMALES	Best model	Goodness of fit	1970 Rate	Cases	1985 Rate	Cases	Cumulative risk 1915	1940	Recent trend
USA									
Bay Area, Black	A1	0.69	6.6	4	6.6	6	3.9	3.9	*-6.2*
Bay Area, Chinese	A1	-0.54	*3.3*	*0*	*3.3*	*1*	2.2	*2.2*	–
Bay Area, White	A2P2	0.71	7.4	51	8.6	60	4.2	7.0	20.8
Connecticut	A2D	2.15	6.9	53	8.1	75	4.5	6.0	*-0.4*
Detroit, Black	A2	0.15	8.8	13	8.8	18	4.9	4.9	*5.4*
Detroit, White	A2P3	-1.68	7.4	62	10.1	85	5.3	8.9	12.5
Iowa	A2D	-1.42	6.1	47	10.1	80	5.0	11.5	16.1
New Orleans, Black	A2	0.33	*7.9*	*4*	7.9	6	4.4	4.4	*23.2*
New Orleans, White	A2	-0.24	*9.8*	*19*	9.8	18	5.9	5.9	*10.7*
Seattle	A2D	-1.03	*6.7*	*36*	9.3	67	4.8	8.3	12.3

* : not enough cases for reliable estimation
– : incomplete or missing data
Best model: polynomial of the given degree in age (A), period (P) or cohort (C), or linear drift (D) model.
Goodness of fit: the normalised likelihood ratio chi-square for the best model (see Method).
Rate: world-standardised truncated rate per 100 000 per year (30-74 years) and number of **cases** are both estimated from the best-fitting model for the single years cited.
Cumulative risk per 1000 (30-74 years) is estimated from the best-fitting *age-cohort* model for cohorts of central birth year cited.
Recent trend: estimated mean percentage change per five-year period in the age-specific rates (30-74 years) over the period 1973-1987.
Italics denote recent trends not significant at 5 per cent level, or other figures which should be interpreted with caution (see Method).

KIDNEY (ICD-9 189)

AMERICAS (USA), INCIDENCE

MALES

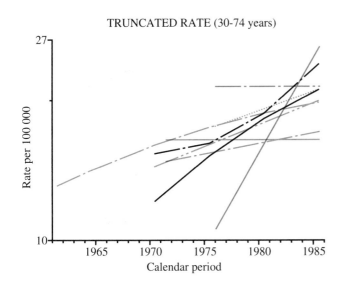

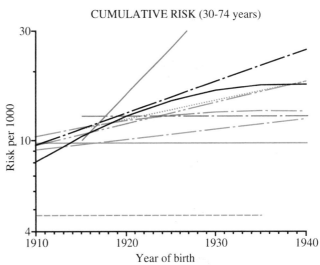

FEMALES

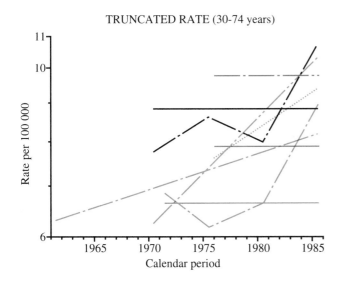

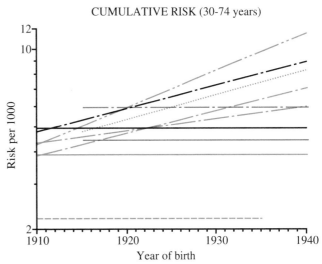

—— BAY AREA Black	·········· SEATTLE
----- BAY AREA Chinese	—— NEW ORLEANS Black
—·— BAY AREA White	—··— NEW ORLEANS White
—··— CONNECTICUT	—— DETROIT Black
—···— IOWA	—··— DETROIT White

KIDNEY (ICD-9 189)

AMERICAS (except USA), INCIDENCE
Percentage change per five-year period, 1973-1987

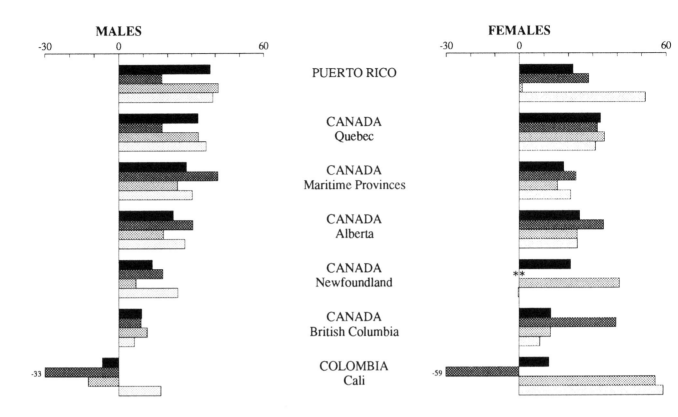

KIDNEY (ICD-9 189)

AMERICAS (USA), INCIDENCE
Percentage change per five-year period, 1973-1987

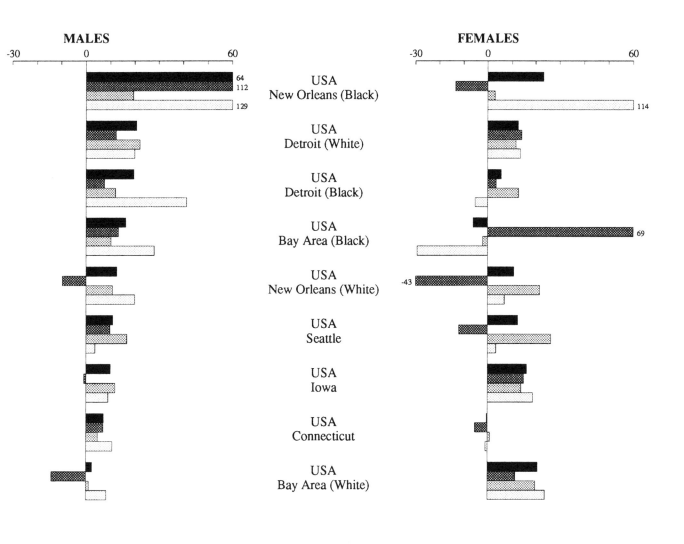

KIDNEY (ICD-9 189)

AMERICAS, MORTALITY

MALES	Best model	Goodness of fit	1965 Rate	1965 Deaths	1985 Rate	1985 Deaths	Cumulative risk 1900	Cumulative risk 1940	Recent trend
CANADA	A2D	0.45	6.7	253	7.4	427	4.1	5.1	*4.0*
CHILE	A2D	0.63	3.8	44	*5.4*	*97*	2.3	*4.6*	–
COSTA RICA	–	–	–	–	–	–	–	–	–
PANAMA	–	–	–	–	–	–	–	–	–
PUERTO RICO	–	–	–	–	–	–	–	–	–
URUGUAY	–	–	–	–	–	–	–	–	–
USA	A8C9	0.62	6.5	2748	7.0	3915	3.9	4.1	1.9
VENEZUELA	A2D	0.91	1.7	15	*2.4*	*42*	0.9	*1.9*	–

FEMALES	Best model	Goodness of fit	1965 Rate	1965 Deaths	1985 Rate	1985 Deaths	Cumulative risk 1900	Cumulative risk 1940	Recent trend
CANADA	A2	-0.69	3.3	130	3.3	217	2.1	2.1	*2.4*
CHILE	A2	0.45	2.2	28	*2.2*	*46*	1.3	*1.3*	–
COSTA RICA	–	–	–	–	–	–	–	–	–
PANAMA	–	–	–	–	–	–	–	–	–
PUERTO RICO	–	–	–	–	–	–	–	–	–
URUGUAY	–	–	–	–	–	–	–	–	–
USA	A4P3C5	0.51	2.9	1398	3.2	2121	1.8	2.0	6.4
VENEZUELA	A2	0.36	1.3	12	*1.3*	*24*	0.7	*0.7*	–

* : not enough deaths for reliable estimation
– : incomplete or missing data
Best model: polynomial of the given degree in age (A), period (P) or cohort (C), or linear drift (D) model.
Goodness of fit: the normalised likelihood ratio chi-square for the best model (see Method).
Rate: world-standardised truncated rate per 100 000 per year (30-74 years) and number of **deaths** are both estimated from the best-fitting model for the single years cited.
Cumulative risk per 1000 (30-74 years) is estimated from the best-fitting *age-cohort* model for cohorts of central birth year cited.
Recent trend: estimated mean percentage change per five-year period in the age-specific rates (30-74 years) over the period 1975-1988.
Italics denote recent trends not significant at 5 per cent level, or other figures which should be interpreted with caution (see Method).

KIDNEY (ICD-9 189)

AMERICAS, MORTALITY

MALES

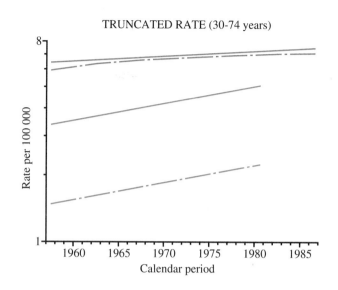

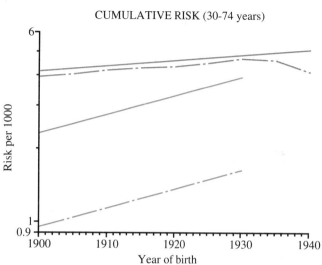

FEMALES

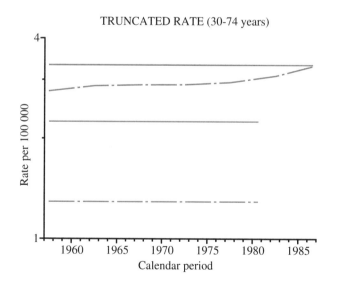

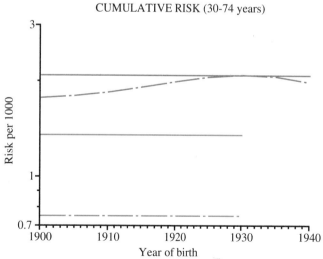

CANADA
USA
CHILE
VENEZUELA

KIDNEY (ICD-9 189)

AMERICAS, MORTALITY
Percentage change per five-year period, 1975-1988

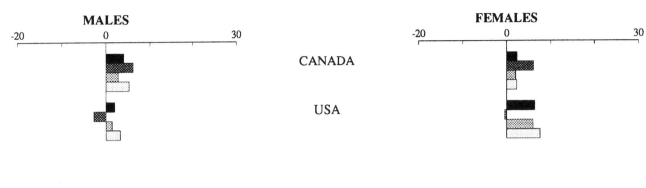

Chapter 25

THYROID

Thyroid cancer is an uncommon tumour in the age range 30-74 years, usually representing less than 2% of all malignant neoplasms. Incidence rates are two or three times higher in females than in males, although this sex ratio declines after middle age. The three main histological types of thyroid carcinoma, follicular, papillary and anaplastic, account for 80% or more of cases. Although divergent secular trends have been noted in the incidence of these types of thyroid carcinoma in several studies[4,235,242], only the trends for all thyroid malignancies combined could be examined with the available data. The disadvantage in loss of detail is compensated to some extent by the availability of comparable mortality data, which are not published for different histological types of thyroid cancer. Although survival from thyroid cancer is good, typically 80% or more at five years, mortality data are a useful adjunct to interpreting the incidence data.

Europe

Among European populations, the highest incidence rates in both sexes have been observed in Switzerland, among Jews in Israel, and in the Nordic countries, particularly in Iceland (data not shown). Incidence has risen still further in the Nordic countries, particularly among females: in Finland, where the rates have been increasing at 20% every five years, the estimated cumulative risk (30-74 years) for females born in the 1940 cohort exceeds 1%. In Geneva (Switzerland), however, where incidence has also been high, there has been a sharp decline, particularly in males: by 1985, it had fallen to less than half the rate recorded around 1970.

European incidence trends are dominated by the German Democratic Republic (GDR), where there has been a steady increase in incidence in both sexes: it has doubled since the 1960s, and is still increasing at more than 20% every five years. Over 95% of thyroid cancers registered in the GDR in persons aged 30-74 were histologically confirmed during the period 1973-87. These increases are based on large numbers of cases each year; if they continue, cumulative risk (30-74 years) for the 1940 birth cohort will begin to approach the levels seen in Iceland (data not shown) and Hawaii, at around 7 per 1000 in

females and 3 per 1000 in males. The pattern is strikingly different from that seen in Saarland (FRG), where although incidence is still higher than in the GDR, it has changed very little in males, and has increased only slowly in females. Although most of the overall recent trends in incidence are not statistically significant, it is notable that the rates of increase are often highest among younger persons (aged 30-44 years).

The sharp peak in incidence seen among Jews of both sexes in Israel around 1970 seems difficult to explain. The number of cases involved is substantial, and age-specific rates almost doubled in males within five years, before declining almost as rapidly within a further five years, although the overall trend is still upward, with a gradual deceleration. Incidence data for Zaragoza (Spain) and Doubs (France) are irregular, and the recent linear trends for these populations should be discounted.

There has been a marked and general decline in thyroid cancer mortality in Europe, especially in northern and western Europe, exceeding 10% every five years in both sexes in several countries. In Austria and Switzerland, where mortality rates exceeded those in all other European countries (except Iceland) by 2-fold or more in the 1960s, the decline has been the most dramatic, the annual number of deaths falling by 50% over the 20 years to 1985. Mortality in these countries is now similar to that in the rest of Europe, with truncated rates around 1 per 100 000.

The fall in mortality began in the 1960s or earlier in Austria and Switzerland, where rates were the highest, and then in Ireland, Scotland and the Nordic countries. By the 1970s, mortality had also begun to fall in Czechoslovakia (females), France, the Netherlands, Italy and England and Wales. In all these countries the decline affected females earlier and more rapidly than males. Mortality in Hungary, Belgium and Czechoslovakia (males) appears not to have changed at all. The sex difference in mortality trends in Czechoslovakia may reflect different trends in incidence: thyroid cancer increased 22% among Slovak males in the decade 1979-88, but remained unchanged among females[237].

The range of thyroid cancer mortality in Europe narrowed from 10-fold in the 1960s to little more than 2-fold by 1985. A few age-specific or overall increases in mortality have been

continued page 630

THYROID (ICD-9 193)

EUROPE (non-EC), INCIDENCE

MALES	Best model	Goodness of fit	1970 Rate	1970 Cases	1985 Rate	1985 Cases	Cumulative risk 1915	Cumulative risk 1940	Recent trend
FINLAND	A1C3	0.63	2.2	22	3.4	41	1.4	2.8	*8.9*
HUNGARY									
County Vas	A1C2	-0.99	*0.6*	*0*	2.2	1	1.3	1.3	*42.7*
Szabolcs-Szatmar	A1	-0.71	1.0	1	1.0	1	0.6	0.6	*3.0*
ISRAEL									
All Jews	A1P4	0.18	7.2	34	4.4	27	2.4	2.9	*5.1*
Non-Jews	A1	-0.69	*2.3*	*0*	2.3	1	1.2	1.2	*4.8*
NORWAY	A5D	-0.80	2.4	24	3.1	34	1.4	2.2	*4.0*
POLAND									
Warsaw City	A1P2	-0.64	1.9	5	1.9	7	1.0	1.5	*25.6*
ROMANIA									
Cluj	A1	-0.54	*1.4*	*2*	1.4	2	0.8	0.8	*43.4*
SWEDEN	A1D	0.37	2.6	59	3.0	72	1.5	1.9	*2.2*
SWITZERLAND									
Geneva	A1D	0.03	6.2	4	2.1	1	3.4	0.6	*-24.1*
YUGOSLAVIA									
Slovenia	A1D	3.26	2.5	9	1.8	7	1.3	0.7	*-14.3*

FEMALES	Best model	Goodness of fit	1970 Rate	1970 Cases	1985 Rate	1985 Cases	Cumulative risk 1915	Cumulative risk 1940	Recent trend
FINLAND	A8P5C9	-0.26	5.3	66	10.0	137	3.2	10.7	21.2
HUNGARY									
County Vas	A1D	0.72	2.6	2	3.0	2	1.8	2.2	*21.5*
Szabolcs-Szatmar	A1P3	-0.74	1.1	1	3.0	4	1.3	3.6	*-2.7*
ISRAEL									
All Jews	A1P4C2	1.16	13.4	66	10.9	77	4.6	6.2	*0.5*
Non-Jews	A0C2	0.18	3.4	1	4.8	4	1.4	2.1	23.8
NORWAY	A4P2C2	-0.71	6.4	66	9.6	104	3.0	7.8	6.3
POLAND									
Warsaw City	A1P3	0.26	3.0	12	3.0	15	1.8	1.9	*0.7*
ROMANIA									
Cluj	A1	1.08	*3.5*	*6*	3.5	6	1.9	1.9	*18.4*
SWEDEN	A3P3C4	-0.06	6.3	142	7.2	171	3.1	4.3	*0.6*
SWITZERLAND									
Geneva	A0D	-0.04	8.7	7	4.7	5	5.0	1.8	*-5.4*
YUGOSLAVIA									
Slovenia	A1C3	0.07	4.0	19	3.8	21	2.1	2.0	*-4.5*

* : not enough cases for reliable estimation
− : incomplete or missing data
Best model: polynomial of the given degree in age (A), period (P) or cohort (C), or linear drift (D) model.
Goodness of fit: the normalised likelihood ratio chi-square for the best model (see Method).
Rate: world-standardised truncated rate per 100 000 per year (30-74 years) and number of **cases** are both estimated from the best-fitting model for the single years cited.
Cumulative risk per 1000 (30-74 years) is estimated from the best-fitting *age-cohort* model for cohorts of central birth year cited.
Recent trend: estimated mean percentage change per five-year period in the age-specific rates (30-74 years) over the period 1973-1987.
Italics denote recent trends not significant at 5 per cent level, or other figures which should be interpreted with caution (see Method).

THYROID (ICD-9 193)

EUROPE (non-EC), INCIDENCE

MALES

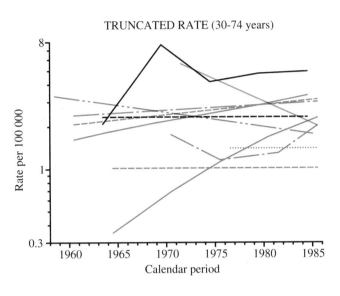

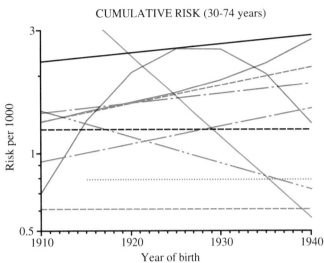

FEMALES

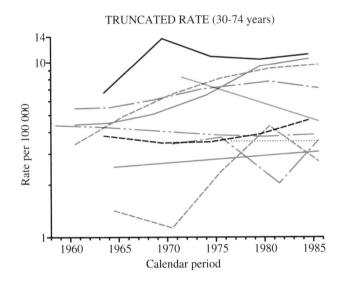

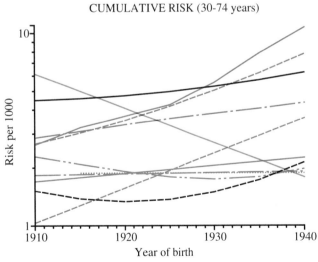

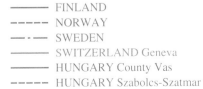

——— FINLAND	—·—· POLAND Warsaw City
- - - - NORWAY	·········· ROMANIA Cluj
—·—· SWEDEN	—··—·· YUGOSLAVIA Slovenia
——— SWITZERLAND Geneva	——— ISRAEL All Jews
——— HUNGARY County Vas	- - - - ISRAEL Non-Jews
- - - - HUNGARY Szabolcs-Szatmar	

THYROID (ICD-9 193)

EUROPE (EC), INCIDENCE

MALES	Best model	Goodness of fit	1970 Rate	1970 Cases	1985 Rate	1985 Cases	Cumulative risk 1915	Cumulative risk 1940	Recent trend
DENMARK	A3C3	0.61	1.4	18	1.8	25	0.8	1.6	2.3
FRANCE									
Bas-Rhin	A1	1.04	2.4	4	2.4	4	1.2	1.2	10.7
Doubs	A8C7	-1.12	0.2	0	2.1	2	0.0	0.0	69.7
GERMANY (FRG)									
Hamburg	A1	0.09	1.5	7	1.5	6	0.8	0.8	–
Saarland	A1	-0.61	2.7	7	2.7	7	1.5	1.5	15.9
GERMANY (GDR)	A1C2	2.58	1.2	52	2.4	90	0.9	3.3	20.3
ITALY									
Varese	A0	-0.53	3.3	5	3.3	6	1.5	1.5	-11.1
SPAIN									
Navarra	*	..	..	..	..	..	..	..	..
Zaragoza	A3P3	0.88	0.4	0	2.0	4	0.7	1.1	-30.7
UK									
Birmingham	A1	-1.53	1.2	15	1.2	16	0.6	0.6	0.4
Scotland	A2C2	0.39	1.1	14	1.5	19	0.6	1.2	13.7
South Thames	A1C4	0.30	1.0	22	1.2	21	0.6	0.7	0.9

FEMALES	Best model	Goodness of fit	1970 Rate	1970 Cases	1985 Rate	1985 Cases	Cumulative risk 1915	Cumulative risk 1940	Recent trend
DENMARK	A2P5C3	-0.86	2.8	39	3.8	56	1.4	2.3	16.9
FRANCE									
Bas-Rhin	A1	-0.27	5.2	13	5.2	12	2.6	2.6	2.5
Doubs	A2	0.44	4.8	4	4.8	5	2.1	2.1	36.2
GERMANY (FRG)									
Hamburg	A1P4	-0.44	2.6	17	0.0	0	1.6	3.1	–
Saarland	A1D	-0.63	5.1	17	6.7	22	2.8	4.3	13.8
GERMANY (GDR)	A3P3C2	-1.15	2.1	127	5.2	249	1.5	7.0	25.9
ITALY									
Varese	A0	1.49	8.9	16	8.9	19	4.0	4.0	9.0
SPAIN									
Navarra	A1D	0.59	1.7	2	8.8	12	2.0	30.0	71.5
Zaragoza	A1P3	-0.54	1.8	3	4.0	9	3.0	1.8	-54.2
UK									
Birmingham	A2	-0.32	2.5	34	2.5	36	1.3	1.3	0.1
Scotland	A2C4	0.85	2.8	44	3.6	49	1.2	2.6	5.7
South Thames	A2C2	-1.14	2.3	61	2.8	52	1.1	1.7	-1.4

* : not enough cases for reliable estimation
– : incomplete or missing data
Best model: polynomial of the given degree in age (A), period (P) or cohort (C), or linear drift (D) model.
Goodness of fit: the normalised likelihood ratio chi-square for the best model (see Method).
Rate: world-standardised truncated rate per 100 000 per year (30-74 years) and number of **cases** are both estimated from the best-fitting model for the single years cited.
Cumulative risk per 1000 (30-74 years) is estimated from the best-fitting *age-cohort* model for cohorts of central birth year cited.
Recent trend: estimated mean percentage change per five-year period in the age-specific rates (30-74 years) over the period 1973-1987.
Italics denote recent trends not significant at 5 per cent level, or other figures which should be interpreted with caution (see Method).

THYROID (ICD-9 193)

EUROPE (EC), INCIDENCE

MALES

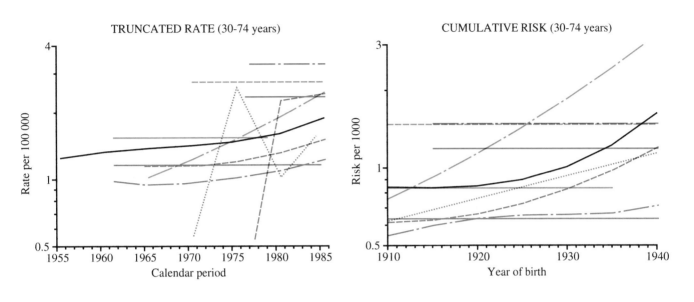

TRUNCATED RATE (30-74 years)

CUMULATIVE RISK (30-74 years)

FEMALES

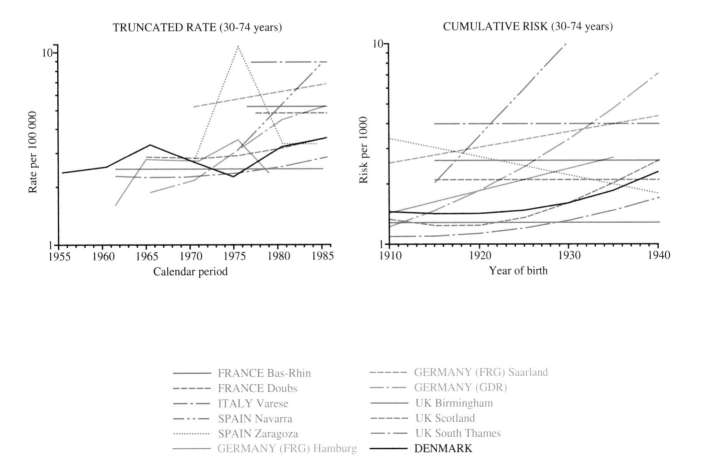

TRUNCATED RATE (30-74 years)

CUMULATIVE RISK (30-74 years)

—————— FRANCE Bas-Rhin	— — — — GERMANY (FRG) Saarland
– – – – FRANCE Doubs	—·—·— GERMANY (GDR)
—·—·— ITALY Varese	—————— UK Birmingham
—··—··— SPAIN Navarra	- - - - - UK Scotland
············ SPAIN Zaragoza	—·—·— UK South Thames
—————— GERMANY (FRG) Hamburg	—————— DENMARK

THYROID (ICD-9 193)

EUROPE (non-EC), INCIDENCE
Percentage change per five-year period, 1973-1987

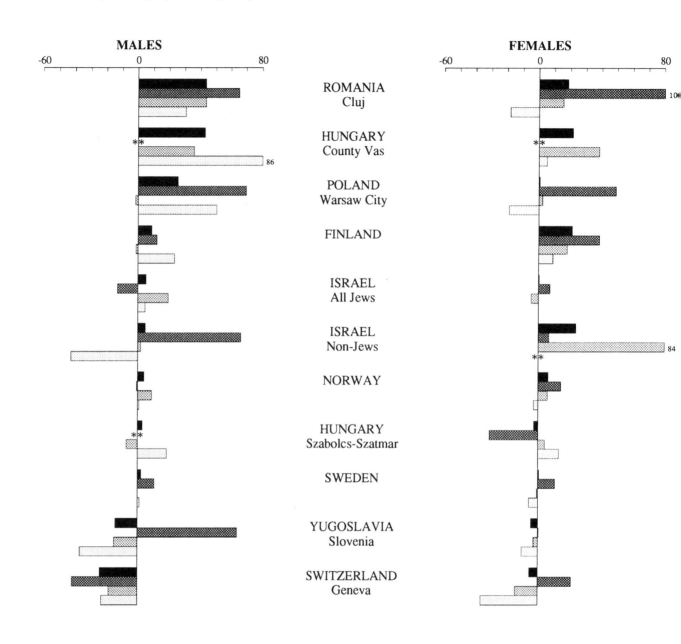

THYROID (ICD-9 193)

EUROPE (EC), INCIDENCE
Percentage change per five-year period, 1973-1987

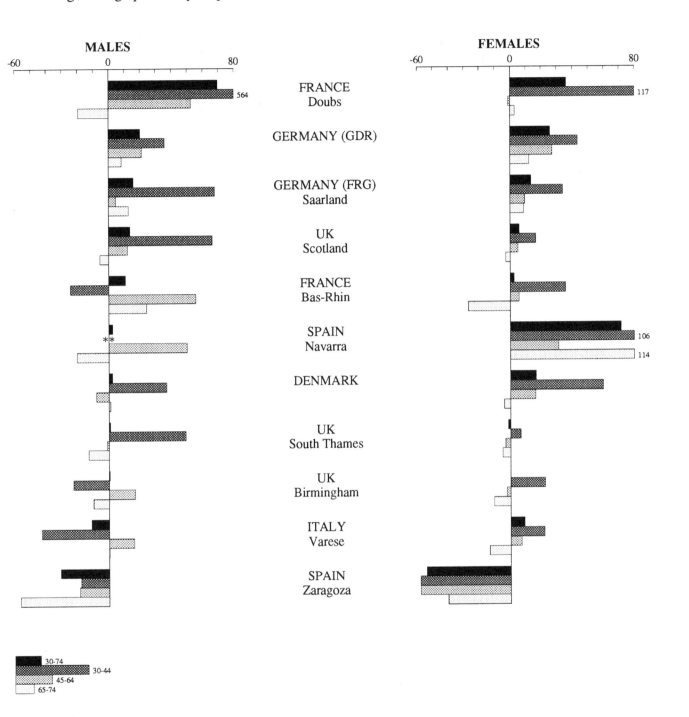

615

EUROPE (non-EC), MORTALITY

MALES	Best model	Goodness of fit	1965 Rate	1965 Deaths	1985 Rate	1985 Deaths	Cumulative risk 1900	Cumulative risk 1940	Recent trend
AUSTRIA	A4P2	-0.28	2.2	42	1.3	23	1.4	0.6	-24.5
CZECHOSLOVAKIA	A2	-0.28	1.0	36	1.0	37	0.6	0.6	*-7.9*
FINLAND	A4C2	0.00	1.1	9	0.9	10	0.7	0.3	*-6.9*
HUNGARY	A2	0.44	*1.1*	*28*	1.1	30	*0.7*	0.7	*3.3*
NORWAY	A1D	0.33	0.9	9	0.6	7	0.6	0.3	*20.3*
POLAND	A2	1.19	0.7	39	*0.7*	*51*	0.4	*0.4*	–
ROMANIA	–	–	–	–	–	–	–	–	–
SWEDEN	A4P2	0.23	1.0	24	0.7	19	0.6	0.5	-17.1
SWITZERLAND	A2D	1.45	2.3	33	1.3	22	1.6	0.5	-14.2
YUGOSLAVIA	A2P3	1.41	0.5	18	0.8	40	0.4	0.8	*-9.2*

FEMALES	Best model	Goodness of fit	1965 Rate	1965 Deaths	1985 Rate	1985 Deaths	Cumulative risk 1900	Cumulative risk 1940	Recent trend
AUSTRIA	A2P2	1.75	2.8	78	1.7	44	1.8	0.8	-19.0
CZECHOSLOVAKIA	A2C2	0.22	1.7	75	1.4	64	1.1	0.6	-13.4
FINLAND	A1C2	-0.32	1.7	21	1.2	20	1.2	0.5	*-15.3*
HUNGARY	A1C4	0.06	*1.4*	*42*	1.5	54	*1.0*	1.4	*-0.2*
NORWAY	A1D	1.72	1.3	15	0.8	12	0.9	0.3	*-14.7*
POLAND	A2C4	-1.74	1.2	93	*1.9*	*189*	0.8	*1.5*	–
ROMANIA	–	–	–	–	–	–	–	–	–
SWEDEN	A1P4	-0.33	1.5	37	0.8	25	1.0	0.4	-29.1
SWITZERLAND	A2P3C2	-0.27	2.6	45	1.2	26	2.0	0.3	-25.9
YUGOSLAVIA	A2C2	-0.02	1.2	50	1.2	71	0.7	0.6	*-6.6*

* : not enough deaths for reliable estimation
– : incomplete or missing data
Best model: polynomial of the given degree in age (A), period (P) or cohort (C), or linear drift (D) model.
Goodness of fit: the normalised likelihood ratio chi-square for the best model (see Method).
Rate: world-standardised truncated rate per 100 000 per year (30-74 years) and number of **deaths** are both estimated from the best-fitting model for the single years cited.
Cumulative risk per 1000 (30-74 years) is estimated from the best-fitting *age-cohort* model for cohorts of central birth year cited.
Recent trend: estimated mean percentage change per five-year period in the age-specific rates (30-74 years) over the period 1975-1988.
Italics denote recent trends not significant at 5 per cent level, or other figures which should be interpreted with caution (see Method).

THYROID (ICD-9 193)

EUROPE (non-EC), MORTALITY

MALES

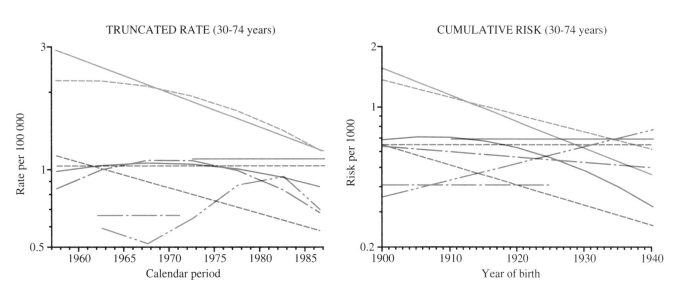

FEMALES

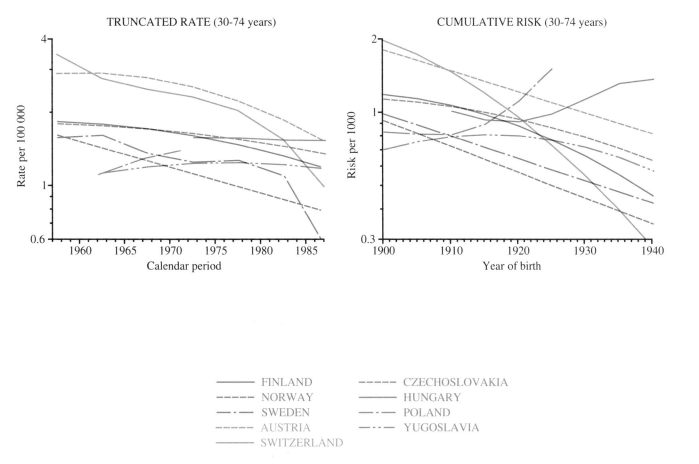

—— FINLAND	----- CZECHOSLOVAKIA
---- NORWAY	—— HUNGARY
—·— SWEDEN	—·— POLAND
----- AUSTRIA	—··— YUGOSLAVIA
—— SWITZERLAND	

THYROID (ICD-9 193)

EUROPE (EC), MORTALITY

MALES	Best model	Goodness of fit	1965 Rate	1965 Deaths	1985 Rate	1985 Deaths	Cumulative risk 1900	Cumulative risk 1940	Recent trend
BELGIUM	A8P6	0.25	0.8	20	0.8	21	0.5	0.4	*25.4*
DENMARK	A1	1.85	0.9	11	0.9	13	0.6	0.6	*-2.3*
FRANCE	A2P2	-0.17	0.7	88	0.8	108	0.4	0.6	*-0.7*
GERMANY (FRG)	A2P3	1.07	1.1	162	1.1	167	0.7	0.7	-7.0
GREECE	A2D	0.07	*0.2*	*3*	0.5	14	*0.1*	1.0	34.6
IRELAND	A1	0.28	0.7	5	0.7	5	0.4	0.4	*1.6*
ITALY	A2P2	1.03	0.9	114	1.0	155	0.5	0.7	-5.9
NETHERLANDS	A2P2	0.81	0.8	22	0.7	24	0.5	0.5	*-4.8*
PORTUGAL	–	–	–	–	–	–	–	–	–
SPAIN	A2D	2.00	0.3	18	0.5	45	0.2	0.5	*11.0*
UK ENGLAND & WALES	A2D	0.27	0.6	80	0.5	76	0.4	0.3	-8.4
UK SCOTLAND	A1C2	-0.27	0.7	9	0.5	7	0.5	0.2	*4.6*

FEMALES	Best model	Goodness of fit	1965 Rate	1965 Deaths	1985 Rate	1985 Deaths	Cumulative risk 1900	Cumulative risk 1940	Recent trend
BELGIUM	A2	2.21	1.1	36	1.1	36	0.7	0.7	*-3.3*
DENMARK	A4D	0.79	1.5	21	1.0	17	1.0	0.5	-17.6
FRANCE	A2P4	-0.12	1.0	157	1.0	160	0.7	0.6	-7.4
GERMANY (FRG)	A2P3C5	-1.56	1.6	338	1.3	298	1.1	0.7	-12.1
GREECE	A1D	0.49	*0.4*	*8*	0.7	21	*0.3*	0.8	*-4.4*
IRELAND	A2C2	0.98	2.0	14	1.2	10	1.3	0.4	*19.6*
ITALY	A2P2C2	2.06	1.5	218	1.3	238	0.9	0.7	-12.6
NETHERLANDS	A2P2	1.12	1.3	41	0.8	34	0.8	0.5	-21.5
PORTUGAL	–	–	–	–	–	–	–	–	–
SPAIN	A2D	1.42	0.5	44	0.7	84	0.3	0.7	*-1.1*
UK ENGLAND & WALES	A2P2	1.73	1.1	184	0.7	124	0.7	0.4	-17.4
UK SCOTLAND	A1D	0.61	1.5	25	0.8	13	1.0	0.3	*-12.5*

* : not enough deaths for reliable estimation
– : incomplete or missing data
Best model: polynomial of the given degree in age (A), period (P) or cohort (C), or linear drift (D) model.
Goodness of fit: the normalised likelihood ratio chi-square for the best model (see Method).
Rate: world-standardised truncated rate per 100 000 per year (30-74 years) and number of **deaths** are both estimated from the best-fitting model for the single years cited.
Cumulative risk per 1000 (30-74 years) is estimated from the best-fitting *age-cohort* model for cohorts of central birth year cited.
Recent trend: estimated mean percentage change per five-year period in the age-specific rates (30-74 years) over the period 1975-1988.
Italics denote recent trends not significant at 5 per cent level, or other figures which should be interpreted with caution (see Method).

THYROID (ICD-9 193)

EUROPE (EC), MORTALITY

MALES

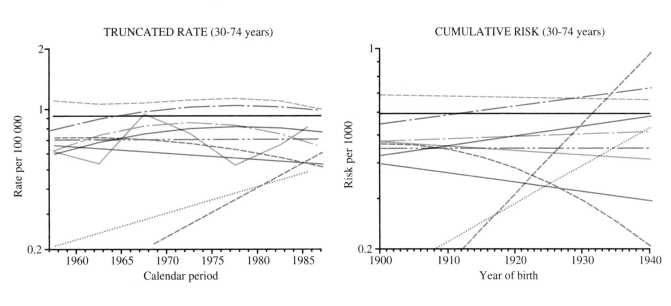

FEMALES

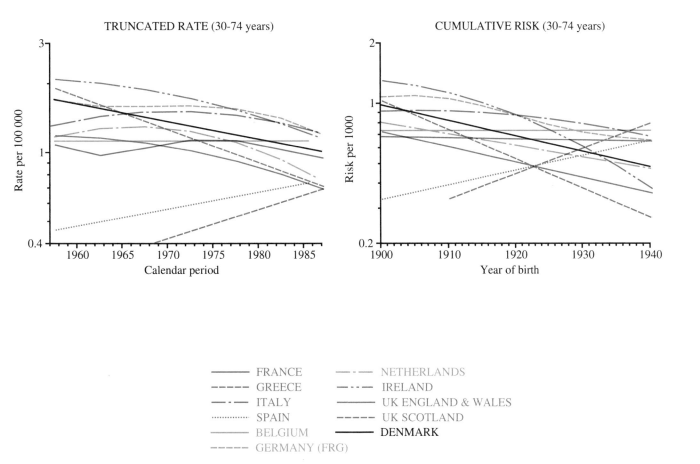

—— FRANCE	—·— NETHERLANDS
---- GREECE	—··— IRELAND
—·— ITALY	—— UK ENGLAND & WALES
···· SPAIN	---- UK SCOTLAND
—— BELGIUM	—— DENMARK
---- GERMANY (FRG)	

THYROID (ICD-9 193)

EUROPE (non-EC), MORTALITY
Percentage change per five-year period, 1975-1988

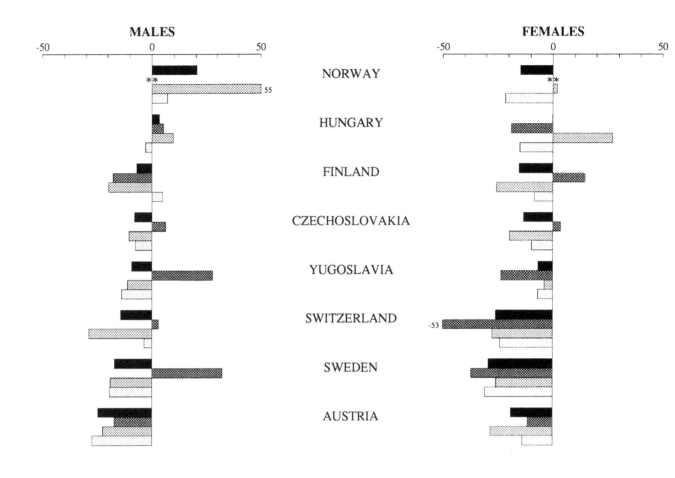

MALES

FEMALES

NORWAY

HUNGARY

FINLAND

CZECHOSLOVAKIA

YUGOSLAVIA

SWITZERLAND

SWEDEN

AUSTRIA

30-74
30-44
45-64
65-74

THYROID (ICD-9 193)

EUROPE (EC), MORTALITY
Percentage change per five-year period, 1975-1988

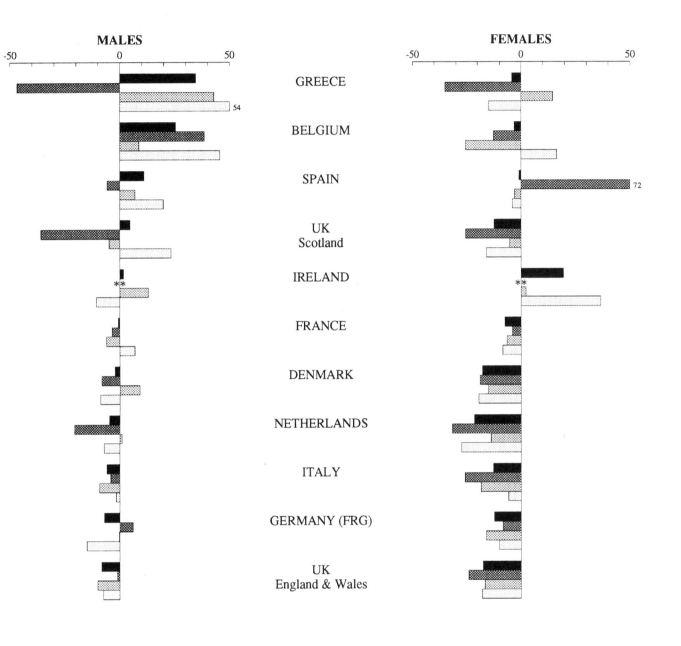

THYROID (ICD-9 193)

ASIA, INCIDENCE

MALES	Best model	Goodness of fit	1970 Rate	1970 Cases	1985 Rate	1985 Cases	Cumulative risk 1915	Cumulative risk 1940	Recent trend
CHINA									
Shanghai	A2P2	-0.83	*25.8*	*321*	1.5	26	13.4	0.6	-47.0
HONG KONG	A2	-0.81	*2.7*	*17*	2.7	32	1.4	1.4	*3.6*
INDIA									
Bombay	A3	0.85	1.4	12	1.4	19	0.8	0.8	*0.2*
JAPAN									
Miyagi	A1D	-0.49	1.5	5	2.4	12	1.0	2.1	23.8
Nagasaki	A8	-0.20	*3.3*	*2*	3.3	3	1.5	1.5	*-13.5*
Osaka	A1D	-1.20	0.9	11	2.0	40	0.9	3.4	34.4
SINGAPORE									
Chinese	A1D	1.19	1.9	4	3.3	11	1.3	3.2	*23.3*
Indian	A1	-1.36	*2.8*	*0*	2.8	1	1.6	1.6	*-13.6*
Malay	A1	0.57	3.2	1	3.2	1	1.8	1.8	*22.0*

FEMALES	Best model	Goodness of fit	1970 Rate	1970 Cases	1985 Rate	1985 Cases	Cumulative risk 1915	Cumulative risk 1940	Recent trend
CHINA									
Shanghai	A6P2C3	-1.32	*34.3*	*484*	3.9	66	27.3	1.6	-40.6
HONG KONG	A1D	-1.97	*6.5*	*42*	10.2	115	3.4	7.2	16.2
INDIA									
Bombay	A2D	-0.61	3.1	17	3.1	32	1.6	1.6	*-0.3*
JAPAN									
Miyagi	A1P2C4	-0.88	3.9	16	10.9	65	2.5	15.9	54.4
Nagasaki	A1	0.26	*11.3*	*11*	11.3	14	5.5	5.5	*-12.1*
Osaka	A1P3C2	-0.01	4.6	69	6.2	144	2.1	7.9	39.5
SINGAPORE									
Chinese	A1P2C2	2.30	8.2	20	9.9	40	3.3	6.2	30.1
Indian	A0P2	0.62	10.5	1	5.7	1	2.8	2.2	*38.3*
Malay	A1	1.15	7.9	2	7.9	4	4.0	4.0	*6.8*

* : not enough cases for reliable estimation
− : incomplete or missing data
Best model: polynomial of the given degree in age (A), period (P) or cohort (C), or linear drift (D) model.
Goodness of fit: the normalised likelihood ratio chi-square for the best model (see Method).
Rate: world-standardised truncated rate per 100 000 per year (30-74 years) and number of **cases** are both estimated from the best-fitting model for the single years cited.
Cumulative risk per 1000 (30-74 years) is estimated from the best-fitting *age-cohort* model for cohorts of central birth year cited.
Recent trend: estimated mean percentage change per five-year period in the age-specific rates (30-74 years) over the period 1973-1987.
Italics denote recent trends not significant at 5 per cent level, or other figures which should be interpreted with caution (see Method).

THYROID (ICD-9 193)

ASIA, INCIDENCE

MALES

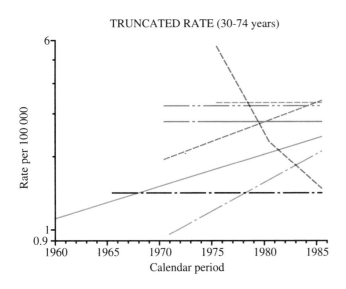

TRUNCATED RATE (30-74 years)

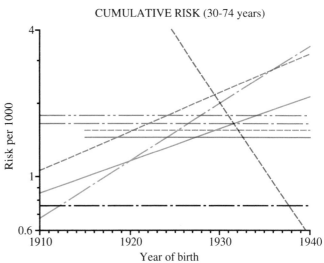

CUMULATIVE RISK (30-74 years)

FEMALES

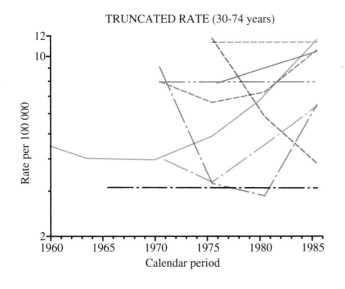

TRUNCATED RATE (30-74 years)

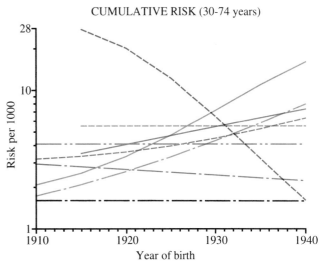

CUMULATIVE RISK (30-74 years)

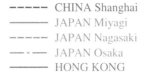

----- CHINA Shanghai	----- SINGAPORE Chinese
——— JAPAN Miyagi	—·— SINGAPORE Indian
- - - JAPAN Nagasaki	—··— SINGAPORE Malay
—·— JAPAN Osaka	—·— INDIA Bombay
——— HONG KONG	

THYROID (ICD-9 193)

OCEANIA, INCIDENCE

MALES	Best model	Goodness of fit	1970 Rate	1970 Cases	1985 Rate	1985 Cases	Cumulative risk 1915	Cumulative risk 1940	Recent trend
AUSTRALIA									
New South Wales	A1	2.79	*2.1*	*21*	2.1	26	1.0	1.0	*13.0*
South	A1	-0.09	*2.2*	*4*	2.2	7	1.1	1.1	*-29.0*
HAWAII									
Caucasian	A0C3	0.57	5.9	2	5.2	3	2.6	2.6	*-10.8*
Chinese	A0	0.98	12.3	1	12.3	1	5.5	5.5	*-8.9*
Filipino	A1	0.82	11.2	2	11.2	3	5.5	5.5	*3.0*
Hawaiian	A1	0.91	10.6	1	10.6	2	5.9	5.9	*-2.6*
Japanese	A1P2	0.95	5.9	2	7.2	5	3.8	7.5	*-8.2*
NEW ZEALAND									
Maori	*	..	..	..	..	..	..	..	..
Non-Maori	A1	1.37	1.9	10	1.9	12	1.0	1.0	*-5.6*

FEMALES	Best model	Goodness of fit	1970 Rate	1970 Cases	1985 Rate	1985 Cases	Cumulative risk 1915	Cumulative risk 1940	Recent trend
AUSTRALIA									
New South Wales	A8P2C7	0.28	*1.5*	*18*	6.5	81	1.6	5.3	22.9
South	A0	2.68	*6.1*	*14*	6.1	20	2.8	2.8	*-13.2*
HAWAII									
Caucasian	A0P3	-1.22	16.8	7	12.9	8	5.4	6.0	*12.6*
Chinese	A0D	1.59	25.0	2	12.9	1	14.6	4.9	*-15.2*
Filipino	A1D	1.06	27.3	3	40.3	11	13.3	25.3	*9.3*
Hawaiian	A8	0.79	23.4	4	23.4	7	11.1	11.1	*-21.3*
Japanese	A1	-0.08	10.5	5	10.5	8	5.1	5.1	*-3.3*
NEW ZEALAND									
Maori	A1	0.62	8.6	2	8.6	3	4.3	4.3	-31.4
Non-Maori	A1C2	1.68	4.3	24	5.4	38	2.1	3.0	*2.9*

* : not enough cases for reliable estimation
− : incomplete or missing data
Best model: polynomial of the given degree in age (A), period (P) or cohort (C), or linear drift (D) model.
Goodness of fit: the normalised likelihood ratio chi-square for the best model (see Method).
Rate: world-standardised truncated rate per 100 000 per year (30-74 years) and number of **cases** are both estimated from the best-fitting model for the single years cited.
Cumulative risk per 1000 (30-74 years) is estimated from the best-fitting *age-cohort* model for cohorts of central birth year cited.
Recent trend: estimated mean percentage change per five-year period in the age-specific rates (30-74 years) over the period 1973-1987.
Italics denote recent trends not significant at 5 per cent level, or other figures which should be interpreted with caution (see Method).

624

THYROID (ICD-9 193)

OCEANIA, INCIDENCE

MALES

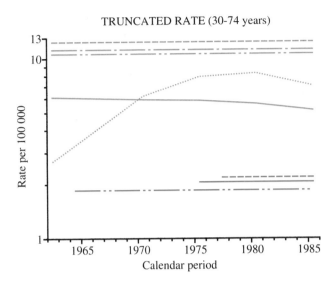

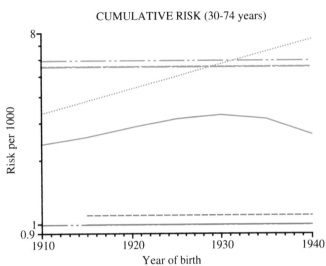

FEMALES

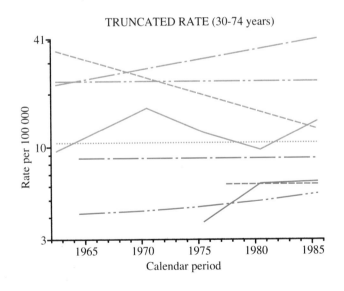

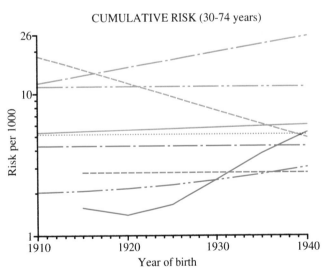

———— AUSTRALIA New South Wales
– – – – AUSTRALIA South
–·–·– NEW ZEALAND Maori
–··–··– NEW ZEALAND Non-Maori
———— HAWAII Caucasian

– – – – HAWAII Chinese
–·–·– HAWAII Filipino
–··–··– HAWAII Hawaiian
··············· HAWAII Japanese

THYROID (ICD-9 193)

ASIA, INCIDENCE
Percentage change per five-year period, 1973-1987

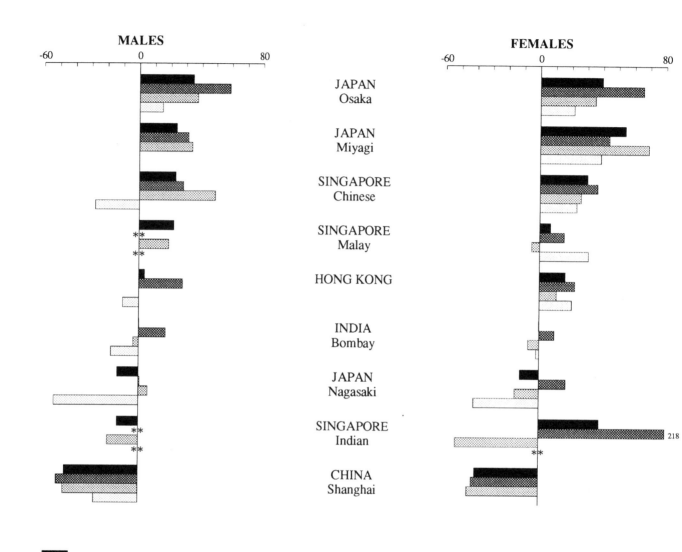

MALES

FEMALES

JAPAN
Osaka

JAPAN
Miyagi

SINGAPORE
Chinese

SINGAPORE
Malay

HONG KONG

INDIA
Bombay

JAPAN
Nagasaki

SINGAPORE
Indian

CHINA
Shanghai

30-74
30-44
45-64
65-74

THYROID (ICD-9 193)

OCEANIA, INCIDENCE
Percentage change per five-year period, 1973-1987

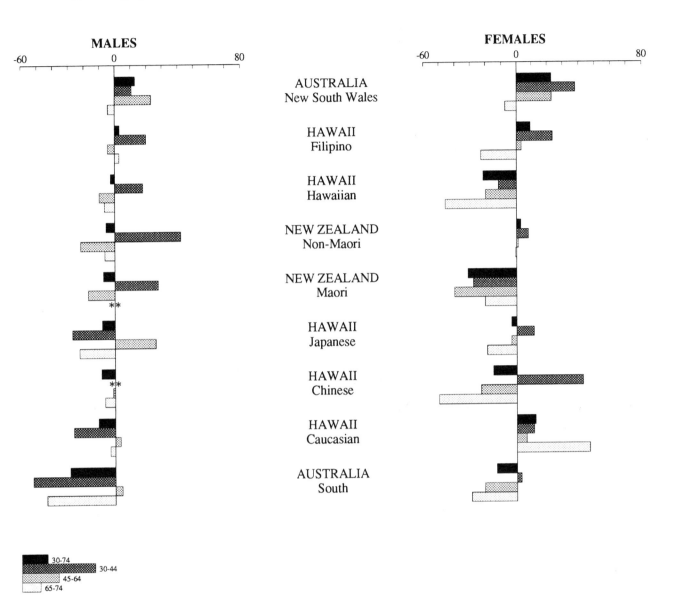

THYROID (ICD-9 193)

ASIA and OCEANIA, MORTALITY

MALES	Best model	Goodness of fit	1965 Rate	1965 Deaths	1985 Rate	1985 Deaths	Cumulative risk 1900	Cumulative risk 1940	Recent trend
AUSTRALIA	A2D	-0.74	0.6	13	0.4	15	0.4	0.2	*-8.3*
HONG KONG	A2	-1.19	*0.7*	*2*	0.7	6	*0.4*	0.4	*-12.3*
JAPAN	A2P3C3	-2.00	0.5	91	0.6	162	0.3	0.4	*0.0*
MAURITIUS	*	..	..	..	..	..	..	..	..
NEW ZEALAND	A1	0.20	0.7	3	0.7	5	0.4	0.4	*-15.7*
SINGAPORE	A1	0.02	0.9	1	0.9	2	*0.5*	0.5	–

FEMALES	Best model	Goodness of fit	1965 Rate	1965 Deaths	1985 Rate	1985 Deaths	Cumulative risk 1900	Cumulative risk 1940	Recent trend
AUSTRALIA	A1D	0.21	0.9	24	0.7	27	0.6	0.3	*-4.1*
HONG KONG	A4	-0.21	*1.3*	*5*	1.3	10	*0.9*	0.9	*-2.0*
JAPAN	A2P2C3	-0.53	0.9	186	0.9	325	0.6	0.4	-8.7
MAURITIUS	A1	-0.63	*0.8*	*0*	*0.8*	*0*	*0.5*	0.5	*54.8*
NEW ZEALAND	A2D	-0.35	1.2	7	0.8	6	0.8	0.4	*-10.2*
SINGAPORE	A1	1.17	1.7	2	1.7	4	*0.9*	0.9	–

* : not enough deaths for reliable estimation
– : incomplete or missing data
Best model: polynomial of the given degree in age (A), period (P) or cohort (C), or linear drift (D) model.
Goodness of fit: the normalised likelihood ratio chi-square for the best model (see Method).
Rate: world-standardised truncated rate per 100 000 per year (30-74 years) and number of **deaths** are both estimated from the best-fitting model for the single years cited.
Cumulative risk per 1000 (30-74 years) is estimated from the best-fitting *age-cohort* model for cohorts of central birth year cited.
Recent trend: estimated mean percentage change per five-year period in the age-specific rates (30-74 years) over the period 1975-1988.
Italics denote recent trends not significant at 5 per cent level, or other figures which should be interpreted with caution (see Method).

THYROID (ICD-9 193)

ASIA and OCEANIA, MORTALITY

MALES

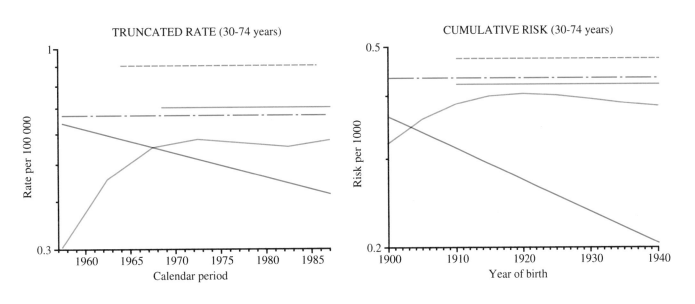

FEMALES

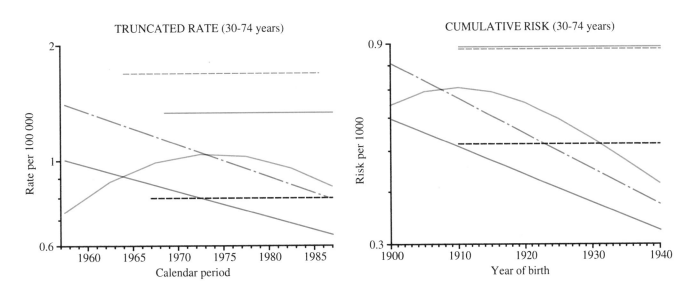

AUSTRALIA   HONG KONG
NEW ZEALAND   SINGAPORE
JAPAN   MAURITIUS

THYROID (ICD-9 193)

ASIA and OCEANIA, MORTALITY
Percentage change per five-year period, 1975-1988

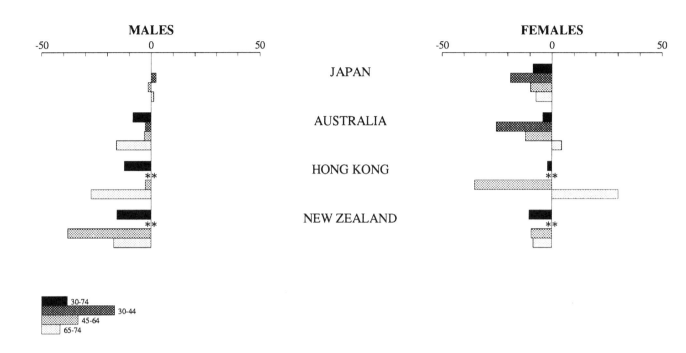

from page 609

observed, but none is significant, with the exception of that for males in Greece (35% every five years, two standard errors). In Greece and Spain, mortality was very much lower in both sexes than in other European countries in the 1960s, and it is still quite low by European standards, though now in the same range (truncated rates 0.5-1.3 per 100 000).

Asia and Oceania

Thyroid cancer incidence in the various ethnic groups in Hawaii is among the highest in the world, at 10 or more per 100 000 in both sexes, but there has been little overall change. The recent decline of 21% every five years among Hawaiian females is not significant, and is based on some seven cases a year. Females in Miyagi and Osaka (Japan) show large recent rates of increase of 54% and 40% every five years, respectively, with a marked cohort effect. In Miyagi, the recent rate of increase in females aged between 30 and 44 years is greater than 40% every five years (4 standard errors), while in the same age group in Osaka, incidence is increasing by 66% every five

years (8 standard errors). The lifetime risk (30-74 years) for the 1940 birth cohort for females in these populations is now around 1%, similar to the risk in Finland. Large increases in thyroid cancer incidence have also been observed in Japanese males, both in Japan and in Hawaii.

Incidence rates in the Caucasian populations of Australia and New Zealand are very similar to those of European populations, at around 5 and 2 per 100 000 in females and males, respectively. There has been little change in incidence except among females in New South Wales, where the abrupt increase after 1973-77 did not continue.

Mortality has declined steadily in Australia and New Zealand, particularly in females, and truncated rates are now 2 per 100 000 or less in all Asian and American populations included here. In Japan, the large increases in incidence observed in the prefectures of Miyagi and Osaka contrast sharply with the national trends in mortality. There was a peak in mortality in the early 1970s in both sexes, followed by a decline in females; these peaks correspond to a peak in the cumulative risk of 0.7 per 1000 for Japanese females born around 1910 and 0.4 per 1000 for Japanese males born around 1920.

Americas

Incidence has been increasing in both sexes in many North American populations. In Alberta (Canada) and Puerto Rico, incidence rates of 2-4 per 100 000 in males and 5-9 in females are now similar to those in other American populations, whereas 25 years ago they were 50% lower. Incidence in Connecticut (USA) and Quebec (Canada) has increased too, but more slowly; the increase in Iowa (USA) is confined to females. In these populations, recent increases in incidence have been 10-30% every five years. In most other American populations there has been little change, except in Cali (Colombia), where the decline in males is based on very few cases. In these American populations, cumulative risks for the 1940 birth cohort are now 2-5 per 1000 in females and 1-3 per 1000 in males.

Mortality has fallen steadily by some 50% since the 1960s in the USA and Canada, to truncated rates of 0.5 per 100 000 per year, and age-specific mortality patterns suggest this decline will continue. Mortality has not changed in Chile or Venezuela.

Comment

Observations of increasing thyroid cancer incidence in adults, particularly younger adults, with more recent flattening or reversal of the trend, have been made in Norway[4,111], Sweden[235] and Connecticut (USA)[242], where the increases affected mainly papillary and follicular carcinomas, and anaplastic carcinoma has become less common. Similar patterns have also been observed in England and Wales[89]. The decline in mortality in Japan has also been noted[198]. The incidence of thyroid cancer in children has apparently declined in Turin (Italy)[194].

The increase in Norway from 1970 to 1985 was due to primarily to thyroid cancers diagnosed in stage I (localised tumour), but was not considered to be an artefact of better diagnosis, and the incidence of stage I tumours is now falling. Radio-iodine contamination from fallout due to atmospheric nuclear weapons testing was considered an unlikely explanation for the spatial and temporal patterns observed in Norway[111]. Radio-iodine was considered a possible explanation for the patterns in England and Wales, however, where a peak risk was seen for women born in 1952-55, but unidentified and longstanding environmental factors, also associated with benign thyroid disease, were judged to be a more likely explanation[89]. In Vaud (Switzerland)[164], there was a decline in incidence during the period 1979-88, as in Geneva, but it was greater in females (15.5%) than in males (3.2%), the converse of the pattern in Geneva. Incidence among Chinese females in Singapore was reported as increasing at a rate equivalent to 8% every five years during the period 1968-82[154]; this rate now appears to have accelerated, averaging 30% every five years (five standard errors) in the 15 years to 1987, and even more in younger females. Substantial recent increases in thyroid cancer in both sexes have been observed in Ontario (Canada), attributed to the use of irradiation for benign conditions of the head and neck[182].

Devesa *et al.*[77] pointed out that survival in the USA was better in females, and that the decline in mortality up to 1984 was larger in middle than older age groups. The analyses presented here for the USA in the period up to 1987 confirm and extend these observations, with recent linear rates of decline in the age range 45-74 years of 17% and 9% every five years in females and males, respectively, and 11% and 6% at 75 years and over (data not shown).

Increased diagnosis of clinically occult or biologically benign lesions and further improvements in survival due to better treatment have been suggested as likely explanations for the divergent trends in incidence and mortality[286], especially in the USA, where the association between increasing incidence and stable or declining mortality has also been noted. This explanation is attractive, but some aspects of the international pattern of thyroid cancer do not easily fit into it. These include the recent decline in incidence of early (stage I) thyroid cancer in Norway, the widespread differences in the rate of change of mortality between the sexes, and the large increases in incidence in countries such as Japan and the GDR.

THYROID (ICD-9 193)

AMERICAS (except USA), INCIDENCE

MALES	Best model	Goodness of fit	1970 Rate	1970 Cases	1985 Rate	1985 Cases	Cumulative risk 1915	Cumulative risk 1940	Recent trend
BRAZIL									
Sao Paulo	A1	0.86	2.5	18	*2.5*	*23*	1.1	*1.1*	–
CANADA									
Alberta	A1D	0.63	1.6	5	3.9	19	1.1	4.8	30.2
British Columbia	A1D	0.49	1.8	8	2.8	19	0.9	1.9	22.0
Maritime Provinces	A1D	1.18	1.5	4	2.6	9	0.9	2.3	*17.7*
Newfoundland	A1D	-0.29	1.7	1	3.3	3	1.1	3.2	*32.5*
Quebec	A1C2	0.33	1.8	20	2.8	42	1.0	2.3	11.5
COLOMBIA									
Cali	A3D	-1.38	4.7	3	2.4	3	2.2	0.7	*10.6*
CUBA	A1	-0.81	1.3	20	1.3	26	0.6	*0.6*	–
PUERTO RICO	A2D	1.29	1.3	6	2.2	14	0.8	1.9	*15.4*

FEMALES	Best model	Goodness of fit	1970 Rate	1970 Cases	1985 Rate	1985 Cases	Cumulative risk 1915	Cumulative risk 1940	Recent trend
BRAZIL									
Sao Paulo	A2C3	-0.59	5.6	48	*12.5*	*139*	2.2	*12.6*	–
CANADA									
Alberta	A1D	0.50	4.8	14	9.6	48	2.5	7.9	28.0
British Columbia	A0	0.91	6.0	27	6.0	43	2.7	2.7	*7.7*
Maritime Provinces	A1	0.03	5.9	17	5.9	21	2.7	2.7	*4.0*
Newfoundland	A8P5C9	0.40	4.6	3	4.1	4	2.4	3.8	*-18.8*
Quebec	A2C3	-1.84	4.3	52	6.0	100	2.0	4.2	18.3
COLOMBIA									
Cali	A1	1.53	10.2	10	10.2	20	5.3	5.3	*-0.5*
CUBA	A4	0.15	5.4	77	5.4	113	2.5	*2.5*	–
PUERTO RICO	A0D	-1.09	4.5	21	5.7	43	2.0	3.0	*6.0*

* : not enough cases for reliable estimation
– : incomplete or missing data
Best model: polynomial of the given degree in age (A), period (P) or cohort (C), or linear drift (D) model.
Goodness of fit: the normalised likelihood ratio chi-square for the best model (see Method).
Rate: world-standardised truncated rate per 100 000 per year (30-74 years) and number of **cases** are both estimated from the best-fitting model for the single years cited.
Cumulative risk per 1000 (30-74 years) is estimated from the best-fitting *age-cohort* model for cohorts of central birth year cited.
Recent trend: estimated mean percentage change per five-year period in the age-specific rates (30-74 years) over the period 1973-1987.
Italics denote recent trends not significant at 5 per cent level, or other figures which should be interpreted with caution (see Method).

THYROID (ICD-9 193)

AMERICAS (except USA), INCIDENCE

MALES

TRUNCATED RATE (30-74 years)

CUMULATIVE RISK (30-74 years)

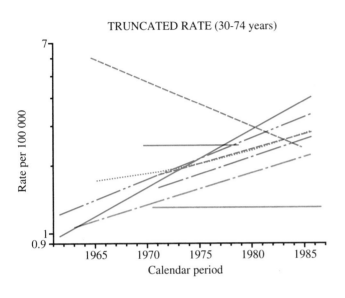

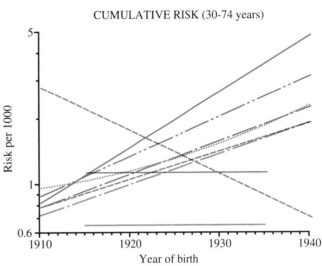

FEMALES

TRUNCATED RATE (30-74 years)

CUMULATIVE RISK (30-74 years)

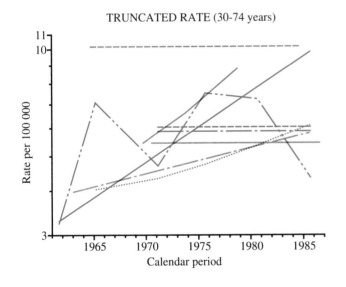

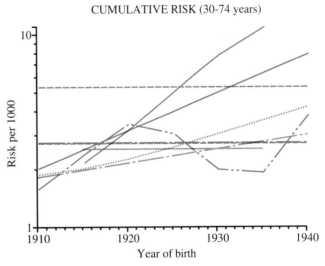

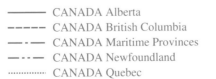

——— CANADA Alberta	——— CUBA
– – – CANADA British Columbia	–·–·– PUERTO RICO
–··–··– CANADA Maritime Provinces	——— BRAZIL Sao Paulo
–··–··– CANADA Newfoundland	– – – – COLOMBIA Cali
············· CANADA Quebec	

THYROID (ICD-9 193)

AMERICAS (USA), INCIDENCE

MALES	Best model	Goodness of fit	1970 Rate	1970 Cases	1985 Rate	1985 Cases	Cumulative risk 1915	Cumulative risk 1940	Recent trend
USA									
Bay Area, Black	A1	1.65	2.6	1	2.6	2	1.4	1.4	*-38.0*
Bay Area, Chinese	A0	0.78	5.4	1	*5.4*	*2*	2.4	*2.4*	–
Bay Area, White	A1	-1.26	5.1	29	5.1	33	2.4	2.4	*-1.3*
Connecticut	A8P5C9	0.12	2.2	14	3.4	25	1.0	2.6	*0.5*
Detroit, Black	A1	-0.19	2.7	3	2.7	4	1.4	1.4	*17.1*
Detroit, White	A1D	0.94	3.2	23	5.1	35	1.7	3.7	16.6
Iowa	A1	0.59	2.9	17	2.9	19	1.4	1.4	*8.5*
New Orleans, Black	A1	0.16	*2.4*	*1*	2.4	1	1.4	1.4	*27.2*
New Orleans, White	A1	-1.56	*4.4*	*6*	4.4	6	2.2	2.2	*6.6*
Seattle	A0C2	1.56	*3.0*	*13*	4.0	27	1.4	2.2	*8.1*

FEMALES	Best model	Goodness of fit	1970 Rate	1970 Cases	1985 Rate	1985 Cases	Cumulative risk 1915	Cumulative risk 1940	Recent trend
USA									
Bay Area, Black	A0	0.46	5.6	3	5.6	5	2.5	2.5	*0.8*
Bay Area, Chinese	A0P2	-0.98	5.2	1	*0.7*	*0*	7.2	*2.7*	–
Bay Area, White	A3	-0.01	10.0	61	10.0	67	4.4	4.4	*-7.6*
Connecticut	A0D	1.71	5.7	40	8.1	67	2.5	4.5	10.3
Detroit, Black	A1	-0.69	6.5	9	6.5	14	3.1	3.1	*-3.1*
Detroit, White	A0D	0.61	8.4	65	10.5	79	3.7	5.4	8.4
Iowa	A0D	0.52	5.4	34	8.9	61	2.4	5.7	23.8
New Orleans, Black	A1	-0.28	*6.1*	*3*	6.1	5	3.0	3.0	*17.8*
New Orleans, White	A0D	-0.56	*5.5*	*9*	10.7	18	2.6	7.8	25.7
Seattle	A0D	-0.60	*4.8*	*22*	9.3	67	2.3	6.8	25.8

* : not enough cases for reliable estimation
– : incomplete or missing data
Best model: polynomial of the given degree in age (A), period (P) or cohort (C), or linear drift (D) model.
Goodness of fit: the normalised likelihood ratio chi-square for the best model (see Method).
Rate: world-standardised truncated rate per 100 000 per year (30-74 years) and number of **cases** are both estimated from the best-fitting model for the single years cited.
Cumulative risk per 1000 (30-74 years) is estimated from the best-fitting *age-cohort* model for cohorts of central birth year cited.
Recent trend: estimated mean percentage change per five-year period in the age-specific rates (30-74 years) over the period 1973-1987.
Italics denote recent trends not significant at 5 per cent level, or other figures which should be interpreted with caution (see Method).

THYROID (ICD-9 193)

AMERICAS (USA), INCIDENCE

MALES

TRUNCATED RATE (30-74 years)

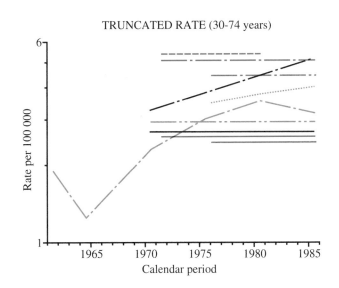

CUMULATIVE RISK (30-74 years)

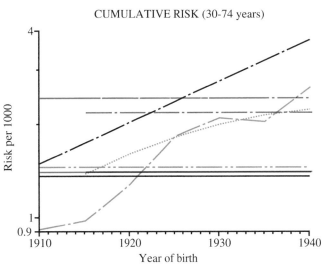

FEMALES

TRUNCATED RATE (30-74 years)

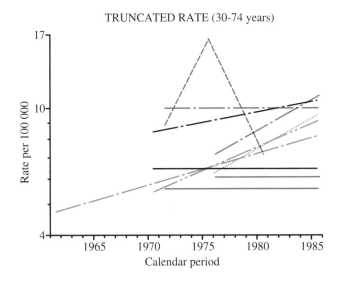

CUMULATIVE RISK (30-74 years)

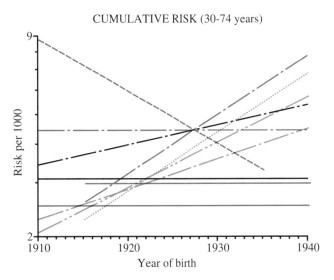

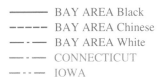

———— BAY AREA Black	·········· SEATTLE	
– – – – BAY AREA Chinese	———— NEW ORLEANS Black	
–·—·— BAY AREA White	–··—··— NEW ORLEANS White	
–··—··— CONNECTICUT	———— DETROIT Black	
–···—···— IOWA	–··—··— DETROIT White	

THYROID (ICD-9 193)

AMERICAS (except USA), INCIDENCE
Percentage change per five-year period, 1973-1987

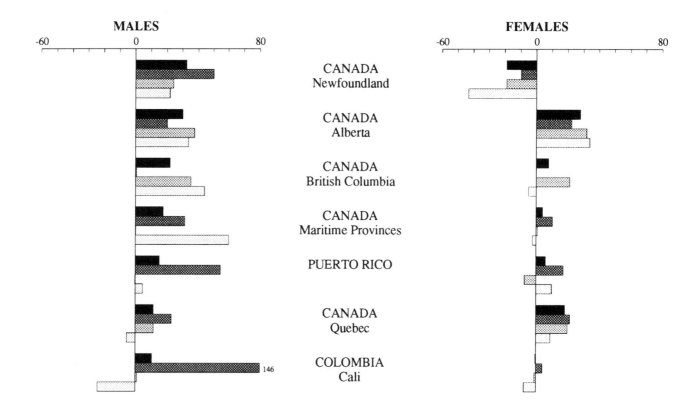

THYROID (ICD-9 193)

AMERICAS (USA), INCIDENCE
Percentage change per five-year period, 1973-1987

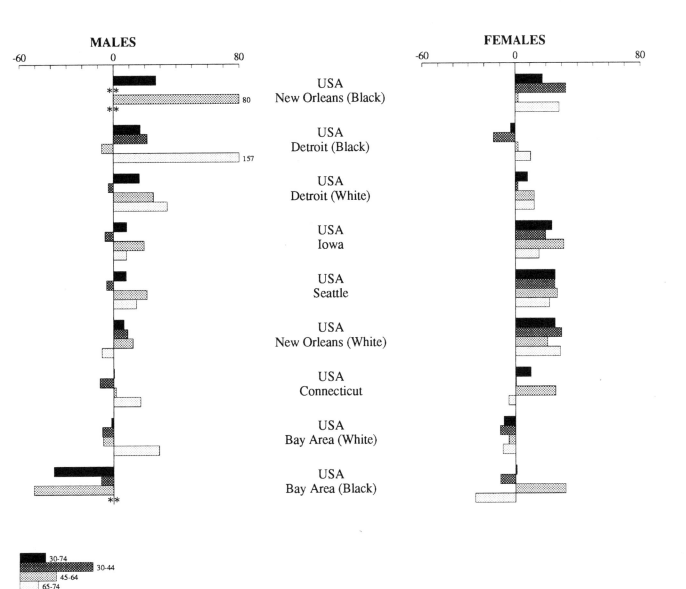

THYROID (ICD-9 193)

AMERICAS, MORTALITY

MALES	Best model	Goodness of fit	1965 Rate	1965 Deaths	1985 Rate	1985 Deaths	Cumulative risk 1900	Cumulative risk 1940	Recent trend
CANADA	A2D	2.04	0.7	26	0.5	27	0.5	0.2	-7.3
CHILE	A1	-0.89	0.7	8	0.7	13	0.5	0.5	–
COSTA RICA	–	–	–	–	–	–	–	–	–
PANAMA	–	–	–	–	–	–	–	–	–
PUERTO RICO	–	–	–	–	–	–	–	–	–
URUGUAY	–	–	–	–	–	–	–	–	–
USA	A2D	-0.25	0.6	265	0.4	237	0.4	0.2	-8.3
VENEZUELA	A2	1.00	0.5	4	0.5	8	0.3	0.3	–

FEMALES	Best model	Goodness of fit	1965 Rate	1965 Deaths	1985 Rate	1985 Deaths	Cumulative risk 1900	Cumulative risk 1940	Recent trend
CANADA	A2P2	-0.52	1.1	44	0.5	35	0.7	0.2	-18.8
CHILE	A2	0.25	1.4	18	1.4	30	1.0	1.0	–
COSTA RICA	–	–	–	–	–	–	–	–	–
PANAMA	–	–	–	–	–	–	–	–	–
PUERTO RICO	–	–	–	–	–	–	–	–	–
URUGUAY	–	–	–	–	–	–	–	–	–
USA	A2C4	-0.50	0.9	444	0.5	311	0.6	0.2	-13.8
VENEZUELA	A2	1.15	1.2	10	1.2	19	0.8	0.8	–

* : not enough deaths for reliable estimation
– : incomplete or missing data
Best model: polynomial of the given degree in age (A), period (P) or cohort (C), or linear drift (D) model.
Goodness of fit: the normalised likelihood ratio chi-square for the best model (see Method).
Rate: world-standardised truncated rate per 100 000 per year (30-74 years) and number of **deaths** are both estimated from the best-fitting model for the single years cited.
Cumulative risk per 1000 (30-74 years) is estimated from the best-fitting *age-cohort* model for cohorts of central birth year cited.
Recent trend: estimated mean percentage change per five-year period in the age-specific rates (30-74 years) over the period 1975-1988.
Italics denote recent trends not significant at 5 per cent level, or other figures which should be interpreted with caution (see Method).

THYROID (ICD-9 193)

AMERICAS, MORTALITY

MALES

TRUNCATED RATE (30-74 years)

CUMULATIVE RISK (30-74 years)

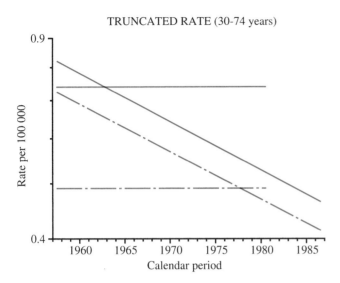

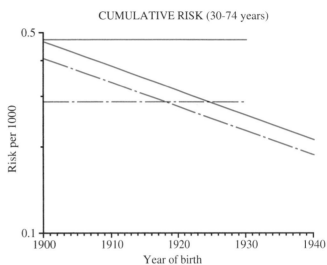

FEMALES

TRUNCATED RATE (30-74 years)

CUMULATIVE RISK (30-74 years)

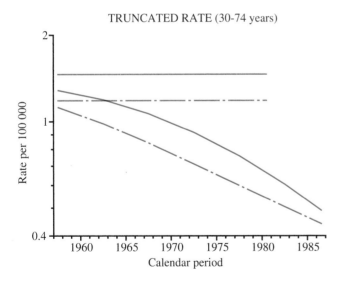

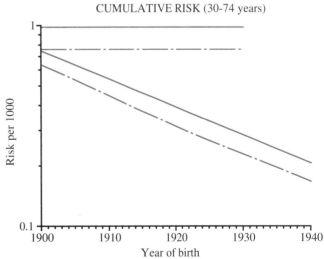

——— CANADA
—·—· USA
——— CHILE
—··—··— VENEZUELA

THYROID (ICD-9 193)

AMERICAS, MORTALITY
Percentage change per five-year period, 1975-1988

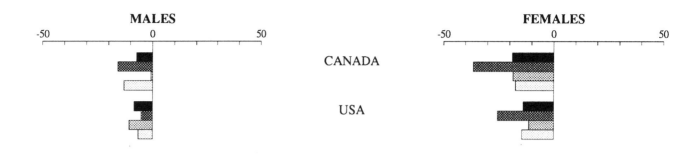

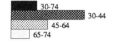

Chapter 26
NON-HODGKIN LYMPHOMA

Lymphomas as a group ranked ninth among all cancers world-wide around 1980, accounting for about 3.7% of new cases; the rank order is the same in both developed and developing countries[219].

Malignant lymphomas other than Hodgkin's disease (ICD-9 201) are a heterogeneous group comprising lymphosarcoma, reticulosarcoma and Burkitt's lymphoma (ICD-9 200) and other malignant neoplasms of lymphoid tissue (ICD-9 202), including mycosis fungoides. About 20% of lymphomas arise outside lymph nodes, in organs such as stomach, bone, bowel and brain. ICD coding rules require malignant lymphomas to be assigned to the rubrics 200-202, but some cancer registries assign extra-nodal lymphomas to the organ in which they arise[196]. The morphology codes enable them to be distinguished from other tumours at the same site in data submitted as anonymised case listings. Since the 1970s there has been a fall in the incidence of neoplasms assigned to the rubric 200 and a corresponding rise in those assigned to the rubric 202[18,80], probably due to changes in the way pathologists have classified the lymphomas[196]. Changes in classification of the lymphomas and in the precision of diagnosis complicate the interpretation of trends[18]. For these reasons, and in common with other studies of non-Hodgkin lymphoma, trends have been examined for all malignant lymphomas (except Hodgkin's disease) combined, even though this category is clearly not a single disease entity. Unlike Hodgkin's disease, the incidence of non-Hodgkin lymphoma in adults increases with age at least as a power function, as for epithelial cancers. Incidence is generally 1.5- to 2-fold higher in males than females.

For the period 1963-65 (volume II), data on Hodgkin's disease for Connecticut (USA) were included with those for other lymphomas in a single category, and were thus excluded from analysis: the data for 1960-62, presented separately, were included.

Europe

Incidence has been rising steadily in both sexes and in almost all parts of Europe since the 1960s, particularly in the European Community and the Nordic countries, and recent rates of increase have been in the range 15-40% or more every five years. Most data sets are well described by models with linear drift or period effects, and the rates of increase are similar at all ages in the range 30-74 years. Incidence is substantially higher among Jews in Israel than among non-Jews, and is increasing in both sexes. Incidence in Hungary, Poland and Romania is lower than elsewhere, and has risen very little in the past 20 years. In Slovenia, however, incidence has increased substantially, and rates are now intermediate between those of eastern and western Europe.

Mortality in Europe has also been increasing, although less rapidly than incidence, and there is evidence of further flattening of the rate of increase in Scotland and the Nordic countries. These patterns are largely consistent, and suggest that progressive improvements in treatment and survival have partially attenuated the increases in mortality which would otherwise have arisen from the substantial increases in incidence. Recorded mortality from non-Hodgkin lymphoma in Switzerland in 1975-79 dipped sharply but transiently in both sexes to about half the previous level, while incidence in Geneva rose steadily. Mortality from Hodgkin's disease increased transiently by a similar amount in both sexes during the same period. Examination of the data suggests an error of coding between ICD-9 rubrics 200 and 201; it is unlikely that a change in death certification practice would be so sudden, and so sharply reversed.

The declines in mortality in Hungary and Yugoslavia are in sharp contrast to the general trend. The data for Hungary are well fitted by a simple cohort model, and the recent linear decline is similar in both sexes at 9% every five years. In Yugoslavia, the decline is less marked, and the small recent linear trend is not significant. Both trends are difficult to reconcile with the patterns of incidence observed in Szabolcs-Szatmar and Vas (Hungary) and in Slovenia, respectively, although in each country the registry data only cover about 8% of the national populations (Table 2.8). Over-certification of death due to non-Hodgkin lymphoma in previous decades may be a partial explanation. In Yugoslavia, some deaths from non-Hodgkin lymphoma may have been misclassified as due to Hodgkin's disease, for which the inverse pattern

continued page 662

NON-HODGKIN LYMPHOMA (ICD-9 200, 202)

EUROPE (non-EC), INCIDENCE

MALES	Best model	Goodness of fit	1970 Rate	1970 Cases	1985 Rate	1985 Cases	Cumulative risk 1915	Cumulative risk 1940	Recent trend
FINLAND	A8P5	-0.16	7.3	74	12.9	153	6.8	24.2	33.2
HUNGARY									
County Vas	A1	2.51	7.2	5	7.2	5	4.0	4.0	*4.1*
Szabolcs-Szatmar	A1	0.47	5.0	6	5.0	6	3.0	3.0	*4.6*
ISRAEL									
All Jews	A1P2	2.86	14.4	65	16.8	97	8.9	13.5	*4.3*
Non-Jews	A1D	0.92	11.7	4	7.2	5	5.9	2.6	*-18.6*
NORWAY	A3P2	0.21	8.3	87	14.0	161	6.4	13.5	23.3
POLAND									
Warsaw City	A2D	1.83	4.2	11	5.6	21	2.9	4.7	*1.9*
ROMANIA									
Cluj	A1	-0.30	*4.6*	*7*	4.6	8	2.5	2.5	*-19.6*
SWEDEN	A2D	-0.02	9.4	223	15.7	397	7.5	17.7	18.9
SWITZERLAND									
Geneva	A1D	4.14	13.3	10	19.8	18	9.7	18.7	*5.3*
YUGOSLAVIA									
Slovenia	A2P2	-0.04	4.5	16	8.5	37	3.6	7.4	28.1

FEMALES	Best model	Goodness of fit	1970 Rate	1970 Cases	1985 Rate	1985 Cases	Cumulative risk 1915	Cumulative risk 1940	Recent trend
FINLAND	A1P4	-1.19	3.4	45	10.3	159	4.8	24.5	44.9
HUNGARY									
County Vas	*	..	..	..	..	..	..	..	..
Szabolcs-Szatmar	A1D	0.94	1.5	2	3.9	6	1.6	7.3	*29.6*
ISRAEL									
All Jews	A1D	2.25	11.2	50	13.7	87	7.2	10.2	7.3
Non-Jews	A1	0.06	6.3	2	6.3	4	3.3	3.3	*7.7*
NORWAY	A4D	0.65	6.0	68	10.6	132	4.7	12.1	27.3
POLAND									
Warsaw City	A1	0.09	3.4	14	3.4	17	2.0	2.0	*13.3*
ROMANIA									
Cluj	–	–	–	–	–	–	–	–	–
SWEDEN	A2D	-1.33	6.9	177	10.3	283	5.1	10.0	15.5
SWITZERLAND									
Geneva	A1D	0.16	6.4	6	10.9	12	5.3	12.6	*16.7*
YUGOSLAVIA									
Slovenia	A1P2	1.17	2.8	13	5.9	33	2.5	6.6	30.1

* : not enough cases for reliable estimation
– : incomplete or missing data
Best model: polynomial of the given degree in age (A), period (P) or cohort (C), or linear drift (D) model.
Goodness of fit: the normalised likelihood ratio chi-square for the best model (see Method).
Rate: world-standardised truncated rate per 100 000 per year (30-74 years) and number of **cases** are both estimated from the best-fitting model for the single years cited.
Cumulative risk per 1000 (30-74 years) is estimated from the best-fitting *age-cohort* model for cohorts of central birth year cited.
Recent trend: estimated mean percentage change per five-year period in the age-specific rates (30-74 years) over the period 1973-1987.
Italics denote recent trends not significant at 5 per cent level, or other figures which should be interpreted with caution (see Method).

NON-HODGKIN LYMPHOMA (ICD-9 200, 202)

EUROPE (non-EC), INCIDENCE

MALES

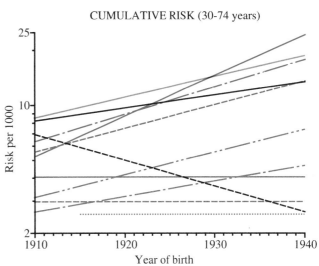

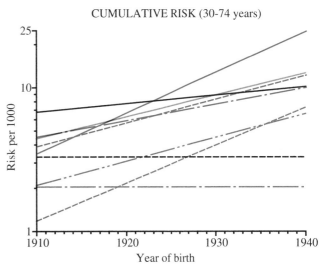

FEMALES

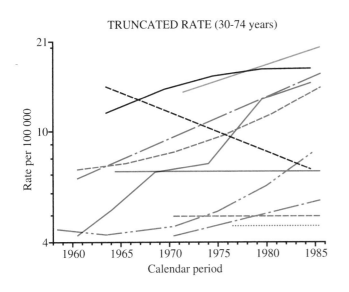

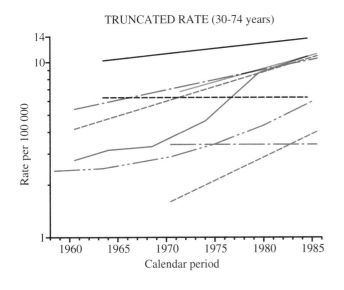

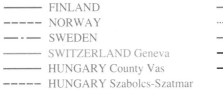

—— FINLAND	—·— POLAND Warsaw City
---- NORWAY	·········· ROMANIA Cluj
—·— SWEDEN	—··— YUGOSLAVIA Slovenia
—— SWITZERLAND Geneva	—— ISRAEL All Jews
—— HUNGARY County Vas	----- ISRAEL Non-Jews
----- HUNGARY Szabolcs-Szatmar	

EUROPE (EC), INCIDENCE

MALES	Best model	Goodness of fit	1970 Rate	Cases	1985 Rate	Cases	Cumulative risk 1915	1940	Recent trend
DENMARK	A5D	2.40	7.6	99	14.0	197	6.2	16.9	22.1
FRANCE									
Bas-Rhin	A1D	-1.34	*4.1*	*9*	21.6	44	8.6	129.2	74.8
Doubs	A8C7	0.50	*6.5*	*6*	9.3	10	1.8	29.7	*13.0*
GERMANY (FRG)									
Hamburg	A3P3	0.09	6.1	31	*65.9*	*263*	3.4	*1.3*	–
Saarland	A2D	0.97	7.8	21	11.6	32	5.5	10.8	13.9
GERMANY (GDR)	A4P4C2	0.58	7.4	313	10.2	378	4.9	7.2	16.8
ITALY									
Varese	A1D	-0.01	*11.1*	*14*	19.9	40	9.0	23.7	22.3
SPAIN									
Navarra	A1D	-0.95	*4.6*	*5*	11.9	16	4.4	21.1	38.0
Zaragoza	A2D	1.04	4.6	8	9.2	20	3.6	11.5	40.2
UK									
Birmingham	A2P5C2	1.04	7.7	100	11.6	165	5.5	8.6	13.9
Scotland	A1P3	-1.56	9.5	124	15.2	202	6.8	18.2	23.8
South Thames	A1P4C4	-1.59	5.7	134	14.7	266	5.5	14.9	49.5

FEMALES	Best model	Goodness of fit	1970 Rate	Cases	1985 Rate	Cases	Cumulative risk 1915	1940	Recent trend
DENMARK	A8P6	0.92	6.4	93	12.9	202	4.6	14.5	34.0
FRANCE									
Bas-Rhin	A1D	0.81	*4.9*	*14*	9.7	24	4.1	12.6	24.9
Doubs	A1	-0.91	*7.3*	*5*	7.3	8	4.2	4.2	*15.9*
GERMANY (FRG)									
Hamburg	A1P3	0.43	4.4	32	*50.3*	*269*	2.0	*0.8*	–
Saarland	A1D	0.39	4.2	15	8.0	29	3.6	10.5	19.3
GERMANY (GDR)	A3P2C2	-0.54	4.6	294	6.6	354	3.3	5.3	15.7
ITALY									
Varese	A1D	0.56	*5.0*	*7*	12.1	30	4.9	21.4	32.6
SPAIN									
Navarra	A1D	1.79	*2.8*	*3*	7.6	11	3.0	15.5	39.3
Zaragoza	A8P3C8	-0.04	2.3	5	7.8	20	2.5	13.6	93.8
UK									
Birmingham	A2C3	1.30	5.2	76	7.4	114	3.6	5.9	11.5
Scotland	A1C2	2.09	6.1	99	11.6	186	5.3	13.8	24.9
South Thames	A1P4	0.03	3.8	111	9.8	209	3.8	11.5	44.4

* : not enough cases for reliable estimation
– : incomplete or missing data
Best model: polynomial of the given degree in age (A), period (P) or cohort (C), or linear drift (D) model.
Goodness of fit: the normalised likelihood ratio chi-square for the best model (see Method).
Rate: world-standardised truncated rate per 100 000 per year (30-74 years) and number of **cases** are both estimated from the best-fitting model for the single years cited.
Cumulative risk per 1000 (30-74 years) is estimated from the best-fitting *age-cohort* model for cohorts of central birth year cited.
Recent trend: estimated mean percentage change per five-year period in the age-specific rates (30-74 years) over the period 1973-1987.
Italics denote recent trends not significant at 5 per cent level, or other figures which should be interpreted with caution (see Method).

NON-HODGKIN LYMPHOMA (ICD-9 200, 202)

EUROPE (EC), INCIDENCE

MALES

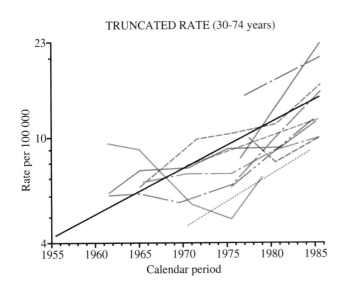

TRUNCATED RATE (30-74 years)

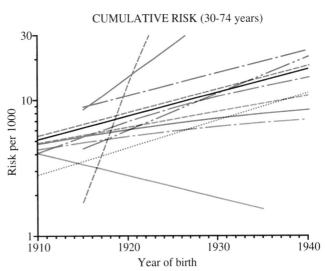

CUMULATIVE RISK (30-74 years)

FEMALES

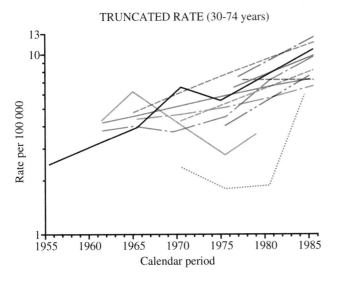

TRUNCATED RATE (30-74 years)

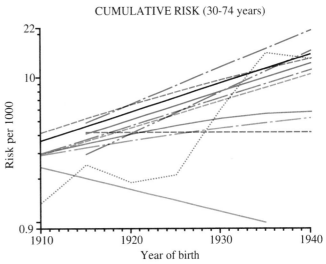

CUMULATIVE RISK (30-74 years)

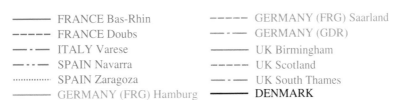

—— FRANCE Bas-Rhin	------ GERMANY (FRG) Saarland
- - - FRANCE Doubs	—·—·— GERMANY (GDR)
—·—·— ITALY Varese	—— UK Birmingham
—··—··— SPAIN Navarra	------ UK Scotland
·········· SPAIN Zaragoza	—·—·— UK South Thames
—— GERMANY (FRG) Hamburg	—— DENMARK

NON-HODGKIN LYMPHOMA (ICD-9 200, 202)

EUROPE (non-EC), INCIDENCE
Percentage change per five-year period, 1973-1987

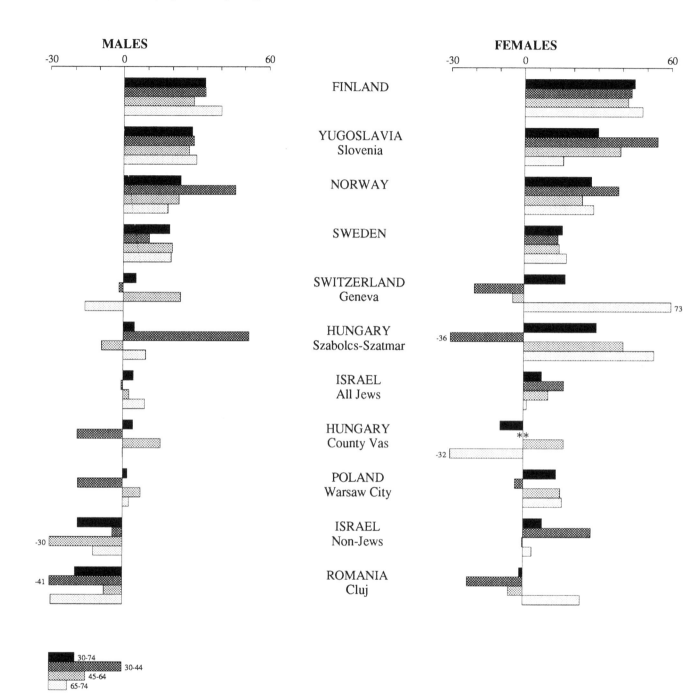

MALES

-30   0   60

FEMALES

-30   0   60

FINLAND

YUGOSLAVIA
Slovenia

NORWAY

SWEDEN

SWITZERLAND
Geneva

HUNGARY
Szabolcs-Szatmar

ISRAEL
All Jews

HUNGARY
County Vas

POLAND
Warsaw City

ISRAEL
Non-Jews

ROMANIA
Cluj

Legend:
30-74
30-44
45-64
65-74

NON-HODGKIN LYMPHOMA (ICD-9 200, 202)

EUROPE (EC), INCIDENCE
Percentage change per five-year period, 1973-1987

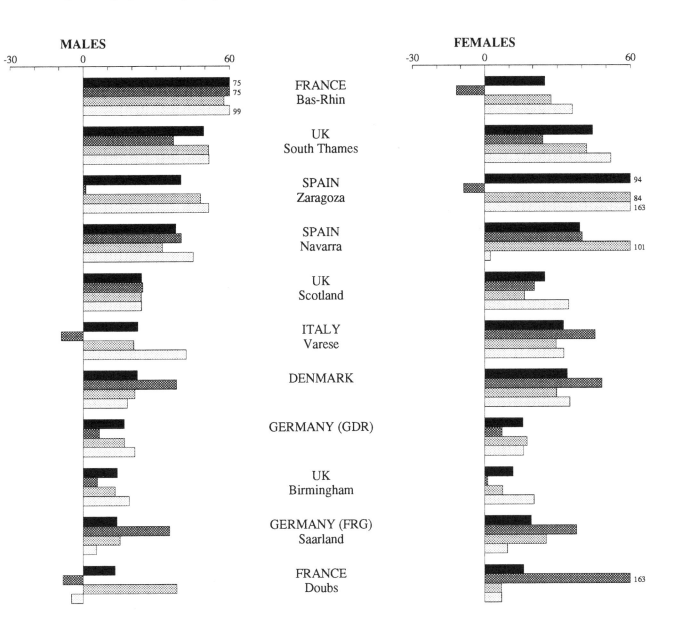

NON-HODGKIN LYMPHOMA (ICD-9 200, 202)

EUROPE (non-EC), MORTALITY

MALES	Best model	Goodness of fit	1965 Rate	Deaths	1985 Rate	Deaths	Cumulative risk 1900	1940	Recent trend
AUSTRIA	A2D	0.04	*3.5*	*67*	5.3	97	*2.1*	4.7	11.0
CZECHOSLOVAKIA	A3P3C2	1.31	4.6	160	5.9	215	2.3	4.0	14.8
FINLAND	A3P2	-0.50	5.3	49	7.6	90	3.1	7.5	*3.1*
HUNGARY	A2C2	0.70	*7.6*	*193*	6.0	164	*4.5*	2.5	-9.5
NORWAY	A1P3C2	0.53	5.7	57	6.7	79	3.2	4.1	14.2
POLAND	A3D	-0.64	2.0	124	*6.3*	*503*	1.0	*9.7*	–
ROMANIA	*	..	..	..	..	..	..	..	..
SWEDEN	A3P2C3	0.14	4.8	109	7.0	184	3.0	5.4	*1.8*
SWITZERLAND	A3P6C2	-1.48	4.6	64	15.0	261	3.1	4.0	55.8
YUGOSLAVIA	A3P5C2	-2.22	3.9	148	2.5	124	2.0	1.1	*-1.4*

FEMALES	Best model	Goodness of fit	1965 Rate	Deaths	1985 Rate	Deaths	Cumulative risk 1900	1940	Recent trend
AUSTRIA	A1P3C2	-1.60	*2.4*	*62*	3.7	94	*1.0*	3.6	20.6
CZECHOSLOVAKIA	A1P3C3	-0.79	2.6	110	3.0	137	1.5	2.1	6.6
FINLAND	A1C2	-0.96	2.7	33	4.9	78	1.7	4.5	15.5
HUNGARY	A3C2	0.68	*4.2*	*127*	3.5	122	2.4	1.3	-9.2
NORWAY	A1D	-1.95	3.1	34	4.1	55	1.9	3.4	11.7
POLAND	A3D	-0.85	1.0	79	*2.4*	*236*	0.5	*3.0*	–
ROMANIA	*	..	..	..	..	..	..	..	..
SWEDEN	A1C3	0.02	3.5	84	4.7	136	2.1	3.6	7.6
SWITZERLAND	A2P6C2	-0.82	3.0	51	7.5	153	1.9	2.2	52.1
YUGOSLAVIA	A3P3C2	-0.62	2.1	91	1.6	94	1.1	0.6	*1.9*

* : not enough deaths for reliable estimation
– : incomplete or missing data
Best model: polynomial of the given degree in age (A), period (P) or cohort (C), or linear drift (D) model.
Goodness of fit: the normalised likelihood ratio chi-square for the best model (see Method).
Rate: world-standardised truncated rate per 100 000 per year (30-74 years) and number of **deaths** are both estimated from the best-fitting model for the single years cited.
Cumulative risk per 1000 (30-74 years) is estimated from the best-fitting *age-cohort* model for cohorts of central birth year cited.
Recent trend: estimated mean percentage change per five-year period in the age-specific rates (30-74 years) over the period 1975-1988.
Italics denote recent trends not significant at 5 per cent level, or other figures which should be interpreted with caution (see Method).

NON-HODGKIN LYMPHOMA (ICD-9 200, 202)

EUROPE (non-EC), MORTALITY

MALES

TRUNCATED RATE (30-74 years)

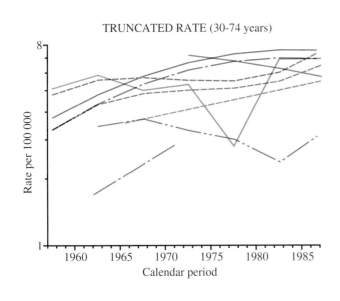

CUMULATIVE RISK (30-74 years)

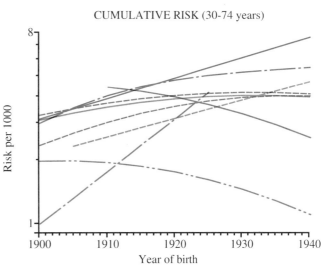

FEMALES

TRUNCATED RATE (30-74 years)

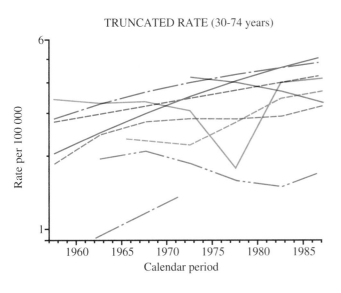

CUMULATIVE RISK (30-74 years)

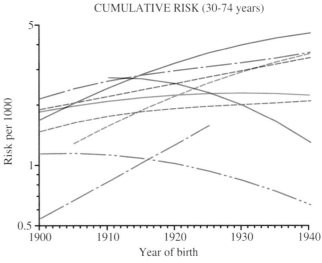

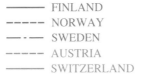

FINLAND — CZECHOSLOVAKIA
NORWAY — HUNGARY
SWEDEN — POLAND
AUSTRIA — YUGOSLAVIA
SWITZERLAND

NON-HODGKIN LYMPHOMA (ICD-9 200, 202)

EUROPE (EC), MORTALITY

MALES	Best model	Goodness of fit	1965 Rate	1965 Deaths	1985 Rate	1985 Deaths	Cumulative risk 1900	Cumulative risk 1940	Recent trend
BELGIUM	A3P4C3	0.64	3.4	86	5.1	136	2.1	2.9	*7.1*
DENMARK	A2D	0.80	5.8	72	6.5	93	3.4	4.4	10.8
FRANCE	A8P5C2	1.07	3.2	384	6.0	819	1.6	4.4	29.2
GERMANY (FRG)	A3P4C8	2.10	*3.9*	*583*	5.3	830	*1.9*	4.7	32.1
GREECE	A3C2	0.35	*2.0*	*38*	3.1	82	*1.0*	2.2	16.6
IRELAND	A1C2	0.79	3.2	22	6.8	53	1.7	6.9	26.6
ITALY	A2P6C9	2.58	4.9	592	6.6	1006	2.5	2.6	30.9
NETHERLANDS	A3P4C2	-1.59	5.2	142	8.0	282	3.0	5.3	16.4
PORTUGAL	–	–	–	–	–	–	–	–	–
SPAIN	A5P4C2	-0.71	1.9	130	3.9	370	0.8	4.0	24.4
UK ENGLAND & WALES	A3P4C3	2.33	4.8	609	7.3	1028	2.5	5.6	22.3
UK SCOTLAND	A2C2	-0.33	5.6	72	7.4	100	3.1	4.7	12.3

FEMALES	Best model	Goodness of fit	1965 Rate	1965 Deaths	1985 Rate	1985 Deaths	Cumulative risk 1900	Cumulative risk 1940	Recent trend
BELGIUM	A1C6	1.68	1.9	54	2.8	86	1.0	2.0	35.5
DENMARK	A1D	-0.89	3.5	49	4.2	69	2.2	3.2	15.0
FRANCE	A8P6C9	1.08	1.5	222	3.9	619	0.8	3.0	35.9
GERMANY (FRG)	A1P4C7	0.78	*2.2*	*440*	3.3	724	*1.1*	3.0	33.7
GREECE	A3D	1.04	*1.1*	*24*	1.7	51	*0.6*	1.5	*13.0*
IRELAND	A2P5C3	1.83	2.2	16	5.0	42	1.0	5.1	43.0
ITALY	A3P6C6	0.22	2.3	334	3.6	658	1.2	1.7	34.4
NETHERLANDS	A8P6C9	1.87	3.5	107	4.4	183	1.8	3.5	12.5
PORTUGAL	–	–	–	–	–	–	–	–	–
SPAIN	A3C2	0.78	0.9	70	2.4	260	0.4	3.1	33.8
UK ENGLAND & WALES	A3P3C6	0.69	2.9	452	4.7	757	1.6	3.7	20.6
UK SCOTLAND	A2P4C2	-0.29	4.2	67	5.7	96	2.2	3.7	23.9

* : not enough deaths for reliable estimation
– : incomplete or missing data
Best model: polynomial of the given degree in age (A), period (P) or cohort (C), or linear drift (D) model.
Goodness of fit: the normalised likelihood ratio chi-square for the best model (see Method).
Rate: world-standardised truncated rate per 100 000 per year (30-74 years) and number of **deaths** are both estimated from the best-fitting model for the single years cited.
Cumulative risk per 1000 (30-74 years) is estimated from the best-fitting *age-cohort* model for cohorts of central birth year cited.
Recent trend: estimated mean percentage change per five-year period in the age-specific rates (30-74 years) over the period 1975-1988.
Italics denote recent trends not significant at 5 per cent level, or other figures which should be interpreted with caution (see Method).

NON-HODGKIN LYMPHOMA (ICD-9 200, 202)

EUROPE (EC), MORTALITY

MALES

TRUNCATED RATE (30-74 years)

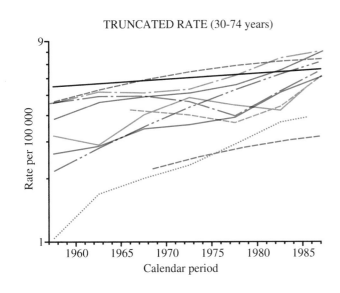

CUMULATIVE RISK (30-74 years)

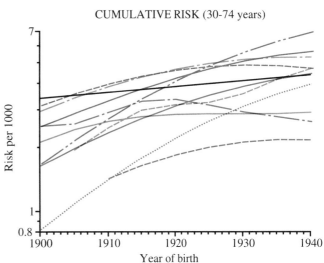

FEMALES

TRUNCATED RATE (30-74 years)

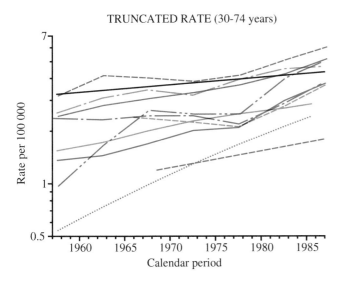

CUMULATIVE RISK (30-74 years)

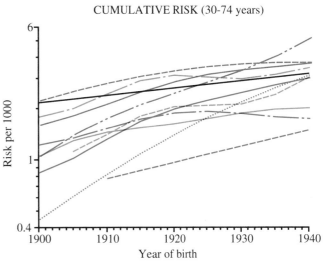

FRANCE
GREECE
ITALY
SPAIN
BELGIUM
GERMANY (FRG)
NETHERLANDS
IRELAND
UK ENGLAND & WALES
UK SCOTLAND
DENMARK

NON-HODGKIN LYMPHOMA (ICD-9 200, 202)

EUROPE (non-EC), MORTALITY
Percentage change per five-year period, 1975-1988

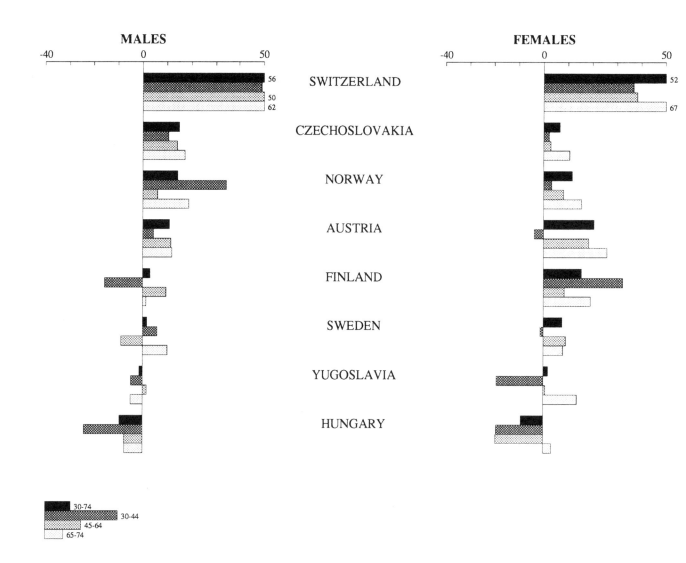

NON-HODGKIN LYMPHOMA (ICD-9 200, 202)

EUROPE (EC), MORTALITY
Percentage change per five-year period, 1975-1988

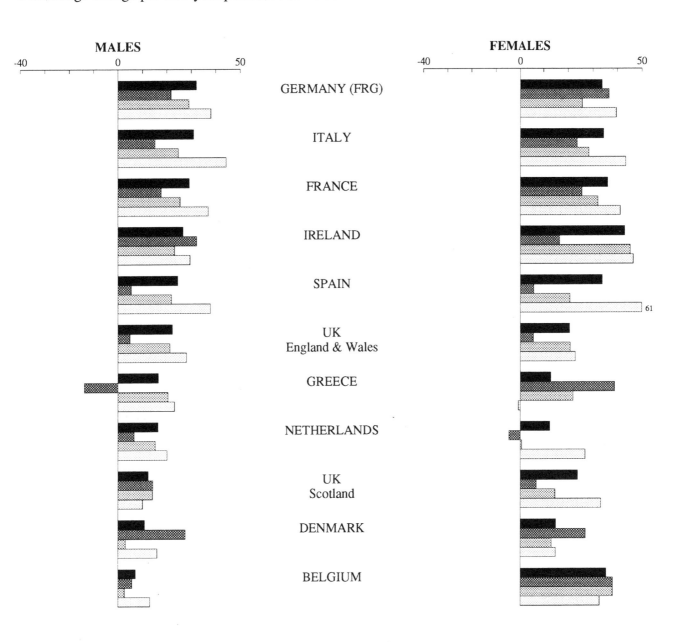

NON-HODGKIN LYMPHOMA (ICD-9 200, 202)

ASIA, INCIDENCE

MALES	Best model	Goodness of fit	1970 Rate	1970 Cases	1985 Rate	1985 Cases	Cumulative risk 1915	Cumulative risk 1940	Recent trend
CHINA									
Shanghai	A1C2	-1.57	*4.1*	*46*	6.5	110	3.0	5.7	13.8
HONG KONG	A1C2	1.99	*6.1*	*37*	13.9	163	5.5	19.9	27.8
INDIA									
Bombay	A1P4	1.03	3.2	26	5.2	67	2.8	4.8	15.1
JAPAN									
Miyagi	A1P3	1.53	4.6	16	7.4	39	3.9	5.6	*6.0*
Nagasaki	A2D	-0.44	*31.5*	*26*	13.1	14	15.5	3.6	-25.7
Osaka	A2D	0.61	5.6	71	10.0	195	4.7	12.6	22.3
SINGAPORE									
Chinese	A3D	0.57	5.0	10	10.1	33	4.4	14.5	31.0
Indian	A1P2	0.71	*0.0*	*0*	4.0	1	2.9	3.5	*6.9*
Malay	A1D	0.30	5.2	1	10.7	5	5.1	16.6	*22.9*

FEMALES	Best model	Goodness of fit	1970 Rate	1970 Cases	1985 Rate	1985 Cases	Cumulative risk 1915	Cumulative risk 1940	Recent trend
CHINA									
Shanghai	A3	-0.43	*3.7*	*44*	3.7	65	1.9	1.9	*0.3*
HONG KONG	A1P2	1.67	*1.9*	*11*	10.0	114	3.7	15.5	32.8
INDIA									
Bombay	A2D	0.94	2.6	13	4.0	37	1.9	3.8	22.1
JAPAN									
Miyagi	A8P5C9	0.75	2.2	9	3.1	18	2.1	5.0	19.6
Nagasaki	A2D	0.87	*21.1*	*21*	7.3	9	10.1	1.7	-29.7
Osaka	A2C3	0.12	2.6	39	5.1	115	2.5	5.0	23.7
SINGAPORE									
Chinese	A1D	-1.83	2.7	6	6.8	24	3.1	13.7	33.3
Indian	A1	0.15	*5.3*	*0*	5.3	1	3.0	3.0	*27.8*
Malay	A8C8	-1.20	4.2	1	7.8	3	3.4	3.3	*19.8*

* : not enough cases for reliable estimation
− : incomplete or missing data
Best model: polynomial of the given degree in age (A), period (P) or cohort (C), or linear drift (D) model.
Goodness of fit: the normalised likelihood ratio chi-square for the best model (see Method).
Rate: world-standardised truncated rate per 100 000 per year (30-74 years) and number of **cases** are both estimated from the best-fitting model for the single years cited.
Cumulative risk per 1000 (30-74 years) is estimated from the best-fitting *age-cohort* model for cohorts of central birth year cited.
Recent trend: estimated mean percentage change per five-year period in the age-specific rates (30-74 years) over the period 1973-1987.
Italics denote recent trends not significant at 5 per cent level, or other figures which should be interpreted with caution (see Method).

654

NON-HODGKIN LYMPHOMA (ICD-9 200, 202)

ASIA, INCIDENCE

MALES

TRUNCATED RATE (30-74 years)

CUMULATIVE RISK (30-74 years)

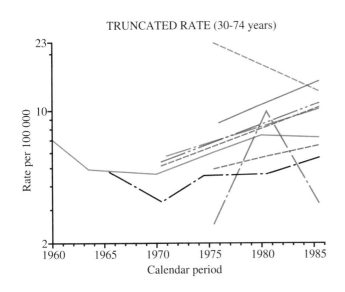
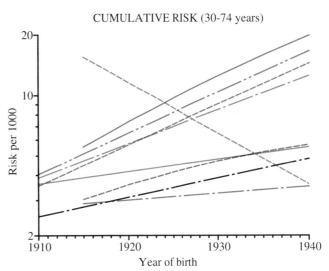

FEMALES

TRUNCATED RATE (30-74 years)

CUMULATIVE RISK (30-74 years)

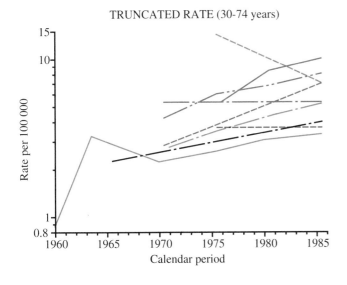
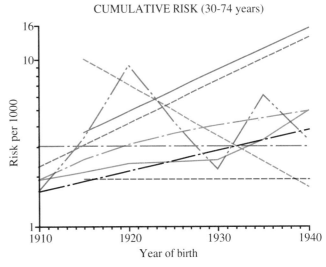

----- CHINA Shanghai
—— JAPAN Miyagi
----- JAPAN Nagasaki
—·— JAPAN Osaka
—— HONG KONG

----- SINGAPORE Chinese
—·— SINGAPORE Indian
—··— SINGAPORE Malay
—··— INDIA Bombay

OCEANIA, INCIDENCE

MALES	Best model	Goodness of fit	1970 Rate	Cases	1985 Rate	Cases	Cumulative risk 1915	1940	Recent trend
AUSTRALIA									
New South Wales	A2D	-0.75	*11.6*	*121*	18.2	241	8.8	18.4	16.0
South	A1	-0.15	*19.1*	*36*	19.1	66	11.2	11.2	*14.3*
HAWAII									
Caucasian	A3C2	0.05	13.1	4	21.5	14	8.6	36.5	*13.2*
Chinese	A1C3	0.37	10.2	1	10.2	1	7.4	0.4	*9.5*
Filipino	A1C3	0.89	11.6	3	13.8	5	7.6	9.6	*8.3*
Hawaiian	A1	0.65	16.9	2	16.9	4	9.9	9.9	*-5.1*
Japanese	A1	0.88	10.6	5	10.6	9	6.4	6.4	32.2
NEW ZEALAND									
Maori	A3	0.74	11.5	2	11.5	3	7.0	7.0	*35.3*
Non-Maori	A3D	1.21	10.6	59	14.5	101	7.4	12.6	10.4

FEMALES	Best model	Goodness of fit	1970 Rate	Cases	1985 Rate	Cases	Cumulative risk 1915	1940	Recent trend
AUSTRALIA									
New South Wales	A2D	0.35	*9.0*	*106*	14.2	199	6.8	14.6	16.3
South	A1	-0.36	*15.0*	*29*	15.0	56	8.8	8.8	*9.2*
HAWAII									
Caucasian	A2	2.10	11.9	4	11.9	7	6.9	6.9	*19.3*
Chinese	A1	-1.06	10.1	1	10.1	1	6.5	6.5	*4.6*
Filipino	A1	0.39	*9.3*	*0*	9.3	2	5.7	5.7	*32.2*
Hawaiian	A1	0.53	11.3	1	11.3	3	6.7	6.7	*2.3*
Japanese	A1C2	1.77	6.4	3	10.5	10	6.2	8.3	*14.2*
NEW ZEALAND									
Maori	A1	0.14	8.4	1	8.4	2	5.2	5.2	*3.1*
Non-Maori	A1P3	1.02	8.8	54	10.3	78	5.5	8.8	*7.1*

* : not enough cases for reliable estimation
− : incomplete or missing data
Best model: polynomial of the given degree in age (A), period (P) or cohort (C), or linear drift (D) model.
Goodness of fit: the normalised likelihood ratio chi-square for the best model (see Method).
Rate: world-standardised truncated rate per 100 000 per year (30-74 years) and number of **cases** are both estimated from the best-fitting model for the single years cited.
Cumulative risk per 1000 (30-74 years) is estimated from the best-fitting *age-cohort* model for cohorts of central birth year cited.
Recent trend: estimated mean percentage change per five-year period in the age-specific rates (30-74 years) over the period 1973-1987.
Italics denote recent trends not significant at 5 per cent level, or other figures which should be interpreted with caution (see Method).

NON-HODGKIN LYMPHOMA (ICD-9 200, 202)

OCEANIA, INCIDENCE

MALES

TRUNCATED RATE (30-74 years)

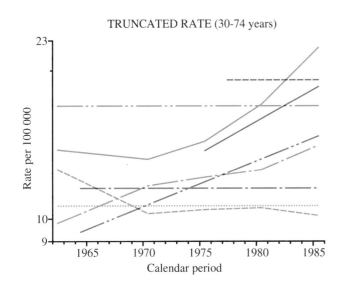

CUMULATIVE RISK (30-74 years)

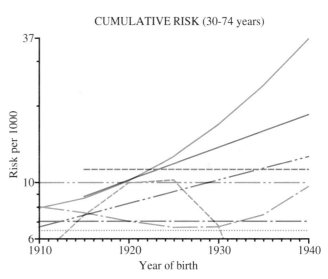

FEMALES

TRUNCATED RATE (30-74 years)

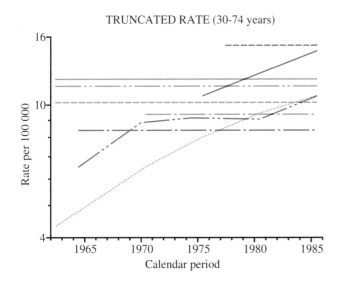

CUMULATIVE RISK (30-74 years)

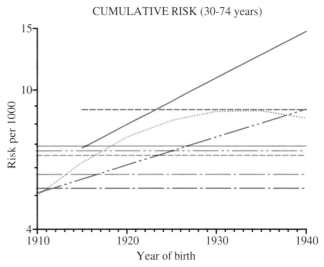

———— AUSTRALIA New South Wales
– – – – AUSTRALIA South
–·–·– NEW ZEALAND Maori
–··–··– NEW ZEALAND Non-Maori
———— HAWAII Caucasian

– – – – HAWAII Chinese
–·–·– HAWAII Filipino
–··–··– HAWAII Hawaiian
············ HAWAII Japanese

NON-HODGKIN LYMPHOMA (ICD-9 200, 202)

ASIA, INCIDENCE
Percentage change per five-year period, 1973-1987

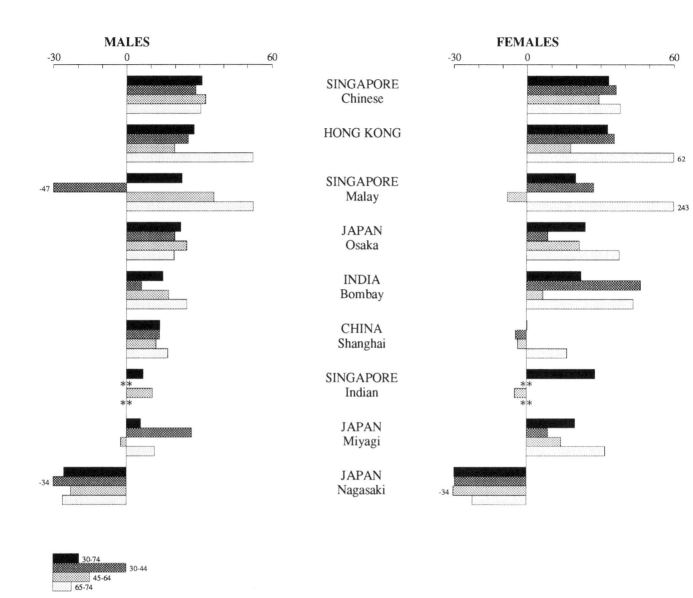

NON-HODGKIN LYMPHOMA (ICD-9 200, 202)

OCEANIA, INCIDENCE
Percentage change per five-year period, 1973-1987

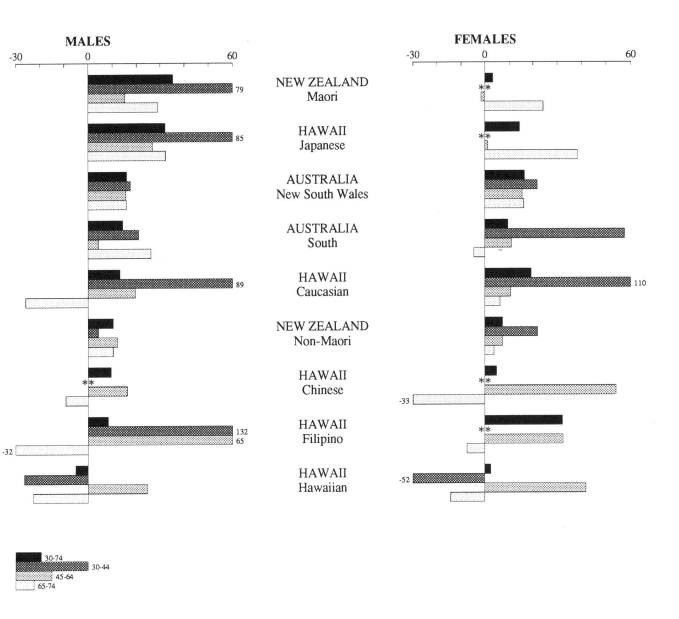

NON-HODGKIN LYMPHOMA (ICD-9 200, 202)

ASIA and OCEANIA, MORTALITY

MALES	Best model	Goodness of fit	1965 Rate	1965 Deaths	1985 Rate	1985 Deaths	Cumulative risk 1900	Cumulative risk 1940	Recent trend
AUSTRALIA	A2P3C2	1.48	7.1	174	8.7	321	3.9	5.8	14.1
HONG KONG	A1C2	1.03	*3.5*	*17*	5.7	56	*1.8*	4.4	*-3.4*
JAPAN	A8P6C9	-0.14	3.3	607	5.9	1733	1.7	4.3	6.0
MAURITIUS	A2	-0.09	*1.3*	*0*	1.3	1	*0.9*	0.9	*-36.0*
NEW ZEALAND	A3C2	3.56	7.0	37	6.9	51	4.3	3.8	*-0.3*
SINGAPORE	A1P4	0.07	4.6	8	6.6	19	*1.8*	6.0	–

FEMALES	Best model	Goodness of fit	1965 Rate	1965 Deaths	1985 Rate	1985 Deaths	Cumulative risk 1900	Cumulative risk 1940	Recent trend
AUSTRALIA	A3C2	1.50	4.7	124	6.1	248	2.8	4.0	10.4
HONG KONG	A1C2	0.53	*2.1*	*12*	3.4	31	*1.0*	2.4	*-0.6*
JAPAN	A4P3C3	3.02	1.7	344	3.0	1063	0.9	2.4	6.7
MAURITIUS	A1	-0.12	*0.7*	*0*	*0.7*	*0*	*0.4*	0.4	*21.9*
NEW ZEALAND	A4D	1.57	4.6	27	5.4	44	2.9	3.9	*-6.3*
SINGAPORE	A1D	1.10	2.0	3	3.2	9	*1.1*	2.7	–

* : not enough deaths for reliable estimation
– : incomplete or missing data
Best model: polynomial of the given degree in age (A), period (P) or cohort (C), or linear drift (D) model.
Goodness of fit: the normalised likelihood ratio chi-square for the best model (see Method).
Rate: world-standardised truncated rate per 100 000 per year (30-74 years) and number of **deaths** are both estimated from the best-fitting model for the single years cited.
Cumulative risk per 1000 (30-74 years) is estimated from the best-fitting *age-cohort* model for cohorts of central birth year cited.
Recent trend: estimated mean percentage change per five-year period in the age-specific rates (30-74 years) over the period 1975-1988.
Italics denote recent trends not significant at 5 per cent level, or other figures which should be interpreted with caution (see Method).

NON-HODGKIN LYMPHOMA (ICD-9 200, 202)

ASIA and OCEANIA, MORTALITY

MALES

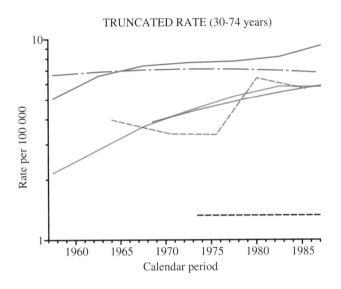

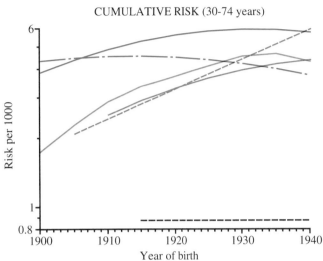

FEMALES

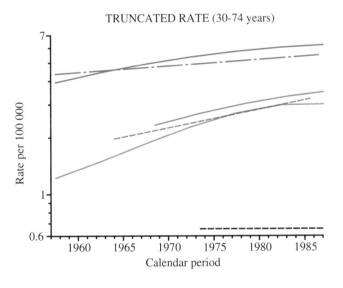

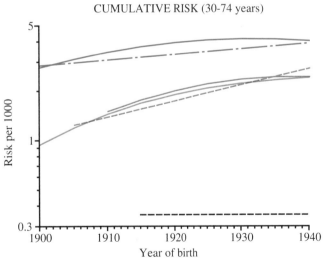

——— AUSTRALIA	——— HONG KONG
—·—·— NEW ZEALAND	- - - - SINGAPORE
——— JAPAN	- - - - MAURITIUS

NON-HODGKIN LYMPHOMA (ICD-9 200, 202)

ASIA and OCEANIA, MORTALITY
Percentage change per five-year period, 1975-1988

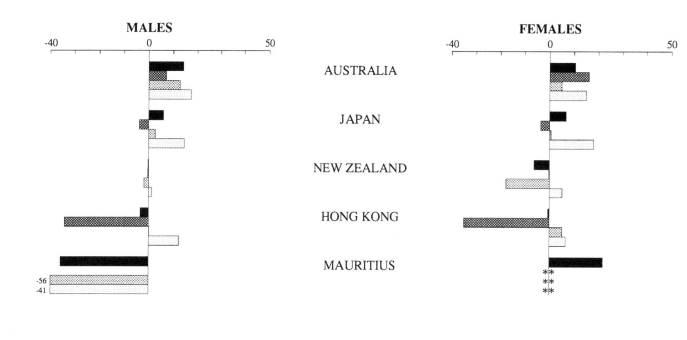

from page 641

is observed: an increase in mortality in both sexes, with a concurrent decline in incidence in Slovenia.

Asia and Oceania

The incidence of non-Hodgkin lymphoma is lower in Asian than in European populations, especially among Indians in Bombay and Singapore. Incidence has been increasing in most Asian and Caucasian populations, although trends among the ethnic groups in Hawaii with small populations are unstable. Incidence among Japanese has increased substantially in Osaka and Miyagi, particularly among females, and recent trends remain strongly positive at around 20% every five years. In Nagasaki, truncated incidence rates for the rubrics 200 and 202 combined were the highest on record for the period around 1975 in both males and females, at 22.4 and 13.0 per 100 000; incidence has fallen steadily since then at all ages in both sexes, at more than 25% (3 standard errors) every five years. Chinese populations in Shanghai (China), Hong Kong and Singapore mostly reflect rapid increases in incidence in

both sexes, at 15-30% every five years: females in Shanghai are an exception. In New Zealand, incidence of non-Hodgkin lymphoma was similar in non-Maoris and Maoris in the 1970s, but has diverged since, with an increase among non-Maoris; similar increases have been observed for both Australian populations, though the rise in South Australia does not quite reach significance.

Mortality in Australia is increasing somewhat less rapidly than incidence (10-14% versus 16% every five years), a pattern similar to that seen in Caucasian populations in Europe. For New Zealand, the overall trend is small, and the age-cohort model fits the data poorly. The age-specific trends are not significant, and mortality from lymphoma should be considered stable in this population.

Americas

Incidence has been increasing rapidly in most populations over much of the period since 1960. Recent rates of increase range from 15% to 50% every five years for Canadians of both sexes and US males, somewhat less for US females and for

662

Puerto Ricans. There is no systematic difference in the trends in the USA by race. In North America, cumulative risks (30-74 years) for the 1940 birth cohort range from 2% to 4% in males and 1% to 3% in females. Little change in incidence has occurred among South American males in São Paulo (Brazil), Cali (Colombia) or Cuba, though upward trends are seen among females in all these populations. Most data sets are fitted well by linear drift or period effects.

Mortality in Canada and the USA has increased too, but as elsewhere, much more slowly than incidence. Mortality in Chile and Venezuela has risen substantially from very low levels recorded in the 1960s, and is now approaching the rates observed in North America.

Comment

The patterns of increasing incidence and mortality from non-Hodgkin lymphoma reported here are coherent with previous reports from France[128], Slovakia[237], the UK, Singapore and the USA[77,84]. Barnes et al.[18] concluded, after extensive review of pathological specimens, that the increase in incidence over 20 years in Yorkshire (UK) was genuine, despite weaknesses in the registration data. Lee et al.[154] attributed the rapid increase in Singapore Chinese to a cohort effect, particularly in males, but speculated that improvements in diagnosis might be responsible. The brief report from Kingston and St Andrew (Jamaica)[42] concludes that there was no overall increase in lymphoma between 1958 and 1987, although in fact the data provided show that the world-standardised rate for non-Hodgkin lymphoma almost doubled in both sexes. Devesa et al.[77] showed that incidence in the USA more than doubled in both sexes between 1947 and 1987, especially in persons over 65 years of age, which they attributed partly to more aggressive diagnostic techniques in the elderly and to primary or acquired immunosuppression.

Although AIDS has undoubtedly increased the risk of certain types of non-Hodgkin lymphoma greatly in young US males[123,248], the increases reported here are very widespread, and they antedate the AIDS epidemic. A shift in the distribution of non-Hodgkin lymphoma sub-types toward higher-grade tumours with extra-nodal presentation has been observed during the period 1977-82 among young (20-49 years) males in Atlanta (USA), where AIDS was probably uncommon[32]. Eby et al.[92] showed that primary malignant lymphoma of brain in the USA, accounting for less than 1% of non-Hodgkin lymphoma, had increased more rapidly than lymphoma at all other sites, and that this was unlikely to be due to AIDS, better diagnosis or changes in classification. The increases in non-Hodgkin lymphoma are too large and too long-standing to be explained by AIDS[32] or by Epstein-Barr virus-associated lymphoma in immunosuppressed transplant recipients[83]; other causes should now be sought.

NON-HODGKIN LYMPHOMA (ICD-9 200, 202)

AMERICAS (except USA), INCIDENCE

MALES	Best model	Goodness of fit	1970 Rate	1970 Cases	1985 Rate	1985 Cases	Cumulative risk 1915	Cumulative risk 1940	Recent trend
BRAZIL									
Sao Paulo	A1	1.82	9.1	60	*9.1*	*75*	5.2	*5.2*	–
CANADA									
Alberta	A2C2	0.19	10.2	31	19.4	89	8.9	22.9	19.8
British Columbia	A2P2	0.11	14.0	65	21.4	151	9.4	23.9	30.5
Maritime Provinces	A2D	0.04	10.5	32	18.1	64	8.0	19.6	28.8
Newfoundland	A1P2	1.59	5.2	4	11.4	13	4.8	11.5	51.2
Quebec	A8P4C9	0.33	8.3	92	23.6	345	9.3	35.9	48.7
COLOMBIA									
Cali	A3	-1.09	7.9	6	7.9	13	4.3	4.3	*-13.6*
CUBA	A1P2	1.40	5.5	83	5.9	121	3.5	*3.6*	–
PUERTO RICO	A1D	0.56	6.4	29	11.1	74	5.0	12.5	16.6

FEMALES	Best model	Goodness of fit	1970 Rate	1970 Cases	1985 Rate	1985 Cases	Cumulative risk 1915	Cumulative risk 1940	Recent trend
BRAZIL									
Sao Paulo	A1D	0.06	6.1	42	*11.5*	*108*	5.1	*14.5*	–
CANADA									
Alberta	A3P4	2.85	7.5	22	14.0	67	6.5	18.2	15.8
British Columbia	A2P3	-0.13	11.8	56	14.8	115	7.0	13.9	20.8
Maritime Provinces	A1D	0.39	7.8	25	13.5	53	6.2	15.4	20.7
Newfoundland	A1D	0.01	4.0	3	7.8	9	3.3	9.8	50.7
Quebec	A2P3	1.19	6.0	73	17.5	294	7.1	30.1	45.0
COLOMBIA									
Cali	A1P2	1.64	4.6	3	8.8	15	3.7	6.3	57.1
CUBA	A8C7	-0.01	3.1	42	5.9	116	2.4	*3.8*	–
PUERTO RICO	A1P3	0.98	3.9	18	8.0	61	3.7	10.4	11.1

* : not enough cases for reliable estimation
– : incomplete or missing data
Best model: polynomial of the given degree in age (A), period (P) or cohort (C), or linear drift (D) model.
Goodness of fit: the normalised likelihood ratio chi-square for the best model (see Method).
Rate: world-standardised truncated rate per 100 000 per year (30-74 years) and number of **cases** are both estimated from the best-fitting model for the single years cited.
Cumulative risk per 1000 (30-74 years) is estimated from the best-fitting *age-cohort* model for cohorts of central birth year cited.
Recent trend: estimated mean percentage change per five-year period in the age-specific rates (30-74 years) over the period 1973-1987.
Italics denote recent trends not significant at 5 per cent level, or other figures which should be interpreted with caution (see Method).

NON-HODGKIN LYMPHOMA (ICD-9 200, 202)

AMERICAS (except USA), INCIDENCE

MALES

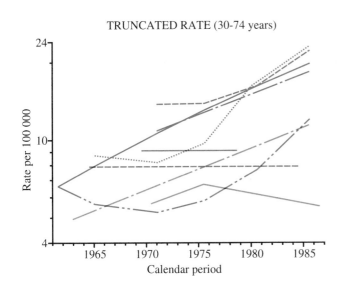

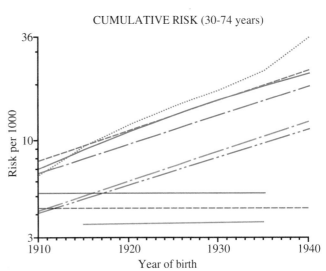

FEMALES

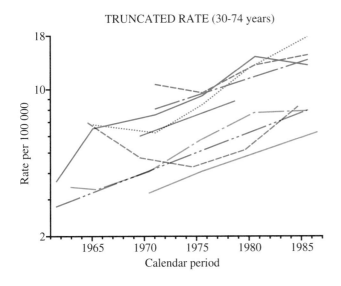

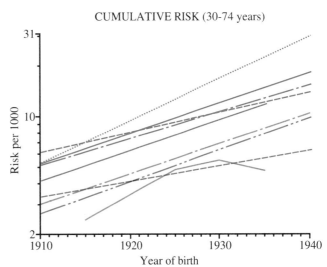

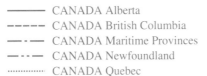

———— CANADA Alberta	———— CUBA
– – – – CANADA British Columbia	–·–·– PUERTO RICO
–··–··– CANADA Maritime Provinces	———— BRAZIL Sao Paulo
–···–···– CANADA Newfoundland	– – – – COLOMBIA Cali
············ CANADA Quebec	

AMERICAS (USA), INCIDENCE

MALES	Best model	Goodness of fit	1970 Rate	1970 Cases	1985 Rate	1985 Cases	Cumulative risk 1915	Cumulative risk 1940	Recent trend
USA									
Bay Area, Black	A1D	-0.10	10.4	5	18.4	15	8.1	21.0	21.9
Bay Area, Chinese	A1	-0.17	12.6	2	*12.6*	*6*	7.2	*7.2*	–
Bay Area, White	A8P3C8	2.05	17.4	103	29.6	190	11.0	38.3	40.8
Connecticut	A2C2	1.26	11.7	76	21.6	171	10.2	23.4	25.1
Detroit, Black	A1D	1.60	9.8	13	15.5	27	7.3	15.6	14.9
Detroit, White	A1C2	-1.07	11.4	84	25.0	178	11.2	36.7	26.0
Iowa	A2D	0.00	13.9	90	23.7	161	10.7	26.0	15.3
New Orleans, Black	A8D	0.82	*5.1*	*2*	15.1	9	4.2	25.6	46.4
New Orleans, White	A1D	0.52	*12.1*	*17*	22.8	35	11.0	31.3	23.0
Seattle	A2D	-0.41	*12.7*	*59*	24.9	166	10.5	31.8	25.7

FEMALES	Best model	Goodness of fit	1970 Rate	1970 Cases	1985 Rate	1985 Cases	Cumulative risk 1915	Cumulative risk 1940	Recent trend
USA									
Bay Area, Black	A1D	0.10	5.1	3	12.2	12	5.5	22.8	34.5
Bay Area, Chinese	A1	-0.09	9.3	1	*9.3*	*5*	5.2	*5.2*	–
Bay Area, White	A2D	0.81	11.4	79	17.0	121	8.4	16.2	15.1
Connecticut	A2D	0.95	8.8	67	17.0	156	7.7	22.8	18.6
Detroit, Black	A1C2	0.70	6.6	9	10.0	21	5.3	7.2	*9.8*
Detroit, White	A2D	1.10	9.1	75	18.0	150	8.1	25.1	22.6
Iowa	A3P3C2	0.18	8.3	61	15.6	126	8.8	13.3	6.7
New Orleans, Black	A1D	-0.82	*3.7*	*2*	9.2	7	3.0	13.5	*35.7*
New Orleans, White	A1	1.39	*14.9*	*29*	14.9	28	9.1	9.1	*11.8*
Seattle	A1D	1.56	*12.0*	*66*	15.6	116	8.2	12.5	10.1

* : not enough cases for reliable estimation
– : incomplete or missing data
Best model: polynomial of the given degree in age (A), period (P) or cohort (C), or linear drift (D) model.
Goodness of fit: the normalised likelihood ratio chi-square for the best model (see Method).
Rate: world-standardised truncated rate per 100 000 per year (30-74 years) and number of **cases** are both estimated from the best-fitting model for the single years cited.
Cumulative risk per 1000 (30-74 years) is estimated from the best-fitting *age-cohort* model for cohorts of central birth year cited.
Recent trend: estimated mean percentage change per five-year period in the age-specific rates (30-74 years) over the period 1973-1987.
Italics denote recent trends not significant at 5 per cent level, or other figures which should be interpreted with caution (see Method).

NON-HODGKIN LYMPHOMA (ICD-9 200, 202)

AMERICAS (USA), INCIDENCE

MALES

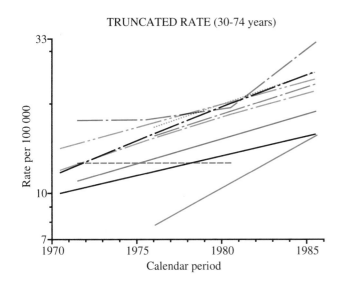

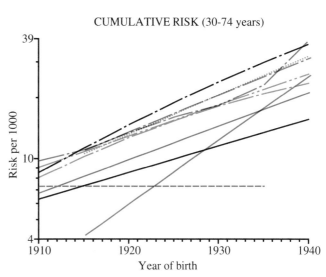

FEMALES

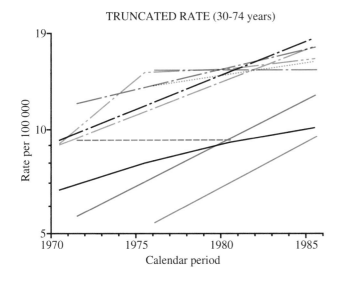

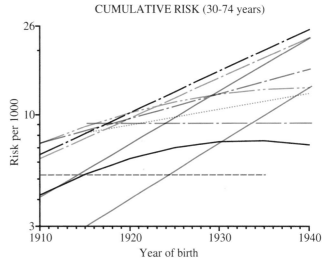

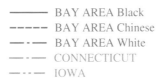

——— BAY AREA Black	·········· SEATTLE
– – – BAY AREA Chinese	——— NEW ORLEANS Black
–·–·– BAY AREA White	–··–··– NEW ORLEANS White
–··–··– CONNECTICUT	——— DETROIT Black
–···–···– IOWA	–·–·– DETROIT White

AMERICAS (except USA), INCIDENCE
Percentage change per five-year period, 1973-1987

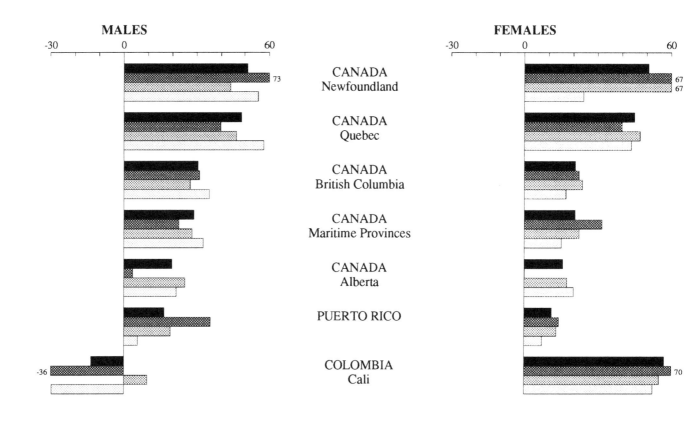

NON-HODGKIN LYMPHOMA (ICD-9 200, 202)

AMERICAS (USA), INCIDENCE
Percentage change per five-year period, 1973-1987

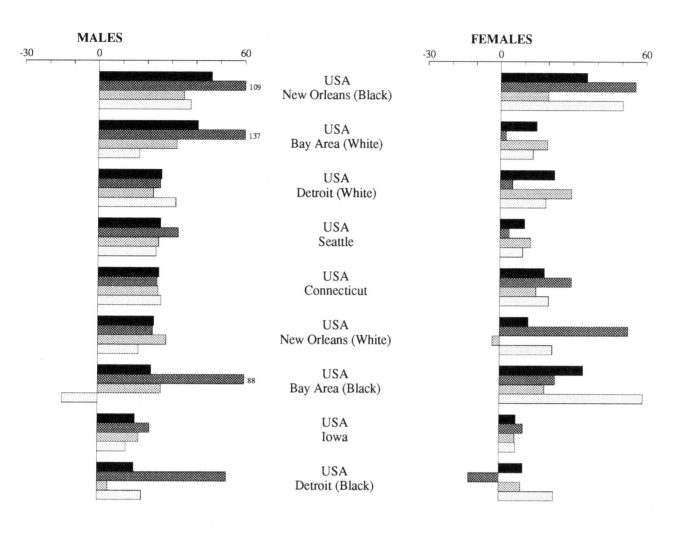

NON-HODGKIN LYMPHOMA (ICD-9 200, 202)

AMERICAS, MORTALITY

MALES	Best model	Goodness of fit	1965 Rate	1965 Deaths	1985 Rate	1985 Deaths	Cumulative risk 1900	Cumulative risk 1940	Recent trend
CANADA	A3P3C2	0.57	6.9	267	8.6	502	3.9	5.6	9.4
CHILE	A1P2	-0.67	3.5	42	*4.5*	*84*	1.8	*6.9*	–
COSTA RICA	–	–	–	–	–	–	–	–	–
PANAMA	*	..	..	..	..	..	..	..	..
PUERTO RICO	–	–	–	–	–	–	–	–	–
URUGUAY	–	–	–	–	–	–	–	–	–
USA	–	–	–	–	–	–	–	–	–
VENEZUELA	A2P2	-0.82	3.0	30	*2.4*	*46*	1.3	*3.9*	–

FEMALES	Best model	Goodness of fit	1965 Rate	1965 Deaths	1985 Rate	1985 Deaths	Cumulative risk 1900	Cumulative risk 1940	Recent trend
CANADA	A3C2	2.01	4.7	186	5.8	386	2.9	3.8	7.3
CHILE	A2D	-0.48	1.8	23	*4.5*	*94*	0.9	*5.7*	–
COSTA RICA	–	–	–	–	–	–	–	–	–
PANAMA	*	..	..	..	..	..	..	..	..
PUERTO RICO	–	–	–	–	–	–	–	–	–
URUGUAY	–	–	–	–	–	–	–	–	–
USA	–	–	–	–	–	–	–	–	–
VENEZUELA	A1P2C2	-0.59	2.5	24	*1.5*	*26*	1.1	*2.1*	–

* : not enough deaths for reliable estimation
– : incomplete or missing data
Best model: polynomial of the given degree in age (A), period (P) or cohort (C), or linear drift (D) model.
Goodness of fit: the normalised likelihood ratio chi-square for the best model (see Method).
Rate: world-standardised truncated rate per 100 000 per year (30-74 years) and number of **deaths** are both estimated from the best-fitting model for the single years cited.
Cumulative risk per 1000 (30-74 years) is estimated from the best-fitting *age-cohort* model for cohorts of central birth year cited.
Recent trend: estimated mean percentage change per five-year period in the age-specific rates (30-74 years) over the period 1975-1988.
Italics denote recent trends not significant at 5 per cent level, or other figures which should be interpreted with caution (see Method).

NON-HODGKIN LYMPHOMA (ICD-9 200, 202)

AMERICAS, MORTALITY

MALES

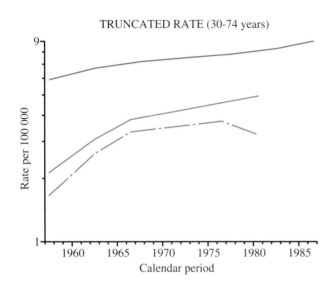

TRUNCATED RATE (30-74 years)

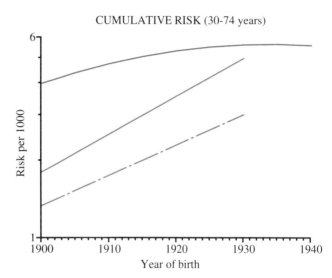

CUMULATIVE RISK (30-74 years)

FEMALES

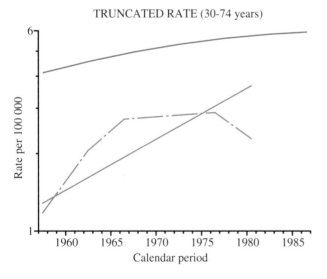

TRUNCATED RATE (30-74 years)

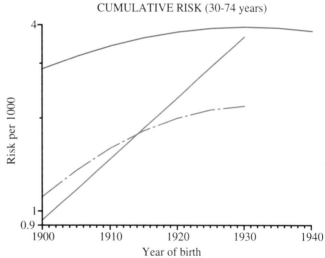

CUMULATIVE RISK (30-74 years)

———— CANADA
———— CHILE
—·—·— VENEZUELA

NON-HODGKIN LYMPHOMA (ICD-9 200, 202)

AMERICAS, MORTALITY
Percentage change per five-year period, 1975-1988

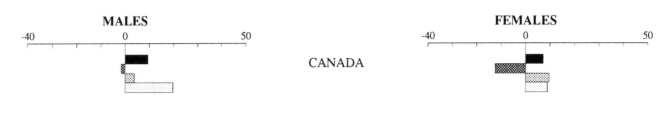

672

Chapter 27

HODGKIN'S DISEASE

Hodgkin's disease is an uncommon lymphoma, morphologically distinguishable from other types of lymphoma by the Reed-Sternberg cell. The age-incidence is unusual, and resembles that of testicular cancer[210]. It occurs in childhood, mainly in developing countries, but in developed countries there is a marked peak in young adults (15-34 years), among whom it is one of the most frequent malignancies. There is a further increase in incidence after the age of 65 years. Classification of the various sub-types of Hodgkin's disease has undergone several revisions since the 1940s. The clinical behaviour and the distribution of sub-types vary greatly with age, and it is likely that Hodgkin's disease comprises two or more aetiologically distinct entities. Incidence varies more than 10-fold, being highest in north Italian populations[221] and lowest in Asian populations, and it is usually greater in males than females. Survival has improved dramatically, particularly in younger patients, with the advent of intensive radiotherapy and chemotherapy around 1970; for example, five-year survival in Scotland increased from less than 30% to 70% or more[46].

For the period 1963-65 (volume II), data on Hodgkin's disease for Connecticut (USA) were included with those for other lymphomas in a single category, and were thus excluded from analysis; the data for 1960-62, presented separately, were included.

Europe

With few exceptions, Hodgkin's disease incidence in Europe is either stable or declining. The highest incidence in Europe in both sexes is seen in Varese (Italy), where, in common with most southern European populations, there has been no significant change in incidence since the mid-1970s. Incidence has been declining steadily since the 1960s in the Nordic countries, and to a lesser extent in Germany and Slovenia. Almost everywhere in Europe, however, increases have been more rapid (or declines less rapid) in younger (15-44 years) than in older subjects, suggesting a shift to the left in the age-incidence curve, or an increase in the relative importance of the young adult form of the disease.

Mortality from Hodgkin's disease has declined dramatically in most parts of Europe since about 1970, with the notable exception of Hungary, Poland and Romania, where there has been little change. Mortality in Czechoslovakia has been falling as rapidly as in western and northern Europe, in contrast to the pattern for most other neoplasms, including non-Hodgkin lymphoma, for which mortality trends in Czechoslovakia are similar to those in Hungary, Poland and Romania. The aberrant peak in mortality in Switzerland in the late 1970s is seen at all ages, and is the converse of that for non-Hodgkin lymphoma (*q.v.*); it is undoubtedly an artefact. The rapid increase in mortality from Hodgkin's disease in Yugoslavia between 1970 and 1985 also appears implausible; incidence rates in Slovenia are in the same range as elsewhere in Europe, and show a continuing decline. Comparison of the age-specific mortality trends for both Hodgkin's disease and non-Hodgkin lymphoma suggests that change in death certification practice may be partly responsible for the discrepancy, with compensating shifts from non-Hodgkin lymphoma to Hodgkin's disease.

Asia and Oceania

Hodgkin's disease is notably less frequent among the nine Asian populations studied than in Europe or North America, with cumulative risks (15-74 years) of 1 per 1000 or less. Incidence has generally been stable in females since 1970. The sharp decline among females in Nagasaki (Japan) is significant, but it depends on very few cases in any five-year period in the age range 15-74 years (3 cases in 1983-87). It should be considered less reliable than the trends in Miyagi and Osaka (Japan), where there has been an increase in incidence among 15-44 year-olds and a decline among older persons. This is reflected in a recent deceleration of the rate of decline in incidence. The cumulative risk (15-74 years) in Miyagi and Osaka is now low (0.2 per 1000), but there is evidence of an increase in risk for those born since 1940-45. This is shown in the cohort risk curves, which incorporate data from much of the early peak in incidence (15-44 years; data up to 1987 for cohort born in 1950). The peak of incidence in 1975 among males in Bombay (India) appears odd: it was not seen in females, and does not seem due to mis-classification of non-Hodgkin lymphoma,

673

continued page 694

EUROPE (non-EC), INCIDENCE

MALES	Best model	Goodness of fit	1970 Rate	1970 Cases	1985 Rate	1985 Cases	Cumulative risk 1915	Cumulative risk 1950	Recent trend
FINLAND	A4P2	1.83	3.7	60	3.2	59	2.4	2.3	*-5.5*
HUNGARY									
County Vas	A0	1.82	3.0	3	3.0	2	1.8	1.8	*39.2*
Szabolcs-Szatmar	A1P3	1.85	2.9	5	1.8	3	1.2	1.4	*-9.9*
ISRAEL									
All Jews	A1C2	0.10	3.1	25	3.5	37	1.9	2.3	*4.9*
Non-Jews	A3D	-1.61	3.7	3	2.4	4	3.3	1.2	*-3.4*
NORWAY	A4P2	1.54	3.7	53	2.8	44	2.5	1.7	-11.8
POLAND									
Warsaw City	A1P3	2.17	2.1	10	2.6	15	2.0	1.9	*-13.9*
ROMANIA									
Cluj	A2	0.77	*2.1*	*5*	2.1	5	1.4	1.4	*-20.7*
SWEDEN	A9P5C9	0.18	3.9	126	2.4	78	3.0	1.7	-18.4
SWITZERLAND									
Geneva	A0	1.01	3.9	4	3.9	5	2.4	2.4	*3.5*
YUGOSLAVIA									
Slovenia	A1P3	1.91	3.4	20	2.7	18	2.0	1.7	*6.9*

FEMALES	Best model	Goodness of fit	1970 Rate	1970 Cases	1985 Rate	1985 Cases	Cumulative risk 1915	Cumulative risk 1950	Recent trend
FINLAND	A4P2	0.65	2.3	41	2.0	39	1.4	1.6	*-7.8*
HUNGARY									
County Vas	A0	-1.51	2.2	2	2.2	2	1.3	1.3	*14.3*
Szabolcs-Szatmar	A0	0.04	1.3	2	1.3	2	0.8	0.8	*-20.5*
ISRAEL									
All Jews	A9P4C9	-1.03	3.3	27	3.0	34	1.8	1.6	*-0.4*
Non-Jews	A0	0.16	1.4	1	1.4	2	0.8	0.8	*-2.7*
NORWAY	A3P2	0.26	2.5	36	1.6	26	1.7	1.0	-16.9
POLAND									
Warsaw City	A4C2	-0.79	2.3	13	2.4	14	1.5	1.1	*-2.6*
ROMANIA									
Cluj	A0	0.52	*1.4*	*3*	1.4	3	0.8	0.8	*1.5*
SWEDEN	A4C3	1.37	2.3	76	2.0	68	1.9	1.0	-10.0
SWITZERLAND									
Geneva	A3	2.00	2.3	3	2.3	3	1.3	1.3	*9.5*
YUGOSLAVIA									
Slovenia	A2P2C2	3.02	2.1	14	1.5	10	1.1	0.9	*-4.1*

* : not enough cases for reliable estimation
− : incomplete or missing data
Best model: polynomial of the given degree in age (A), period (P) or cohort (C), or linear drift (D) model.
Goodness of fit: the normalised likelihood ratio chi-square for the best model (see Method).
Rate: world-standardised truncated rate per 100 000 per year (15-74 years) and number of **cases** are both estimated from the best-fitting model for the single years cited.
Cumulative risk per 1000 (15-74 years) is estimated from the best-fitting *age-cohort* model for cohorts of central birth year cited.
Recent trend: estimated mean percentage change per five-year period in the age-specific rates (15-74 years) over the period 1973-1987.
Italics denote recent trends not significant at 5 per cent level, or other figures which should be interpreted with caution (see Method).

674

HODGKIN'S DISEASE (ICD-9 201)

EUROPE (non-EC), INCIDENCE

MALES

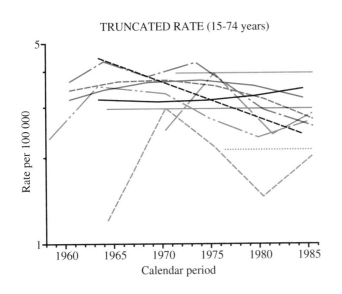

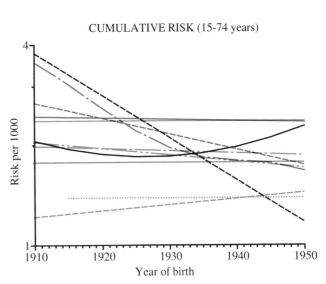

FEMALES

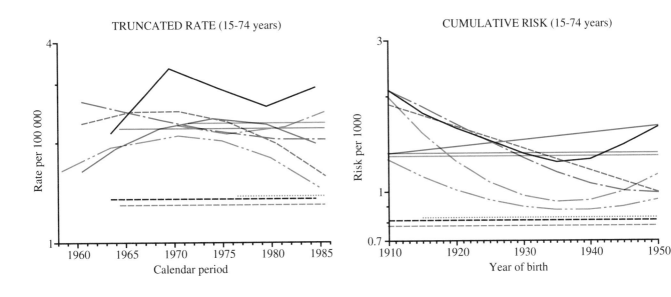

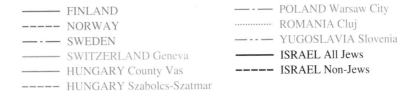

FINLAND

NORWAY

SWEDEN

SWITZERLAND Geneva

HUNGARY County Vas

HUNGARY Szabolcs-Szatmar

POLAND Warsaw City

ROMANIA Cluj

YUGOSLAVIA Slovenia

ISRAEL All Jews

ISRAEL Non-Jews

HODGKIN'S DISEASE (ICD-9 201)

EUROPE (EC), INCIDENCE

MALES	Best model	Goodness of fit	1970 Rate	1970 Cases	1985 Rate	1985 Cases	Cumulative risk 1915	Cumulative risk 1950	Recent trend
DENMARK	*	..	..	..	..	..	..	..	..
FRANCE									
Bas-Rhin	A0	2.62	*3.8*	*12*	3.8	12	2.3	2.3	*4.5*
Doubs	A0	0.01	*3.3*	*5*	3.3	5	2.0	2.0	*7.9*
GERMANY (FRG)									
Hamburg	A1P2	1.98	5.3	35	*1.4*	*8*	3.3	2.0	–
Saarland	A3	0.45	3.6	13	3.6	14	2.4	2.4	*-3.0*
GERMANY (GDR)	A4P3C5	2.04	4.0	237	3.8	219	2.6	2.0	6.1
ITALY									
Varese	A1	-0.18	*5.4*	*13*	5.4	16	3.5	3.5	*-7.5*
SPAIN									
Navarra	A0	2.89	*4.1*	*6*	4.1	7	2.5	2.5	*10.4*
Zaragoza	A3P3	0.31	1.9	5	4.7	14	1.8	4.8	*-4.5*
UK									
Birmingham	A9C9	-1.33	3.6	66	3.6	70	2.4	2.2	*-4.0*
Scotland	A9C9	1.00	3.6	65	3.8	70	2.2	2.4	*-5.0*
South Thames	A5C4	2.32	3.5	108	3.8	91	2.0	2.5	*-0.2*

FEMALES	Best model	Goodness of fit	1970 Rate	1970 Cases	1985 Rate	1985 Cases	Cumulative risk 1915	Cumulative risk 1950	Recent trend
DENMARK	*	..	..	..	..	..	..	..	..
FRANCE									
Bas-Rhin	A0	1.68	*2.7*	*8*	2.7	9	1.6	1.6	*-7.8*
Doubs	A0	0.18	*2.8*	*4*	2.8	4	1.7	1.7	*-7.9*
GERMANY (FRG)									
Hamburg	A4P3	-0.64	3.4	26	*77.6*	*505*	2.7	1.1	–
Saarland	A0P3	0.11	1.2	5	2.1	9	0.8	2.1	*5.9*
GERMANY (GDR)	A4P3C5	1.82	2.5	180	2.6	169	1.8	1.2	*2.5*
ITALY									
Varese	A5	-0.03	*3.6*	*8*	3.6	11	2.2	2.2	*8.5*
SPAIN									
Navarra	A0	0.27	*1.5*	*2*	1.5	2	0.9	0.9	*-8.0*
Zaragoza	A1P3	2.12	1.1	3	3.9	12	1.2	1.7	*-14.8*
UK									
Birmingham	A4P2C2	0.43	2.3	43	2.1	41	1.2	1.5	-11.3
Scotland	A4P3C4	-0.35	2.9	59	2.8	55	1.6	2.0	*-3.8*
South Thames	A6P2C3	0.26	2.3	75	2.3	54	1.4	1.2	*-3.9*

* : not enough cases for reliable estimation
– : incomplete or missing data
Best model: polynomial of the given degree in age (A), period (P) or cohort (C), or linear drift (D) model.
Goodness of fit: the normalised likelihood ratio chi-square for the best model (see Method).
Rate: world-standardised truncated rate per 100 000 per year (15-74 years) and number of **cases** are both estimated from the best-fitting model for the single years cited.
Cumulative risk per 1000 (15-74 years) is estimated from the best-fitting *age-cohort* model for cohorts of central birth year cited.
Recent trend: estimated mean percentage change per five-year period in the age-specific rates (15-74 years) over the period 1973-1987.
Italics denote recent trends not significant at 5 per cent level, or other figures which should be interpreted with caution (see Method).

HODGKIN'S DISEASE (ICD-9 201)

EUROPE (EC), INCIDENCE

MALES

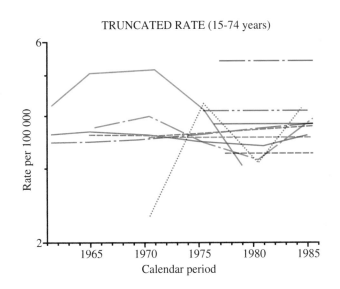

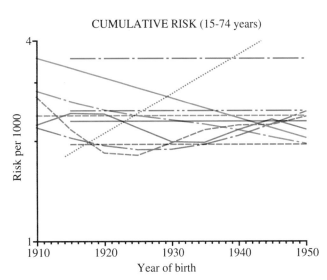

FEMALES

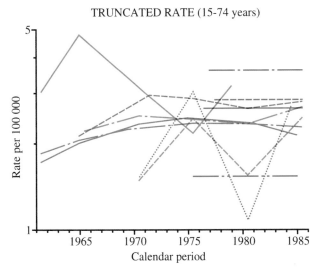

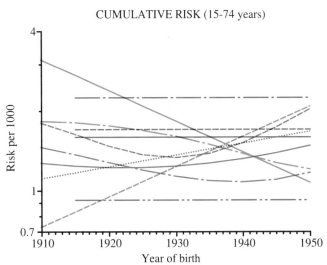

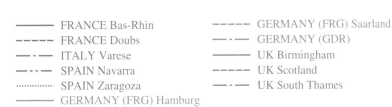

—— FRANCE Bas-Rhin	— — — GERMANY (FRG) Saarland
– – – FRANCE Doubs	—·— GERMANY (GDR)
—··— ITALY Varese	—— UK Birmingham
—·— SPAIN Navarra	— — — UK Scotland
········ SPAIN Zaragoza	—·— UK South Thames
—— GERMANY (FRG) Hamburg	

HODGKIN'S DISEASE (ICD-9 201)

EUROPE (non-EC), INCIDENCE
Percentage change per five-year period, 1973-1987

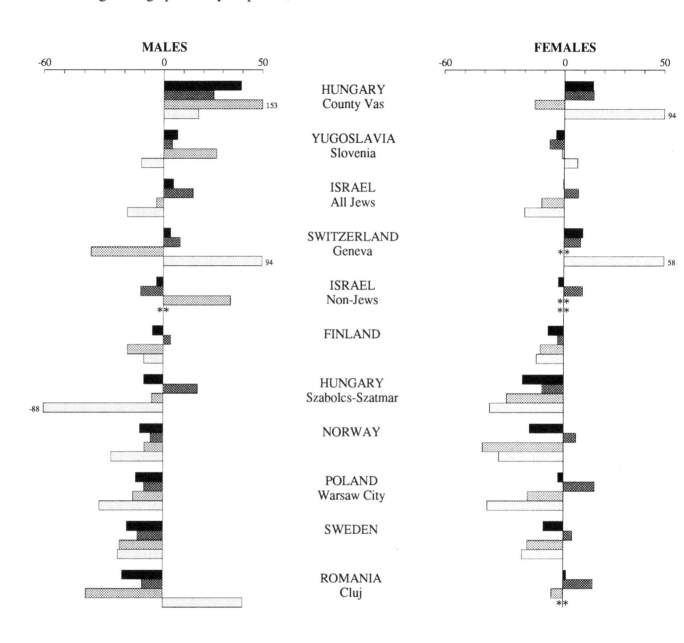

HODGKIN'S DISEASE (ICD-9 201)

EUROPE (EC), INCIDENCE
Percentage change per five-year period, 1973-1987

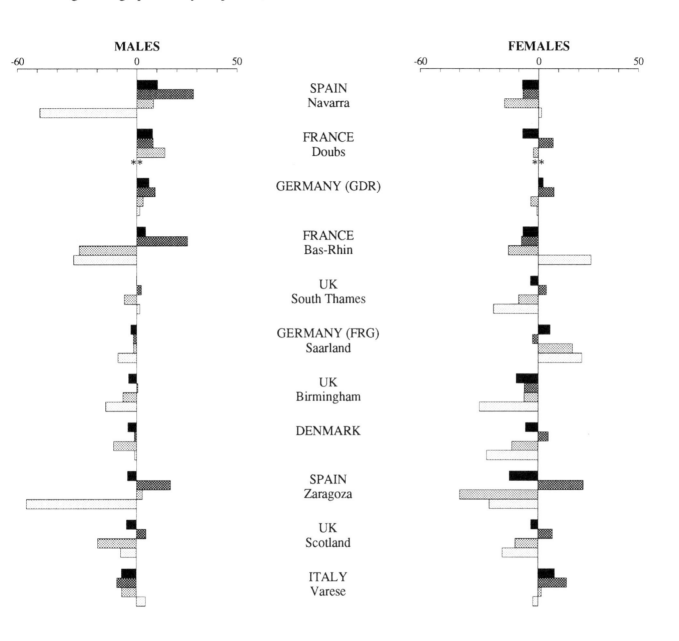

HODGKIN'S DISEASE (ICD-9 201)

EUROPE (non-EC), MORTALITY

MALES	Best model	Goodness of fit	1965 Rate	1965 Deaths	1985 Rate	1985 Deaths	Cumulative risk 1900	Cumulative risk 1950	Recent trend
AUSTRIA	A5P5	2.17	3.3	87	1.8	49	3.1	0.8	*-8.0*
CZECHOSLOVAKIA	A4P3C8	1.43	4.1	214	2.1	115	3.8	0.9	-12.2
FINLAND	A4P2C4	-0.27	2.8	41	1.4	26	3.0	0.8	-20.9
HUNGARY	A1D	-0.24	*1.2*	*44*	1.5	62	*0.8*	1.6	14.0
NORWAY	A3P2C2	0.20	2.6	37	1.0	16	2.9	0.4	-33.2
POLAND	A5C2	0.86	2.2	218	2.1	269	1.4	1.3	–
ROMANIA	A2	1.40	*1.6*	*102*	*1.6*	*128*	*1.1*	1.1	–
SWEDEN	A4P2C2	-1.34	2.7	84	0.8	31	3.2	0.4	-34.0
SWITZERLAND	A7P6C4	0.92	3.3	69	0.9	24	2.7	1.1	-45.8
YUGOSLAVIA	A9P5C9	1.32	1.7	103	2.9	238	1.0	3.5	*-2.8*

FEMALES	Best model	Goodness of fit	1965 Rate	1965 Deaths	1985 Rate	1985 Deaths	Cumulative risk 1900	Cumulative risk 1950	Recent trend
AUSTRIA	A4P3C2	-0.10	2.1	67	0.9	29	2.4	0.4	-13.8
CZECHOSLOVAKIA	A4P3C2	0.07	2.2	126	1.1	70	2.0	0.5	-15.9
FINLAND	A3P2C4	0.17	1.4	25	0.6	13	1.2	0.4	-34.7
HUNGARY	A4D	0.07	*0.6*	*26*	0.9	44	*0.4*	1.2	21.9
NORWAY	A4P2C3	0.41	1.8	27	0.5	8	2.6	0.2	-33.3
POLAND	A6P4C2	0.35	1.2	131	1.1	159	0.6	0.7	–
ROMANIA	A4C2	-0.41	*0.8*	*62*	*0.8*	*69*	*0.8*	0.5	–
SWEDEN	A4P2	0.85	1.5	50	0.5	20	1.9	0.3	-30.6
SWITZERLAND	A4P6C3	1.69	1.9	44	0.5	14	1.7	0.6	-49.4
YUGOSLAVIA	A9P5C9	0.24	1.1	72	1.6	144	0.5	2.1	*-5.3*

∗ : not enough deaths for reliable estimation
– : incomplete or missing data
Best model: polynomial of the given degree in age (A), period (P) or cohort (C), or linear drift (D) model.
Goodness of fit: the normalised likelihood ratio chi-square for the best model (see Method).
Rate: world-standardised truncated rate per 100 000 per year (15-74 years) and number of **deaths** are both estimated from the best-fitting model for the single years cited.
Cumulative risk per 1000 (15-74 years) is estimated from the best-fitting *age-cohort* model for cohorts of central birth year cited.
Recent trend: estimated mean percentage change per five-year period in the age-specific rates (15-74 years) over the period 1975-1988.
Italics denote recent trends not significant at 5 per cent level, or other figures which should be interpreted with caution (see Method).

HODGKIN'S DISEASE (ICD-9 201)

EUROPE (non-EC), MORTALITY

MALES

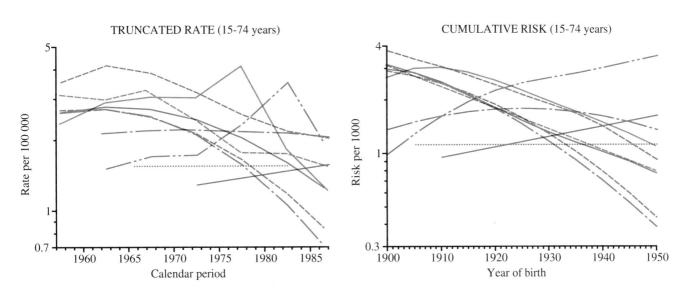

TRUNCATED RATE (15-74 years)

CUMULATIVE RISK (15-74 years)

FEMALES

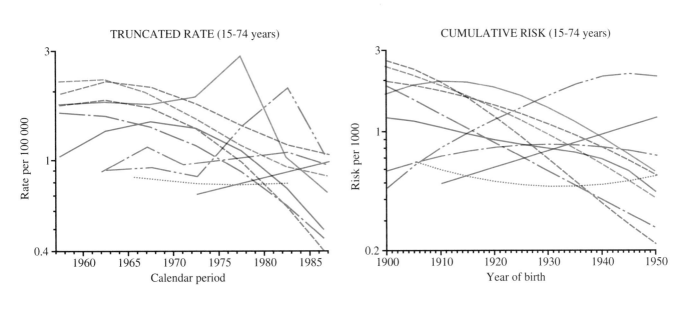

TRUNCATED RATE (15-74 years)

CUMULATIVE RISK (15-74 years)

——— FINLAND	– – – – CZECHOSLOVAKIA	
– – – NORWAY	——— HUNGARY	
– · – · SWEDEN	– · – · POLAND	
– – – AUSTRIA	· · · · · · ROMANIA	
——— SWITZERLAND	– ·· – ·· YUGOSLAVIA	

EUROPE (EC), MORTALITY

MALES	Best model	Goodness of fit	1965 Rate	1965 Deaths	1985 Rate	1985 Deaths	Cumulative risk 1900	Cumulative risk 1950	Recent trend
BELGIUM	A4C2	0.43	3.1	111	1.8	72	3.0	0.8	*-7.4*
DENMARK	A5P3C2	1.39	3.4	59	1.1	23	3.9	0.5	-14.8
FRANCE	A6P2C4	3.96	2.2	392	1.1	222	2.2	0.6	-21.8
GERMANY (FRG)	A5P6C4	6.16	3.0	666	1.6	389	2.8	0.8	-18.7
GREECE	A1P4C4	-0.24	2.1	61	1.6	65	*2.3*	1.2	-21.0
IRELAND	A2C2	0.84	2.8	28	1.9	22	2.3	0.9	*-9.3*
ITALY	A4P2C5	1.41	3.4	646	1.7	382	3.0	0.9	-26.0
NETHERLANDS	A4P3C3	1.58	3.2	133	1.3	72	3.2	0.5	-13.9
PORTUGAL	–	–	–	–	–	–	–	–	–
SPAIN	A4P2C4	0.07	1.8	192	1.1	158	1.3	0.9	-17.9
UK ENGLAND & WALES	A5P4C6	1.24	2.8	494	1.3	250	2.9	0.7	-23.3
UK SCOTLAND	A4P3	-0.18	3.4	63	1.1	21	3.9	0.6	-17.5

FEMALES	Best model	Goodness of fit	1965 Rate	1965 Deaths	1985 Rate	1985 Deaths	Cumulative risk 1900	Cumulative risk 1950	Recent trend
BELGIUM	A4C3	0.97	1.6	62	1.0	42	1.6	0.5	*-5.6*
DENMARK	A4P2C2	2.01	1.8	33	0.5	10	3.1	0.2	-27.8
FRANCE	A9P6C9	0.92	1.3	245	0.6	123	1.7	0.3	-26.6
GERMANY (FRG)	A4P5C2	4.60	1.7	445	1.0	286	1.4	0.4	-18.1
GREECE	A4C2	1.15	1.3	41	0.8	36	*1.2*	0.4	-27.3
IRELAND	A6P2C2	0.57	1.6	16	0.7	9	1.3	0.4	-26.2
ITALY	A4P2C4	3.52	2.0	412	1.0	237	1.9	0.6	-27.4
NETHERLANDS	A6P4C2	0.42	1.7	74	0.6	37	2.1	0.3	-17.0
PORTUGAL	–	–	–	–	–	–	–	–	–
SPAIN	A4P2	2.20	0.8	102	0.6	90	0.6	0.5	-11.7
UK ENGLAND & WALES	A5P2C4	1.14	1.4	283	0.7	145	1.5	0.4	-21.8
UK SCOTLAND	A4P2	-0.78	1.7	35	0.8	16	1.6	0.5	-25.9

* : not enough deaths for reliable estimation
– : incomplete or missing data
Best model: polynomial of the given degree in age (A), period (P) or cohort (C), or linear drift (D) model.
Goodness of fit: the normalised likelihood ratio chi-square for the best model (see Method).
Rate: world-standardised truncated rate per 100 000 per year (15-74 years) and number of **deaths** are both estimated from the best-fitting model for the single years cited.
Cumulative risk per 1000 (15-74 years) is estimated from the best-fitting *age-cohort* model for cohorts of central birth year cited.
Recent trend: estimated mean percentage change per five-year period in the age-specific rates (15-74 years) over the period 1975-1988.
Italics denote recent trends not significant at 5 per cent level, or other figures which should be interpreted with caution (see Method).

HODGKIN'S DISEASE (ICD-9 201)

EUROPE (EC), MORTALITY

MALES

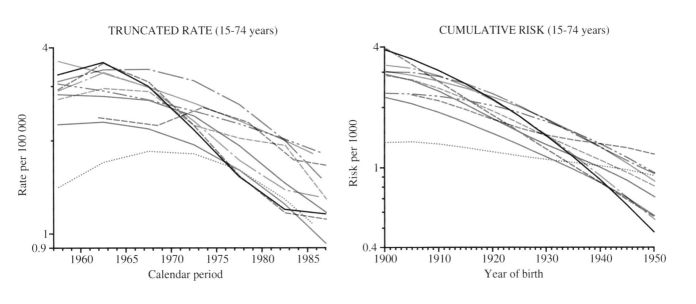

TRUNCATED RATE (15-74 years)

CUMULATIVE RISK (15-74 years)

FEMALES

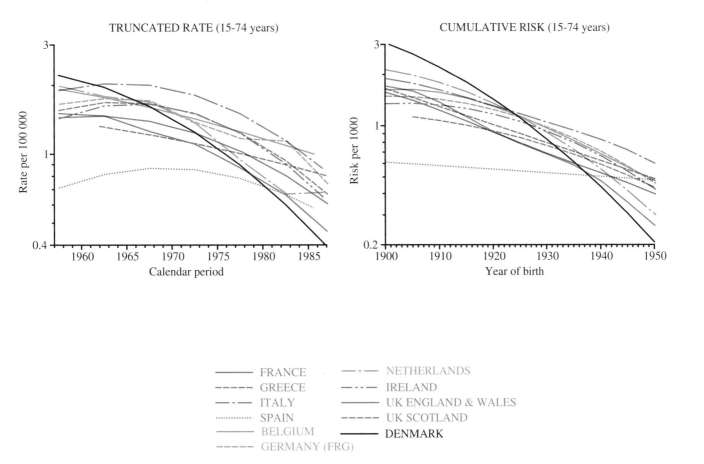

TRUNCATED RATE (15-74 years)

CUMULATIVE RISK (15-74 years)

FRANCE   NETHERLANDS
GREECE   IRELAND
ITALY   UK ENGLAND & WALES
SPAIN   UK SCOTLAND
BELGIUM   DENMARK
GERMANY (FRG)

HODGKIN'S DISEASE (ICD-9 201)

EUROPE (non-EC), MORTALITY
Percentage change per five-year period, 1975-1988

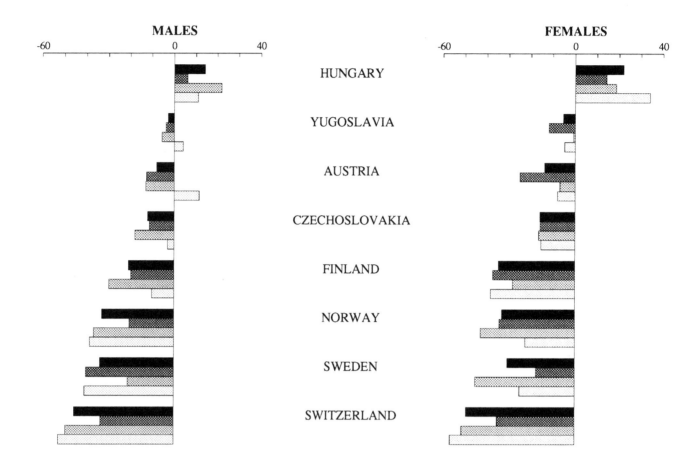

MALES

-60   0   40

FEMALES

-60   0   40

HUNGARY

YUGOSLAVIA

AUSTRIA

CZECHOSLOVAKIA

FINLAND

NORWAY

SWEDEN

SWITZERLAND

15-74
15-44
45-64
65-74

HODGKIN'S DISEASE (ICD-9 201)

EUROPE (EC), MORTALITY
Percentage change per five-year period, 1975-1988

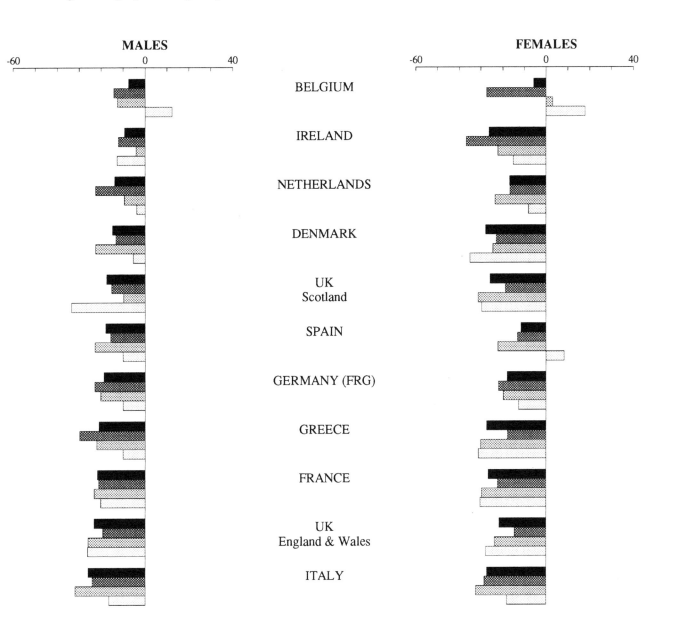

MALES

FEMALES

-60   0   40

-60   0   40

BELGIUM

IRELAND

NETHERLANDS

DENMARK

UK
Scotland

SPAIN

GERMANY (FRG)

GREECE

FRANCE

UK
England & Wales

ITALY

15-74
15-44
45-64
65-74

HODGKIN'S DISEASE (ICD-9 201)

ASIA, INCIDENCE

MALES	Best model	Goodness of fit	1970 Rate	1970 Cases	1985 Rate	1985 Cases	Cumulative risk 1915	Cumulative risk 1950	Recent trend
CHINA									
Shanghai	A1C3	0.75	*1.6*	*28*	0.4	10	7.8	0.1	-40.6
HONG KONG	A1D	1.07	*1.2*	*13*	0.6	13	1.2	0.3	-20.3
INDIA									
Bombay	A9P4	0.64	1.0	18	1.1	31	0.8	1.2	-15.4
JAPAN									
Miyagi	A1C3	0.74	0.7	4	0.6	4	0.7	0.2	*-9.0*
Nagasaki	A1	-0.53	*1.1*	*1*	1.1	1	1.1	1.1	*-33.9*
Osaka	A1C3	1.00	1.0	20	0.6	18	0.9	0.2	*-12.7*
SINGAPORE									
Chinese	A3	0.62	0.9	3	0.9	5	0.8	0.8	*-8.0*
Indian	A0	-0.34	*1.3*	*0*	*1.3*	*0*	0.8	0.8	*-11.1*
Malay	A1	0.27	*1.2*	*0*	1.2	1	0.9	0.9	*42.1*

FEMALES	Best model	Goodness of fit	1970 Rate	1970 Cases	1985 Rate	1985 Cases	Cumulative risk 1915	Cumulative risk 1950	Recent trend
CHINA									
Shanghai	A9C8	0.26	*	*	0.2	7	21.4	0.1	-44.7
HONG KONG	A1	1.11	*0.5*	5	0.5	9	0.4	0.4	*-12.4*
INDIA									
Bombay	A5	1.20	0.7	7	0.7	13	0.5	0.5	*-12.7*
JAPAN									
Miyagi	A2C5	-0.29	0.3	2	0.4	3	0.4	0.2	*7.2*
Nagasaki	A1D	0.45	*2.5*	*4*	*0.3*	*0*	8.2	0.1	-51.6
Osaka	A3	0.90	0.3	8	0.3	11	0.3	0.3	-19.1
SINGAPORE									
Chinese	A1	0.00	0.4	1	0.4	2	0.3	0.3	*-12.6*
Indian	–	–	–	–	–	–	–	–	–
Malay	A0	-1.31	*0.5*	*0*	*0.5*	*0*	0.3	0.3	*-1.9*

* : not enough cases for reliable estimation
– : incomplete or missing data
Best model: polynomial of the given degree in age (A), period (P) or cohort (C), or linear drift (D) model.
Goodness of fit: the normalised likelihood ratio chi-square for the best model (see Method).
Rate: world-standardised truncated rate per 100 000 per year (15-74 years) and number of **cases** are both estimated from the best-fitting model for the single years cited.
Cumulative risk per 1000 (15-74 years) is estimated from the best-fitting *age-cohort* model for cohorts of central birth year cited.
Recent trend: estimated mean percentage change per five-year period in the age-specific rates (15-74 years) over the period 1973-1987.
Italics denote recent trends not significant at 5 per cent level, or other figures which should be interpreted with caution (see Method).

HODGKIN'S DISEASE (ICD-9 201)

ASIA, INCIDENCE

MALES

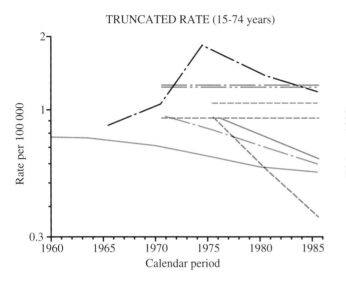

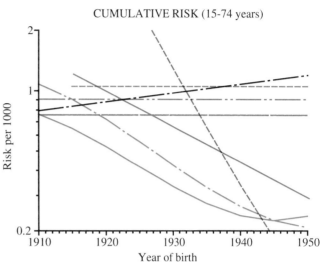

FEMALES

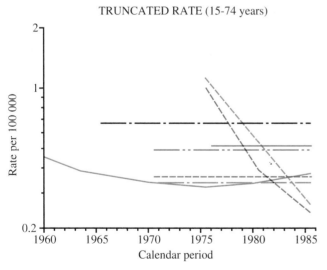

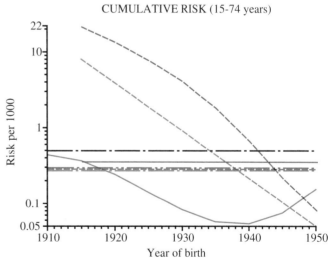

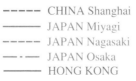

----- CHINA Shanghai	----- SINGAPORE Chinese
——— JAPAN Miyagi	—·—·— SINGAPORE Indian
----- JAPAN Nagasaki	—··—··— SINGAPORE Malay
—·—·— JAPAN Osaka	—··—··— INDIA Bombay
——— HONG KONG	

HODGKIN'S DISEASE (ICD-9 201)

OCEANIA, INCIDENCE

MALES	Best model	Goodness of fit	1970 Rate	1970 Cases	1985 Rate	1985 Cases	Cumulative risk 1915	Cumulative risk 1950	Recent trend
AUSTRALIA									
New South Wales	A1C4	0.77	*3.3*	*54*	2.8	57	2.8	1.6	*-6.6*
South	A0D	0.44	*6.3*	*24*	2.8	14	10.0	1.5	-24.5
HAWAII									
Caucasian	A1	1.63	3.2	2	3.2	3	2.1	2.1	*-7.2*
Chinese	A1	-3.41	*1.2*	*0*	*1.2*	*0*	1.0	1.0	*
Filipino	A0	-0.44	2.2	*0*	2.2	*0*	1.3	1.3	-24.7
Hawaiian	A0D	-0.85	3.1	1	*1.1*	*0*	6.3	0.6	-25.0
Japanese	A1D	0.10	2.1	1	*0.7*	*0*	2.3	0.2	*-41.6*
NEW ZEALAND									
Maori	A1	0.06	2.9	1	2.9	1	2.4	2.4	*4.7*
Non-Maori	A3D	-1.28	4.0	34	3.1	33	3.1	1.7	-17.0

FEMALES	Best model	Goodness of fit	1970 Rate	1970 Cases	1985 Rate	1985 Cases	Cumulative risk 1915	Cumulative risk 1950	Recent trend
AUSTRALIA									
New South Wales	A4C2	0.59	*2.7*	*46*	2.0	39	2.2	0.9	*-7.9*
South	A0P2C3	-0.22	*0.0*	*0*	1.6	8	1.8	1.0	*-18.2*
HAWAII									
Caucasian	A2C3	-0.20	2.3	1	4.0	3	0.8	6.8	*40.8*
Chinese	*	..	..	..	..	..	..	..	..
Filipino	A0D	-2.40	*2.0*	*0*	*0.5*	*0*	7.7	0.3	*
Hawaiian	A0	-0.94	*1.5*	*0*	*1.5*	*0*	0.9	0.9	*-24.1*
Japanese	A0	-0.90	*0.8*	*0*	*0.8*	*0*	0.5	0.5	*-3.7*
NEW ZEALAND									
Maori	A1C2	-1.64	*1.6*	*0*	*1.2*	*0*	1.6	0.3	*-34.7*
Non-Maori	A4C3	-0.13	2.3	20	2.6	28	1.8	1.3	*-7.0*

* : not enough cases for reliable estimation
− : incomplete or missing data
Best model: polynomial of the given degree in age (A), period (P) or cohort (C), or linear drift (D) model.
Goodness of fit: the normalised likelihood ratio chi-square for the best model (see Method).
Rate: world-standardised truncated rate per 100 000 per year (15-74 years) and number of **cases** are both estimated from the best-fitting model for the single years cited.
Cumulative risk per 1000 (15-74 years) is estimated from the best-fitting *age-cohort* model for cohorts of central birth year cited.
Recent trend: estimated mean percentage change per five-year period in the age-specific rates (15-74 years) over the period 1973-1987.
Italics denote recent trends not significant at 5 per cent level, or other figures which should be interpreted with caution (see Method).

HODGKIN'S DISEASE (ICD-9 201)

OCEANIA, INCIDENCE

MALES

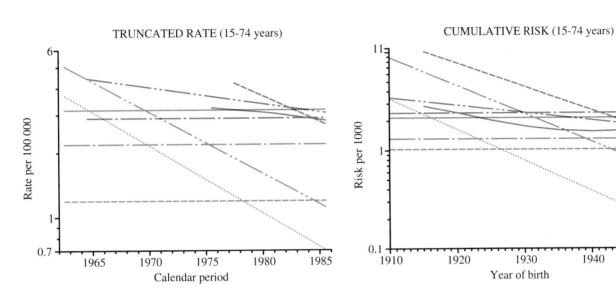

FEMALES

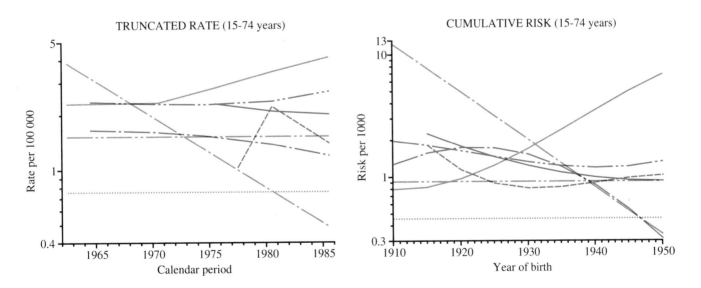

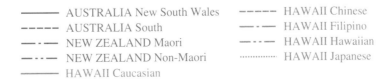

—— AUSTRALIA New South Wales	----- HAWAII Chinese
----- AUSTRALIA South	—·—· HAWAII Filipino
—·—· NEW ZEALAND Maori	—··—·· HAWAII Hawaiian
—··—·· NEW ZEALAND Non-Maori	·········· HAWAII Japanese
—— HAWAII Caucasian	

HODGKIN'S DISEASE (ICD-9 201)

ASIA, INCIDENCE
Percentage change per five-year period, 1973-1987

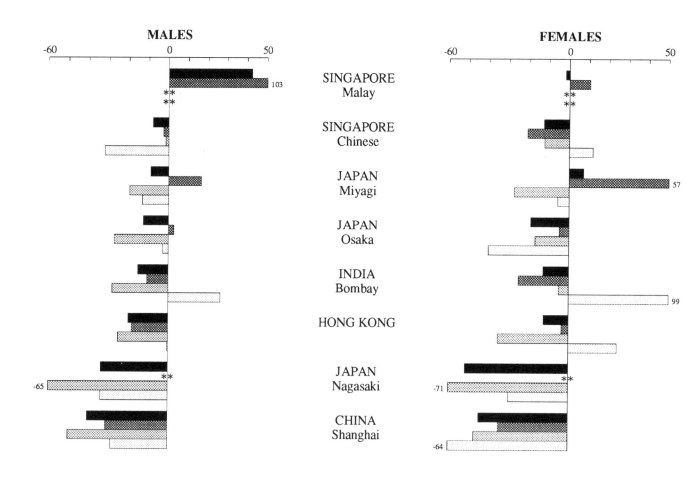

HODGKIN'S DISEASE (ICD-9 201)

OCEANIA, INCIDENCE
Percentage change per five-year period, 1973-1987

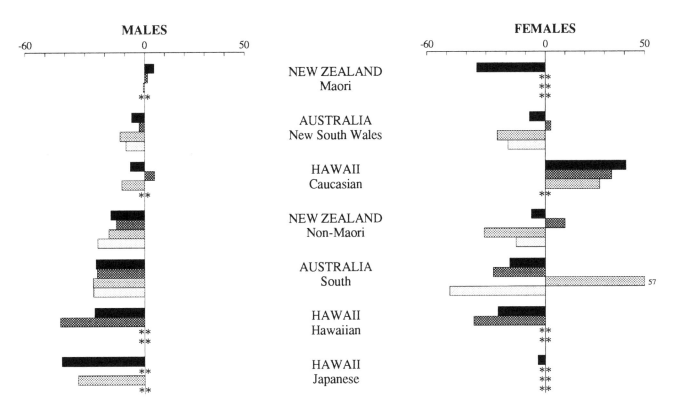

HODGKIN'S DISEASE (ICD-9 201)

ASIA and OCEANIA, MORTALITY

MALES	Best model	Goodness of fit	1965 Rate	1965 Deaths	1985 Rate	1985 Deaths	Cumulative risk 1900	Cumulative risk 1950	Recent trend
AUSTRALIA	A4P2	0.39	2.0	78	0.9	52	2.3	0.5	-19.0
HONG KONG	A1P4	-0.80	0.7	5	0.3	4	*1.0*	0.1	*-28.2*
JAPAN	A4P2C4	0.98	0.9	260	0.2	112	1.2	0.1	-40.7
MAURITIUS	A1P4	0.66	5.0	7	1.3	3	*1.2*	0.3	140.5
NEW ZEALAND	A3P3C2	0.86	2.9	24	1.0	11	2.5	0.5	*-18.0*
SINGAPORE	A2D	-0.04	0.8	3	0.3	2	*1.1*	0.1	–

FEMALES	Best model	Goodness of fit	1965 Rate	1965 Deaths	1985 Rate	1985 Deaths	Cumulative risk 1900	Cumulative risk 1950	Recent trend
AUSTRALIA	A7P3	2.31	1.4	55	0.5	32	1.4	0.3	-24.2
HONG KONG	A1D	0.57	0.3	3	0.1	1	*0.6*	0.0	*-31.8*
JAPAN	A9P6C9	-0.07	0.5	162	0.1	41	0.7	0.0	-43.6
MAURITIUS	A1	-2.10	*0.3*	*0*	*0.3*	*0*	*0.2*	0.2	*-37.4*
NEW ZEALAND	A4P2	-0.09	1.5	13	0.6	7	1.5	0.4	-40.0
SINGAPORE	A1	0.12	*0.3*	*0*	0.3	1	*0.2*	0.2	–

* : not enough deaths for reliable estimation
− : incomplete or missing data
Best model: polynomial of the given degree in age (A), period (P) or cohort (C), or linear drift (D) model.
Goodness of fit: the normalised likelihood ratio chi-square for the best model (see Method).
Rate: world-standardised truncated rate per 100 000 per year (15-74 years) and number of **deaths** are both estimated from the best-fitting model for the single years cited.
Cumulative risk per 1000 (15-74 years) is estimated from the best-fitting *age-cohort* model for cohorts of central birth year cited.
Recent trend: estimated mean percentage change per five-year period in the age-specific rates (15-74 years) over the period 1975-1988.
Italics denote recent trends not significant at 5 per cent level, or other figures which should be interpreted with caution (see Method).

HODGKIN'S DISEASE (ICD-9 201)

ASIA and OCEANIA, MORTALITY

MALES

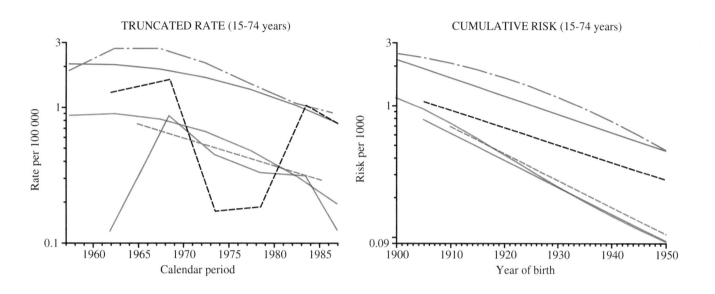

FEMALES

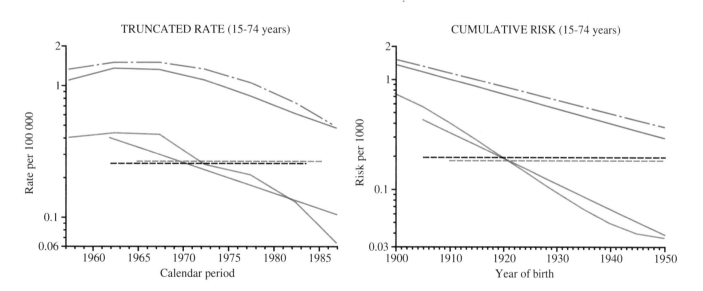

HODGKIN'S DISEASE (ICD-9 201)

ASIA and OCEANIA, MORTALITY
Percentage change per five-year period, 1975-1988

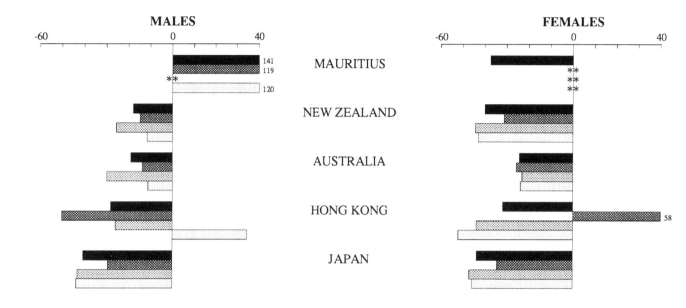

from page 673

which has been increasing steadily in both sexes; it may nevertheless be an artefact in the data. The very rapid decline among both sexes in Shanghai (China) since 1975 is difficult to explain, despite the change in population size covered by the registry since 1983. Substantial mis-classification to non-Hodgkin lymphoma is unlikely, and would need to have affected only males in order to account for the observed trends of the two types of lymphoma in Shanghai.

Incidence has declined in Caucasian populations in Australia and New Zealand, although the rate in younger females (15-44 years) in New Zealand has increased more recently. Caucasian females in Hawaii show an overall increase, particularly in the younger age group, but Hodgkin's disease remains uncommon in all ethnic groups in Hawaii, and the trends depend on very few cases.

Although mortality was already low in Asia and Oceania (truncated rates for 15-74 years of 2 per 100 000 or less in 1965), substantial declines at all ages are clearly seen from 1970 onward in Japan, Hong Kong, Australia and New Zealand. The data are well described by period effects with little or no curvature in cohort, and the recent rate of

decline of 30% every five years clearly demonstrates the impact of improved treatment.

Americas

The incidence of Hodgkin's disease has been fairly stable in most North American populations for some 20 years, with truncated rates (15-74 years) in the range 1-5 per 100 000. There has been no significant increase in either sex among the US or Canadian populations studied here since around 1975, and in Alberta (Canada), incidence has steadily declined at around 15% every five years in both sexes since reaching a plateau in 1975. In Cali (Colombia), incidence in males has fallen by more than half since 1965, and at 2 per 100 000 is among the lowest in the Americas, along with Cuba, where incidence has also fallen in males. Among females, incidence seems to be increasing in São Paulo (Brazil), and in Cuba, with cumulative risks of around 7 per 1000 for the 1950 birth cohort.

Mortality in the Americas has been falling rapidly at all ages since the late 1960s, particularly in the USA and Canada, where rates have fallen by 25-30% every five years since 1975, and the cumulative risk of death (15-74 years) from Hodgkin's disease has now fallen to 0.5 per 1000 or less for the 1950 birth cohort.

Comment

Most other reports are compatible with the results presented here; data from other parts of Switzerland and the UK, however, suggest different trends. The incidence of Hodgkin's disease in the canton of Vaud (Switzerland)[164] fell by about 15% in both sexes between 1979-83 and 1984-88, and world-standardised rates are now lower than those in Geneva, where incidence has not changed significantly since the 1970s. In Yorkshire (UK)[18], the incidence trend appears to have been different from that seen here for Birmingham, South Thames or Scotland: Hodgkin's disease incidence in both sexes combined rose by 29% in the 15 years to 1978-82, there was little change in the distribution of sub-types, and the increase was most marked at age 60 and over. In Slovakia[237], the eastern part of the former Czechoslovakia, Hodgkin's disease incidence changed little between 1979-83 and 1984-88, and with world-standardised rates of 2.3 and 1.7 per 100 000 in males and females, is similar to the levels in nearby County Vas (Hungary) and Slovenia.

In the USA, the increase in Hodgkin's disease in San Francisco County and the Bay Area in men from the mid-1970s up to 1987 has been minor, and does not appear related to the AIDS epidemic, either by marital status or geographical pattern[123,248]. The 5.2% overall rate

of increase every five years up to 1987 reported here among white males aged 30-74 years in the Bay Area is not significant; although the 22% rate of increase in 45-64 year-old white males is just significant (2 standard errors), the increase in younger males (15-44 years), who are more likely to be affected by any AIDS-related increase, is small (4% every five years). In Connecticut[293], where data are available since 1935, Hodgkin's disease incidence among 15-19 year-olds tripled over the three consecutive 15-year periods up to 1979, rising to 43 per million in each sex; recent quinquennial trends, evaluated from a linear model equivalent to the age-drift models used here, were 19% in males and 15% in females. These large increases were not due to changes in registration practice, diagnostic methods or confusion with other lymphomas. Connecticut covers about 1.3% of the US population, however, and among the 10% of the population covered by the SEER registries, including Connecticut, the incidence of Hodgkin's disease among 20-44 year-olds did not increase over the 15-year period ending in 1987[84].

Survival from Hodgkin's disease improved dramatically in the 1970s, increasing from 62% at five years for cases diagnosed in 1973 to 73% for cases diagnosed in 1978[83]. This is reflected in the sharp declines in mortality seen at all ages since 1970 in both Canada and the USA[77], but also in almost all the other countries studied here in Europe, Asia and Oceania.

The incidence of Hodgkin's disease is changing relatively slowly in most countries, and the speed and magnitude of the reduction in mortality, seen almost everywhere, testifies to a major success of cancer therapy.

AMERICAS (except USA), INCIDENCE

MALES	Best model	Goodness of fit	1970		1985		Cumulative risk		Recent trend
			Rate	Cases	Rate	Cases	1915	1950	
BRAZIL									
Sao Paulo	A2P2	-0.20	3.1	53	*0.8*	*15*	1.8	3.5	–
CANADA									
Alberta	A9P5C9	1.26	4.6	23	3.3	29	2.9	2.2	-14.7
British Columbia	A4C2	0.36	5.1	36	3.4	36	5.2	1.5	*-6.0*
Maritime Provinces	A3	0.71	4.2	20	4.2	24	2.7	2.7	*6.0*
Newfoundland	A0	0.63	3.0	4	3.0	6	1.8	1.8	*-2.2*
Quebec	A8P4	0.52	4.3	84	5.4	132	2.5	4.6	*-0.6*
COLOMBIA									
Cali	A1D	-0.62	3.8	6	2.0	6	3.8	0.8	-27.7
CUBA	A2P2	1.45	3.0	75	2.0	69	2.7	1.1	–
PUERTO RICO	A1P3C2	1.27	2.3	17	2.9	30	2.0	1.7	*2.1*

FEMALES	Best model	Goodness of fit	1970		1985		Cumulative risk		Recent trend
			Rate	Cases	Rate	Cases	1915	1950	
BRAZIL									
Sao Paulo	A1D	1.06	1.7	29	*3.8*	*85*	1.0	6.4	–
CANADA									
Alberta	A3P2C2	1.89	2.8	14	2.1	18	1.6	1.2	-17.2
British Columbia	A4P2C3	0.30	4.7	33	2.6	28	5.7	0.9	*11.0*
Maritime Provinces	A2C4	1.45	2.2	11	1.9	11	1.6	1.0	*-1.8*
Newfoundland	A9P5C9	-0.24	0.8	1	0.6	1	1.0	0.8	*-15.1*
Quebec	A4P4	0.95	2.7	54	3.7	94	1.5	3.0	*5.7*
COLOMBIA									
Cali	A2D	1.44	1.9	3	1.0	3	2.0	0.4	*-7.4*
CUBA	A2P2	-0.24	1.5	35	2.7	94	1.1	6.7	–
PUERTO RICO	A2P3C2	0.70	1.5	11	1.6	18	1.2	1.0	*-8.0*

* : not enough cases for reliable estimation
– : incomplete or missing data
Best model: polynomial of the given degree in age (A), period (P) or cohort (C), or linear drift (D) model.
Goodness of fit: the normalised likelihood ratio chi-square for the best model (see Method).
Rate: world-standardised truncated rate per 100 000 per year (15-74 years) and number of **cases** are both estimated from the best-fitting model for the single years cited.
Cumulative risk per 1000 (15-74 years) is estimated from the best-fitting *age-cohort* model for cohorts of central birth year cited.
Recent trend: estimated mean percentage change per five-year period in the age-specific rates (15-74 years) over the period 1973-1987.
Italics denote recent trends not significant at 5 per cent level, or other figures which should be interpreted with caution (see Method).

HODGKIN'S DISEASE (ICD-9 201)

AMERICAS (except USA), INCIDENCE

MALES

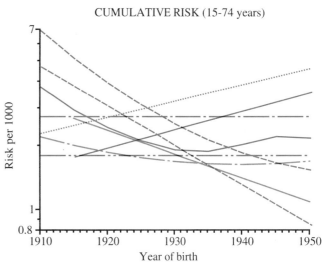

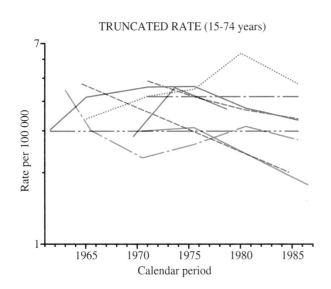

FEMALES

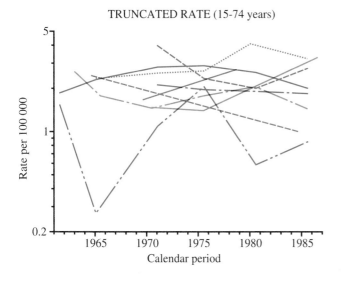

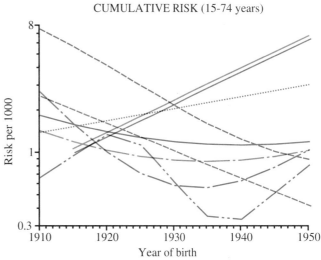

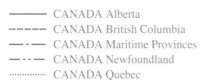

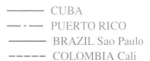

HODGKIN'S DISEASE (ICD-9 201)

AMERICAS (USA), INCIDENCE

MALES	Best model	Goodness of fit	1970 Rate	1970 Cases	1985 Rate	1985 Cases	Cumulative risk 1915	Cumulative risk 1950	Recent trend
USA									
Bay Area, Black	A0	2.18	3.9	4	3.9	6	2.3	2.3	-20.7
Bay Area, Chinese	A0	-1.03	*1.5*	*0*	*1.5*	*1*	0.9	0.9	–
Bay Area, White	A4P2	0.12	7.3	66	4.9	50	4.4	2.4	*5.2*
Connecticut	A5C2	0.53	5.5	53	5.7	65	3.5	3.1	*0.5*
Detroit, Black	A0	0.19	3.4	7	3.4	10	2.0	2.0	*-12.4*
Detroit, White	A4	0.92	4.5	49	4.5	48	2.8	2.8	*3.1*
Iowa	A5D	0.25	5.1	46	3.9	40	4.0	2.1	-7.8
New Orleans, Black	A0	-0.75	2.7	*1*	2.7	3	1.6	1.6	*4.2*
New Orleans, White	A0	-1.22	*4.5*	*9*	4.5	11	2.7	2.7	*8.5*
Seattle	A3	2.26	*4.1*	*26*	4.1	47	2.6	2.6	*-1.3*

FEMALES	Best model	Goodness of fit	1970 Rate	1970 Cases	1985 Rate	1985 Cases	Cumulative risk 1915	Cumulative risk 1950	Recent trend
USA									
Bay Area, Black	A0	0.40	2.0	2	2.0	3	1.2	1.2	*5.0*
Bay Area, Chinese	A0	-1.49	*1.3*	*0*	*1.3*	*1*	0.8	0.8	–
Bay Area, White	A4P2C3	0.09	4.9	46	3.4	34	2.8	1.7	*-1.1*
Connecticut	A5C2	0.30	4.2	44	3.7	43	3.5	1.6	*-1.3*
Detroit, Black	A0	4.17	1.7	4	1.7	5	1.0	1.0	-19.4
Detroit, White	A4C2	0.34	3.2	38	3.8	41	1.9	2.1	*10.5*
Iowa	A4C3	-0.17	3.3	32	3.2	33	3.6	1.1	*2.2*
New Orleans, Black	A0	1.70	*1.5*	*1*	1.5	2	0.9	0.9	46.4
New Orleans, White	A9C8	0.16	*2.2*	*5*	2.8	7	0.7	4.1	22.1
Seattle	A4	0.00	*3.2*	*19*	3.2	36	1.8	1.8	*9.9*

* : not enough cases for reliable estimation
− : incomplete or missing data
Best model: polynomial of the given degree in age (A), period (P) or cohort (C), or linear drift (D) model.
Goodness of fit: the normalised likelihood ratio chi-square for the best model (see Method).
Rate: world-standardised truncated rate per 100 000 per year (15-74 years) and number of **cases** are both estimated from the best-fitting model for the single years cited.
Cumulative risk per 1000 (15-74 years) is estimated from the best-fitting *age-cohort* model for cohorts of central birth year cited.
Recent trend: estimated mean percentage change per five-year period in the age-specific rates (15-74 years) over the period 1973-1987.
Italics denote recent trends not significant at 5 per cent level, or other figures which should be interpreted with caution (see Method).

HODGKIN'S DISEASE (ICD-9 201)

AMERICAS (USA), INCIDENCE

MALES

TRUNCATED RATE (15-74 years)

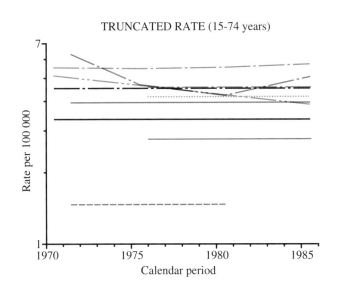

CUMULATIVE RISK (15-74 years)

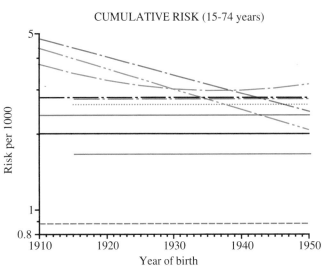

FEMALES

TRUNCATED RATE (15-74 years)

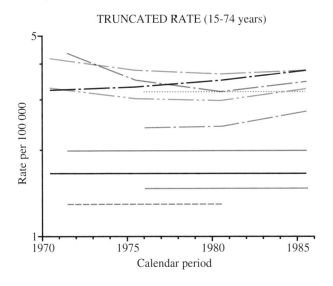

CUMULATIVE RISK (15-74 years)

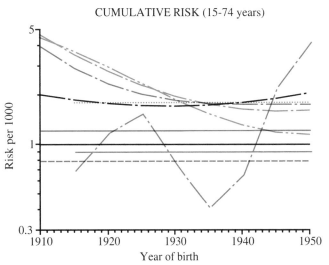

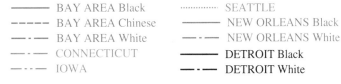

——— BAY AREA Black
- - - - BAY AREA Chinese
—·—·— BAY AREA White
—··— CONNECTICUT
—···— IOWA

·············· SEATTLE
——— NEW ORLEANS Black
—·—·— NEW ORLEANS White
——— DETROIT Black
—··— DETROIT White

HODGKIN'S DISEASE (ICD-9 201)

AMERICAS (except USA), INCIDENCE
Percentage change per five-year period, 1973-1987

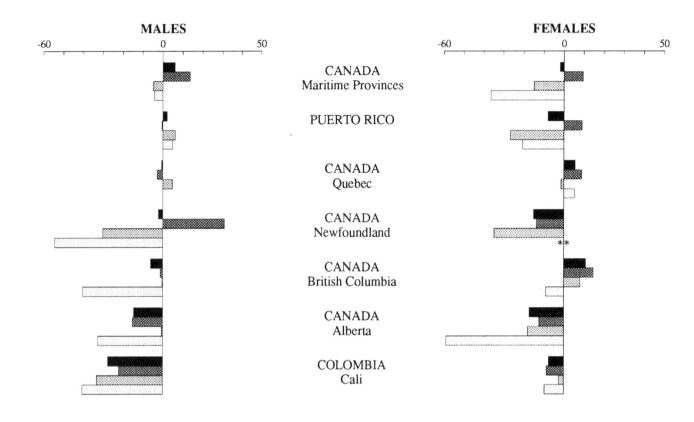

HODGKIN'S DISEASE (ICD-9 201)

AMERICAS (USA), INCIDENCE
Percentage change per five-year period, 1973-1987

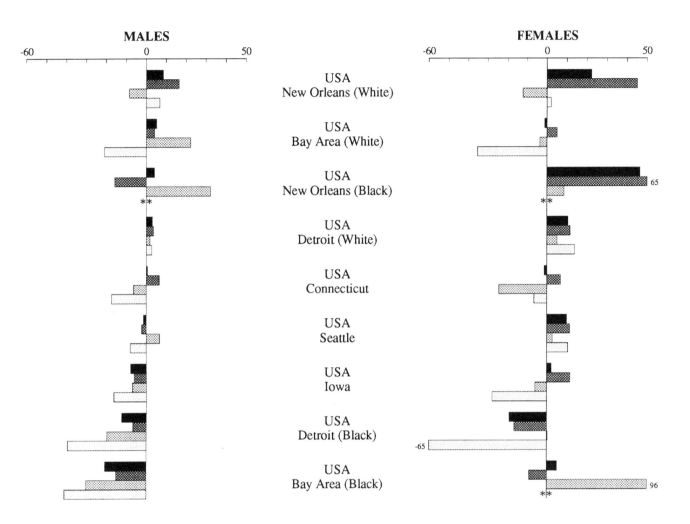

HODGKIN'S DISEASE (ICD-9 201)

AMERICAS, MORTALITY

MALES	Best model	Goodness of fit	1965 Rate	1965 Deaths	1985 Rate	1985 Deaths	Cumulative risk 1900	Cumulative risk 1950	Recent trend
CANADA	A5P5C2	-0.92	2.8	170	1.1	103	2.7	0.5	-17.5
CHILE	A1D	-0.45	1.4	30	*1.0*	*34*	1.3	*0.6*	–
COSTA RICA	–	–	–	–	–	–	–	–	–
PANAMA	–	–	–	–	–	–	–	–	–
PUERTO RICO	–	–	–	–	–	–	–	–	–
URUGUAY	–	–	–	–	–	–	–	–	–
USA	A6P6C6	4.83	2.9	1809	1.1	963	3.7	0.5	-20.3
VENEZUELA	A1	0.77	1.0	19	*1.0*	*38*	0.8	*0.8*	–

FEMALES	Best model	Goodness of fit	1965 Rate	1965 Deaths	1985 Rate	1985 Deaths	Cumulative risk 1900	Cumulative risk 1950	Recent trend
CANADA	A5P4	2.75	1.4	88	0.5	53	1.7	0.3	-23.2
CHILE	A2D	0.11	0.6	13	*0.3*	*11*	0.7	*0.1*	–
COSTA RICA	–	–	–	–	–	–	–	–	–
PANAMA	–	–	–	–	–	–	–	–	–
PUERTO RICO	–	–	–	–	–	–	–	–	–
URUGUAY	–	–	–	–	–	–	–	–	–
USA	A5P6C6	3.36	1.6	1103	0.6	628	2.2	0.3	-20.6
VENEZUELA	A1	0.57	0.6	10	*0.6*	*22*	0.4	*0.4*	–

* : not enough deaths for reliable estimation
– : incomplete or missing data
Best model: polynomial of the given degree in age (A), period (P) or cohort (C), or linear drift (D) model.
Goodness of fit: the normalised likelihood ratio chi-square for the best model (see Method).
Rate: world-standardised truncated rate per 100 000 per year (15-74 years) and number of **deaths** are both estimated from the best-fitting model for the single years cited.
Cumulative risk per 1000 (15-74 years) is estimated from the best-fitting *age-cohort* model for cohorts of central birth year cited.
Recent trend: estimated mean percentage change per five-year period in the age-specific rates (15-74 years) over the period 1975-1988.
Italics denote recent trends not significant at 5 per cent level, or other figures which should be interpreted with caution (see Method).

HODGKIN'S DISEASE (ICD-9 201)

AMERICAS, MORTALITY

MALES

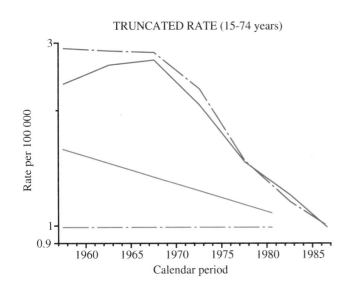

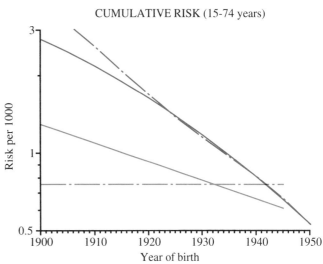

FEMALES

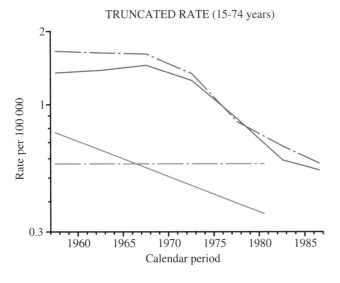

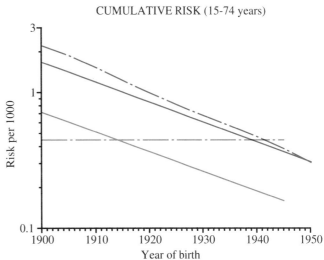

——— CANADA
—·—·— USA
——— CHILE
—··—··— VENEZUELA

HODGKIN'S DISEASE (ICD-9 201)

AMERICAS, MORTALITY
Percentage change per five-year period, 1975-1988

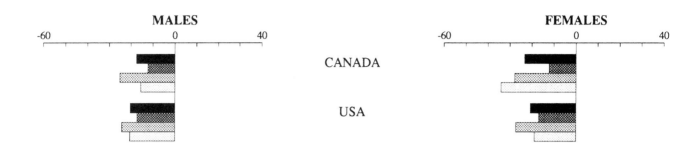

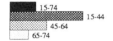

Chapter 28

MYELOMA

Multiple myeloma is a relatively uncommon malignancy, representing less than 1% of all cancers in most populations. It is a malignant proliferation of plasma cells originating in the bone marrow, and causing destruction of bone, particularly in the skull and vertebrae, often with a characteristic radiological appearance. The classical diagnostic elements of radiological appearance and microscopic examination of the bone marrow aspirate were reinforced some 30 years ago by detection of characteristic proteins in the urine (and later the blood). The availability for many years of simple and precise diagnostic techniques for multiple myeloma is of relevance in the interpretation of incidence trends. Survival from myeloma is poor, typically only 20-30% at five years after diagnosis. Mortality statistics may be affected by a change in classification and coding: solitary plasmacytoma was classified with multiple myeloma (ICD-8 203) in the eighth revision of the ICD, but under a separate rubric (ICD-9 238.6) in the ninth revision. In countries where a significant fraction of myelomas were classified as solitary plasmacytoma, a sharp and artefactual decrease in myeloma mortality would be expected when ICD-9 came into force in 1979. This has been observed for Germany and to a lesser extent for Italy[64]. The effect in England and Wales was small[211]. Ionising radiation can cause myeloma, and increased risks of the disease have been observed among survivors of the atomic bomb explosions at Hiroshima and Nagasaki, among women irradiated for treatment of cervical carcinoma and among workers in the nuclear industry.

Myeloma is essentially a malignancy of adults, being very rare in persons under 35 years of age. Males are affected more often than females. Myeloma incidence is highest in black populations in the USA, and in Maoris and Hawaiians, with cumulative risks (30-74 years) around 1%, and lowest in Chinese, Indian and Japanese populations.

Switzerland, and among Jews in Israel, while France, Germany, Austria, Slovenia and populations in the east and south of Europe have had lower rates.

There has been a fairly widespread increase in incidence and mortality from multiple myeloma in most parts of Europe since the 1960s, but the rate of increase has slowed down materially. Significant rates of increase in Finland, the UK and the GDR of about 10% every five years have been observed in the past 15 years, but recent trends elsewhere have been either downward or not significantly upward. There was a marked narrowing of the overall range of incidence and mortality rates by the 1980s, especially in the European Community.

The recent trends in the UK and the GDR exemplify the pattern in higher-risk countries, where there has been a flattening or deceleration of the upward trend in recent years, more clearly seen for males than for females, and there is a consistent decrease in risk for younger persons, suggesting a peak risk for the cohorts born around 1925 to 1935, with a subsequent decline. The rates of increase in the oldest age groups, aged 75 years and over (data not shown) are often larger than those observed among 65-74 year-olds, which is consistent with a cohort effect that has passed its peak.

The effect on mortality is perhaps seen most clearly for the Netherlands, where the overall recent trend in the age range 30-74 years has now been downward since the mid-1970s, and the peak risks of around 3 and 2 per 1000 in males and females, respectively, occurred among persons born in the period 1915-20, with a steady decline in cumulative risk (30-74 years) for persons born later. Mortality in Greece and Yugoslavia is the lowest in Europe, and appears to be following a parallel course, maintaining the relative position with mortality in other countries. Mortality data for Portugal were only available from 1980, and none were available for Romania.

Europe

Myeloma is uncommon in Europe, with truncated incidence rates of up to 8 and 5 per 100 000 in males and females, respectively, and mortality rates up to 5 and 3 per 100 000. The highest rates occur in the Nordic countries, the UK and

Asia and Oceania

Incidence and mortality are increasing rapidly in Japanese of both sexes. Myeloma was evidently diagnosed in Japan only rarely before the 1960s, but increased very rapidly thereafter; this

continued page 726

MULTIPLE MYELOMA (ICD-9 203)

EUROPE (non-EC), INCIDENCE

MALES	Best model	Goodness of fit	1970 Rate	1970 Cases	1985 Rate	1985 Cases	Cumulative risk 1915	Cumulative risk 1940	Recent trend
FINLAND	A2D	0.73	3.9	39	5.6	66	3.2	6.0	14.7
HUNGARY									
County Vas	A1P2	-0.74	*0.6*	*0*	2.4	1	1.6	14.0	*12.5*
Szabolcs-Szatmar	A8C9	-0.97	0.8	1	1.1	1	0.4	0.1	*7.3*
ISRAEL									
All Jews	A2D	0.75	4.0	18	5.5	31	3.1	5.4	*4.8*
Non-Jews	A4	-1.73	*3.1*	*0*	3.1	1	1.9	1.9	75.6
NORWAY	A2P3	-0.53	5.5	61	7.3	89	4.6	6.7	*3.2*
POLAND									
Warsaw City	A2	-0.12	3.1	8	3.1	11	2.0	2.0	*-6.6*
ROMANIA									
Cluj	A4	0.82	*1.9*	*3*	1.9	3	1.1	1.1	*36.4*
SWEDEN	A4D	0.29	5.9	148	6.9	184	4.3	5.5	*3.8*
SWITZERLAND									
Geneva	A1C2	1.07	3.6	2	6.8	6	4.5	4.1	*22.4*
YUGOSLAVIA									
Slovenia	A2C2	-0.03	2.7	10	4.0	16	2.5	2.8	*14.0*

FEMALES	Best model	Goodness of fit	1970 Rate	1970 Cases	1985 Rate	1985 Cases	Cumulative risk 1915	Cumulative risk 1940	Recent trend
FINLAND	A2C2	-0.30	3.1	42	4.0	66	2.6	2.7	*5.7*
HUNGARY									
County Vas	A1D	0.15	1.3	1	3.6	3	1.5	8.3	*50.3*
Szabolcs-Szatmar	A2	-0.37	1.1	1	1.1	1	0.7	0.7	*14.9*
ISRAEL									
All Jews	A2	1.04	3.6	15	3.6	22	2.3	2.3	*8.4*
Non-Jews	A1	-0.08	*1.9*	*0*	1.9	1	1.3	1.3	*-22.5*
NORWAY	A2P2	-1.27	4.1	52	4.6	63	3.0	4.4	*-0.1*
POLAND									
Warsaw City	A2	-0.57	2.8	12	2.8	14	1.8	1.8	*9.9*
ROMANIA									
Cluj	A2	-0.13	*1.4*	*2*	1.4	2	0.8	0.8	*-3.1*
SWEDEN	A3P5	-0.81	4.2	114	4.1	121	2.9	3.7	*-3.3*
SWITZERLAND									
Geneva	A1	0.18	3.6	3	3.6	4	2.5	2.5	*-19.2*
YUGOSLAVIA									
Slovenia	A2C2	0.15	2.2	10	2.7	15	1.7	1.6	*7.0*

* : not enough cases for reliable estimation
− : incomplete or missing data
Best model: polynomial of the given degree in age (A), period (P) or cohort (C), or linear drift (D) model.
Goodness of fit: the normalised likelihood ratio chi-square for the best model (see Method).
Rate: world-standardised truncated rate per 100 000 per year (30-74 years) and number of **cases** are both estimated from the best-fitting model for the single years cited.
Cumulative risk per 1000 (30-74 years) is estimated from the best-fitting *age-cohort* model for cohorts of central birth year cited.
Recent trend: estimated mean percentage change per five-year period in the age-specific rates (30-74 years) over the period 1973-1987.
Italics denote recent trends not significant at 5 per cent level, or other figures which should be interpreted with caution (see Method).

706

MULTIPLE MYELOMA (ICD-9 203)

EUROPE (non-EC), INCIDENCE

MALES

TRUNCATED RATE (30-74 years)

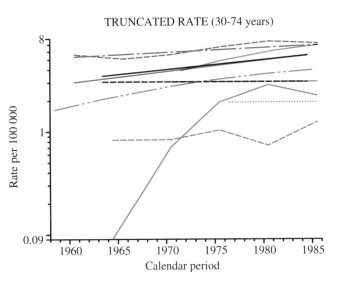

CUMULATIVE RISK (30-74 years)

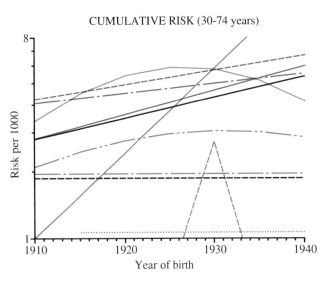

FEMALES

TRUNCATED RATE (30-74 years)

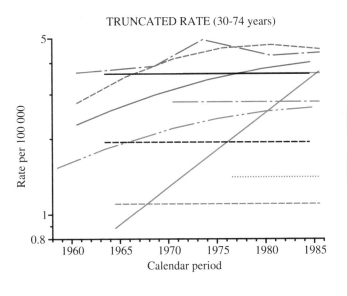

CUMULATIVE RISK (30-74 years)

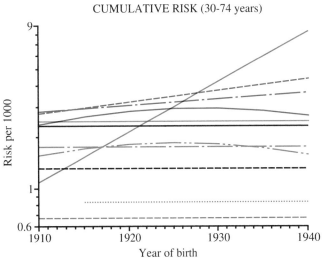

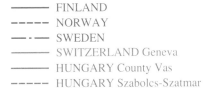

—— FINLAND	—·— POLAND Warsaw City
----- NORWAY	········ ROMANIA Cluj
—··— SWEDEN	—··— YUGOSLAVIA Slovenia
—— SWITZERLAND Geneva	—— ISRAEL All Jews
—— HUNGARY County Vas	----- ISRAEL Non-Jews
----- HUNGARY Szabolcs-Szatmar	

MULTIPLE MYELOMA (ICD-9 203)

EUROPE (EC), INCIDENCE

MALES	Best model	Goodness of fit	1970 Rate	1970 Cases	1985 Rate	1985 Cases	Cumulative risk 1915	Cumulative risk 1940	Recent trend
DENMARK	A2D	1.94	4.9	67	5.4	80	3.4	4.1	*5.6*
FRANCE									
Bas-Rhin	A1P2	1.12	*42.5*	*101*	9.5	19	5.0	118.5	91.3
Doubs	A1	0.28	*3.9*	*2*	3.9	4	2.7	2.7	*36.0*
GERMANY (FRG)									
Hamburg	A1	1.30	3.4	18	*3.4*	*12*	2.2	*2.2*	–
Saarland	A4C3	-0.55	3.4	9	3.1	9	1.8	8.4	*6.4*
GERMANY (GDR)	A4C2	2.30	2.8	125	3.9	142	2.3	3.1	14.1
ITALY									
Varese	A2	1.36	*5.1*	*5*	5.1	10	3.3	3.3	*6.6*
SPAIN									
Navarra	A1	0.23	*4.0*	*4*	4.0	5	2.6	2.6	*21.6*
Zaragoza	A2C3	0.40	1.2	2	3.8	9	2.2	3.9	*13.2*
UK									
Birmingham	A2C2	0.48	3.3	44	5.1	77	3.2	3.7	23.2
Scotland	A2P2C2	0.21	4.2	57	5.6	79	3.7	4.5	*3.5*
South Thames	A2C2	-0.17	3.8	96	5.6	108	3.4	4.7	10.2

FEMALES	Best model	Goodness of fit	1970 Rate	1970 Cases	1985 Rate	1985 Cases	Cumulative risk 1915	Cumulative risk 1940	Recent trend
DENMARK	A2P3	-0.32	3.4	52	4.0	67	2.4	3.1	13.0
FRANCE									
Bas-Rhin	A8D	0.63	*0.8*	*2*	7.0	18	2.8	103.0	109.0
Doubs	A1P2	-0.98	*0.0*	*0*	3.9	4	2.1	2.9	*7.8*
GERMANY (FRG)									
Hamburg	A2	-0.68	2.7	21	*2.7*	*15*	1.7	*1.7*	–
Saarland	A2	-1.06	2.1	8	2.1	8	1.4	1.4	*-13.1*
GERMANY (GDR)	A4D	0.17	2.1	146	2.9	166	1.7	2.9	10.7
ITALY									
Varese	A4	-3.30	*3.8*	*4*	3.8	9	2.4	2.4	*5.6*
SPAIN									
Navarra	A1	-0.59	*2.8*	*4*	2.8	4	1.9	1.9	*21.3*
Zaragoza	A2D	-1.38	0.9	1	3.5	9	1.6	17.1	*34.9*
UK									
Birmingham	A2C2	-0.04	2.4	38	3.1	54	2.1	1.9	10.6
Scotland	A2D	1.78	2.6	46	4.6	79	2.5	6.4	11.9
South Thames	A4C4	-1.10	2.9	94	3.6	84	2.1	3.7	7.6

* : not enough cases for reliable estimation
– : incomplete or missing data
Best model: polynomial of the given degree in age (A), period (P) or cohort (C), or linear drift (D) model.
Goodness of fit: the normalised likelihood ratio chi-square for the best model (see Method).
Rate: world-standardised truncated rate per 100 000 per year (30-74 years) and number of **cases** are both estimated from the best-fitting model for the single years cited.
Cumulative risk per 1000 (30-74 years) is estimated from the best-fitting *age-cohort* model for cohorts of central birth year cited.
Recent trend: estimated mean percentage change per five-year period in the age-specific rates (30-74 years) over the period 1973-1987.
Italics denote recent trends not significant at 5 per cent level, or other figures which should be interpreted with caution (see Method).

MULTIPLE MYELOMA (ICD-9 203)

EUROPE (EC), INCIDENCE

MALES

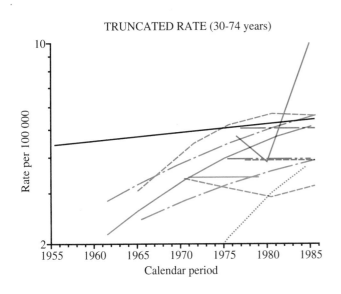

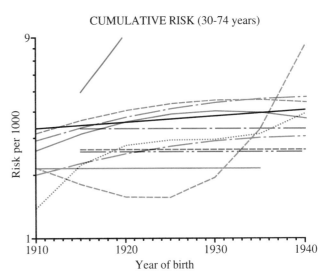

FEMALES

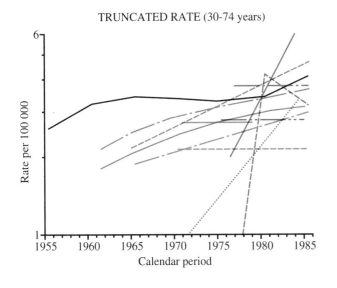

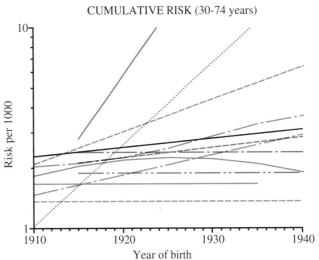

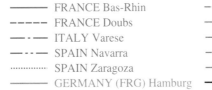

―――― FRANCE Bas-Rhin	‑ ‑ ‑ ‑ GERMANY (FRG) Saarland
‑ ‑ ‑ ‑ FRANCE Doubs	‑·‑·‑ GERMANY (GDR)
‑·‑·‑ ITALY Varese	―――― UK Birmingham
‑··‑··‑ SPAIN Navarra	‑ ‑ ‑ ‑ UK Scotland
············ SPAIN Zaragoza	‑·‑·‑ UK South Thames
―――― GERMANY (FRG) Hamburg	―――― DENMARK

MULTIPLE MYELOMA (ICD-9 203)

EUROPE (non-EC), INCIDENCE
Percentage change per five-year period, 1973-1987

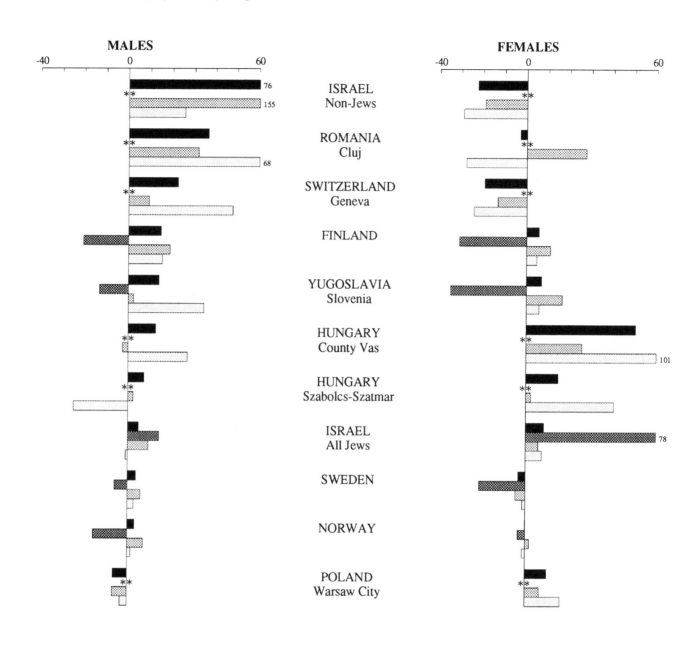

MULTIPLE MYELOMA (ICD-9 203)

EUROPE (EC), INCIDENCE
Percentage change per five-year period, 1973-1987

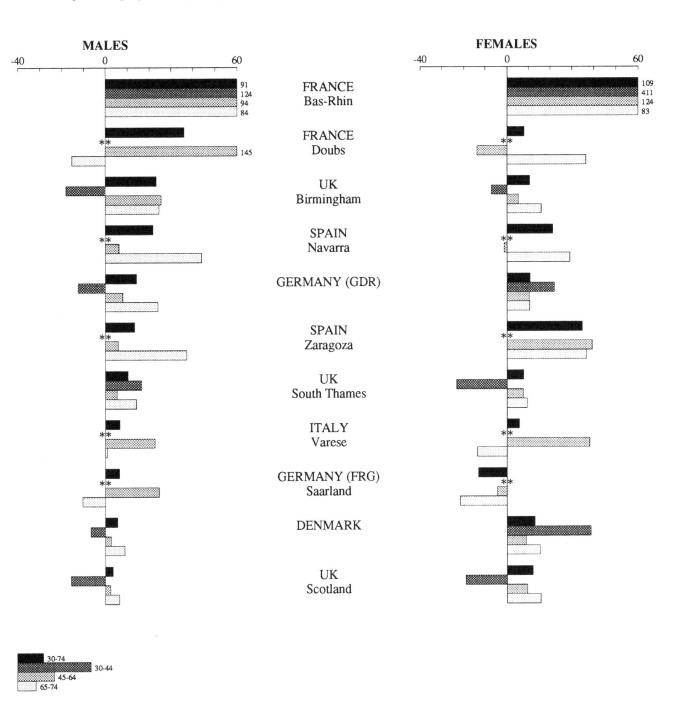

MULTIPLE MYELOMA (ICD-9 203)

EUROPE (non-EC), MORTALITY

MALES	Best model	Goodness of fit	1965 Rate	1965 Deaths	1985 Rate	1985 Deaths	Cumulative risk 1900	Cumulative risk 1940	Recent trend
AUSTRIA	A2D	-0.48	1.8	36	2.8	52	1.2	2.8	10.7
CZECHOSLOVAKIA	A2C2	0.23	1.8	65	3.1	112	1.2	2.6	9.5
FINLAND	A2P3C4	-0.33	3.2	29	3.9	45	2.0	2.7	14.1
HUNGARY	A2P3C2	0.10	7.4	188	3.1	87	0.2	4.5	40.1
NORWAY	A2P2	-0.66	4.4	46	5.7	72	3.1	4.5	5.3
POLAND	A2D	-0.42	0.9	55	3.3	253	0.5	6.7	–
ROMANIA	–	–	–	–	–	–	–	–	–
SWEDEN	A2P2C2	-0.36	4.3	100	4.2	117	2.9	2.2	-9.0
SWITZERLAND	A2C2	-0.04	2.9	41	4.0	70	2.0	2.4	-1.5
YUGOSLAVIA	A2C4	1.14	0.7	27	1.2	59	0.5	0.9	10.4

FEMALES	Best model	Goodness of fit	1965 Rate	1965 Deaths	1985 Rate	1985 Deaths	Cumulative risk 1900	Cumulative risk 1940	Recent trend
AUSTRIA	A2C2	-0.25	1.4	37	2.2	61	0.9	1.5	14.1
CZECHOSLOVAKIA	A2C4	0.17	1.5	62	2.2	104	1.0	1.5	7.4
FINLAND	A2C2	0.33	2.3	28	2.9	49	1.5	1.4	2.1
HUNGARY	A2P2C2	0.06	0.2	6	2.2	77	0.3	4.7	38.6
NORWAY	A2D	-0.18	2.8	32	3.7	51	1.9	3.3	6.1
POLAND	A2C2	0.67	0.6	44	2.6	274	0.4	3.1	–
ROMANIA	–	–	–	–	–	–	–	–	–
SWEDEN	A2C2	0.32	3.1	78	3.0	93	2.1	1.3	-9.2
SWITZERLAND	A2C2	0.53	2.3	40	2.8	60	1.6	1.6	4.2
YUGOSLAVIA	A4P3C2	0.44	0.5	23	0.9	54	0.3	0.7	9.9

* : not enough deaths for reliable estimation
– : incomplete or missing data
Best model: polynomial of the given degree in age (A), period (P) or cohort (C), or linear drift (D) model.
Goodness of fit: the normalised likelihood ratio chi-square for the best model (see Method).
Rate: world-standardised truncated rate per 100 000 per year (30-74 years) and number of **deaths** are both estimated from the best-fitting model for the single years cited.
Cumulative risk per 1000 (30-74 years) is estimated from the best-fitting *age-cohort* model for cohorts of central birth year cited.
Recent trend: estimated mean percentage change per five-year period in the age-specific rates (30-74 years) over the period 1975-1988.
Italics denote recent trends not significant at 5 per cent level, or other figures which should be interpreted with caution (see Method).

MULTIPLE MYELOMA (ICD-9 203)

EUROPE (non-EC), MORTALITY

MALES

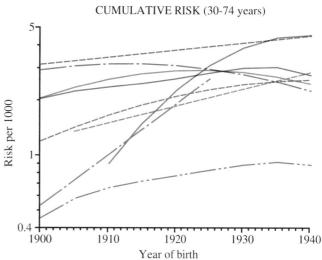

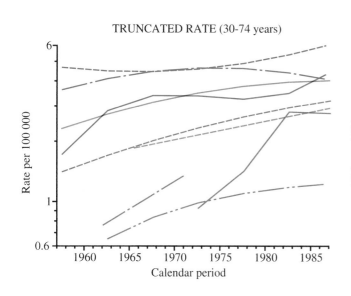

FEMALES

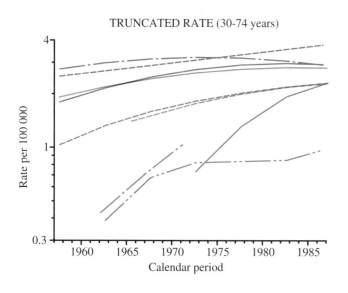

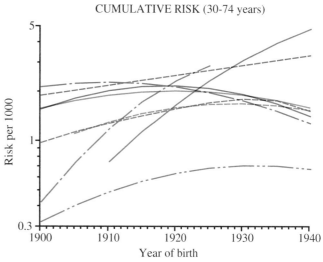

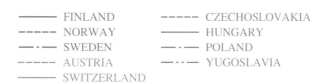

——— FINLAND	----- CZECHOSLOVAKIA
----- NORWAY	——— HUNGARY
—·—· SWEDEN	—··— POLAND
----- AUSTRIA	—···— YUGOSLAVIA
——— SWITZERLAND	

MULTIPLE MYELOMA (ICD-9 203)

EUROPE (EC), MORTALITY

MALES	Best model	Goodness of fit	1965 Rate	1965 Deaths	1985 Rate	1985 Deaths	Cumulative risk 1900	Cumulative risk 1940	Recent trend
BELGIUM	A2C2	0.74	1.9	51	3.7	103	1.3	2.8	*5.1*
DENMARK	A2	0.45	4.0	52	4.0	59	2.7	2.7	*6.2*
FRANCE	A2P3C6	-0.37	1.6	194	3.0	416	1.1	3.0	8.6
GERMANY (FRG)	A2P4C2	2.47	*3.7*	*575*	1.9	308	*1.8*	1.6	*1.7*
GREECE	A2C2	0.60	1.5	28	2.0	56	*1.0*	1.3	*1.5*
IRELAND	A2C4	-1.22	2.7	19	4.8	38	1.8	3.4	*12.7*
ITALY	A2P2C3	0.85	1.6	198	3.2	500	1.0	2.5	7.9
NETHERLANDS	A2P3C2	-0.87	4.3	122	4.4	157	2.8	2.5	*3.7*
PORTUGAL	–	–	–	–	–	–	–	–	–
SPAIN	A4P2C3	-0.26	0.5	33	2.6	253	0.3	5.8	31.4
UK ENGLAND & WALES	A2P2C2	2.60	2.6	333	4.2	616	1.7	2.9	11.0
UK SCOTLAND	A2C2	1.44	2.9	38	4.0	57	1.9	2.1	*6.1*

FEMALES	Best model	Goodness of fit	1965 Rate	1965 Deaths	1985 Rate	1985 Deaths	Cumulative risk 1900	Cumulative risk 1940	Recent trend
BELGIUM	A2C2	-0.50	1.5	48	2.7	88	1.0	2.6	23.2
DENMARK	A2D	2.67	2.7	39	3.0	51	1.8	2.3	*9.6*
FRANCE	A3P3C4	0.24	1.3	202	2.2	381	1.0	2.2	*2.2*
GERMANY (FRG)	A2P4C2	3.90	*2.3*	*506*	1.4	315	*1.3*	0.9	-3.3
GREECE	A2P3C2	0.42	1.1	23	1.8	59	*0.6*	1.3	*6.9*
IRELAND	A8C9	-0.04	2.0	14	3.2	26	1.1	1.1	17.7
ITALY	A2P2C3	1.85	1.3	183	2.3	449	0.8	1.9	6.8
NETHERLANDS	A2P2C2	-2.33	2.7	87	3.0	129	1.8	1.9	*-0.8*
PORTUGAL	–	–	–	–	–	–	–	–	–
SPAIN	A2P2C4	0.58	0.4	31	1.9	221	0.3	4.3	27.6
UK ENGLAND & WALES	A3P2C3	1.88	2.0	328	2.8	492	1.4	2.0	7.6
UK SCOTLAND	A2P3C2	-0.22	2.3	39	2.6	47	1.4	1.5	*10.4*

* : not enough deaths for reliable estimation
– : incomplete or missing data
Best model: polynomial of the given degree in age (A), period (P) or cohort (C), or linear drift (D) model.
Goodness of fit: the normalised likelihood ratio chi-square for the best model (see Method).
Rate: world-standardised truncated rate per 100 000 per year (30-74 years) and number of **deaths** are both estimated from the best-fitting model for the single years cited.
Cumulative risk per 1000 (30-74 years) is estimated from the best-fitting *age-cohort* model for cohorts of central birth year cited.
Recent trend: estimated mean percentage change per five-year period in the age-specific rates (30-74 years) over the period 1975-1988.
Italics denote recent trends not significant at 5 per cent level, or other figures which should be interpreted with caution (see Method).

MULTIPLE MYELOMA (ICD-9 203)

EUROPE (EC), MORTALITY

MALES

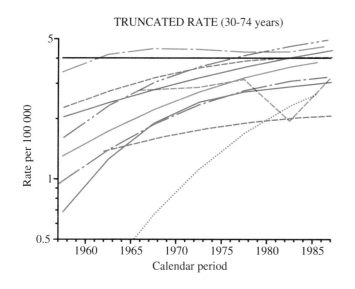

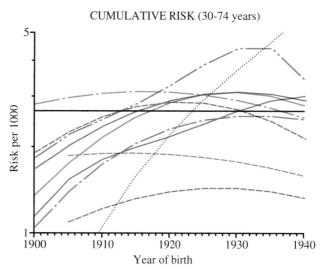

FEMALES

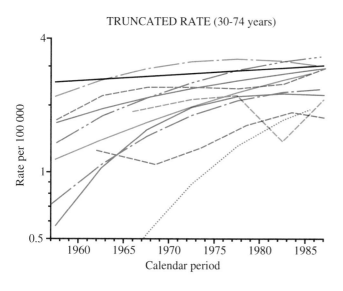

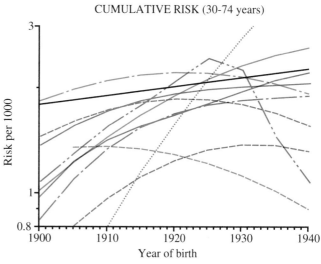

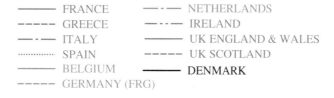

FRANCE

GREECE

ITALY

SPAIN

BELGIUM

GERMANY (FRG)

NETHERLANDS

IRELAND

UK ENGLAND & WALES

UK SCOTLAND

DENMARK

MULTIPLE MYELOMA (ICD-9 203)

EUROPE (non-EC), MORTALITY
Percentage change per five-year period, 1975-1988

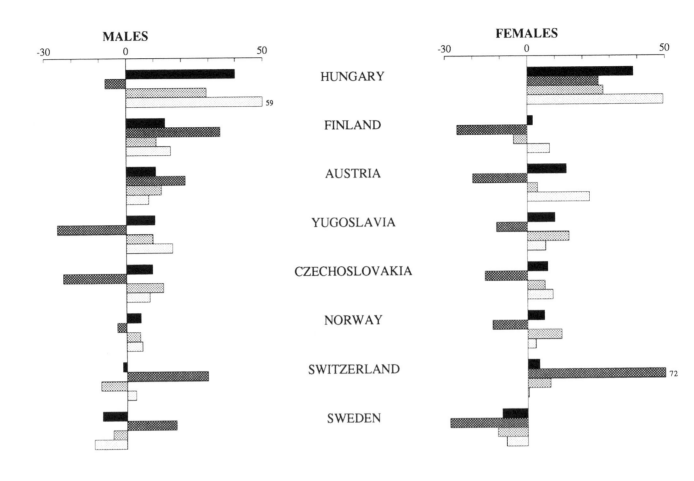

MULTIPLE MYELOMA (ICD-9 203)

EUROPE (EC), MORTALITY
Percentage change per five-year period, 1975-1988

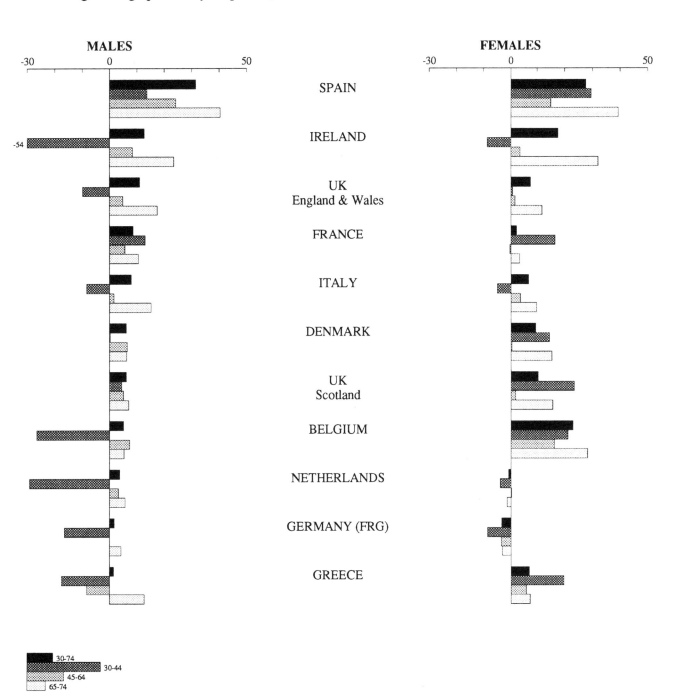

ASIA, INCIDENCE

MALES	Best model	Goodness of fit	1970 Rate	1970 Cases	1985 Rate	1985 Cases	Cumulative risk 1915	Cumulative risk 1940	Recent trend
CHINA									
Shanghai	A2D	1.51	*0.9*	*9*	1.8	30	0.8	2.4	22.5
HONG KONG	A2D	0.36	*1.8*	*9*	3.2	36	1.5	4.1	19.2
INDIA									
Bombay	A5P4	0.73	0.8	6	1.4	16	0.9	1.7	-14.8
JAPAN									
Miyagi	A2P2	-0.60	1.4	4	2.8	14	1.7	6.6	*9.7*
Nagasaki	A1	-0.34	*3.3*	*2*	3.3	3	2.2	2.2	*-3.7*
Osaka	A2C2	0.53	1.2	15	2.6	47	1.7	2.9	20.0
SINGAPORE									
Chinese	A2D	1.36	1.1	2	2.4	7	1.1	4.3	35.8
Indian	A1	0.51	*4.4*	*0*	4.4	1	3.3	3.3	*38.0*
Malay	A2D	-1.74	*0.7*	*0*	3.9	2	0.6	9.7	91.0

FEMALES	Best model	Goodness of fit	1970 Rate	1970 Cases	1985 Rate	1985 Cases	Cumulative risk 1915	Cumulative risk 1940	Recent trend
CHINA									
Shanghai	A2D	3.13	*0.4*	*4*	1.1	20	0.5	2.4	38.2
HONG KONG	A1P2	1.18	*4.2*	*19*	2.0	24	1.2	4.0	27.6
INDIA									
Bombay	A2P3C2	0.62	0.9	4	2.0	16	1.1	1.3	*1.8*
JAPAN									
Miyagi	A2C2	0.25	1.1	4	2.4	15	1.5	1.4	24.1
Nagasaki	A1D	-1.71	*8.1*	*8*	1.9	2	2.8	0.2	-38.7
Osaka	A2P2	2.06	0.6	8	1.7	37	1.0	2.4	14.7
SINGAPORE									
Chinese	A2	0.08	1.3	3	1.3	4	0.8	0.8	*13.1*
Indian	*	..	..	..	..	..	..	..	..
Malay	A1C2	-1.55	*0.7*	*0*	*2.0*	*0*	1.7	0.1	*80.5*

* : not enough cases for reliable estimation
− : incomplete or missing data
Best model: polynomial of the given degree in age (A), period (P) or cohort (C), or linear drift (D) model.
Goodness of fit: the normalised likelihood ratio chi-square for the best model (see Method).
Rate: world-standardised truncated rate per 100 000 per year (30-74 years) and number of **cases** are both estimated from the best-fitting model for the single years cited.
Cumulative risk per 1000 (30-74 years) is estimated from the best-fitting *age-cohort* model for cohorts of central birth year cited.
Recent trend: estimated mean percentage change per five-year period in the age-specific rates (30-74 years) over the period 1973-1987.
Italics denote recent trends not significant at 5 per cent level, or other figures which should be interpreted with caution (see Method).

MULTIPLE MYELOMA (ICD-9 203)

ASIA, INCIDENCE

MALES

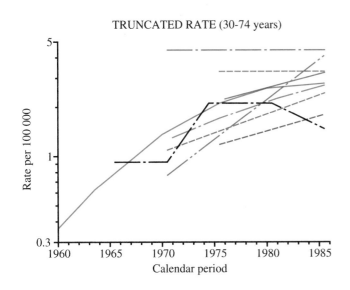

TRUNCATED RATE (30-74 years)

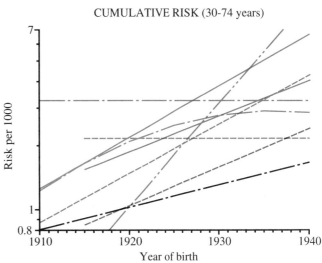

CUMULATIVE RISK (30-74 years)

FEMALES

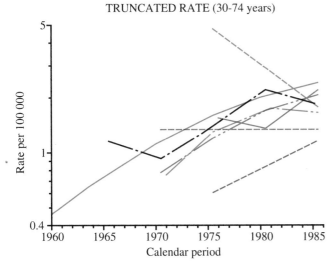

TRUNCATED RATE (30-74 years)

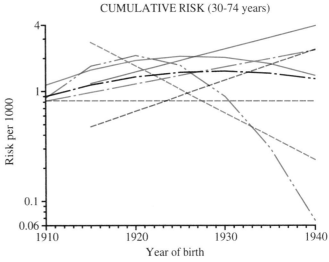

CUMULATIVE RISK (30-74 years)

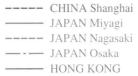

------ CHINA Shanghai	------ SINGAPORE Chinese
——— JAPAN Miyagi	—·—·— SINGAPORE Indian
------ JAPAN Nagasaki	—··—··— SINGAPORE Malay
—·—·— JAPAN Osaka	—··—··— INDIA Bombay
——— HONG KONG	

MULTIPLE MYELOMA (ICD-9 203)

OCEANIA, INCIDENCE

MALES	Best model	Goodness of fit	1970 Rate	1970 Cases	1985 Rate	1985 Cases	Cumulative risk 1915	Cumulative risk 1940	Recent trend
AUSTRALIA									
New South Wales	A2D	-1.50	*4.2*	*43*	6.3	84	3.6	7.2	14.5
South	A2	0.55	*6.2*	*9*	6.2	22	4.1	4.1	*-10.7*
HAWAII									
Caucasian	A1	-0.79	5.5	1	5.5	3	3.5	3.5	*4.3*
Chinese	A1	-2.38	*2.5*	*0*	2.5	0	1.7	1.7	*20.9*
Filipino	A1P3	0.11	9.4	2	4.7	1	3.1	2.4	*17.3*
Hawaiian	A2	-1.26	7.8	1	7.8	1	4.4	4.4	*-30.9*
Japanese	A1	0.36	*1.9*	*0*	1.9	1	1.2	1.2	*67.5*
NEW ZEALAND									
Maori	A1	-1.05	11.2	2	11.2	3	7.6	7.6	*-12.4*
Non-Maori	A2D	0.32	5.3	29	6.6	46	4.0	5.8	10.5

FEMALES	Best model	Goodness of fit	1970 Rate	1970 Cases	1985 Rate	1985 Cases	Cumulative risk 1915	Cumulative risk 1940	Recent trend
AUSTRALIA									
New South Wales	A2D	1.43	*2.8*	*34*	4.4	64	2.5	5.2	15.8
South	A3	-0.06	*4.3*	*8*	4.3	16	2.7	2.7	*-0.9*
HAWAII									
Caucasian	A2	-0.56	4.1	1	4.1	2	2.6	2.6	*-22.9*
Chinese	*	..	..	..	..	..	..	..	..
Filipino	A1	-1.57	*4.6*	*0*	4.6	1	3.3	3.3	*-15.0*
Hawaiian	A1P2	-0.49	*4.8*	*0*	6.1	1	4.9	10.6	*-24.6*
Japanese	A8P4	0.77	*1.6*	*0*	1.9	1	1.2	1.6	*19.0*
NEW ZEALAND									
Maori	A8C9	0.35	4.8	1	8.8	2	6.2	0.9	*19.0*
Non-Maori	A2D	-1.35	3.6	22	4.5	35	2.7	3.9	*7.9*

* : not enough cases for reliable estimation
− : incomplete or missing data
Best model: polynomial of the given degree in age (A), period (P) or cohort (C), or linear drift (D) model.
Goodness of fit: the normalised likelihood ratio chi-square for the best model (see Method).
Rate: world-standardised truncated rate per 100 000 per year (30-74 years) and number of **cases** are both estimated from the best-fitting model for the single years cited.
Cumulative risk per 1000 (30-74 years) is estimated from the best-fitting *age-cohort* model for cohorts of central birth year cited.
Recent trend: estimated mean percentage change per five-year period in the age-specific rates (30-74 years) over the period 1973-1987.
Italics denote recent trends not significant at 5 per cent level, or other figures which should be interpreted with caution (see Method).

MULTIPLE MYELOMA (ICD-9 203)

OCEANIA, INCIDENCE

MALES

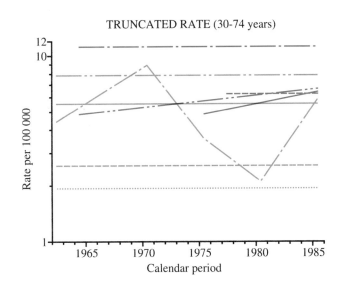

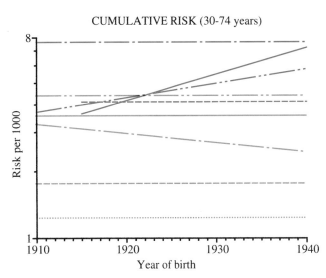

FEMALES

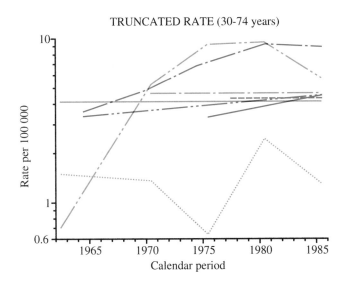

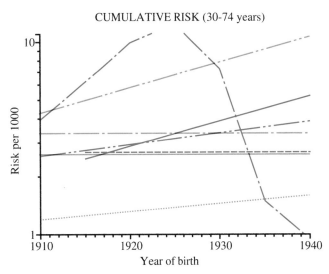

——— AUSTRALIA New South Wales	— — — HAWAII Chinese
– – – AUSTRALIA South	—·—·— HAWAII Filipino
—·—·— NEW ZEALAND Maori	—··—··— HAWAII Hawaiian
—··—··— NEW ZEALAND Non-Maori	············ HAWAII Japanese
——— HAWAII Caucasian	

MULTIPLE MYELOMA (ICD-9 203)

ASIA, INCIDENCE
Percentage change per five-year period, 1973-1987

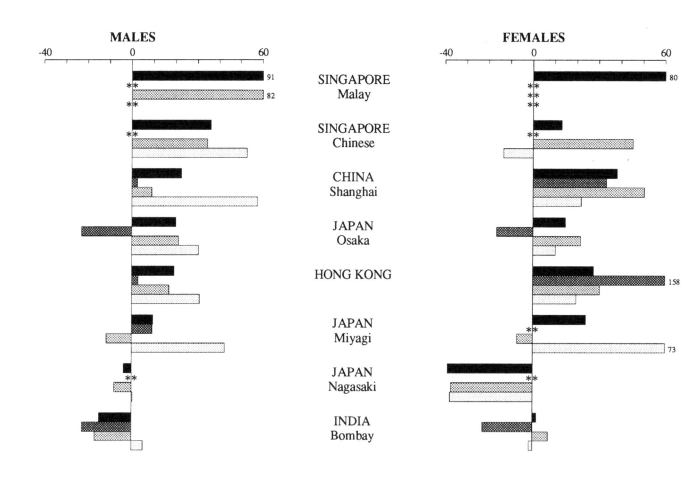

MULTIPLE MYELOMA (ICD-9 203)

OCEANIA, INCIDENCE
Percentage change per five-year period, 1973-1987

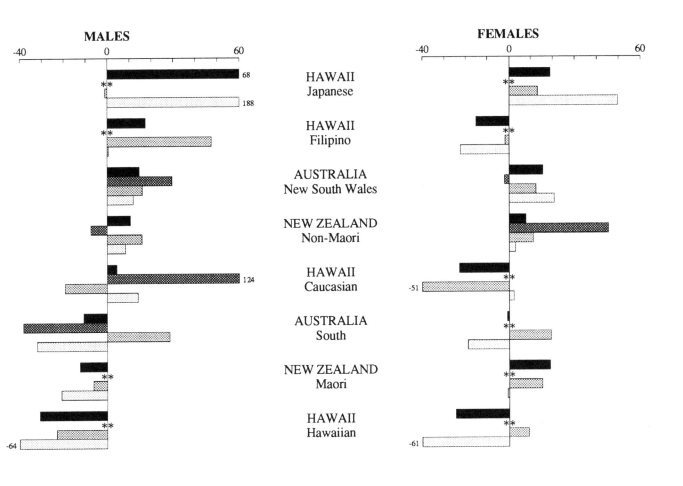

MULTIPLE MYELOMA (ICD-9 203)

ASIA and OCEANIA, MORTALITY

MALES	Best model	Goodness of fit	1965 Rate	Deaths	1985 Rate	Deaths	Cumulative risk 1900	1940	Recent trend
AUSTRALIA	A2C3	0.40	2.5	60	3.6	136	1.8	3.4	13.0
HONG KONG	A1D	1.01	0.6	2	1.4	12	*0.4*	2.3	*26.4*
JAPAN	A3P4C6	1.80	0.8	152	2.0	582	0.5	1.7	7.1
MAURITIUS	*	..	..	..	..	..	..	..	..
NEW ZEALAND	A2D	0.17	3.3	17	4.7	35	2.2	4.6	25.9
SINGAPORE	A7P4C8	-1.77	*0.1*	*0*	0.4	1	*0.0*	8.5	–

FEMALES	Best model	Goodness of fit	1965 Rate	Deaths	1985 Rate	Deaths	Cumulative risk 1900	1940	Recent trend
AUSTRALIA	A2P3C2	-0.01	1.9	52	2.5	106	1.2	1.8	15.2
HONG KONG	A2D	-0.86	0.4	1	0.9	7	*0.3*	1.5	*29.7*
JAPAN	A2P4C6	0.48	0.6	116	1.5	521	0.3	1.1	9.6
MAURITIUS	*	..	..	..	..	..	..	..	..
NEW ZEALAND	A3D	0.45	2.4	14	3.2	26	1.6	2.9	*3.2*
SINGAPORE	A1	0.37	*0.8*	*0*	0.8	1	*0.4*	0.4	–

* : not enough deaths for reliable estimation
– : incomplete or missing data
Best model: polynomial of the given degree in age (A), period (P) or cohort (C), or linear drift (D) model.
Goodness of fit: the normalised likelihood ratio chi-square for the best model (see Method).
Rate: world-standardised truncated rate per 100 000 per year (30-74 years) and number of **deaths** are both estimated from the best-fitting model for the single years cited.
Cumulative risk per 1000 (30-74 years) is estimated from the best-fitting *age-cohort* model for cohorts of central birth year cited.
Recent trend: estimated mean percentage change per five-year period in the age-specific rates (30-74 years) over the period 1975-1988.
Italics denote recent trends not significant at 5 per cent level, or other figures which should be interpreted with caution (see Method).

MULTIPLE MYELOMA (ICD-9 203)

ASIA and OCEANIA, MORTALITY

MALES

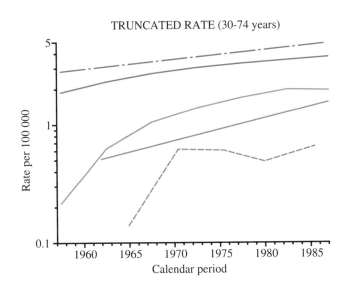

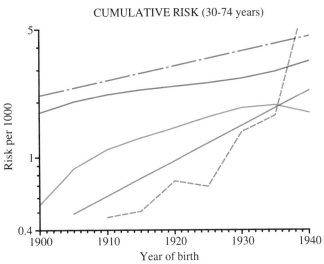

FEMALES

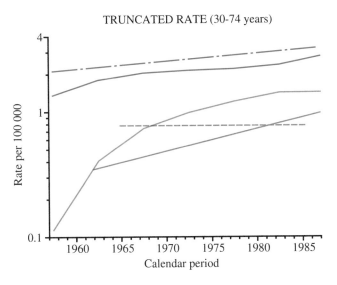

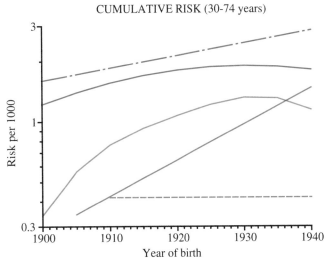

AUSTRALIA   HONG KONG
NEW ZEALAND --- SINGAPORE
JAPAN

MULTIPLE MYELOMA (ICD-9 203)

ASIA and OCEANIA, MORTALITY
Percentage change per five-year period, 1975-1988

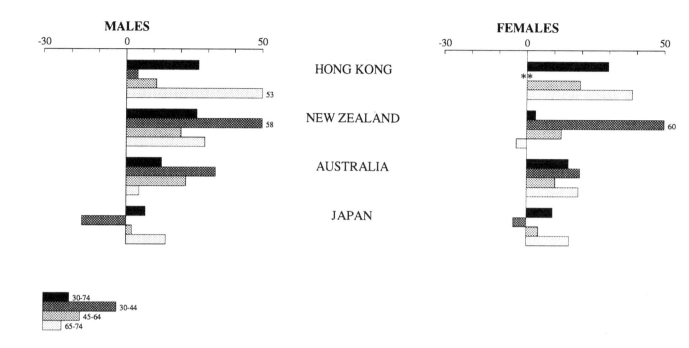

from page 705

was presumably due at least in part to improved diagnosis and certification of death in cases of myeloma. The rate of increase has decelerated since the 1970s, and although it is still increasing quite fast, at 20% every five years, the rates of incidence and mortality are now declining in males and females under the age of 45, and those born around 1935 would appear to represent the cohort at highest risk.

The highest incidence rates are seen among Maoris in New Zealand and among Hawaiians in Hawaii in both sexes (7-10 per 100 000 in males and 5-7 in females). There are fewer than 50 000 persons aged 30-74 of each sex in these populations, however, and the increasing trends are unstable, due to the small number of cases observed in each time period. Significant increases in incidence and mortality from myeloma have been occurring in both sexes among non-Maoris in New Zealand and among Australians. The apparent deceleration of the increase in mortality among Australian females should be viewed with caution, however, since the death rate in younger females is still increasing at 19% every five years, albeit not significantly.

Americas

Myeloma is more than twice as frequent among blacks than among whites in the USA, with truncated rates of 12-15 per 100 000 in males and about 10 per 100 000 in females. For black males in Detroit, there has been a steady increase in myeloma of about 10% every five years; although this trend is not quite significant over the last 15 years, it is nevertheless a fair estimate of the trend in this population, since the age-drift model fits the data well, showing a significant linear increase in the rate with time over the full 19 years of data available since 1969. There has been no real change in incidence in the other black populations examined, however.

Among white populations in the USA there has been a slight overall increase in incidence between the ages of 30 and 74 years. Not all of the changes in the elderly (65-74 years) are upward, however, and the same is true for persons aged 75 years and over (Table 28.1). Among the 10 populations for which data were examined in the continental United States, none of the recent trends in incidence at ages 75 and over is significant in males, and only half are increases. For females

726

Table 28.1   Recent linear trends in the incidence of multiple myeloma in the elderly, by age and sex, USA, 1973-87: trend[a] and ratio of trend to its standard error (β/SE)

		65-74 years		75 years and over	
		Trend	β/SE	Trend	β/SE
Bay Area, Black	M	21.0	1.1	-5.2	-0.3
	F	31.1	1.5	2.6	0.1
Bay Area, White	M	-2.0	-0.2	-2.9	-0.4
	F	-0.4	-0.1	3.8	0.5
Connecticut	M	-8.1	-1.2	-5.3	-0.8
	F	-9.2	-1.4	-4.2	-0.7
Detroit, Black	M	18.1	1.7	19.0	1.3
	F	-1.4	-0.1	4.4	0.4
Detroit, White	M	14.6	1.9	8.8	1.1
	F	-7.5	-1.1	25.2	3.2
Iowa	M	11.0	1.7	10.9	1.7
	F	6.6	0.9	5.7	0.9
New Orleans, Black	M	8.2	0.4	-2.7	-0.1
	F	2.1	0.1	-5.0	-0.2
New Orleans, White	M	-27.5	-1.5	-7.7	0.3
	F	22.9	1.2	23.4	1.2
Seattle	M	3.3	0.4	7.6	0.9
	F	-6.4	0.7	23.7	2.4

[a] Percentage change every five years (see Chapter 3).   Chinese in San Francisco Bay Area excluded.

aged 75 and over, there has been a significant recent increase of around 22% every five years in Seattle and among white females in Detroit.

Mortality from myeloma in Canada and the USA has been increasing slowly but steadily for 25 years or more, at around 5% every five years. There has been a flattening of the rate of increase in both sexes in each country since about 1980. The increases are similar in each of the broad age groups examined between 35 and 74 years of age, but at 75 years and above (data not shown), the increases in mortality have been significant and much larger, at 15-18% every five years. These trends in mortality at the oldest ages are difficult to reconcile with the patterns of incidence, unless survival in the elderly has declined sharply, which seems unlikely, or else the populations for which incidence has been examined here are not at all representative of the USA in general, a possibility which is not supported by the coherence of incidence and mortality data from the USA for other cancers.

continued page 736

MULTIPLE MYELOMA (ICD-9 203)

AMERICAS (except USA), INCIDENCE

MALES	Best model	Goodness of fit	1970 Rate	Cases	1985 Rate	Cases	Cumulative risk 1915	1940	Recent trend
BRAZIL									
Sao Paulo	A1C5	0.24	1.1	9	*	*	1.4	0.2	–
CANADA									
Alberta	A2D	0.57	4.1	12	7.1	31	3.9	9.7	23.0
British Columbia	A2P2	2.64	5.6	26	5.7	42	3.5	4.7	16.1
Maritime Provinces	A1P2	2.30	5.4	17	7.0	26	3.9	8.8	30.7
Newfoundland	A2D	0.47	3.0	2	4.7	5	2.6	5.4	-1.2
Quebec	A2D	-0.37	3.7	39	6.1	89	3.3	7.7	24.8
COLOMBIA									
Cali	A1	-1.30	3.1	1	3.1	3	2.1	2.1	-14.4
CUBA	A2P2	0.77	2.6	39	3.6	74	2.2	3.2	–
PUERTO RICO	A2D	0.11	3.9	17	5.8	39	3.2	6.3	16.7

FEMALES	Best model	Goodness of fit	1970 Rate	Cases	1985 Rate	Cases	Cumulative risk 1915	1940	Recent trend
BRAZIL									
Sao Paulo	A1D	0.46	0.7	4	7.2	69	1.2	60.7	–
CANADA									
Alberta	A2C3	-1.19	3.5	10	4.3	20	2.8	4.3	11.3
British Columbia	A8	-0.41	3.7	17	3.7	30	2.4	2.4	12.4
Maritime Provinces	A3	2.07	3.5	11	3.5	14	2.2	2.2	0.5
Newfoundland	A1C5	-1.19	2.9	2	5.4	6	3.6	9.8	12.4
Quebec	A2P2	0.74	2.5	30	4.8	82	2.5	6.9	30.8
COLOMBIA									
Cali	A2	-1.38	2.1	1	2.1	3	1.3	1.3	-9.2
CUBA	A2C2	0.48	2.3	29	4.0	83	2.5	3.5	–
PUERTO RICO	A2C2	0.19	3.3	14	4.1	32	2.7	2.3	-2.1

* : not enough cases for reliable estimation
– : incomplete or missing data
Best model: polynomial of the given degree in age (A), period (P) or cohort (C), or linear drift (D) model.
Goodness of fit: the normalised likelihood ratio chi-square for the best model (see Method).
Rate: world-standardised truncated rate per 100 000 per year (30-74 years) and number of **cases** are both estimated from the best-fitting model for the single years cited.
Cumulative risk per 1000 (30-74 years) is estimated from the best-fitting *age-cohort* model for cohorts of central birth year cited.
Recent trend: estimated mean percentage change per five-year period in the age-specific rates (30-74 years) over the period 1973-1987.
Italics denote recent trends not significant at 5 per cent level, or other figures which should be interpreted with caution (see Method).

MULTIPLE MYELOMA (ICD-9 203)

AMERICAS (except USA), INCIDENCE

MALES

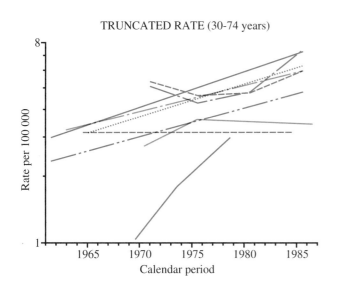

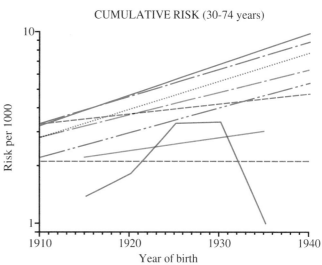

FEMALES

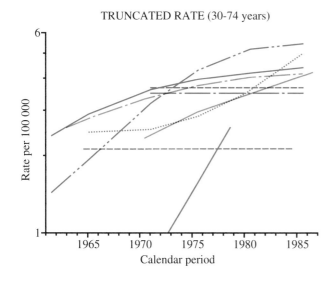

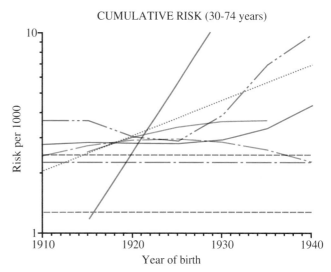

——— CANADA Alberta	——— CUBA
– – – CANADA British Columbia	–·–·– PUERTO RICO
–··–··– CANADA Maritime Provinces	——— BRAZIL Sao Paulo
–···–···– CANADA Newfoundland	– – – – COLOMBIA Cali
··········· CANADA Quebec	

MULTIPLE MYELOMA (ICD-9 203)

AMERICAS (USA), INCIDENCE

MALES	Best model	Goodness of fit	1970 Rate	Cases	1985 Rate	Cases	Cumulative risk 1915	1940	Recent trend
USA									
Bay Area, Black	A2	0.25	14.8	7	14.8	12	9.0	9.0	-2.8
Bay Area, Chinese	A0	-0.39	*2.1*	*0*	2.1	*1*	0.9	*0.9*	–
Bay Area, White	A5	-1.48	5.8	34	5.8	36	3.7	3.7	*6.0*
Connecticut	A2P2	0.97	5.1	33	5.6	45	3.5	5.1	*-4.6*
Detroit, Black	A2D	-0.24	11.6	15	17.1	30	9.1	17.4	*10.4*
Detroit, White	A2C2	0.00	5.2	38	6.5	47	4.2	3.8	*4.2*
Iowa	A2D	-0.07	5.4	37	7.5	54	4.6	7.9	*9.2*
New Orleans, Black	A1	-0.56	*12.6*	*6*	12.6	7	8.4	8.4	*-4.3*
New Orleans, White	A2	0.08	*5.2*	*7*	5.2	8	3.3	3.3	*-14.2*
Seattle	A3	-0.34	*7.1*	*34*	7.1	47	4.6	4.6	*1.9*

FEMALES	Best model	Goodness of fit	1970 Rate	Cases	1985 Rate	Cases	Cumulative risk 1915	1940	Recent trend
USA									
Bay Area, Black	A1	-0.98	10.3	6	10.3	10	6.7	6.7	*11.9*
Bay Area, Chinese	A1	-0.25	*3.5*	*0*	3.5	*2*	2.4	*2.4*	–
Bay Area, White	A2	1.04	4.3	30	4.3	32	2.8	2.8	*11.5*
Connecticut	A2P3	-0.61	3.8	29	4.2	41	2.9	3.7	-8.8
Detroit, Black	A2	-0.03	10.1	14	10.1	21	6.2	6.2	*8.2*
Detroit, White	A2	1.03	4.3	35	4.3	37	2.8	2.8	-3.6
Iowa	A4	-0.04	4.6	37	4.6	39	3.0	3.0	*4.9*
New Orleans, Black	A1P2	-0.68	*148.5*	*99*	10.1	8	6.4	9.5	*9.3*
New Orleans, White	A1	0.73	*3.9*	*8*	3.9	7	2.6	2.6	*1.3*
Seattle	A2	-0.50	*4.6*	*27*	4.6	35	3.0	3.0	-7.8

* : not enough cases for reliable estimation
– : incomplete or missing data
Best model: polynomial of the given degree in age (A), period (P) or cohort (C), or linear drift (D) model.
Goodness of fit: the normalised likelihood ratio chi-square for the best model (see Method).
Rate: world-standardised truncated rate per 100 000 per year (30-74 years) and number of **cases** are both estimated from the best-fitting model for the single years cited.
Cumulative risk per 1000 (30-74 years) is estimated from the best-fitting *age-cohort* model for cohorts of central birth year cited.
Recent trend: estimated mean percentage change per five-year period in the age-specific rates (30-74 years) over the period 1973-1987.
Italics denote recent trends not significant at 5 per cent level, or other figures which should be interpreted with caution (see Method).

MULTIPLE MYELOMA (ICD-9 203)

AMERICAS (USA), INCIDENCE

MALES

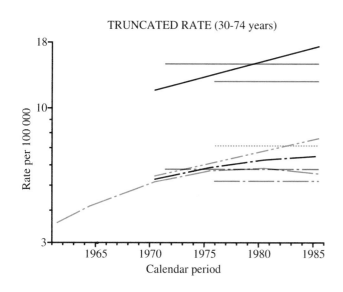

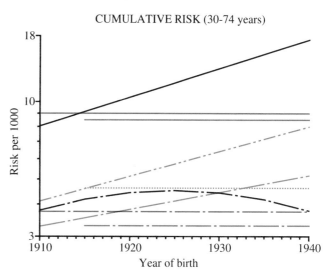

FEMALES

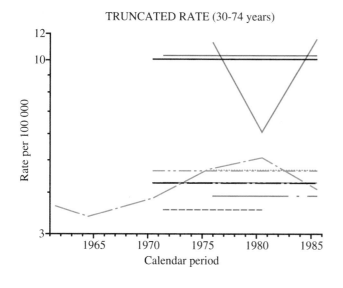

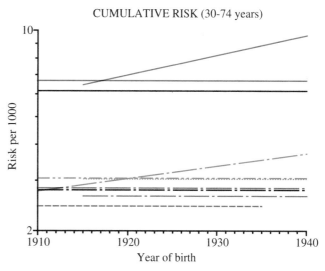

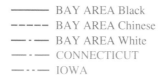

—— BAY AREA Black	············· SEATTLE
----- BAY AREA Chinese	—— NEW ORLEANS Black
—·—· BAY AREA White	—··— NEW ORLEANS White
—·—· CONNECTICUT	—— DETROIT Black
—··— IOWA	—··— DETROIT White

MULTIPLE MYELOMA (ICD-9 203)

AMERICAS (except USA), INCIDENCE
Percentage change per five-year period, 1973-1987

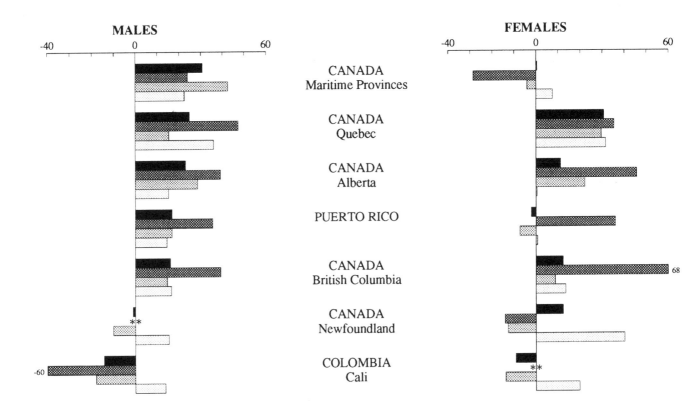

MULTIPLE MYELOMA (ICD-9 203)

AMERICAS (USA), INCIDENCE
Percentage change per five-year period, 1973-1987

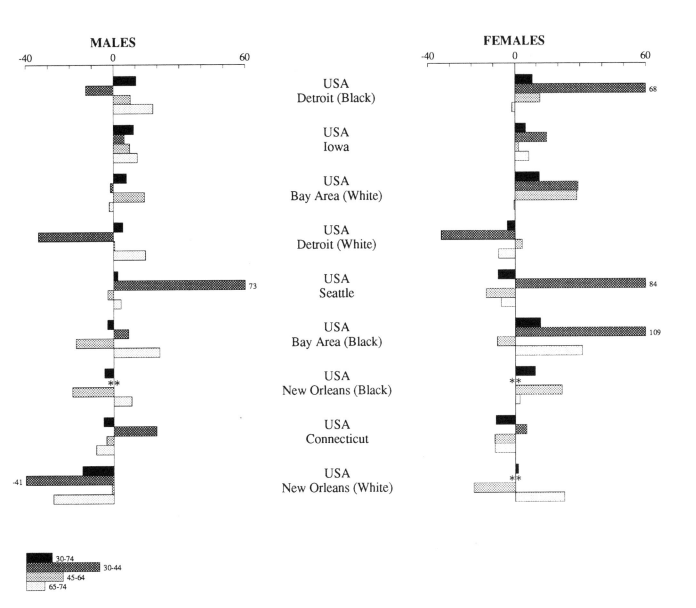

MULTIPLE MYELOMA (ICD-9 203)

AMERICAS, MORTALITY

MALES	Best model	Goodness of fit	1965 Rate	1965 Deaths	1985 Rate	1985 Deaths	Cumulative risk 1900	Cumulative risk 1940	Recent trend
CANADA	A4C2	2.44	3.3	123	4.2	244	2.2	2.8	10.1
CHILE	A2P2C2	-0.77	1.1	12	*4.0*	*68*	0.8	*1.3*	–
COSTA RICA	–	–	–	–	–	–	–	–	–
PANAMA	–	–	–	–	–	–	–	–	–
PUERTO RICO	–	–	–	–	–	–	–	–	–
URUGUAY	–	–	–	–	–	–	–	–	–
USA	A3P5C4	2.40	3.4	1450	4.3	2443	2.4	2.9	3.8
VENEZUELA	A1C2	-0.66	1.0	9	*2.7*	*37*	0.7	*2.4*	–

FEMALES	Best model	Goodness of fit	1965 Rate	1965 Deaths	1985 Rate	1985 Deaths	Cumulative risk 1900	Cumulative risk 1940	Recent trend
CANADA	A2C2	1.09	2.4	93	2.9	193	1.6	1.8	7.2
CHILE	A3D	-1.03	0.9	11	*3.4*	*69*	0.6	*8.1*	–
COSTA RICA	–	–	–	–	–	–	–	–	–
PANAMA	–	–	–	–	–	–	–	–	–
PUERTO RICO	–	–	–	–	–	–	–	–	–
URUGUAY	–	–	–	–	–	–	–	–	–
USA	A3P2C4	2.61	2.5	1211	3.1	2109	1.7	2.0	4.3
VENEZUELA	A4P3	1.52	0.9	8	*0.1*	*1*	0.5	*2.9*	–

* : not enough deaths for reliable estimation
– : incomplete or missing data
Best model: polynomial of the given degree in age (A), period (P) or cohort (C), or linear drift (D) model.
Goodness of fit: the normalised likelihood ratio chi-square for the best model (see Method).
Rate: world-standardised truncated rate per 100 000 per year (30-74 years) and number of **deaths** are both estimated from the best-fitting model for the single years cited.
Cumulative risk per 1000 (30-74 years) is estimated from the best-fitting *age-cohort* model for cohorts of central birth year cited.
Recent trend: estimated mean percentage change per five-year period in the age-specific rates (30-74 years) over the period 1975-1988.
Italics denote recent trends not significant at 5 per cent level, or other figures which should be interpreted with caution (see Method).

MULTIPLE MYELOMA (ICD-9 203)

AMERICAS, MORTALITY

MALES

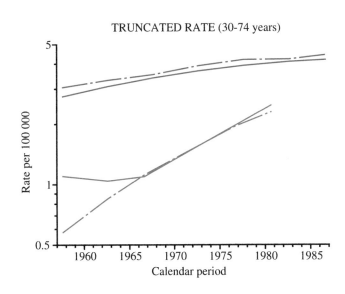

TRUNCATED RATE (30-74 years)

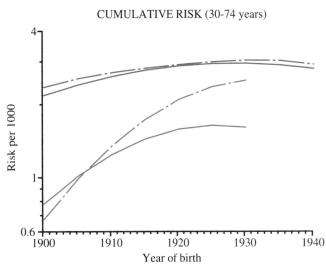

CUMULATIVE RISK (30-74 years)

FEMALES

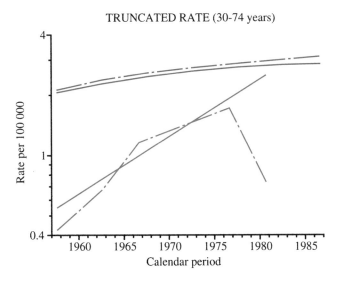

TRUNCATED RATE (30-74 years)

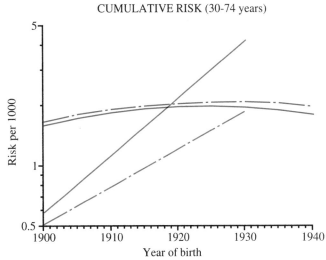

CUMULATIVE RISK (30-74 years)

———— CANADA
—·—·— USA
———— CHILE
—··—··— VENEZUELA

AMERICAS, MORTALITY
Percentage change per five-year period, 1975-1988

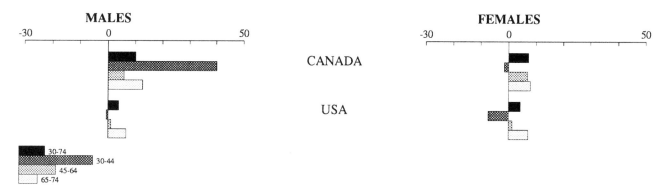

from page 727

Comment

Several artefacts complicate the interpretation of European trends in myeloma. The very rapid increases in Bas-Rhin and Doubs (France) are based on only three data sets, collected since the mid-1970s among small populations (less than 250 000 in the age range 30-74 years), and thus on relatively few cases. The trends are much steeper than those in neighbouring countries, and are not reflected by the national patterns in mortality, the rate of increase in which has tapered off more markedly in France since the 1970s than in any other country in the European Community. The rapid increases in County Vas (Hungary) and in Zaragoza (Spain) also suggest under-ascertainment in the 1970s. The increase in recorded mortality in Spain since the 1960s appears too dramatic to be entirely plausible. Mortality was lower than incidence in 1970, and has been increasing more rapidly; this may be due at least in part to more precise diagnosis and certification of death. Recent analyses of the mortality trends in Spain confirm this evaluation, but increasing incidence is thought to underlie some of the continuing recent increase in mortality[238]. The sharp dip in mortality in Germany during the mid-1980s is an artefact of mortality coding in the ninth revision of the ICD (see Chapter 2).

The results of other studies of trends in multiple myeloma are generally compatible with these results. The trends in Vaud (Switzerland) over the 10[161] or 11[164] years to 1987 are similar to those in Geneva, showing little change in incidence among males or females aged 65 and over. A similar pattern was reported from Doubs (France) over the decade 1979-86[260]; over the slightly longer period 1977-87 represented in these analyses, the trend among elderly males in Doubs is slightly negative

(-15% per five-year period among 65-74 year-olds, +41% among males aged 75 and over), but neither trend is significant. The increases in incidence recorded in Slovakia[237] during the decade 1979-88, 24% and 18% every five years in males and females, respectively, are similar to those in Vas (Hungary), but much larger than the increases in Szabolcs-Szatmar (Hungary) or Slovenia.

It seems at least plausible that improved diagnosis and certification of death from myeloma in old age is partly responsible for the observed patterns of incidence and mortality[59,238], since the trends in incidence and mortality up to the age of 75 appear compatible. Even if artefact were excluded, the analyses reported here suggest that the observed trends in incidence and mortality of myeloma among elderly persons in the USA and other industrial countries do not represent an alarming increase of the disease requiring aggressive investigation[62,64,66], but are rather the outcome of a (still unexplained) increase in risk, affecting both sexes in successive birth cohorts, which has already reached its apogee and started to decline, the cumulative risk (30-74 years) in cohorts born since 1930 showing no further increase. The implications for public health are thus somewhat more reassuring than previous interpretations.

The chief exception to this statement appears to be Japan, where the two large prefectural registries report substantial increases in incidence since 1970, from levels that were previously very low, and mortality has increased in similar measure. Even in Japan, however, there has clearly been a recent deceleration of the rate of increase in incidence and mortality, with the greatest increases confined to older persons, and a suggestion that recent birth cohorts may have a lower lifetime risk than earlier cohorts.

Chapter 29

LEUKAEMIA

The leukaemias are a group of malignancies of the blood precursor cells. The different types of leukaemia can be distinguished by their clinical behaviour and their cell type of origin as acute or chronic and myeloid or lymphocytic, and subtypes can now be defined by cell-surface markers[20]. The different types of leukaemia also have different epidemiological characteristics, but they are not separable in routine vital statistics prior to 1968, when the main types of leukaemia were assigned separate three-digit rubrics (ICD-8 204-207) for the first time in the eighth revision of the International Classification of Diseases, and for this reason they are considered together here. Leukaemias comprise about 3% of all malignancies world-wide. The age-incidence curve in most populations is bimodal, with an early peak in childhood at 2-4 years of age, low levels in adolescence and early adulthood, and a steady increase after about 30 years of age. The childhood peak is essentially due to acute lymphocytic leukaemia, the most common childhood malignancy. Chronic lymphocytic leukaemia is rare before age 50, but is generally the most common type of leukaemia in old age. Rates are generally 1.5- to 2-fold higher in males than in females. Ionising radiation, benzene and certain drugs and industrial exposures are known to be leukaemogenic, but the known causes are unlikely to account for a large proportion of cases either in adults or in children. Viral infections may also play a role in some leukaemias. Genetic conditions such as Down's syndrome and certain chromosomal abnormalities are associated with increased leukaemia risk, and the rarity of chronic lymphocytic leukaemia in Asian populations also suggests a genetic component of risk.

Europe

The range of incidence is narrow, with truncated rates (30-74 years) of 8-12 per 100 000 in males and 4-8 in females. In Warsaw City (Poland) a significant recent decline has occurred in both sexes since 1970: truncated rates were typical for Europe in 1970 (9 and 7 per 100 000), but have since fallen on average 10-15% every five years, and are now among the lowest in Europe. Rates also fell to similar levels in Cracow City (Poland)[202,221]. In marked contrast, incidence has been rising quickly, particularly in males, in both County Vas and Szabolcs-Szatmar (Hungary), from rates that were much lower than elsewhere in Europe in the 1970s to levels that are at least as high, with every prospect of exceeding the rates in other European countries shortly. Incidence in Cluj (Romania) has also been rising quickly among females.

There have been steady increases from the relatively low levels of incidence recorded in both sexes around 1970 in Germany, Spain, Scotland and, more recently, in Birmingham and South Thames (UK). The steady increase of 7-8% every five years in both sexes in Scotland is attributable to a cohort effect. It is based on large numbers of cases, and despite the recent flattening of the rate of increase in risk, Scottish males born after 1935 appear likely to have a higher cumulative risk (30-74 years) of leukaemia than other European populations, around 9 per 1000.

Leukaemia incidence is high in Denmark, at around 15 and 9 per 100 000 in males and females, respectively, and it has been continuing to increase slowly since the mid-1960s in both sexes. Incidence has not changed significantly in Norway, Sweden or Finland, however, and there is a small but consistent decline in females in these populations, particularly among 30-44 year-olds.

There have been impressive declines in leukaemia mortality, which has been falling slowly but steadily in both sexes in the Netherlands, Switzerland, Ireland, Scotland and in the Nordic countries (except Denmark) since about 1970, and in Greece and England and Wales since about 1975. In Denmark, mortality remains the highest in Europe, with no evidence of change. Mortality has more than doubled since 1960 in both sexes in Spain and Portugal, levelling off more recently; this pattern suggests improvement in death certification. The increases in mortality in Hungary are consonant with the rise in incidence recorded in Vas and Szabolcs-Szatmar; the increase in mortality in Poland, however, although it reached a peak in 1985, does not reflect the steady decline in incidence seen in the capital city, Warsaw, and in Cracow (data not shown). Similarly, the level and trend of leukaemia mortality in Romania appears too low, unless leukaemia incidence in County Cluj is much higher than in Romania as a whole.

The declines in mortality in Europe are large, and affected many western European nations at

continued page 758

LEUKAEMIA (ICD-9 204-208)

EUROPE (non-EC), INCIDENCE

MALES	Best model	Goodness of fit	1970 Rate	1970 Cases	1985 Rate	1985 Cases	Cumulative risk 1915	Cumulative risk 1940	Recent trend
FINLAND	A3C2	-0.44	10.1	102	10.5	126	6.6	6.4	2.6
HUNGARY									
County Vas	A1D	0.64	6.8	5	12.0	8	5.7	14.6	29.0
Szabolcs-Szatmar	A3P2	-0.54	3.5	4	8.0	11	3.2	8.1	56.0
ISRAEL									
All Jews	A1P3	-0.93	10.7	47	10.3	57	6.8	5.2	-2.8
Non-Jews	A1	2.24	9.0	3	9.0	5	5.3	5.3	-1.7
NORWAY	A3	-0.69	9.9	106	9.9	117	6.1	6.1	-1.5
POLAND									
Warsaw City	A3C2	2.37	9.1	26	7.3	28	5.6	2.7	-11.3
ROMANIA									
Cluj	A3	1.31	9.4	15	9.4	16	5.4	5.4	6.2
SWEDEN	A3P2C3	-0.24	11.6	280	12.2	320	7.4	6.5	1.9
SWITZERLAND									
Geneva	A1	0.74	10.5	8	10.5	9	6.6	6.6	17.8
YUGOSLAVIA									
Slovenia	A1D	1.78	8.6	32	9.7	42	5.6	6.8	3.1

FEMALES	Best model	Goodness of fit	1970 Rate	1970 Cases	1985 Rate	1985 Cases	Cumulative risk 1915	Cumulative risk 1940	Recent trend
FINLAND	A2C2	-2.62	7.2	94	6.5	101	4.3	3.2	-3.7
HUNGARY									
County Vas	A1D	0.98	4.7	3	7.2	6	2.8	5.8	6.5
Szabolcs-Szatmar	A1D	2.09	3.4	5	5.0	8	2.3	4.3	24.1
ISRAEL									
All Jews	A1D	1.74	8.9	39	7.7	49	4.9	3.9	-2.3
Non-Jews	A1P4C2	1.66	3.2	1	5.8	3	3.5	1.2	15.9
NORWAY	A4C3	-0.62	6.8	80	6.1	80	4.0	3.1	-2.7
POLAND									
Warsaw City	A1D	1.55	7.4	31	4.7	24	3.7	1.7	-15.3
ROMANIA									
Cluj	A1D	1.55	3.6	6	7.5	15	2.8	9.6	26.8
SWEDEN	A1P2	0.46	8.0	203	7.6	209	4.6	3.7	-2.0
SWITZERLAND									
Geneva	A1	0.14	7.9	8	7.9	8	4.7	4.7	22.7
YUGOSLAVIA									
Slovenia	A1C3	-0.57	6.3	30	6.2	35	3.9	3.2	5.5

* : not enough cases for reliable estimation
− : incomplete or missing data
Best model: polynomial of the given degree in age (A), period (P) or cohort (C), or linear drift (D) model.
Goodness of fit: the normalised likelihood ratio chi-square for the best model (see Method).
Rate: world-standardised truncated rate per 100 000 per year (30-74 years) and number of **cases** are both estimated from the best-fitting model for the single years cited.
Cumulative risk per 1000 (30-74 years) is estimated from the best-fitting *age-cohort* model for cohorts of central birth year cited.
Recent trend: estimated mean percentage change per five-year period in the age-specific rates (30-74 years) over the period 1973-1987.
Italics denote recent trends not significant at 5 per cent level, or other figures which should be interpreted with caution (see Method).

LEUKAEMIA (ICD-9 204-208)

EUROPE (non-EC), INCIDENCE

MALES

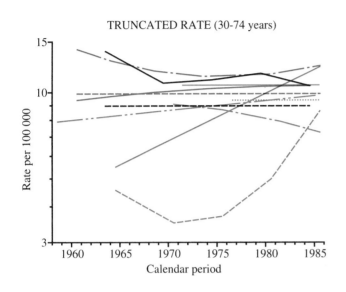

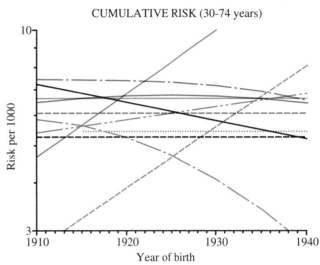

FEMALES

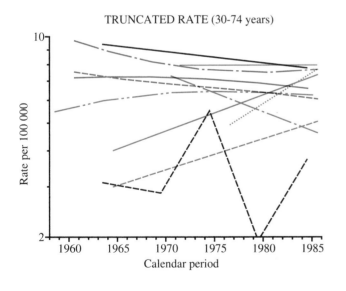

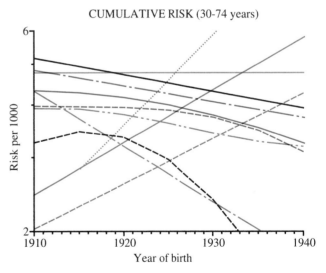

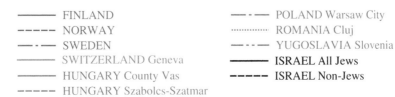

———— FINLAND	—·—·— POLAND Warsaw City
— — — NORWAY	·········· ROMANIA Cluj
—··—··— SWEDEN	—···—··· YUGOSLAVIA Slovenia
———— SWITZERLAND Geneva	———— ISRAEL All Jews
———— HUNGARY County Vas	— — — ISRAEL Non-Jews
— — — HUNGARY Szabolcs-Szatmar	

LEUKAEMIA (ICD-9 204-208)

EUROPE (EC), INCIDENCE

MALES	Best model	Goodness of fit	1970 Rate	1970 Cases	1985 Rate	1985 Cases	Cumulative risk 1915	Cumulative risk 1940	Recent trend
DENMARK	A8P6C9	0.30	13.1	175	15.5	228	8.4	8.2	11.9
FRANCE									
Bas-Rhin	A1	0.59	*13.7*	*32*	13.7	27	8.4	8.4	*4.1*
Doubs	A1	1.05	*13.5*	*9*	13.5	14	8.2	8.2	*17.4*
GERMANY (FRG)									
Hamburg	A8C9	0.63	9.0	46	*64.1*	292	7.3	*4.1*	–
Saarland	A4	-0.32	10.3	28	10.3	28	6.2	6.2	*3.2*
GERMANY (GDR)	A3C7	1.12	10.0	446	10.2	381	6.4	6.9	*1.7*
ITALY									
Varese	A1	-0.84	*13.7*	*16*	13.7	28	8.5	8.5	*2.2*
SPAIN									
Navarra	A1	-0.20	*9.5*	*11*	9.5	13	5.9	5.9	*16.5*
Zaragoza	A2D	1.96	5.4	10	9.2	21	4.3	10.4	*5.7*
UK									
Birmingham	A2P3C2	1.28	8.4	110	9.8	144	5.5	5.8	9.9
Scotland	A3C2	-1.75	7.4	97	10.5	144	5.9	8.9	8.5
South Thames	A8P5C9	0.17	8.0	196	8.4	158	4.9	4.6	*3.1*

FEMALES	Best model	Goodness of fit	1970 Rate	1970 Cases	1985 Rate	1985 Cases	Cumulative risk 1915	Cumulative risk 1940	Recent trend
DENMARK	A3P2	-1.17	7.4	109	8.7	138	4.8	5.5	6.1
FRANCE									
Bas-Rhin	A1C2	-0.26	*10.5*	*27*	6.7	16	6.1	2.0	*-14.0*
Doubs	A1	-0.15	*7.3*	*5*	7.3	8	4.3	4.3	*14.7*
GERMANY (FRG)									
Hamburg	A1D	-0.91	6.5	47	*7.8*	*41*	4.1	*5.7*	–
Saarland	A1	0.75	6.9	25	6.9	25	4.0	4.0	*3.1*
GERMANY (GDR)	A1C3	0.74	6.9	432	7.0	373	4.2	3.8	*2.2*
ITALY									
Varese	A1P2	0.29	*0.5*	*0*	8.6	21	5.9	3.7	*-9.5*
SPAIN									
Navarra	A5D	-0.21	*3.1*	*4*	6.7	10	3.1	11.3	29.8
Zaragoza	A1D	1.85	4.2	9	5.0	12	2.6	3.4	*-8.9*
UK									
Birmingham	A4P4	0.42	5.4	80	6.7	104	3.2	3.7	13.5
Scotland	A2C2	-0.82	5.0	81	6.5	107	3.6	4.9	7.2
South Thames	A2P5	0.72	5.5	162	5.5	119	3.3	3.5	*4.9*

* : not enough cases for reliable estimation
– : incomplete or missing data
Best model: polynomial of the given degree in age (A), period (P) or cohort (C), or linear drift (D) model.
Goodness of fit: the normalised likelihood ratio chi-square for the best model (see Method).
Rate: world-standardised truncated rate per 100 000 per year (30-74 years) and number of **cases** are both estimated from the best-fitting model for the single years cited.
Cumulative risk per 1000 (30-74 years) is estimated from the best-fitting *age-cohort* model for cohorts of central birth year cited.
Recent trend: estimated mean percentage change per five-year period in the age-specific rates (30-74 years) over the period 1973-1987.
Italics denote recent trends not significant at 5 per cent level, or other figures which should be interpreted with caution (see Method).

LEUKAEMIA (ICD-9 204-208)

EUROPE (EC), INCIDENCE

MALES

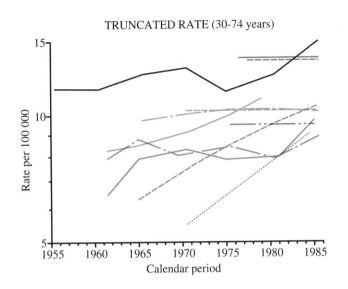

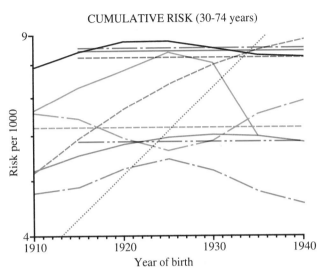

FEMALES

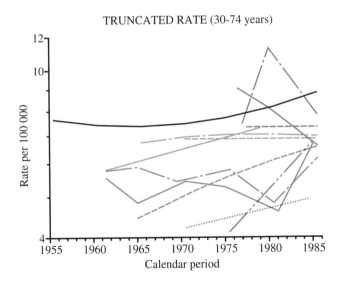

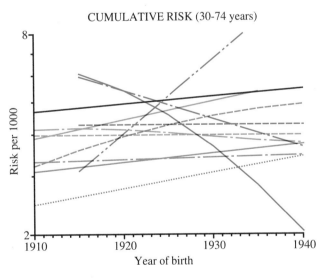

——— FRANCE Bas-Rhin	– – – GERMANY (FRG) Saarland
– – – FRANCE Doubs	–·–·– GERMANY (GDR)
–·–·– ITALY Varese	——— UK Birmingham
–··–··– SPAIN Navarra	– – – UK Scotland
········· SPAIN Zaragoza	–·–·– UK South Thames
——— GERMANY (FRG) Hamburg	——— DENMARK

LEUKAEMIA (ICD-9 204-208)

EUROPE (non-EC), INCIDENCE
Percentage change per five-year period, 1973-1987

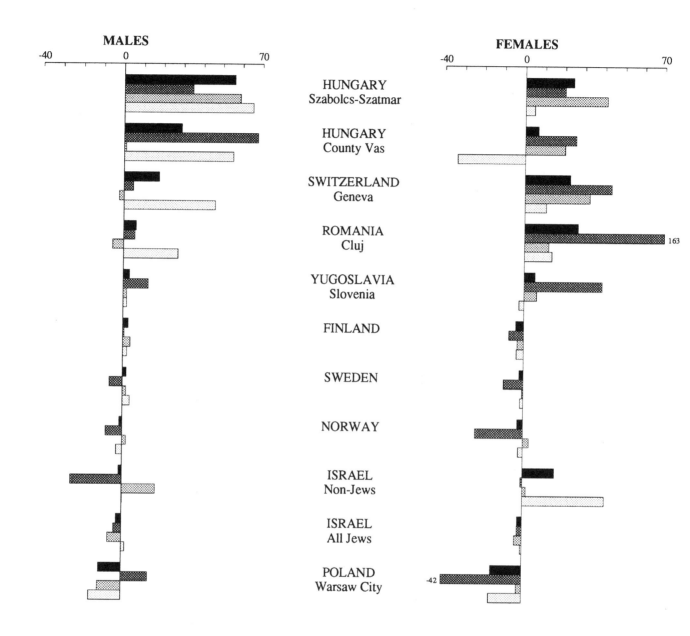

LEUKAEMIA (ICD-9 204-208)

EUROPE (EC), INCIDENCE
Percentage change per five-year period, 1973-1987

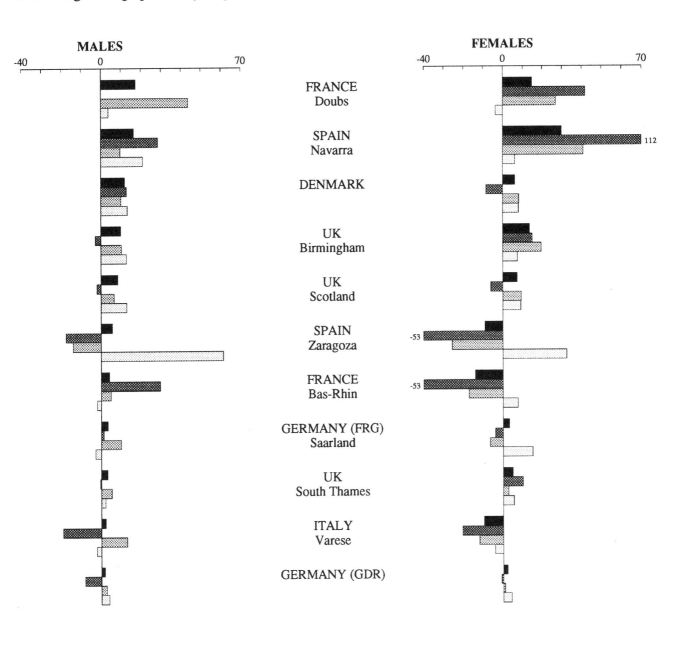

LEUKAEMIA (ICD-9 204-208)

EUROPE (non-EC), MORTALITY

MALES	Best model	Goodness of fit	1965 Rate	Deaths	1985 Rate	Deaths	Cumulative risk 1900	1940	Recent trend
AUSTRIA	A3C2	0.83	8.5	161	8.5	158	5.2	4.8	*-2.5*
CZECHOSLOVAKIA	A3P6C3	0.13	9.9	342	9.7	358	5.9	5.9	*-3.4*
FINLAND	A2C3	-0.38	9.0	83	8.2	98	5.7	4.1	-7.0
HUNGARY	A3P3C3	1.26	8.9	226	10.9	302	5.1	6.9	11.2
NORWAY	A2D	1.16	9.1	93	7.8	92	5.7	4.1	*-4.5*
POLAND	A3C3	-0.55	7.1	437	8.8	692	4.0	4.9	*1.0*
ROMANIA	A4C2	2.68	6.2	259	*6.4*	*338*	3.3	3.3	—
SWEDEN	A3P4C3	1.86	9.8	222	7.3	192	6.0	3.6	-12.6
SWITZERLAND	A2C2	0.30	8.4	117	7.8	138	5.2	3.9	*-0.1*
YUGOSLAVIA	A4P5C2	1.78	6.7	251	4.9	241	3.4	2.6	*3.0*

FEMALES	Best model	Goodness of fit	1965 Rate	Deaths	1985 Rate	Deaths	Cumulative risk 1900	1940	Recent trend
AUSTRIA	A3C5	0.91	5.9	149	5.5	138	3.6	3.2	-5.9
CZECHOSLOVAKIA	A3C3	1.07	6.2	254	6.6	295	3.6	3.7	*1.2*
FINLAND	A3C4	1.20	6.8	82	5.6	86	4.2	2.8	*-6.1*
HUNGARY	A8C9	-0.57	6.2	186	7.0	242	3.4	3.9	*2.4*
NORWAY	A2D	0.56	6.5	72	5.0	65	4.1	2.4	*-4.9*
POLAND	A8C9	-0.06	4.9	373	5.6	545	2.6	3.0	*-0.5*
ROMANIA	A3C2	0.15	4.4	208	*4.3*	*263*	2.1	2.1	—
SWEDEN	A2C2	0.84	6.7	161	5.5	154	4.1	2.6	-7.4
SWITZERLAND	A4C3	-0.24	5.7	95	5.3	105	3.4	2.6	*-2.0*
YUGOSLAVIA	A1P5C3	2.76	5.3	231	3.2	188	2.4	1.6	-6.1

* : not enough deaths for reliable estimation
− : incomplete or missing data
Best model: polynomial of the given degree in age (A), period (P) or cohort (C), or linear drift (D) model.
Goodness of fit: the normalised likelihood ratio chi-square for the best model (see Method).
Rate: world-standardised truncated rate per 100 000 per year (30-74 years) and number of **deaths** are both estimated from the best-fitting model for the single years cited.
Cumulative risk per 1000 (30-74 years) is estimated from the best-fitting *age-cohort* model for cohorts of central birth year cited.
Recent trend: estimated mean percentage change per five-year period in the age-specific rates (30-74 years) over the period 1975-1988. Italics denote recent trends not significant at 5 per cent level, or other figures which should be interpreted with caution (see Method).

LEUKAEMIA (ICD-9 204-208)

EUROPE (non-EC), MORTALITY

MALES

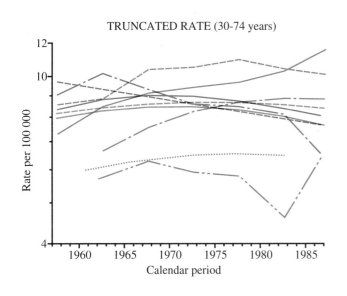

TRUNCATED RATE (30-74 years)

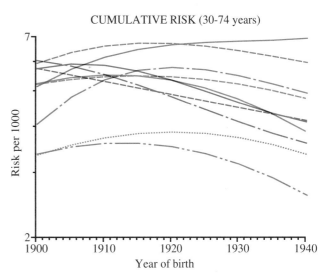

CUMULATIVE RISK (30-74 years)

FEMALES

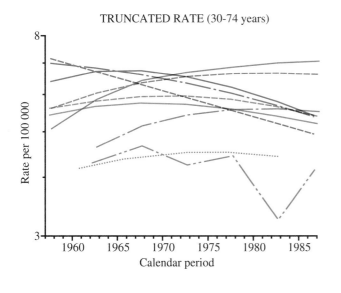

TRUNCATED RATE (30-74 years)

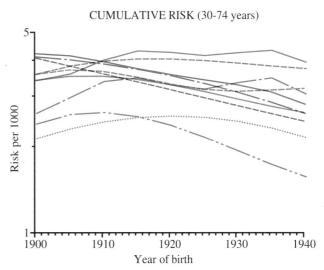

CUMULATIVE RISK (30-74 years)

—— FINLAND	----- CZECHOSLOVAKIA
- - - NORWAY	—— HUNGARY
-·-·- SWEDEN	-··-··- POLAND
--- AUSTRIA	········ ROMANIA
—— SWITZERLAND	-··-··- YUGOSLAVIA

LEUKAEMIA (ICD-9 204-208)

EUROPE (EC), MORTALITY

MALES	Best model	Goodness of fit	1965 Rate	Deaths	1985 Rate	Deaths	Cumulative risk 1900	1940	Recent trend
BELGIUM	A3C3	0.58	8.5	217	8.6	231	5.2	4.6	*-3.2*
DENMARK	A3	0.85	10.1	127	10.1	147	6.3	6.3	*4.7*
FRANCE	A4P4C4	3.12	9.3	1115	8.8	1222	5.7	4.8	-4.8
GERMANY (FRG)	A8P5C3	4.95	8.3	1246	8.3	1311	5.3	4.6	-4.6
GREECE	A3C3	0.00	9.4	178	8.9	245	*5.9*	4.3	-6.4
IRELAND	A1P3C3	2.17	8.4	60	8.0	64	4.6	4.3	*7.3*
ITALY	A4P5C6	4.46	9.2	1117	9.7	1498	5.1	5.6	*-0.4*
NETHERLANDS	A3C3	0.66	9.3	258	8.0	287	6.0	3.7	-6.6
PORTUGAL	A2P2C2	1.28	6.2	114	7.1	174	3.1	4.2	*-4.0*
SPAIN	A8C9	0.39	4.9	343	7.0	659	2.7	5.1	10.1
UK ENGLAND & WALES	A5C5	-1.09	7.5	940	7.5	1064	4.5	4.1	*0.7*
UK SCOTLAND	A2C2	0.53	7.2	92	6.7	92	4.4	3.5	*-3.2*

FEMALES	Best model	Goodness of fit	1965 Rate	Deaths	1985 Rate	Deaths	Cumulative risk 1900	1940	Recent trend
BELGIUM	A2C2	-0.51	5.9	173	5.2	161	3.5	2.3	*-0.9*
DENMARK	A1	0.78	6.6	91	6.6	105	3.9	3.9	*-3.2*
FRANCE	A2P4C5	0.95	6.2	891	5.6	889	3.6	2.8	-5.6
GERMANY (FRG)	A3P4C3	6.52	6.1	1212	5.8	1249	3.6	2.8	-4.5
GREECE	A3C2	0.70	6.2	136	5.6	172	*3.7*	2.7	*-4.8*
IRELAND	A1C3	1.61	5.2	37	4.8	40	3.1	2.4	*-1.5*
ITALY	A4P4C4	4.03	6.2	883	6.1	1079	3.4	3.4	-3.5
NETHERLANDS	A2C3	0.01	6.4	195	5.0	203	4.0	2.3	-6.5
PORTUGAL	A1P5C3	3.79	5.3	118	5.8	164	2.5	2.8	-6.0
SPAIN	A8P6C9	0.79	4.0	326	4.8	512	1.8	3.1	*2.8*
UK ENGLAND & WALES	A2P4C3	-0.49	5.2	782	5.0	790	2.9	2.6	*0.1*
UK SCOTLAND	A1P3	0.23	5.1	82	4.6	74	2.8	2.7	*2.5*

* : not enough deaths for reliable estimation
– : incomplete or missing data
Best model: polynomial of the given degree in age (A), period (P) or cohort (C), or linear drift (D) model.
Goodness of fit: the normalised likelihood ratio chi-square for the best model (see Method).
Rate: world-standardised truncated rate per 100 000 per year (30-74 years) and number of **deaths** are both estimated from the best-fitting model for the single years cited.
Cumulative risk per 1000 (30-74 years) is estimated from the best-fitting *age-cohort* model for cohorts of central birth year cited.
Recent trend: estimated mean percentage change per five-year period in the age-specific rates (30-74 years) over the period 1975-1988.
Italics denote recent trends not significant at 5 per cent level, or other figures which should be interpreted with caution (see Method).

LEUKAEMIA (ICD-9 204-208)

EUROPE (EC), MORTALITY

MALES

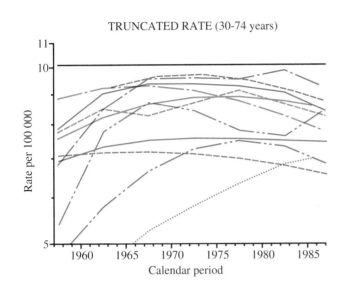

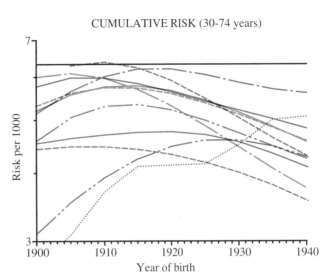

FEMALES

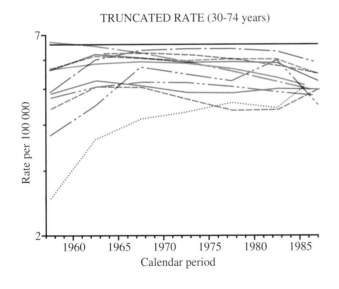

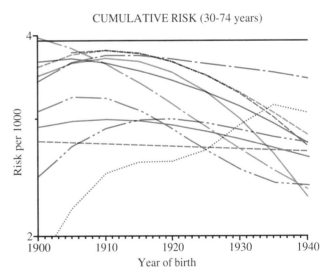

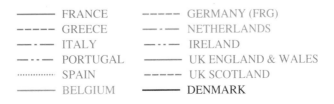

—— FRANCE	----- GERMANY (FRG)
----- GREECE	—·—· NETHERLANDS
—··— ITALY	—···— IRELAND
—·—· PORTUGAL	—— UK ENGLAND & WALES
········· SPAIN	----- UK SCOTLAND
—— BELGIUM	—— DENMARK

LEUKAEMIA (ICD-9 204-208)

EUROPE (non-EC), MORTALITY
Percentage change per five-year period, 1975-1988

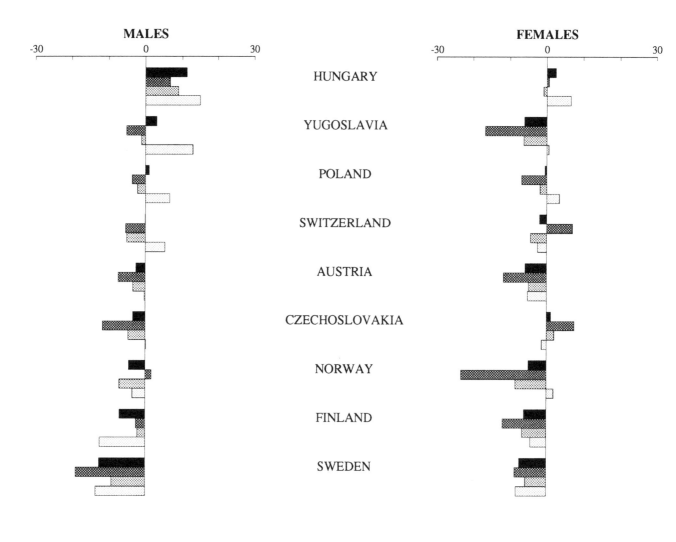

LEUKAEMIA (ICD-9 204-208)

EUROPE (EC), MORTALITY
Percentage change per five-year period, 1975-1988

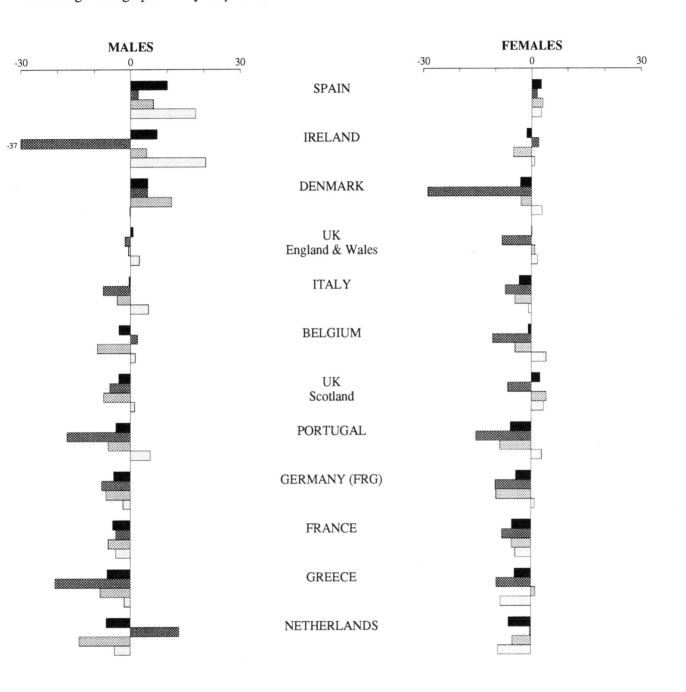

MALES

FEMALES

-30   0   30

-30   0   30

-37

SPAIN

IRELAND

DENMARK

UK
England & Wales

ITALY

BELGIUM

UK
Scotland

PORTUGAL

GERMANY (FRG)

FRANCE

GREECE

NETHERLANDS

30-74
30-44
45-64
65-74

LEUKAEMIA (ICD-9 204-208)

ASIA, INCIDENCE

MALES	Best model	Goodness of fit	1970 Rate	1970 Cases	1985 Rate	1985 Cases	Cumulative risk 1915	Cumulative risk 1940	Recent trend
CHINA									
Shanghai	A2P2	0.84	2.4	27	6.6	113	3.5	3.6	-0.3
HONG KONG	A4C2	0.36	2.8	20	8.7	103	3.0	16.4	36.7
INDIA									
Bombay	A8C9	0.64	3.4	35	4.5	59	2.5	2.6	2.5
JAPAN									
Miyagi	A1C2	-0.48	5.7	21	7.7	41	3.6	5.3	12.1
Nagasaki	A1P2	-1.68	3.3	2	7.1	7	6.8	2.7	-17.5
Osaka	A2C3	-1.12	4.5	66	7.3	147	3.4	5.5	11.4
SINGAPORE									
Chinese	A1	0.15	5.6	12	5.6	19	3.0	3.0	16.0
Indian	A1	0.58	6.3	2	6.3	2	3.4	3.4	-2.7
Malay	A1	0.76	5.6	2	5.6	3	2.9	2.9	24.9

FEMALES	Best model	Goodness of fit	1970 Rate	1970 Cases	1985 Rate	1985 Cases	Cumulative risk 1915	Cumulative risk 1940	Recent trend
CHINA									
Shanghai	A1P2	1.42	1.1	13	5.4	93	2.5	3.1	3.5
HONG KONG	A1D	1.43	2.6	16	7.3	82	2.1	11.9	40.9
INDIA									
Bombay	A1	0.17	3.8	22	3.8	41	2.0	2.0	-1.0
JAPAN									
Miyagi	A1C2	-0.46	4.2	18	4.9	30	2.4	2.7	0.7
Nagasaki	A1	-1.60	4.8	4	4.8	6	2.5	2.5	-4.5
Osaka	A1D	1.77	3.6	56	4.7	107	2.1	3.1	4.3
SINGAPORE									
Chinese	A2D	1.25	5.4	12	3.9	15	2.9	1.7	-10.0
Indian	A3	-0.19	5.6	0	5.6	1	2.9	2.9	1.5
Malay	A0	1.11	4.1	1	4.1	2	1.8	1.8	8.3

* : not enough cases for reliable estimation
− : incomplete or missing data
Best model: polynomial of the given degree in age (A), period (P) or cohort (C), or linear drift (D) model.
Goodness of fit: the normalised likelihood ratio chi-square for the best model (see Method).
Rate: world-standardised truncated rate per 100 000 per year (30-74 years) and number of **cases** are both estimated from the best-fitting model for the single years cited.
Cumulative risk per 1000 (30-74 years) is estimated from the best-fitting *age-cohort* model for cohorts of central birth year cited.
Recent trend: estimated mean percentage change per five-year period in the age-specific rates (30-74 years) over the period 1973-1987.
Italics denote recent trends not significant at 5 per cent level, or other figures which should be interpreted with caution (see Method).

LEUKAEMIA (ICD-9 204-208)

ASIA, INCIDENCE

MALES

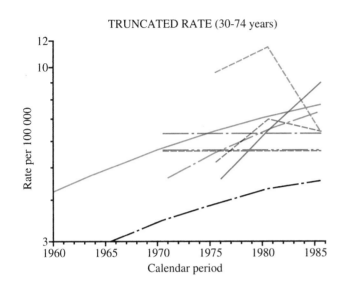

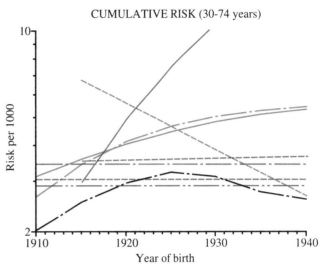

FEMALES

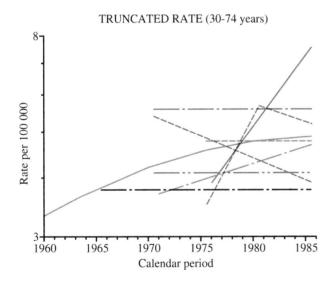

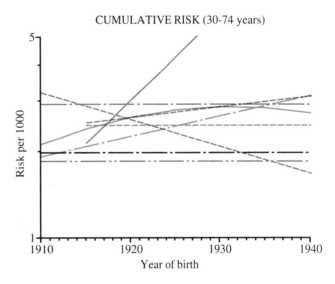

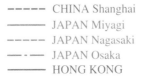

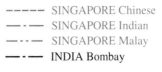

----- CHINA Shanghai

——— JAPAN Miyagi

----- JAPAN Nagasaki

—·—· JAPAN Osaka

——— HONG KONG

----- SINGAPORE Chinese

—·—· SINGAPORE Indian

—··— SINGAPORE Malay

——— INDIA Bombay

LEUKAEMIA (ICD-9 204-208)

OCEANIA, INCIDENCE

MALES	Best model	Goodness of fit	1970 Rate	1970 Cases	1985 Rate	1985 Cases	Cumulative risk 1915	Cumulative risk 1940	Recent trend
AUSTRALIA									
New South Wales	A2D	0.50	*9.8*	*102*	13.3	178	7.5	12.3	10.4
South	A3	1.75	*14.9*	*24*	14.9	53	9.4	9.4	*9.5*
HAWAII									
Caucasian	A1	1.42	11.2	4	11.2	7	7.0	7.0	*-7.0*
Chinese	A1	0.73	10.3	1	10.3	1	5.9	5.9	*45.5*
Filipino	A1	0.46	8.5	2	8.5	3	5.3	5.3	*23.8*
Hawaiian	A8C9	0.74	11.5	1	11.4	3	2.3	8.7	*11.1*
Japanese	A1	0.66	8.0	3	8.0	6	4.5	4.5	*-13.0*
NEW ZEALAND									
Maori	A1C3	0.50	11.5	2	9.2	3	7.9	2.6	*-11.3*
Non-Maori	A2	0.77	11.2	62	11.2	80	7.1	7.1	*-0.8*

FEMALES	Best model	Goodness of fit	1970 Rate	1970 Cases	1985 Rate	1985 Cases	Cumulative risk 1915	Cumulative risk 1940	Recent trend
AUSTRALIA									
New South Wales	A2D	0.55	*5.0*	*59*	8.0	113	3.9	8.5	16.6
South	A1	0.33	*8.0*	*15*	8.0	30	4.8	4.8	*-3.3*
HAWAII									
Caucasian	A1	0.52	7.4	2	7.4	4	4.7	4.7	*16.1*
Chinese	A0	-0.37	*5.8*	*0*	*5.8*	*0*	2.6	2.6	*-35.7*
Filipino	*	..	..	..	..	..	..	..	..
Hawaiian	A1	-0.72	*6.6*	*0*	6.6	1	4.1	4.1	*28.1*
Japanese	A1	-0.12	5.5	2	5.5	4	2.9	2.9	*-3.3*
NEW ZEALAND									
Maori	A2	0.94	10.0	1	10.0	3	6.5	6.5	*-4.4*
Non-Maori	A2	-1.37	7.1	43	7.1	54	4.3	4.3	*-0.2*

* : not enough cases for reliable estimation
– : incomplete or missing data
Best model: polynomial of the given degree in age (A), period (P) or cohort (C), or linear drift (D) model.
Goodness of fit: the normalised likelihood ratio chi-square for the best model (see Method).
Rate: world-standardised truncated rate per 100 000 per year (30-74 years) and number of **cases** are both estimated from the best-fitting model for the single years cited.
Cumulative risk per 1000 (30-74 years) is estimated from the best-fitting *age-cohort* model for cohorts of central birth year cited.
Recent trend: estimated mean percentage change per five-year period in the age-specific rates (30-74 years) over the period 1973-1987.
Italics denote recent trends not significant at 5 per cent level, or other figures which should be interpreted with caution (see Method).

LEUKAEMIA (ICD-9 204-208)

OCEANIA, INCIDENCE

MALES

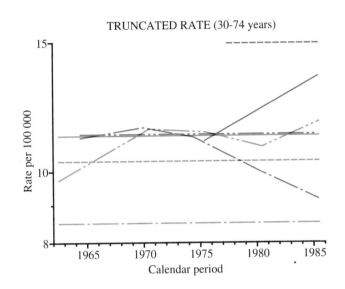

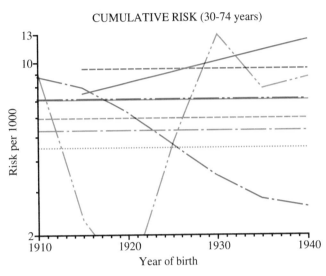

FEMALES

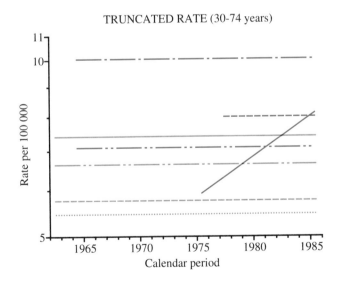

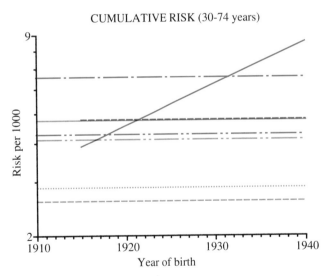

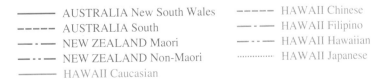

—— AUSTRALIA New South Wales	– – – HAWAII Chinese
– – – AUSTRALIA South	–·–·– HAWAII Filipino
–·–·– NEW ZEALAND Maori	–··–··– HAWAII Hawaiian
–··–··– NEW ZEALAND Non-Maori	············ HAWAII Japanese
—— HAWAII Caucasian	

LEUKAEMIA (ICD-9 204-208)

ASIA, INCIDENCE
Percentage change per five-year period, 1973-1987

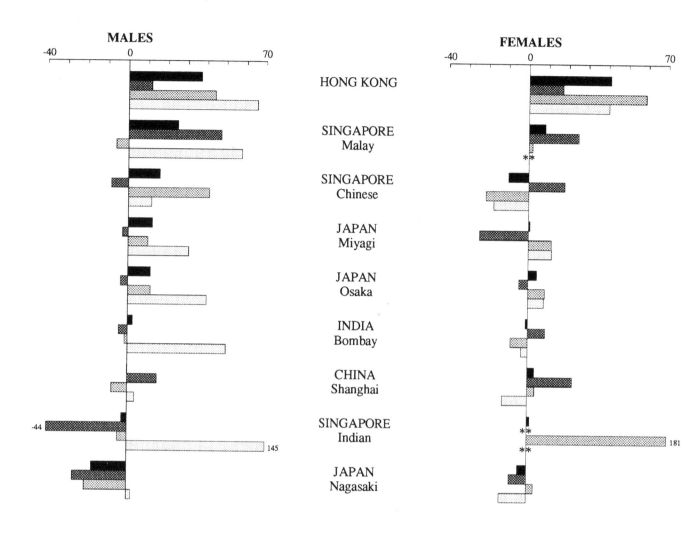

LEUKAEMIA (ICD-9 204-208)

OCEANIA, INCIDENCE
Percentage change per five-year period, 1973-1987

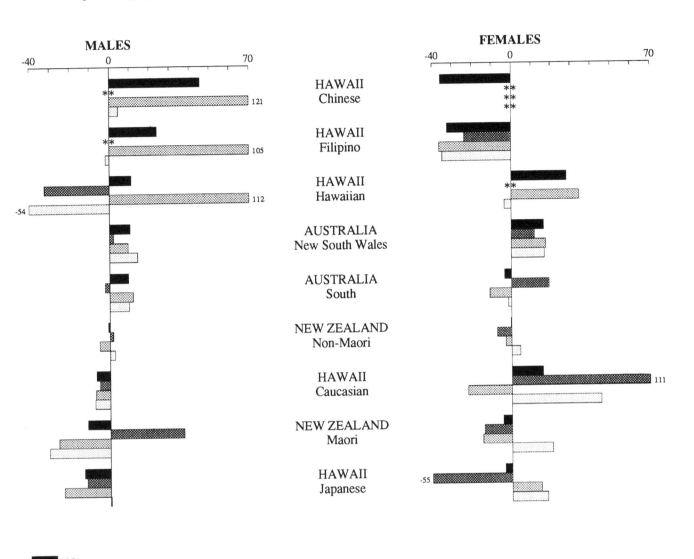

LEUKAEMIA (ICD-9 204-208)

ASIA and OCEANIA, MORTALITY

MALES	Best model	Goodness of fit	1965 Rate	1965 Deaths	1985 Rate	1985 Deaths	Cumulative risk 1900	Cumulative risk 1940	Recent trend
AUSTRALIA	A3C2	0.39	8.4	204	8.4	314	5.2	4.7	*3.2*
HONG KONG	A1D	0.95	3.9	20	4.9	52	*1.9*	3.0	*-3.6*
JAPAN	A2C4	4.42	4.3	837	6.5	1961	1.9	4.3	6.9
MAURITIUS	A1D	1.67	1.4	1	3.5	4	*0.7*	4.5	*40.9*
NEW ZEALAND	A4	0.67	8.4	44	8.4	62	5.3	5.3	-7.4
SINGAPORE	A3D	-0.65	*3.6*	*8*	4.8	19	*1.4*	2.5	–

FEMALES	Best model	Goodness of fit	1965 Rate	1965 Deaths	1985 Rate	1985 Deaths	Cumulative risk 1900	Cumulative risk 1940	Recent trend
AUSTRALIA	A2C2	1.82	5.6	148	5.2	207	3.3	2.8	*1.1*
HONG KONG	A8P5C9	-0.43	4.4	28	3.8	34	*1.4*	2.2	*6.1*
JAPAN	A8P6C9	3.73	3.3	719	4.3	1470	1.3	2.4	2.9
MAURITIUS	A1D	-0.52	1.1	1	3.1	4	*0.4*	3.4	*36.0*
NEW ZEALAND	A2P2	0.59	6.1	36	6.0	48	3.9	3.0	13.6
SINGAPORE	A2D	1.02	*2.7*	*5*	4.0	15	*1.0*	2.3	–

* : not enough deaths for reliable estimation
– : incomplete or missing data
Best model: polynomial of the given degree in age (A), period (P) or cohort (C), or linear drift (D) model.
Goodness of fit: the normalised likelihood ratio chi-square for the best model (see Method).
Rate: world-standardised truncated rate per 100 000 per year (30-74 years) and number of **deaths** are both estimated from the best-fitting model for the single years cited.
Cumulative risk per 1000 (30-74 years) is estimated from the best-fitting *age-cohort* model for cohorts of central birth year cited.
Recent trend: estimated mean percentage change per five-year period in the age-specific rates (30-74 years) over the period 1975-1988.
Italics denote recent trends not significant at 5 per cent level, or other figures which should be interpreted with caution (see Method).

LEUKAEMIA (ICD-9 204-208)

ASIA and OCEANIA, MORTALITY

MALES

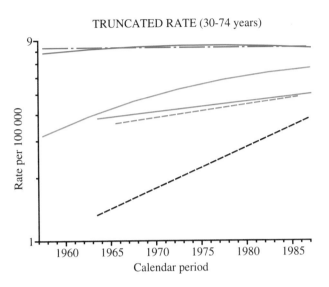

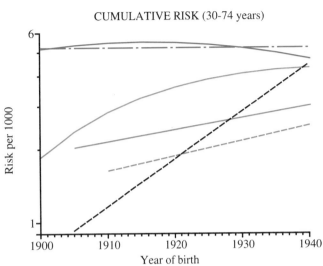

FEMALES

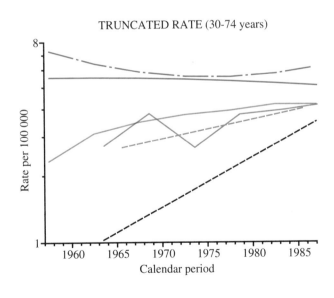

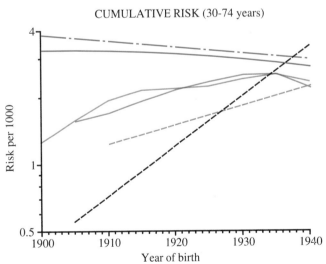

———— AUSTRALIA	———— HONG KONG
—·—·— NEW ZEALAND	– – – SINGAPORE
———— JAPAN	----- MAURITIUS

LEUKAEMIA (ICD-9 204-208)

ASIA and OCEANIA, MORTALITY
Percentage change per five-year period, 1975-1988

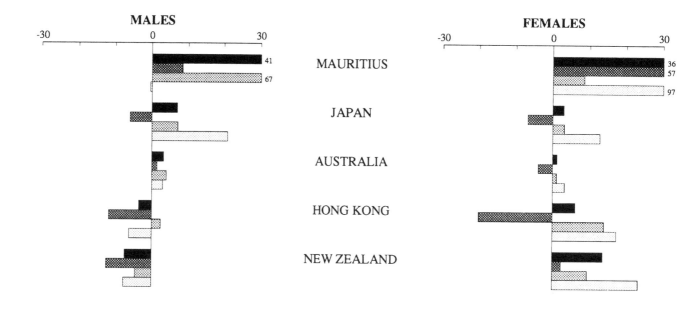

from page 737

about the same time, around 1970-75. Eastern European nations have seen a plateau in mortality, but little evidence of decline. The patterns are consistent with the major improvements in survival brought about by intensive chemotherapy.

Asia and Oceania

Leukaemia incidence in Asian populations is less than half of that in Caucasian populations. There have been substantial increases in both sexes in the large prefectural populations of Miyagi and Osaka (Japan), particularly among males, in whom rates have almost doubled since the 1960s to around 7 per 100 000, and are still rising by 10% every five years. The pattern of age-specific trends is similar in both sexes, with increases at older ages (65-74 years) and declines at younger ages (30-44 years). These patterns are well fitted by cohort models suggesting a peak in lifetime risk (30-74 years) of around 5 and 3 per 1000 among males and females born around 1940, with a decline for those born subsequently. Leukaemia risks in the city of Nagasaki have conver-

ged with those in Miyagi and Osaka. These increases in leukaemia incidence are reflected in a steady but slower increase in leukaemia mortality in Japan, to rates of 6 and 4 per 100 000 in 1985 among males and females, respectively, approaching the levels in Australia and New Zealand. The mortality trends precisely mirror those for incidence at all ages. Leukaemia incidence rates in Hong Kong had reached 9 and 7 per 100 000 in 1985, levels similar to those of Caucasian populations in Europe. The recent rate of increase appears too rapid to be entirely plausible, and is likely to be due in part to the inclusion in 1983-87 of cases registered only at death (see Chapter 2). Although the past trend in incidence in Hong Kong may be partly due to artefact, however, the current incidence rates are plausible; leukaemia mortality has also been rising less rapidly than incidence, and the incidence-to-mortality ratios are now similar to those seen elsewhere.

The incidence of leukaemia in New South Wales (Australia) has increased steadily in both sexes since 1975 by some 10-15% every five years, and now approaches the rates in South Australia (15 and 8 per 100 000 in males and females, respectively), which have changed very little. At least part of the increase in the recorded incidence of leukaemia in New South Wales may be due to improved ascertainment, since mortality from leukaemia in Australia has changed very little since the 1960s, and New South Wales includes about a third of the national population. Although the recent increase in incidence of 28% every five years in younger males in New Zealand is statistically significant, the overall trend in leukaemia mortality in both Australia and New Zealand is slightly downward. Leukaemia mortality has been very similar in Australia and New Zealand for 30 years.

Americas

Leukaemia incidence has been increasing quite quickly in four of the five Canadian populations studied. In Quebec, the largest of these populations, where the recent increase has been most rapid, the rates reached 18 and 10 per 100 000 in males and females, respectively, in 1985, and rates are high across Canada[221]. There has been little change in leukaemia incidence in Central or South America.

In the USA, the range of incidence is narrow, and there is little difference between blacks and whites in New Orleans or the San Francisco Bay Area. The Chinese population in San Francisco has about half the risk of other ethnic groups in the USA. Incidence trends in the 10 US populations studied have generally been small, and contrast sharply with trends in Canada. The only significant increase in males has occurred among whites in Detroit, where an age-cohort model fits well and suggests that the risk of leukaemia reached a peak for males born around 1930, declining for later cohorts, while incidence in black males did not increase. Among females, the risk of leukaemia is increasing for both blacks and whites in Detroit, and among whites in the Bay Area. In Connecticut, the data are well fitted by an age-period-cohort model showing that the truncated rate reached a peak between 1975 and 1980.

The slight but consistent increase in leukaemia mortality in Canadian males since 1960 has now reached a plateau. In the last 15 years, leukaemia mortality has not changed significantly in Canada or the USA, but there are clear signs of improvement in both countries. In the USA, there are small but significant rates of decline in mortality of around 4-7% every five years among males and females aged 30-44 years, and larger rates of decline in 15-29 year-olds (9-10%, data not shown). The equivalent figures for Canada are

10-14% every five years for 30-44 year-olds and 6-14% for 15-29 year-olds. These figures translate into a 20-25% reduction in the lifetime (30-74 years) risk of death from leukaemia for the 1940 birth cohort relative to those born around 1900. With more than 9000 adult leukaemia deaths a year in 1985 in the USA, this risk reduction represents a large public health gain. In view of the absence of any major change in incidence, the improvement in mortality would appear to reflect a significant improvement in the management of leukaemia on a national scale in the USA. Mortality among the elderly (75 years and over) has been increasing fairly rapidly (10% or more every five years) among both sexes in Central and South America, and smaller rates of increase (2-5%) are seen in Canada and the USA (data not shown). Mortality from leukaemia is also declining steadily among males, but not females, in Puerto Rico and Uruguay, particularly among younger persons (30-44 years); the changes in Puerto Rico closely match those seen in incidence.

Comment

The results reported here are generally similar to those in previous reports for Europe[80,116,128,149,164,237,260], Singapore Chinese[154] and the USA[77,144]. The trends in leukaemia incidence recorded since 1975 for Shanghai (China) may reflect improvements in diagnosis and registration, but there have also been increases in leukaemia mortality of about 25% in Henan province (China), world-standardised rates increasing from about 2.5 to 3.0 per 100 000 between 1975 and 1985[169].

Adult leukaemia trends are not in general dramatic, and underlying trends are probably veiled to some extent by improvements in diagnosis, registration and death certification, particularly among older persons. The observed trends appear to reflect a complex pattern in which incidence is generally either stable or increasing slowly, while mortality is stable or declining. Improvements in mortality are generally more marked in younger than in older persons. These trends undoubtedly reflect improvements in treatment and survival, overcoming or attenuating the increase in incidence.

Improvements in diagnosis and registration seem unlikely explanations for all the long-term increases in leukaemia incidence observed in countries as diverse as Scotland, Denmark, Spain, Hungary, Japan and Canada, however, and these trends merit further investigation.

LEUKAEMIA (ICD-9 204-208)

AMERICAS (except USA), INCIDENCE

MALES	Best model	Goodness of fit	1970 Rate	1970 Cases	1985 Rate	1985 Cases	Cumulative risk 1915	Cumulative risk 1940	Recent trend
BRAZIL									
Sao Paulo	A3D	0.56	4.2	32	*10.9*	*108*	2.6	*12.5*	–
CANADA									
Alberta	A1D	0.01	11.4	35	14.8	67	8.2	12.6	*6.6*
British Columbia	A4P2	0.93	13.6	63	12.8	93	7.0	9.2	20.7
Maritime Provinces	A1P2	0.31	11.2	35	10.7	39	5.7	7.1	17.4
Newfoundland	A1D	-0.49	6.3	5	8.5	9	4.4	7.3	*4.2*
Quebec	A3P4C2	0.75	9.2	100	17.7	260	8.6	18.7	29.3
COLOMBIA									
Cali	A1	0.07	7.1	5	7.1	11	3.9	3.9	*-11.9*
CUBA	A8C7	-0.04	6.0	93	6.3	131	3.5	*2.9*	–
PUERTO RICO	A2C2	0.81	6.8	31	7.0	47	4.2	3.9	*-3.8*

FEMALES	Best model	Goodness of fit	1970 Rate	1970 Cases	1985 Rate	1985 Cases	Cumulative risk 1915	Cumulative risk 1940	Recent trend
BRAZIL									
Sao Paulo	A1	-0.46	4.7	38	*4.7*	*51*	2.1	*2.1*	–
CANADA									
Alberta	A1D	0.47	6.5	19	9.2	44	4.7	8.2	11.9
British Columbia	A1P2	1.67	8.5	40	7.2	55	3.8	4.1	15.5
Maritime Provinces	A1P2	-0.24	6.2	20	7.0	27	3.2	5.2	21.1
Newfoundland	A3	0.65	6.2	5	6.2	7	3.5	3.5	*-16.2*
Quebec	A2P4	1.47	5.8	70	10.5	178	4.5	11.6	30.3
COLOMBIA									
Cali	A1D	-0.34	4.8	4	5.5	10	2.8	3.6	*13.6*
CUBA	A2P2	-1.33	5.3	72	6.9	142	3.2	*5.6*	–
PUERTO RICO	A1	0.50	5.4	25	5.4	41	2.9	2.9	*10.9*

* : not enough cases for reliable estimation
– : incomplete or missing data
Best model: polynomial of the given degree in age (A), period (P) or cohort (C), or linear drift (D) model.
Goodness of fit: the normalised likelihood ratio chi-square for the best model (see Method).
Rate: world-standardised truncated rate per 100 000 per year (30-74 years) and number of **cases** are both estimated from the best-fitting model for the single years cited.
Cumulative risk per 1000 (30-74 years) is estimated from the best-fitting *age-cohort* model for cohorts of central birth year cited.
Recent trend: estimated mean percentage change per five-year period in the age-specific rates (30-74 years) over the period 1973-1987.
Italics denote recent trends not significant at 5 per cent level, or other figures which should be interpreted with caution (see Method).

LEUKAEMIA (ICD-9 204-208)

AMERICAS (except USA), INCIDENCE

MALES

TRUNCATED RATE (30-74 years)

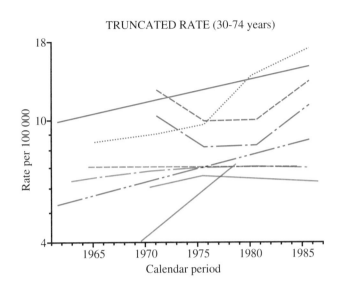

CUMULATIVE RISK (30-74 years)

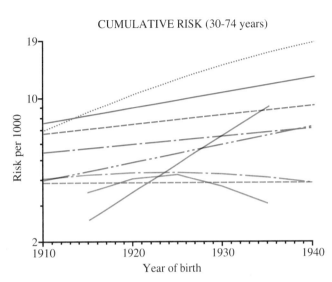

FEMALES

TRUNCATED RATE (30-74 years)

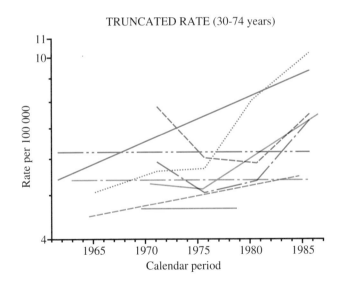

CUMULATIVE RISK (30-74 years)

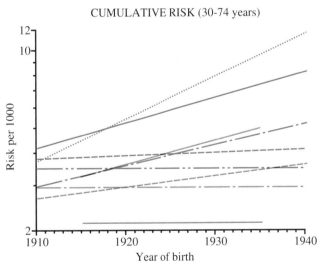

―――――― CANADA Alberta
------ CANADA British Columbia
―・―・― CANADA Maritime Provinces
―・・―・・ CANADA Newfoundland
·········· CANADA Quebec

―――――― CUBA
―・―・― PUERTO RICO
―――――― BRAZIL Sao Paulo
------ COLOMBIA Cali

LEUKAEMIA (ICD-9 204-208)

AMERICAS (USA), INCIDENCE

MALES	Best model	Goodness of fit	1970 Rate	1970 Cases	1985 Rate	1985 Cases	Cumulative risk 1915	Cumulative risk 1940	Recent trend
USA									
Bay Area, Black	A1	2.00	13.9	7	13.9	11	8.4	8.4	*3.9*
Bay Area, White	A3	-0.14	12.4	73	12.4	79	7.8	7.8	*2.5*
Connecticut	A4	1.38	13.6	89	13.6	110	8.6	8.6	*-5.4*
Detroit, Black	A1	0.61	14.0	18	14.0	24	8.4	8.4	*0.9*
Detroit, White	A8C8	0.21	13.6	99	16.8	122	9.4	10.7	9.3
Iowa	A3	0.70	16.4	111	16.4	117	10.4	10.4	*2.8*
New Orleans, Black	A3	1.47	*11.6*	*6*	11.6	7	6.8	6.8	*-3.8*
New Orleans, White	A1	0.08	*11.4*	*16*	11.4	18	7.3	7.3	*-11.0*
Seattle	A1	0.16	*14.1*	*68*	14.1	96	8.7	8.7	*3.0*

FEMALES	Best model	Goodness of fit	1970 Rate	1970 Cases	1985 Rate	1985 Cases	Cumulative risk 1915	Cumulative risk 1940	Recent trend
USA									
Bay Area, Black	A1	0.38	9.0	5	9.0	8	5.3	5.3	*6.6*
Bay Area, White	A1C2	1.64	7.4	52	9.0	65	4.7	8.1	*7.2*
Connecticut	A1P2	0.05	8.2	62	7.9	74	4.8	5.3	*-6.0*
Detroit, Black	A1P2	-0.28	6.8	10	9.4	20	5.4	6.5	*-3.0*
Detroit, White	A1D	-0.41	7.9	65	9.5	81	5.3	7.3	*5.5*
Iowa	A3	-0.43	9.3	72	9.3	76	5.7	5.7	*-5.6*
New Orleans, Black	A1	1.17	*8.6*	*5*	8.6	6	5.1	5.1	*8.7*
New Orleans, White	A1	-0.67	*7.5*	*14*	7.5	14	4.6	4.6	*4.5*
Seattle	A1	-1.02	*8.5*	*47*	8.5	63	5.0	5.0	*6.0*

* : not enough cases for reliable estimation
− : incomplete or missing data
Best model: polynomial of the given degree in age (A), period (P) or cohort (C), or linear drift (D) model.
Goodness of fit: the normalised likelihood ratio chi-square for the best model (see Method).
Rate: world-standardised truncated rate per 100 000 per year (30-74 years) and number of **cases** are both estimated from the best-fitting model for the single years cited.
Cumulative risk per 1000 (30-74 years) is estimated from the best-fitting *age-cohort* model for cohorts of central birth year cited.
Recent trend: estimated mean percentage change per five-year period in the age-specific rates (30-74 years) over the period 1973-1987.
Italics denote recent trends not significant at 5 per cent level, or other figures which should be interpreted with caution (see Method).

LEUKAEMIA (ICD-9 204-208)

AMERICAS (USA), INCIDENCE

MALES

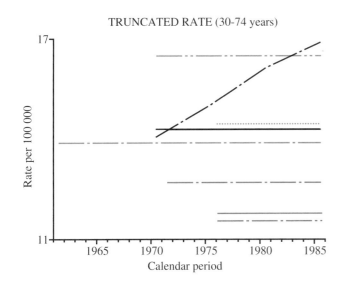

TRUNCATED RATE (30-74 years)

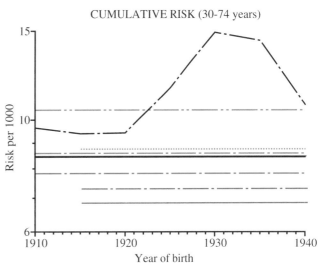

CUMULATIVE RISK (30-74 years)

FEMALES

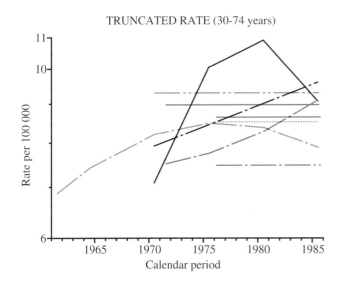

TRUNCATED RATE (30-74 years)

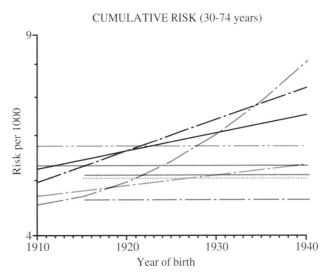

CUMULATIVE RISK (30-74 years)

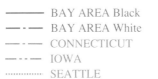

BAY AREA Black
BAY AREA White
CONNECTICUT
IOWA
SEATTLE
NEW ORLEANS Black
NEW ORLEANS White
DETROIT Black
DETROIT White

LEUKAEMIA (ICD-9 204-208)

AMERICAS (except USA), INCIDENCE
Percentage change per five-year period, 1973-1987

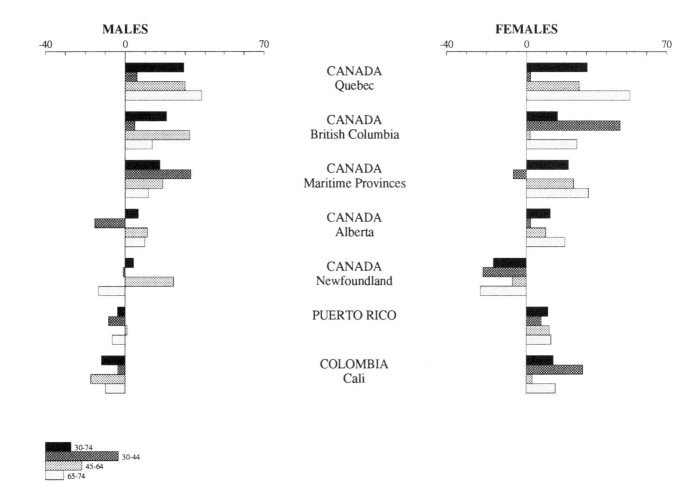

MALES

FEMALES

-40   0   70

CANADA
Quebec

CANADA
British Columbia

CANADA
Maritime Provinces

CANADA
Alberta

CANADA
Newfoundland

PUERTO RICO

COLOMBIA
Cali

30-74
30-44
45-64
65-74

LEUKAEMIA (ICD-9 204-208)

AMERICAS (USA), INCIDENCE
Percentage change per five-year period, 1973-1987

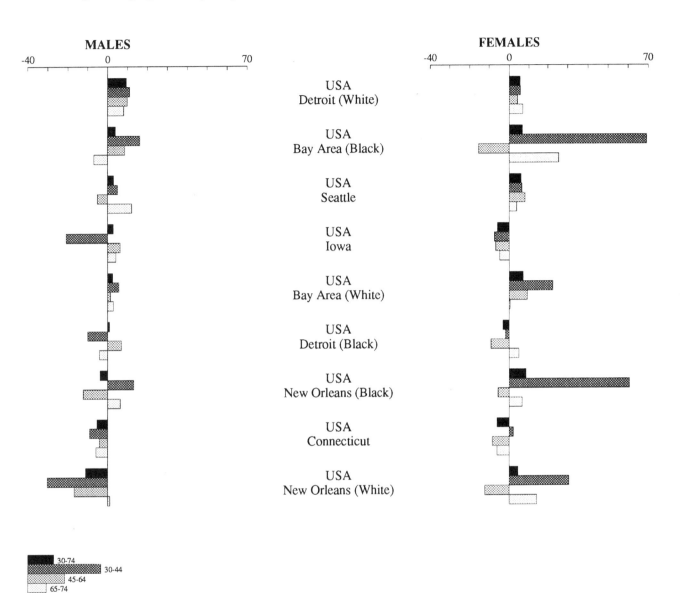

LEUKAEMIA (ICD-9 204-208)

AMERICAS, MORTALITY

MALES	Best model	Goodness of fit	1965 Rate	Deaths	1985 Rate	Deaths	Cumulative risk 1900	1940	Recent trend
CANADA	A3C4	-0.28	9.0	347	9.2	540	5.6	5.8	*0.1*
CHILE	A8P6C9	0.39	4.4	56	5.3	101	2.0	2.4	*5.7*
COSTA RICA	A2P4	-1.29	*5.7*	*9*	5.9	19	*2.7*	5.8	*-1.7*
PANAMA	A2D	0.83	3.8	6	5.3	17	2.1	4.0	–
PUERTO RICO	A2C4	0.24	6.3	26	5.8	28	*3.9*	3.3	-15.9
URUGUAY	A4C4	1.92	8.6	51	7.1	51	5.6	3.8	*-5.2*
USA	A5P5C5	1.59	10.5	4470	9.5	5400	6.6	5.1	-2.1
VENEZUELA	A2C4	-1.47	3.7	38	*5.3*	*98*	2.1	4.3	–

FEMALES	Best model	Goodness of fit	1965 Rate	Deaths	1985 Rate	Deaths	Cumulative risk 1900	1940	Recent trend
CANADA	A3C4	-2.39	6.0	240	5.5	360	3.6	3.1	*-2.1*
CHILE	A2C2	1.50	3.9	54	4.3	94	2.0	2.4	*7.6*
COSTA RICA	A1	0.58	*5.4*	*8*	5.4	16	*2.9*	2.9	*-2.5*
PANAMA	A1	-0.20	2.9	4	2.9	8	1.5	1.5	–
PUERTO RICO	A1	-0.29	5.4	23	5.4	32	*2.9*	2.9	*3.0*
URUGUAY	A1P3	-0.72	6.9	42	5.5	43	3.4	2.9	*-3.7*
USA	A3P5C8	-0.63	6.6	3169	5.9	3882	4.0	3.0	*1.0*
VENEZUELA	A1D	0.68	3.2	33	*4.1*	*87*	1.6	2.7	–

* : not enough deaths for reliable estimation
– : incomplete or missing data
Best model: polynomial of the given degree in age (A), period (P) or cohort (C), or linear drift (D) model.
Goodness of fit: the normalised likelihood ratio chi-square for the best model (see Method).
Rate: world-standardised truncated rate per 100 000 per year (30-74 years) and number of **deaths** are both estimated from the best-fitting model for the single years cited.
Cumulative risk per 1000 (30-74 years) is estimated from the best-fitting *age-cohort* model for cohorts of central birth year cited.
Recent trend: estimated mean percentage change per five-year period in the age-specific rates (30-74 years) over the period 1975-1988.
Italics denote recent trends not significant at 5 per cent level, or other figures which should be interpreted with caution (see Method).

LEUKAEMIA (ICD-9 204-208)

AMERICAS, MORTALITY

MALES

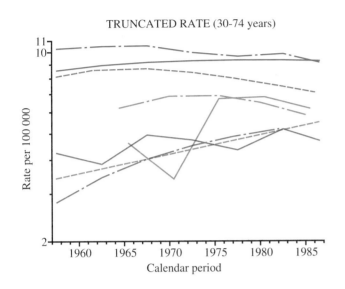

TRUNCATED RATE (30-74 years)

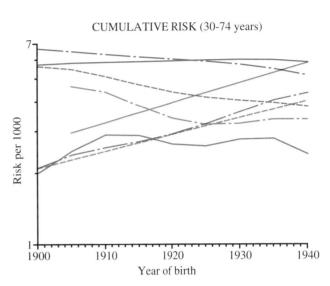

CUMULATIVE RISK (30-74 years)

FEMALES

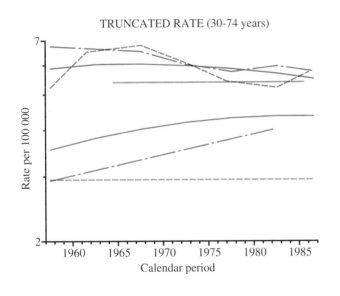

TRUNCATED RATE (30-74 years)

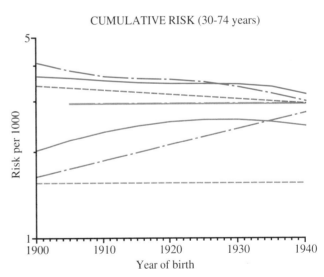

CUMULATIVE RISK (30-74 years)

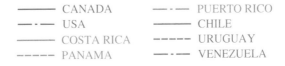

—— CANADA		—·— PUERTO RICO	
—·— USA		—— CHILE	
—— COSTA RICA		---- URUGUAY	
---- PANAMA		—··— VENEZUELA	

LEUKAEMIA (ICD-9 204-208)

AMERICAS, MORTALITY
Percentage change per five-year period, 1975-1988

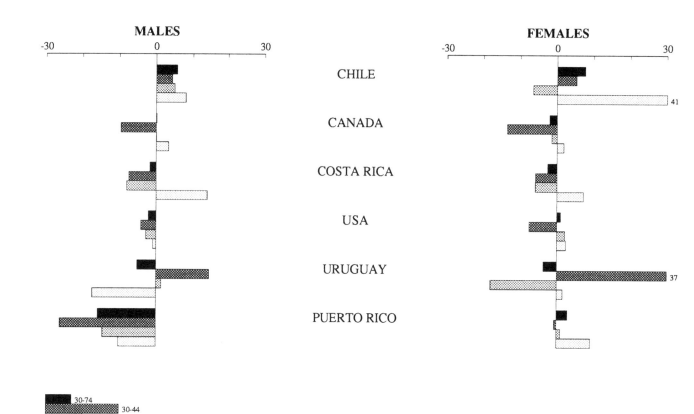

Chapter 30

CHILDHOOD CANCER

The scope of this chapter is narrower than that of the chapters devoted to time trends in adult cancers. The analytic approach was constrained by the nature of the information available for this monograph, and by the greater statistical fluctuation of the rates for childhood cancer. Cancer is a rare disease in childhood, and it is difficult to model trends in each type of cancer with sufficient reliability. Even for leukaemia, the most frequent malignancy, trends could not be reliably modelled for individual cancer registries. The main axis of the ICD classification used in the available data is anatomical, and this coding system is not well suited to the study of childhood cancers, which are often defined on the basis of morphology. It was considered important, however, to examine trends in the incidence of cancer in children, as currently recorded by cancer registries in various parts of the world, and especially to examine trends in mortality from childhood cancer, which reflects one of the outstanding successes in the fight against cancer. For the reasons referred to above, the strategy adopted for adult cancers was not considered appropriate for childhood cancer, and a simplified approach was used.

Method of analysis and presentation of results

The populations for which data were available were grouped by geographical proximity, taking account of their economic development. In some cases, geography took precedence over the level of economic development, producing groups which were heterogeneous for cancer risk: the heterogeneity was analysed, and is commented upon where appropriate. The population groupings ('regions') also took into consideration the calendar period for which data were available, since the presentation of data within each region was inevitably limited to the shortest duration available for any population in the region. The result of this exercise is shown in Table 30.1.

For each region so defined, and for each sex, the cumulative risk (0-14 years) was estimated from the five-year age-specific incidence or mortality rates by assuming a common age effect within the region for both sexes. More precisely, a regression model incorporating age and sex by period interactions was fitted to the data, assum-

ing a Poisson error. The homogeneity of the risks and time trends between populations or registries within a given region was then tested. The addition of the factor "registry" to the model enabled estimation of the standardised morbidity or mortality ratio (SMR) for each population, relative to the region as a whole, and of the standard error of the SMR. Assessment of the interaction between registry and period was then carried out to test the homogeneity of the trends. In performing this test for interaction, the factor "period" was considered as a continuous variable in order to retain sufficient statistical power.

Leukaemia

Leukaemias are the most frequent neoplasm in children, accounting for a third of all childhood cancer. Acute lymphocytic leukaemia is the most frequent sub-type in children, and it is also the type of leukaemia which shows the greatest geographical variation; it usually accounts for more than three quarters of acute leukaemias, except in some populations in Asia and Oceania, where the non-lymphocytic type may account for more than a third. Leukaemia is rarer among black populations in the USA, and it is also believed to be rare among blacks in Africa. In all populations, the disease is slightly more frequent in males than in females[223]. Very little is known about the aetiology of leukaemia in children.

Europe

The incidence of leukaemia has increased significantly among males in central Europe, and in both sexes in the UK; among females, it has increased in Nordic countries and decreased in western Europe.

Detailed analysis of these incidence data shows that Varese (Italy) is at highest risk in western Europe (SMR=132), and Bas-Rhin (France) at lowest risk (SMR=76); other SMRs are not significant. The large and significant decrease seen in females in western Europe is mainly due to the large risk (over 1000) observed in Varese around 1975, and the low risk (300-400) around 1985 in Bas-Rhin, Varese and Saarland (FRG). In the UK, Scotland is at high risk (SMR=107), and South Thames at lower risk (SMR=90): the peak

Table 30.1 Groups of populations (regions) used in the analysis of trends in childhood cancer

REGION	INCIDENCE	MORTALITY
Europe		
Central	Hungary (Vas, Szabolcs), Germany (GDR), Poland (Warsaw City), Slovenia	Austria, Czechoslovakia, Hungary, Poland, Yugoslavia
Nordic	Denmark, Finland, Norway, Sweden	Denmark, Finland, Norway, Sweden
UK (& Ireland)	England (Birmingham, South Thames), Scotland	England and Wales, Scotland, Ireland
Western	France (Bas-Rhin, Doubs), FRG (Saarland), Italy (Varese), Spain (Navarra, Zaragoza), Switzerland (Geneva)	France, Germany, Italy, Netherlands, Portugal, Switzerland
Asia and Oceania		
Australia	New South Wales, South Australia	Australia
China	Shanghai	-
Hawaii	Caucasian, Chinese, Filipino, Hawaiian, Japanese	-
Hong Kong	Hong Kong	Hong Kong
India	Bombay	-
Japan	Miyagi, Osaka	Japan
Singapore	Chinese, Malay, Indian	Singapore
New Zealand	Maori, non-Maori	New Zealand
Americas		
Canada	Alberta, British Columbia, Maritime Provinces, Newfoundland, Quebec	Canada
Colombia	Cali	-
Chile	-	Chile
Costa Rica	-	Costa Rica
Puerto Rico	Puerto Rico	Puerto Rico
Uruguay	-	Uruguay
USA white	Bay Area whites, Connecticut, Detroit whites, Iowa, New Orleans whites, Seattle	-
USA black	Bay Area blacks, Detroit blacks, New Orleans blacks	-
USA	-	USA
Venezuela	-	Venezuela

seen about 1975 in males is present in all three UK populations. The risks reported in Hungary are much lower than elsewhere in central Europe (SMR=71 in Vas and 53 in Szabolcs-Szatmar). The increasing trends are different in different populations, the largest increase being observed in County Vas. The risks are homogeneous in Nordic countries, but the increasing trend in females is mainly seen in Finland, and to a lesser extent in Sweden.

Mortality has decreased dramatically in all regions of Europe. There are, however, some disparities within regions. In western Europe, the risk of death is higher in Italy (SMR=117), and lower in the Netherlands (SMR=93) and Germany (SMR=95). The decline in risk is steeper in Switzerland and in the Netherlands than in France and Italy, but very small in Portugal. In the UK, mortality is lower in Scotland, while mortality in Ireland is at the average level for the region: the trend is the same in the three countries. In central Europe, mortality is greater in Czechoslovakia (SMR=107) and in Poland (SMR=104), and the trends in the various countries are clearly distinct: while the decline is about 20% every five years in Austria, it is less than 10% in the other countries in the region. In these countries, the decline is significantly greater for females than for males. In contrast to the rest of Europe, the risks of death from leukaemia in children and the time trends in the risk are remarkably homogeneous in the four Nordic countries.

Asia and Oceania

The most striking observation is the contrast in risk between Bombay (India) and other Asian countries, especially Hong Kong. Risks are homogeneous within Australia, Hawaii, Japan and New Zealand, and no significant disparities between trends are seen within these groups of populations. The only significant increases are seen in Bombay, Hong Kong and New Zealand in males.

Mortality is falling in Australia, New Zealand and Japan, but substantially less steeply for males in New Zealand. No significant decrease is seen in Hong Kong or Singapore.

Americas

The incidence of leukaemia is similar in the countries for which data are available, but there is a marked difference between blacks and whites in the USA. The apparent decrease among black females in the USA is mainly due to a large but non-significant decrease in Detroit. The risks are homogeneous in all US populations and stable

over time. In Canada, the risk is greater in Quebec (SMR=114) and lower in the Maritime Provinces (SMR=85); the trends also vary between provinces, the increase in risk being limited to Quebec. Mortality is falling quickly in Canada, Puerto Rico and the USA. In South and Central America, no significant decrease has been observed, except for females in Uruguay and Venezuela. In these two countries, the risk of death from leukaemia observed in females in 1980-84 was similar to that in Canada.

All sites

In developed countries, childhood malignancies comprise mainly leukaemia (30%), tumours of the brain and central nervous system (20%), lymphoma (10%), and neuroblastoma (8%). In some developing countries this ranking is different, lymphoma, retinoblastoma and Wilm's tumour playing a more important role. As explained earlier, the analysis carried out in this monograph is limited; more details may be found in *International Incidence of Childhood Cancer*[223].

Europe

The heterogeneity seen in western Europe for leukaemia is still more marked for all cancers combined. The risk is also highest in Varese (Italy) (SMR=113), the only population that is significantly different from the average. The trends are not significant in any of the populations in western Europe.

In the UK, Scotland is at higher risk (SMR=108), while the South Thames region is at lower risk (SMR=92). The risk is increasing significantly for both males and females, and the increase is steeper in Scotland. In central Europe, the risk is greater in Warsaw City (Poland) (SMR=138) and lower in the two Hungarian populations (SMR=72 in Vas and 64 in Szabolcs-Szatmar). In contrast to the increasing trend elsewhere in central Europe, the risk is decreasing in Warsaw City. In the Nordic countries, the risk is higher in Sweden (SMR=106), but the increasing trends seen in the graphs are the same in all four countries.

The risk of death is different in the various countries of western Europe, where it is significantly greater in Portugal (SMR=112) and Italy (SMR=113); the lowest risks are seen in France and Germany (SMR=90). The trends are also very different, the decrease being very small in Portugal and less steep in France and Italy than in the Netherlands and Switzerland; this pattern has already been noted for leukaemias, which may dominate the fall in mortality.

Mortality is greater in England and Wales (SMR=106) than in Ireland (SMR=96) or Scotland (SMR=98). The trends are also different, the decrease being significantly greater in England and Wales and Scotland than in Ireland. In central Europe, mortality is significantly lower in Yugoslavia (SMR=87) and in Austria (SMR=94). The decreasing trend, however, is seen mainly in Austria, where the decline is 13% every five years, a figure similar to that in the Netherlands and Switzerland. In all other countries, the decrease is small, and slightly faster for females than for males. In the Nordic countries, the risk is lower in Sweden (SMR=97) and greater in Denmark (SMR=104), but the range is small. The decreasing trend is steeper in Norway, but identical in the other Nordic countries.

Asia and Oceania

The incidence of childhood cancer is low in Bombay (India) and high in Australia, New Zealand and Hong Kong. In New Zealand, the incidence is higher for Maoris (SMR=106) than non-Maoris; the incidence is also higher among Caucasians in Hawaii than in other ethnic groups (SMR=139). There is no significant heterogeneity of trends within the regions in Asia and Oceania.

Mortality has fallen in all countries for which data are available, except in Singapore, where a non-significant increase is observed. In Hong Kong, the decrease is not significant in females. The cumulative risk of dying from cancer before age 15 was still high (over 1000) in Singapore and in New Zealand in the late 1980s.

Americas

In the USA, incidence differs significantly between blacks and whites. There is also marked heterogeneity within groups. Incidence is higher among blacks in San Francisco (SMR=110) than among blacks in Detroit, and higher among whites in San Francisco (SMR=115) than in other populations. Incidence is lower than average in Connecticut (SMR=93). The trends, however, are homogeneous within the groups defined here.

Incidence varies between the provinces of Canada, with a very low recorded incidence in the Maritime Provinces (SMR=79). The highest incidence rates are recorded in British Columbia (SMR=114) and Quebec (SMR=111). The trend also varies significantly between provinces: in Quebec, the increase is steeper than in other provinces, and in the Maritime Provinces it is decreasing. The incidence of childhood cancer increased significantly in Puerto Rico and in Cali (Colombia).

Childhood mortality from cancer has fallen quite remarkably in Canada, Puerto Rico and the USA. In South and Central America, the decline has been small, except for females in Uruguay. The risk of dying from cancer before age 15 was especially high in Costa Rica (over 1000) in the late 1980s, and it was also high in Uruguay in 1980-84.

Comment

The foregoing brief description reflects the wide geographical variation in the risk of cancer in childhood, reported in more detail in *International Incidence of Childhood Cancer*[223]. There is also considerable geographical variation in the trends of these risks over time. It is likely that completeness of registration, which varies with registry and tends to improve over time for a given registry, explains part of the heterogeneity in risk and the variation in time trends. Since few environmental causes of childhood cancer have been identified, observations of changing cancer risk in children are difficult to interpret, and the literature in this field is rather limited. Change in exposure to ionising radiation is probably the most frequently discussed aspect of environmental aetiology, but no convincing evidence of its effect on the risk of leukaemia is available. Electromagnetic fields have also been suspected as a risk factor for leukaemia and brain tumours in childhood[166], but this is still controversial.

Several reports on trends in childhood cancer in the United Kingdom have been published. An increasing incidence of carcinoma in north-west England has been reported[23], thought to be due to environmental factors; change in case ascertainment with time was excluded as an explanation for this trend. The peak in leukaemia incidence seen around 1975 in the UK has been described in more detail for South Thames[19]; the increase was most marked in boys aged 0-4 years. In contrast, no significant change was seen in the northern region of the UK during the period 1968-82[58], either for individual cancers or for all cancers combined. Trends in childhood cancer have been reported for the province of Torino (Italy)[194]. No important change in incidence was observed, except for an increased incidence of brain tumours, attributed to improved diagnostic procedures. In a detailed analysis of childhood cancer incidence in the Czech regions of Bohemia and Moravia (the western part of former Czechoslovakia) over the period 1963-1985[11], no significant trend was found for males or females. This confirms the heterogeneity of the trend in central Europe discussed above.

An analysis of childhood leukaemia in Hawaii over the period 1960-84[112] showed an increase in incidence among females, and a higher risk among Japanese males in the 1960s. The latter observation is consistent with a peak in the cumulative risk (1230 per million) seen among Japanese in Hawaii in the data analysed here for the period 1968-77. Overall, however, the risk is not high among Japanese. An increasing incidence in males during the period 1973-1988 was reported from Queensland (Australia)[184], while no significant change was found in the data reported here for the registries of New South Wales and South Australia. The increase among males in Queensland was seen only for non-lymphocytic leukaemia and non-Hodgkin lymphoma, while Hodgkin's disease declined. The fact that the increase was confined to males makes it less likely that the observed change could be explained by improved ascertainment.

A detailed analysis of age-specific trends in childhood cancer over the period 1935-79 in Connecticut (USA) showed a clear increase in incidence for several sites of cancer, especially at younger ages[293]. The changes were most evident for acute lymphocytic leukaemia and tumours of the brain and central nervous system, and for Hodgkin's disease. In the opinion of the authors, these trends cannot be attributed to improved ascertainment or to improved diagnostic techniques, except perhaps for brain tumours. Changes in exposure to unknown environmental factors were considered to be responsible for the increasing incidence. The difference in risk of leukaemia between blacks and whites has been analysed for the USA[244], showing a wide difference in the age distribution of the disease between the two racial groups. The large difference in incidence seen for 3-5 year-olds is not reflected in the mortality rates, which were similar in blacks and whites in the 1980s.

The almost universal decrease in cancer mortality among children does not need extensive comment here; the speed of the decline varies between populations[143], and is not the same for all ethnic groups[244]. The change in mortality is attributable to major advances in therapy, which are unfortunately not accessible to all children with cancer, depending on various factors, including the hospital of treatment[58]. Survival for childhood cancer has been analysed for a population-based series of over 15 000 children in Great Britain over the period 1971-1985[275]. Although the prognosis is still poor for many childhood tumours, it has improved for all cancers. The change in five-year survival from 37% to 70% for acute lymphocytic leukaemia, the most frequent neoplasm in children, has certainly made the greatest contribution to the decline in mortality from cancer among children.

LEUKAEMIA (ICD-9 204-208)
EUROPE, CUMULATIVE RISK (0-14 YEARS)
INCIDENCE

Sex	Region	Central year of the period						Linear trend
		1960	1965	1970	1975	1980	1985	
Male								
	Nordic	679	658	692	690	641	727	0.7
	Central		441	529	520	498	559	3.7
	Western				673	650	713	3.0
	UK		456	529	665	577	569	5.2
Female								
	Nordic	561	554	534	522	585	706	4.2
	Central		398	389	481	440	437	3.0
	Western				687	471	447	-22.8
	UK		365	432	467	451	516	7.3

MORTALITY

Sex	Region	Initial year of the period							Linear trend
		1955	1960	1965	1970	1975	1980	1985	
Male									
	Nordic	677	675	664	593	449	363	295	-12.8
	Central		490	480	464	414	365	312	-8.5
	Western	621	616	579	537	458	365	278	-11.5
	UK & Ireland	531	540	493	435	415	319	225	-11.7
Female									
	Nordic	530	539	482	454	325	255	198	-14.9
	Central		387	387	350	313	272	225	-10.4
	Western	506	512	482	439	339	270	214	-13.3
	UK & Ireland	434	427	395	347	269	239	188	-13.4

Regions as defined in Table 30.1
Cumulative risk per million calculated from age-specific rates in each calendar period
Period as defined in Table 2.3 for incidence and Table 2.7 for mortality
Linear trend: percentage change in risk every five years over the entire data period (see text)

CHILDHOOD CANCER

LEUKAEMIA (ICD-9 204-208)
EUROPE, CUMULATIVE RISK (0-14 YEARS)

MALES

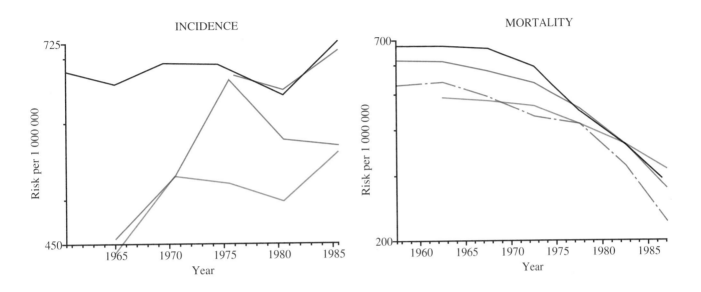

FEMALES

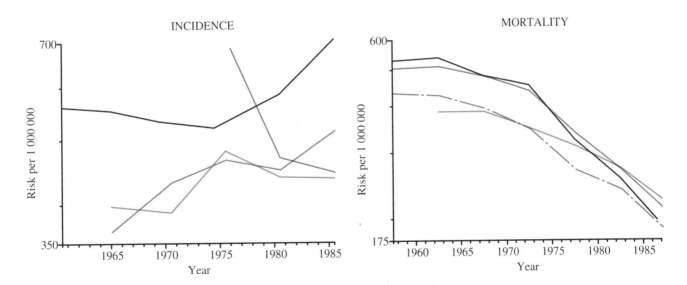

———— WESTERN EUROPE   —·—·— U.K. & IRELAND

———— CENTRAL EUROPE   ———— NORDIC COUNTRIES

———— U.K.

CHILDHOOD CANCER

LEUKAEMIA (ICD-9 204-208)
ASIA and OCEANIA, CUMULATIVE RISK (0-14 YEARS)
INCIDENCE

Sex	Region	Central year of the period						Linear trend
		1960	1965	1970	1975	1980	1985	
Male								
	Australia				654	878	763	4.8
	New Zealand		645	703	733	734	914	8.0
	Hawaii	802		653	850	459	762	-4.6
	India, Bombay		304	357	360	421	503	12.2
	China, Shanghai				685	648	675	1.7
	Hong Kong				835	1172	1212	18.1
	Japan			626	528	648	633	4.1
	Singapore			693	676	543	689	-2.4
Female								
	Australia				642	623	541	-6.3
	New Zealand		610	563	550	508	633	0.1
	Hawaii	613		447	730	576	963	11.6
	India, Bombay		223	285	238	228	284	2.1
	China, Shanghai				535	639	588	-0.8
	Hong Kong				800	700	912	6.1
	Japan			471	464	531	516	4.3
	Singapore			545	469	296	618	0.1

MORTALITY

Sex	Region	Initial year of the period							Linear trend
		1955	1960	1965	1970	1975	1980	1985	
Male									
	Australia	599	560	572	530	355	345	253	-14.3
	New Zealand	626	518	541	506	478	434	469	-8.1
	Hong Kong		378	423	375	362	306		-5.5
	Japan	457	524	522	501	461	375	304	-5.7
	Singapore			567	430	526	446	523	-1.7
Female									
	Australia	500	539	448	458	341	269	182	-13.6
	New Zealand	458	541	587	442	274	260	258	-10.0
	Hong Kong		358	348	320	405	261		-3.9
	Japan	343	410	433	421	370	273	234	-6.2
	Singapore			437	351	414	286	444	-1.8

Regions as defined in Table 30.1
Cumulative risk per million calculated from age-specific rates in each calendar period
Period as defined in Table 2.3 for incidence and Table 2.7 for mortality
Linear trend: percentage change in risk every five years over the entire data period (see text)

CHILDHOOD CANCER

LEUKAEMIA (ICD-9 204-208)
ASIA and OCEANIA, CUMULATIVE RISK (0-14 YEARS)

MALES

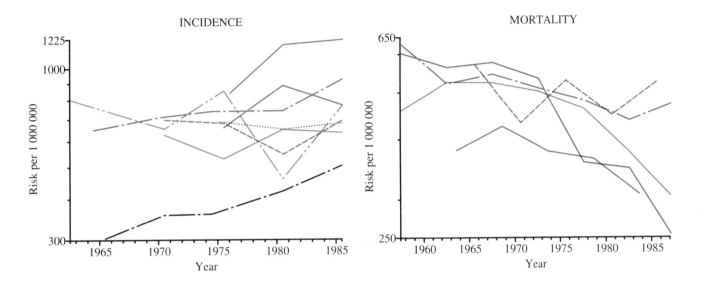

FEMALES

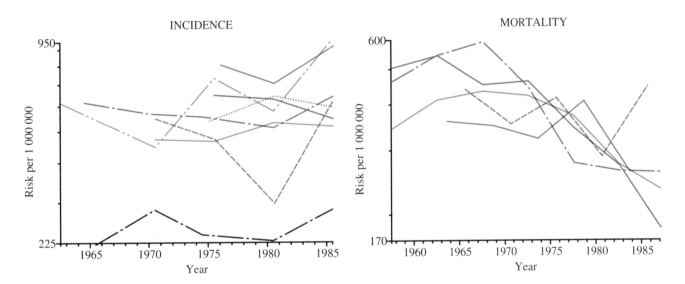

AUSTRALIA		CHINA, Shanghai
NEW ZEALAND		HONG KONG
HAWAII		SINGAPORE
JAPAN		INDIA, Bombay

CHILDHOOD CANCER

LEUKAEMIA (ICD-9 204-208)
AMERICAS, CUMULATIVE RISK (0-14 YEARS)
INCIDENCE

Sex	Region	Central year of the period						Linear trend
		1960	1965	1970	1975	1980	1985	
Male								
	Canada			649	619	586	808	6.9
	USA, White			726	758	649	668	-4.1
	USA, Black			367	304	316	423	6.5
	Puerto Rico			555	423	605	634	6.6
	Colombia, Cali			399	729	773	590	7.8
Female								
	Canada			574	519	589	650	5.3
	USA, White			525	511	592	599	5.5
	USA, Black			440	393	405	348	-6.6
	Puerto Rico			446	462	548	608	12.6
	Colombia, Cali			503	426	535	589	8.8

MORTALITY

Sex	Region	Initial year of the period							Linear trend
		1955	1960	1965	1970	1975	1980	1985	
Male									
	Canada	554	602	568	534	427	313	289	-11.2
	USA	611	596	529	440	342	267	224	-16.9
	Puerto Rico			421	447	314	378	194	-17.6
	Chile	402	431	539	469	434	377	344	-1.8
	Costa Rica			605	464	451	509	486	-2.2
	Uruguay	545	652	683	474	489	535		-3.9
	Venezuela	358	426	458	423	420	374		-0.6
Female									
	Canada	495	460	448	404	348	257	234	-12.0
	USA	498	480	421	342	257	196	171	-18.4
	Puerto Rico			382	403	272	237	209	-15.8
	Chile	285	363	377	428	403	342	346	-0.3
	Costa Rica			337	486	432	455	408	-0.6
	Uruguay	554	475	424	451	397	252		-12.1
	Venezuela	296	412	368	345	402	247		-5.1

Regions as defined in Table 30.1
Cumulative risk per million calculated from age-specific rates in each calendar period
Period as defined in Table 2.3 for incidence and Table 2.7 for mortality
Linear trend: percentage change in risk every five years over the entire data period (see text)

CHILDHOOD CANCER

LEUKAEMIA (ICD-9 204-208)
AMERICAS, CUMULATIVE RISK (0-14 YEARS)

MALES

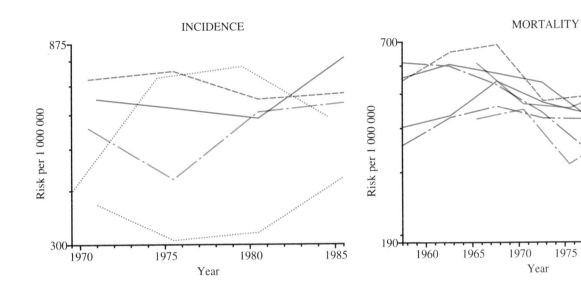

FEMALES

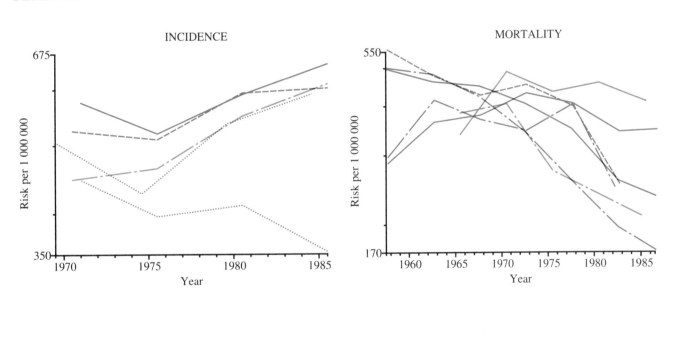

ALL SITES (ICD-9 140-208)
EUROPE, CUMULATIVE RISK (0-14 YEARS)
INCIDENCE

Sex	Region	Central year of the period						Linear trend
		1960	1965	1970	1975	1980	1985	
Male								
	Nordic	1938	1880	2035	2098	2176	2406	3.4
	Central		1654	1776	1772	1850	1929	3.3
	Western				2306	2153	2499	4.2
	UK		1647	1594	1896	1727	1789	2.6
Female								
	Nordic	1627	1720	1676	1756	1806	2153	4.8
	Central		1304	1398	1611	1497	1623	4.6
	Western				1668	1173	1820	4.3
	UK		1221	1313	1481	1470	1591	6.5

MORTALITY

Sex	Region	Initial year of the period							Linear trend
		1955	1960	1965	1970	1975	1980	1985	
Male									
	Nordic	1358	1353	1334	1230	1029	819	772	-9.5
	Central		1108	1164	1147	1091	1083	911	-3.1
	Western	1242	1261	1236	1148	1018	883	729	-8.0
	UK & Ireland	1224	1234	1467	1050	964	765	617	-10.8
Female									
	Nordic	1113	1136	1010	1009	754	637	579	-11.2
	Central		841	918	880	843	811	722	-3.0
	Western	986	1010	984	898	772	667	567	-8.8
	UK & Ireland	986	989	922	798	701	640	561	-9.8

Regions as defined in Table 30.1
Cumulative risk per million calculated from age-specific rates in each calendar period
Period as defined in Table 2.3 for incidence and Table 2.7 for mortality
Linear trend: percentage change in risk every five years over the entire data period (see text)

CHILDHOOD CANCER

ALL SITES (ICD-9 140-208)
EUROPE, CUMULATIVE RISK (0-14 YEARS)

MALES

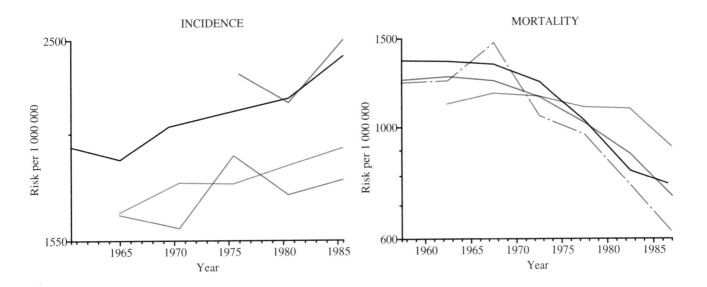

FEMALES

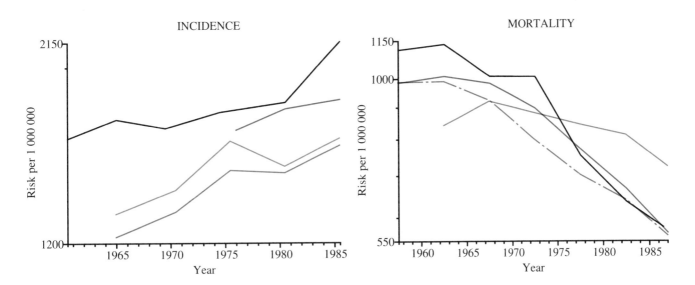

——— WESTERN EUROPE   — · — · U.K. & IRELAND
——— CENTRAL EUROPE   ——— NORDIC COUNTRIES
——— U.K.

CHILDHOOD CANCER

ALL SITES (ICD-9 140-208)
ASIA and OCEANIA, CUMULATIVE RISK (0-14 YEARS)
INCIDENCE

Sex	Region	Central year of the period						Linear trend
		1960	1965	1970	1975	1980	1985	
Male								
	Australia				2024	2470	2133	2.2
	New Zealand		1938	1907	2081	2235	2667	8.4
	Hawaii	1746		1741	2243	1692	2754	9.1
	India, Bombay		1001	1104	1410	1268	1372	7.5
	China, Shanghai				1966	1705	1817	-4.4
	Hong Kong				2456	2658	2779	9.8
	Japan		1523	1599	1859	2014		10.4
	Singapore		1554	1566	1438	1717		2.3
Female								
	Australia				1814	1833	1629	-5.6
	New Zealand		1706	1530	1870	1833	2132	6.4
	Hawaii	1365		1356	1501	1304	2473	12.5
	India, Bombay		734	823	737	793	898	2.6
	China, Shanghai				1752	1503	1454	-3.1
	Hong Kong				1861	1671	2331	7.4
	Japan			1184	1332	1480	1715	12.4
	Singapore			1163	1352	1193	1671	10.2

MORTALITY

Sex	Region	Initial year of the period							Linear trend
		1955	1960	1965	1970	1975	1980	1985	
Male									
	Australia	1309	1284	1258	1153	836	852	682	-11.0
	New Zealand	1501	1400	1295	1237	1155	1034	1073	-7.5
	Hong Kong		944	1031	1010	973	758		-4.5
	Japan	791	904	938	902	859	748	647	-3.0
	Singapore			989	930	1099	894	1081	1.5
Female									
	Australia	1028	1028	946	945	719	641	513	-10.9
	New Zealand	1144	1212	1155	984	947	656	773	-7.8
	Hong Kong		767	831	764	852	703		-1.3
	Japan	597	713	748	743	676	577	504	-2.9
	Singapore			758	652	878	679	915	4.2

Regions as defined in Table 30.1
Cumulative risk per million calculated from age-specific rates in each calendar period
Period as defined in Table 2.3 for incidence and Table 2.7 for mortality
Linear trend: percentage change in risk every five years over the entire data period (see text)

CHILDHOOD CANCER

ALL SITES (ICD-9 140-208)
ASIA and OCEANIA, CUMULATIVE RISK (0-14 YEARS)

MALES

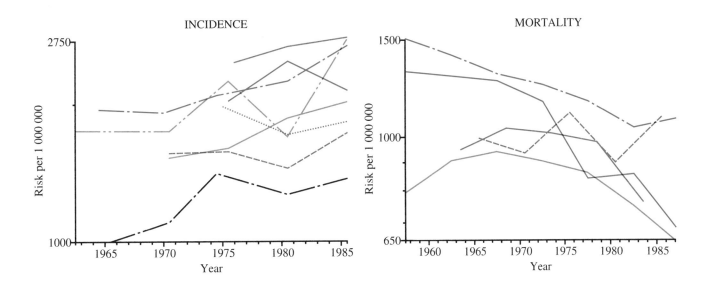

FEMALES

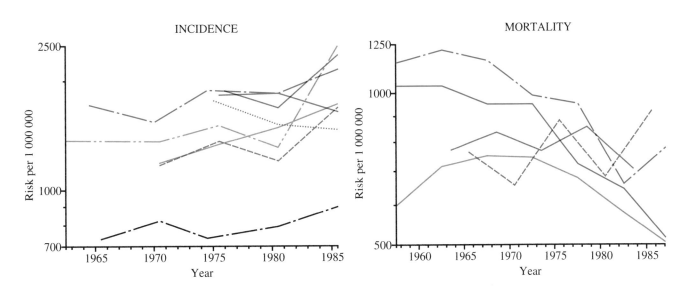

AUSTRALIA
NEW ZEALAND
HAWAII
JAPAN
CHINA, Shanghai
HONG KONG
SINGAPORE
INDIA, Bombay

CHILDHOOD CANCER

ALL SITES (ICD-9 140-208)
AMERICAS, CUMULATIVE RISK (0-14 YEARS)
INCIDENCE

Sex	Region	Central year of the period						Linear trend
		1960	1965	1970	1975	1980	1985	
Male								
	Canada			1970	1812	1986	2487	8.6
	USA, White			2087	2098	2097	2322	3.2
	USA, Black			1540	1460	1866	1487	*1.4*
	Puerto Rico			1558	1323	1832	1732	8.4
	Colombia, Cali			1474	1749	1917	2016	10.6
Female								
	Canada			1700	1494	1767	2014	7.2
	USA, White			1719	1698	2016	1969	5.8
	USA, Black			1674	1459	1610	1429	*-3.5*
	Puerto Rico			1242	1208	1429	1787	11.0
	Colombia, Cali			1203	1354	1592	1652	9.9

MORTALITY

Sex	Region	Initial year of the period							Linear trend
		1955	1960	1965	1970	1975	1980	1985	
Male									
	Canada	1322	1293	1240	1138	912	797	715	-10.3
	USA	1335	1272	1132	971	790	683	578	-14.2
	Puerto Rico			829	910	667	812	471	-13.7
	Chile	951	985	1016	995	961	860	751	-2.5
	Costa Rica			1229	1085	1038	1038	1001	*-2.8*
	Uruguay	1180	1501	1295	1052	1016	1017		-4.7
	Venezuela	754	828	896	861	823	763		*-0.9*
Female									
	Canada	1052	1020	970	894	713	630	535	-11.2
	USA	1078	1033	929	766	605	532	462	-14.8
	Puerto Rico			813	843	510	488	483	-13.6
	Chile	690	792	812	819	792	722	652	-2.2
	Costa Rica			806	853	837	823	756	*-4.2*
	Uruguay	1045	1018	808	834	793	571		-11.8
	Venezuela	608	746	741	660	744	478		-5.2

Regions as defined in Table 30.1
Cumulative risk per million calculated from age-specific rates in each calendar period
Period as defined in Table 2.3 for incidence and Table 2.7 for mortality
Linear trend: percentage change in risk every five years over the entire data period (see text)

CHILDHOOD CANCER

ALL SITES (ICD-9 140-208)
AMERICAS, CUMULATIVE RISK (0-14 YEARS)

MALES

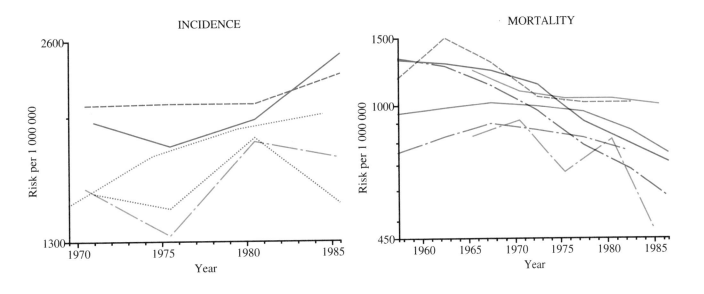

FEMALES

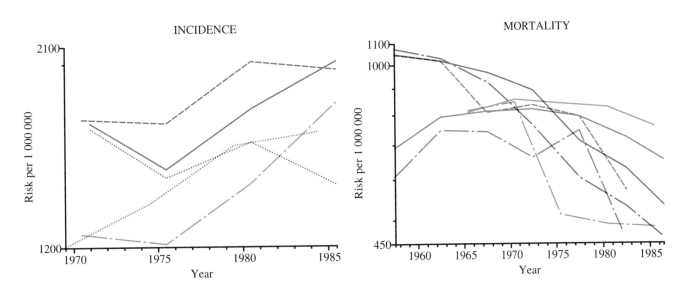

—— CANADA	—·— PUERTO RICO
—·— USA	—— CHILE
— — USA, White	·········· COLOMBIA, Cali
·········· USA, Black	— — URUGUAY
—— COSTA RICA	—··— VENEZUELA

Chapter 31

SUMMARY

Time trends in cancer risk have often been summarised by the observation that mortality from cancers associated with tobacco is increasing rapidly, while mortality from all other cancers is either stable or falling slightly, this slight decline being dominated by the decrease in mortality from stomach cancer. Until recently, and with some variation between the sexes, this simple summary of cancer mortality trends would have been broadly correct for a number of developed countries, and it remains useful in dismissing claims of an impending and unexplained epidemic of cancer, but it does not apply to all countries, and in some there have recently been striking changes in the trends in mortality from cancers associated with tobacco.

Cancer mortality has been widely accepted as the most important measure of progress against cancer, since it reflects the impact of cancer on people, and has been considered less subject to distortion than incidence or survival, although this is open to question. Cancer mortality also reflects trends in incidence and survival to a greater or lesser extent. There has been controversy, however, over how cancer mortality trends should be interpreted, as well as over which measures should be used to assess progress in cancer control. An overall summary of trends in mortality from all cancers combined is of limited value in assessing progress against cancer, in any case. Increases in a common lethal cancer may numerically dominate overall mortality trends, perhaps concealing declines in less common or less lethal cancers, while opposite trends in cancers of the lung and stomach, for example, might lead to an overall impression that little has changed. Further, up to a third of cancer patients will not die of cancer, and cancer mortality statistics do not reflect their experience at all. Cancer mortality trends only indirectly reflect trends in the number of people who are diagnosed with cancer in a given year, and those who do die of cancer in a given year may have been diagnosed more than 3 years previously, even though many die earlier: this blurs the responsiveness of routine cancer mortality statistics as a measure of recent progress, and alternative measures have been proposed[100]. Trends in competing risks of death, especially at higher ages, may also complicate the interpretation of cancer mortality trends[167].

The chance of developing cancer, and in that event, the chances of surviving it, are of direct interest to individuals. Trends in the occurrence of cancer and in the duration and quality of survival after diagnosis are also of interest to governments in reviewing priorities for prevention and research, and for health care planners in assessing the likely burden of patients requiring treatment. Trends in cancer incidence and survival must therefore be considered essential components of any comprehensive evaluation of progress against cancer.

Overall cancer mortality trends in the USA and other industrialised countries have been used to argue that little or no progress has been made against cancer[12,14] or that the increases are so great that intensive investigation of the causes is required[62,129]. More sanguine interpretations have been reached from alternative analyses of essentially the same data[38,84,253], in particular by concentrating attention on favourable trends in mortality at younger ages. It is not our intention to enter this debate here, but it was with the controversy over interpretation of cancer trends in mind that we have tried to provide several quantitative descriptions of incidence and mortality trends for each major cancer in previous chapters, in order to help other scientists reach their own judgement.

One point on which protagonists on both sides of the debate do appear to agree is that there should be an increasing emphasis on research into discovering avoidable causes of cancer, and into the means of implementing primary prevention based on such knowledge[13,14,38,45,82,197,280]. In reviewing progress towards cancer control, Breslow and Cumberland[38], for example, expressed this as follows: "Understanding biological mechanisms can be useful but is not essential for important progress in disease control. ... Hence, research aimed directly at cancer prevention and promoting use of available knowledge for cancer prevention is highly desirable in the present state of cancer control." They add: "In reviewing progress against cancer, reliance on summary statistics that combine death rates for all age groups or that merge all cancers can be misleading"; Muir et al.[198] take a similar view.

Depending on how the trends are assessed, different or even contradictory conclusions may be reached. Figure 31.1 shows trends in summary measures of sex-specific mortality from all malignant neoplasms combined in the USA and

787

Canada, by year of death and by year of birth. Interpretation of the trends in cross-sectional mortality in successive time periods (graphs at upper and lower left) is incomplete without examination of the trends in longitudinal mortality in successive birth cohorts (graphs at upper and lower right): the former may be judged disappointing, the latter encouraging. The data are the same, the presentation is different.

There is, however, one geographical contrast in time trends for mortality from all cancers combined that is unlikely to be seriously misleading. For most cancers reviewed here, but with important exceptions by site and country discussed in earlier chapters, trends in incidence and mortality are more unfavourable in Poland, Hungary, Czechoslovakia, Romania and Yugoslavia than in other European countries to the west and north, and this is reflected by the ranking of recent linear trends for mortality in Figure 31.2.

In general, however, the pattern of trends varies widely between countries, and within countries by type of cancer, and we have felt it unwise to present summary tables and graphics for all cancers combined of the kind presented for each cancer in preceding chapters. Such summaries often conceal more than they reveal[198]. The validity of applying age-period-cohort models to combined data sets of such diversity must be open to doubt. Some of the individual analyses in previous chapters were also constrained to include more than one clinical entity, such as those for cancers of the bone, thyroid and testis, colorectal cancer, lymphoma, Hodgkin's disease and leukaemia. Given the extremely wide variation between the various cancers in incidence and mortality by age, and in their trends over time, the interpretation of trends for all cancers combined would be still more difficult than for individual cancers. Detailed tables of results are available for each cancer, showing changes over time in the truncated rates, the numbers of cases or deaths and the cumulative risks, and age-specific recent linear trends with their standard errors, for each of the 60 populations in 29 countries covered by cancer registries for cancer incidence, and for most cancers, in each of 36 countries for cancer mortality[60].

In attempting to summarise the trend analyses for individual cancer sites presented in this book, as well as some of the geographical variation in those trends, we have found it helpful to borrow the proposal of the Extramural Committee to Assess Measures of Progress against Cancer[100] to group the various cancers into three categories: (a) cancers which are largely preventable; (b) cancers for which secondary prevention (screening and early detection) is practicable, and (c) cancers

for which there is effective treatment, or for which major improvements in therapy have been achieved. Although some cancers may belong to more than one category, and for some cancers the categorisation would not be the same in all countries, this seemed a natural approach to evaluating the success of the three basic approaches to reducing the burden of cancer: primary prevention, early detection, and treatment.

Observed trends in the incidence and mortality of cancers amenable to primary or secondary prevention described here may be compared with estimates of their theoretical preventability, discussed by Tomatis *et al.*[286].

Cancers for which primary prevention is feasible

On present knowledge, the most effective way of preventing cancer would be the elimination of tobacco smoking and chewing, and a reduction in alcohol consumption. This would greatly reduce the incidence of lung cancer and of nearly all cancers of the mouth, larynx and pharynx and, in many countries, the oesophagus. The most visible evidence of the reduction in tobacco smoking is the remarkable decline in lung cancer risk in successive generations among males in several European countries, and to a lesser extent in the USA. This achievement is especially impressive in Finland and in the UK, where the decline is already visible in the cross-sectional data. Even this success among males has not been achieved in many populations, however, and with the exception of the UK there is as yet little evidence of such trends among females. The size of the decline in risk in some populations makes the contrast with others even more stark: in eastern European countries, the continuing increase in cancers of the lung, oral cavity, pharynx and oesophagus is cause for serious concern. Given the numerical importance of lung cancer, and its lethality, this trend has a marked effect on overall cancer incidence and mortality trends in these countries.

On the basis of current knowledge of risk factors, trends for bladder cancer might be expected to resemble those for lung cancer. This is qualitatively true for mortality, but not generally for incidence, for which the less favourable trends may be affected by changes in the definition of the disease (Chapter 23). On the basis of the mortality trends, it may be concluded that the risk of bladder cancer has decreased to some extent where tobacco control has been effective; reduction of occupational chemical exposures may also have played a role.

MALES

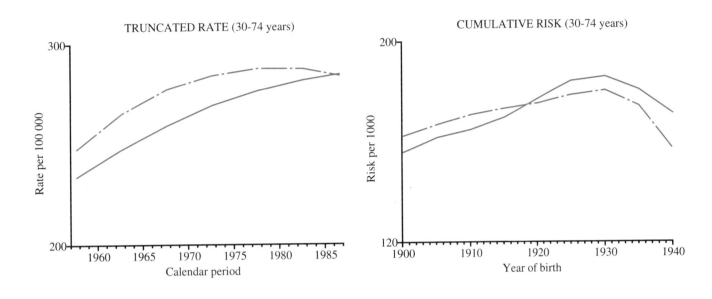

FEMALES

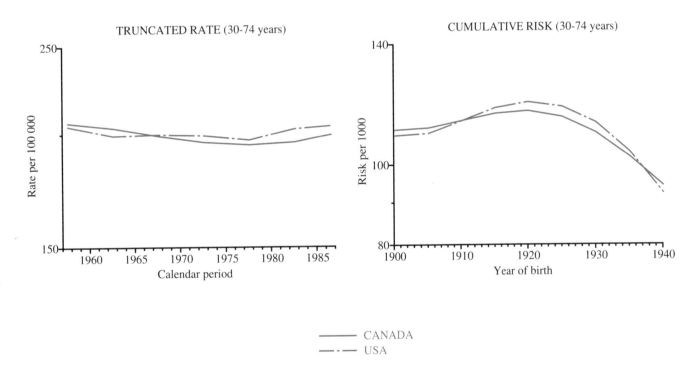

Figure 31.1: Cancer mortality, all malignancies (excluding non-melanoma skin cancer), males and females, USA and Canada: trends in truncated rate (30-74 years) by year of death and in cohort cumulative risk (30-74 years) by year of birth.

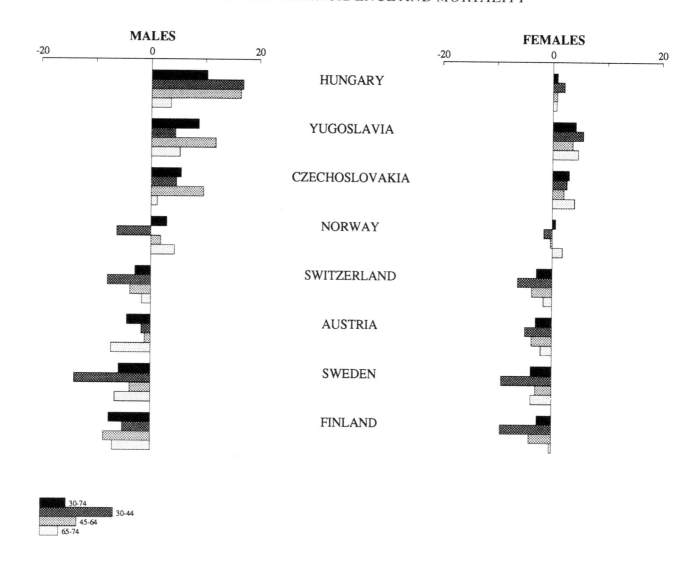

Figure 31.2: Recent linear trends in cancer mortality, all malignancies (excluding non-melanoma skin cancer), males and females, Europe (except EC member states): percentage change in truncated rates per five-year period, by age.

A large proportion of cancers of the oral cavity, pharynx and oesophagus could also be prevented by effective tobacco control; this has been achieved in Finland and, to a lesser extent, in England and Wales. In some countries, alcohol is likely to play a more important role than tobacco in determining the risk of cancers of the upper aerodigestive tract, and time trends in the rate of these cancers do not parallel the trends for lung cancer. A rapid increase in the risk of these cancers is now occurring in several European countries, particularly in Germany, Denmark and eastern European countries. In the countries at highest risk of these cancers, limited progress has been made. In France, where the same shape in the curve of decline in risk by birth cohort is seen for all alcohol-related cancers, this is by reduction of alcohol consumption, and in Bombay (India), probably by reduction of betel chewing.

Stomach cancer falls into the category of preventable cancers, even though its causes are not well understood. The remarkably widespread decline in its incidence, with the possible but important exception of China, is likely to reflect improvements in nutrition and the quality of food, but it is a welcome and unexpected effect of these changes, rather than the result of public health policy. It is notable that in most populations the decline is more rapid among females. Despite the continuing decline, stomach cancer remains an important problem in most countries, and it is still the most frequent cancer in Japan. Survival is poor, and has improved very little. Research into the causes of stomach cancer remains a high priority, as the basis of a more active strategy to reduce its impact still further.

Among cancers for which primary preventive measures are currently feasible, oesophageal cancer has a special position, since its causes are different in different regions of the world. In Asia, the large decreases observed in Singapore, Shanghai (China) and Hong Kong suggest that oesophageal cancer may be preventable by changes in life-style linked to economic development, particularly nutrition. The difficulty here is similar to that associated with stomach cancer, for which the decline in risk is also impressive, and far more widespread, but precise information about specific risk factors to enable more active measures of primary prevention is not available.

Among the malignant neoplasms examined here, the other main candidate for primary prevention is malignant melanoma of the skin. Although the precise mechanism of its induction also remains uncertain, patterns of exposure to sunlight are clearly involved, and primary prevention should be feasible, by changing public behaviour to reduce sun exposure. Little progress is yet apparent here, since in most populations there is still a rapid exponential increase in incidence which cannot be ascribed to changing definitions of disease, and there is at best only a small deceleration in the rate of increase in mortality, which may be ascribable to earlier diagnosis and better treatment. The deceleration of the continuing increase in incidence seen in some populations offers some hope, but since melanoma has now become one of the ten most frequent malignancies in many populations, understanding the reasons behind these trends is increasingly important. Melanoma is also a possible candidate for screening, since survival is strongly related to the thickness of the tumour at diagnosis, but evidence that screening reduces mortality is not yet available[187].

Cancers for which secondary prevention is plausible

The most convincing example of success in screening for cancer is provided by cervical cancer. The decrease in the incidence of invasive cancer of the cervix has been universal in countries where efficient and widespread screening programmes have been implemented. The benefit may be summarised by a 75% decrease in incidence over the last 15 years in most of these countries.

The second example is breast cancer, for which the efficacy of screening has been convincingly demonstrated in controlled trials. No clear benefit of secondary prevention for breast cancer has yet been seen, however, in the mortality data reported here. For example, breast cancer incidence rates in Canada and the USA are changing at different speeds, while mortality rates are decreasing almost identically by birth cohort, suggesting that the more rapid increase in breast cancer incidence in the USA may be partly due to over-diagnosis (diagnosis as invasive breast cancer of some lesions that would not have presented clinically) by more intensive use of mammography in the USA than in Canada. In several other countries, especially Sweden, Norway and Switzerland, declines in mortality by birth cohort have been observed, but these cannot readily be attributed to screening, because the age-distribution of the decline varies, and there has been an upturn in risk for the most recent generations in Sweden and Norway. It is possible that population-based screening for breast cancer has not yet been in operation in any country long enough to have produced clear reductions in mortality[187]. A satisfactory explanation of the observed trends in breast cancer, still the most frequent cancer in women, will require further careful monitoring of incidence and mortality.

Despite several efforts to assess the efficacy of screening for colorectal cancer in randomised controlled trials, no conclusive evidence is yet available. In Germany (FRG), screening by digital examination and by faecal occult blood test has been public health policy since the 1970s, while in the USA, sigmoidoscopy is widely used for early diagnosis. It is possible that these practices have had some impact on incidence and mortality from colorectal cancer. Mortality is generally decreasing in successive birth cohorts in northern and western Europe and in North America, especially in females, while incidence is slightly increasing. In the absence of organised screening programmes, this pattern is consistent with better management of the disease due to earlier diagnosis and/or better treatment. By contrast, both incidence and mortality are generally increasing in eastern Europe and in Asia, suggesting that the prevalence of risk factors for colorectal cancer has been changing adversely.

Screening for stomach cancer in Japan started in the 1960s. Millions of individuals are screened each year, and a shift toward earlier stage of disease at diagnosis has been detected[187]. Incidence in Japan has decreased only slowly, while mortality is falling at the same speed as in Hong Kong or Singapore, and it remains difficult to ascribe the decline in mortality in Japan to screening. The data suggest rather that screening for stomach cancer in Japan may lead to diagnosis of some lesions which would not have been diagnosed clinically. In Venezuela, where screening has been undertaken in a high risk area, national mortality from stomach cancer is decreasing at a similar rate to other countries in the Americas.

The incidence of prostate cancer has increased in several parts of the world; in some countries a substantial part of this increase may be attributable to detection of tumours that would not have presented clinically. Mortality has been stable or increasing, however, and part of the observed increase in incidence is probably real. Miller *et al.*[187] noted that there are contra-indications to large-scale organised screening programmes for prostatic cancer, given the likelihood of over-treatment.

On the basis of the time trends analysed here, there is as yet little evidence that screening for cancer has had a large effect, except for cancer of the cervix. Screening for breast cancer is known to be effective from clinical trials, but it may take longer for any benefits of national screening programmes to become evident in mortality trends.

Cancers for which treatment has improved

The quite dramatic decline in mortality from Hodgkin's disease seen in many populations since about 1970 is clearly due to improvements in treatment and survival. Incidence has been broadly stable.

The treatment of leukaemia in adults has improved, and survival has increased, but while mortality is beginning to decline in many countries, incidence is generally rising. Improvements in the quality of diagnosis, the completeness of registration and the accuracy of death certification have probably all contributed to the observed trends to a greater or lesser extent in each country. The overall patterns of temporal trend in leukaemia somewhat resemble those for testicular cancer, in that a rise in recorded incidence has coincided with a fall in recorded mortality, and although improvements in diagnosis and death certification are likely to have had a greater effect on observed leukaemia trends than those for testicular cancer, the steady increase in the incidence of leukaemia in a number of developed countries seems unlikely to be explicable solely as an artefact.

There have also been great improvements in treatment and survival for leukaemia in childhood, particularly acute lymphocytic leukaemia in the first five years of life. These are reflected in substantial rates of decline in mortality in many regions, although incidence has been broadly stable or increasing in most populations.

The substantial and widespread decline in mortality from testicular cancer represents another considerable therapeutic advance, and data from Finland suggest that this is not due simply to earlier diagnosis. Survival at five years now often exceeds 90%. Testicular cancer exemplifies the danger of relying solely on mortality data to evaluate progress: there is a widespread increase in the occurrence of this disease, for which known risk factors appear to provide only a partial explanation. Since testicular cancer is a leading malignancy among young men, the trends should stimulate further research. The unexplained drop in risk seen in three populations for the 1935-45 cohort, representing a transient reversal of the upward trend, may be of interest here, as are the unexpectedly low and stable risk in Spain and the differences in trend between white, black and Chinese ethnic groups.

Trends in ovarian cancer vary widely. A reduction in risk in successive birth cohorts in the most industrialised countries may be partly explained by trends toward lower parity and wider use of oral contraceptives, which would tend to reduce incidence; earlier diagnosis and improvements in treatment, with longer survival, may also have contributed to the concurrent declines in mortality, while increasingly precise diagnosis during life may have been responsible for some of the earlier and more rapid apparent increases in mortality seen in some countries. The recent increase in ovarian cancer in Japan is cause for some concern. Uterine cancer trends are broadly similar to those for cancer of the ovary; again, the risk is increasing in Japan.

Trends in the incidence of colorectal cancer vary considerably around the world, but many of the populations studied have experienced increases. Mortality in these countries is either rising less rapidly or falling, particularly in the most industrialised nations, and these changes are likely to reflect both true increases in incidence and the benefits of earlier diagnosis and more successful treatment.

Geographical variation in incidence trends for thyroid cancer is quite marked, and in some populations the trends differ markedly between males and females. Mortality is more generally either stable or falling, and better treatment is the most probable explanation.

Conclusion

This examination of trends in cancer incidence and mortality has revealed wide variation in trends for many cancers, both between different regions of the world and, often enough, between males and females or between racial groups within a region. The causes of some of these trends are known, and particularly for tobacco-related cancers in females, they confirm the urgent need for rapid improvements in tobacco control. Progress in controlling cancers associated with alcohol is not so clear as that seen in some regions for tobacco-related cancers in males, and in some countries the rates for alcohol-related cancers are increasing quickly. Screening has had a major impact on incidence and mortality from cervical cancer in a few countries with effective screening programmes, and these benefits could be achieved more widely; for breast cancer, the substantial reduction in mortality which screening can deliver is not yet apparent. Improvements in treatment have transformed the prognosis for patients with some of the less common non-epithelial cancers, particularly leukaemia in childhood, Hodgkin's disease and testicular cancer, but since these malignancies principally affect younger individuals, the gains in person-years of life are substantial. Less spectacular gains from improved therapy are apparent for some of the common cancers, such as breast and colon cancer, and adult leukaemia, but the net gains in life years are probably much larger.

For some malignancies, the analyses reported here confirm the existence of widespread trends for which there is, as yet, no completely satisfactory explanation. These include an increase in the incidence of non-Hodgkin lymphoma, testicular cancer and leukaemia, and the decline in both stomach cancer and, in some developing countries, oesophageal cancer. These cancers are likely to have environmental causes amenable to prevention.

REFERENCES

1. Adami, H.-O., Bergström, R., Persson, I. & Sparén, P. (1990) The incidence of ovarian cancer in Sweden, 1960-1984. *Am. J. Epidemiol.*, **132**, 446-452

2. Adami, H.-O., Bergström, R., Sparén, P. & Baron, J. (1993) Increasing cancer risk in younger birth cohorts in Sweden. *Lancet*, **341**, 773-777

3. Adami, H.-O., Sparén, P., Bergström, R., Holmberg, L., Krusemo, U.B. & Pontén, J. (1989) Increasing survival trend after cancer diagnosis in Sweden: 1960-1984. *J. Natl. Cancer Inst.*, **81**, 1640-1647

4. Akslen, L.A., Haldorsen, T., Thoresen, S.O. & Glattre, E. (1990) Incidence of thyroid cancer in Norway 1970-1985. Population review on time trend, sex, age, histological type and tumour stage in 2625 cases. *Acta Pathol. Microbiol. Immunol. Scand.*, **98**, 549-558

5. Alderson, M.R. & Meade, T.W. (1967) Accuracy of diagnosis on death certificates compared with that in hospital records. *Br. J. Prev. Soc. Med.*, **21**, 22-29

6. Alfonso Sanchez, J.L., Gil Mary, A., Cortes Vizcaino, C. & Cortina Greus, P. (1988) Tendencias actuales de la mortalidad por cáncer de próstata en España (1951-1982). *Arch. Esp. Urol.*, **41**, 581-584

7. Alfonso, J.L., Cortes, C., Gimenez, F. & Cortina, P. (1989) Cáncer de testículo: factores de riesgo y evolución de la mortalidad en España (1951-1983). *Arch. Esp. Urol.*, **42**, 755-760

8. Angst, E., Bisig, B., Tschopp, A., Sigg, C., Schüler, G., Gutzwiller, F. & Schnyder, U.W. (1989) Melanoma mortality in Switzerland 1970-1986. *Schweiz. Med. Wochenschr.*, **119**, 1591-1598

9. Anon. (1989) Changing trends in malignant melanoma in New York State. *N. Y. State J. Med.*, **89**, 239-241

10. Arraiz, G.A., Wigle, D.T. & Mao, Y. (1990) Is cervical cancer increasing among young women in Canada? *Can. J. Public Health*, **81**, 396-397

11. Augustin, J., Kolcová, V. & Wotke, R. (1989) Epidemiological aspects of childhood cancer incidence in Czech regions. *Neoplasma*, **36**, 387-392

12. Bailar, J.C. (1990) Death from all cancers. Trends in sixteen countries. *Ann. N. Y. Acad. Sci.*, **609**, 49-57

13. Bailar, J.C. (1990) Recent trends in cancer. *Ann. N. Y. Acad. Sci.*, **610**, 205-211

14. Bailar, J.C. & Smith, E.M. (1986) Progress against cancer? *N. Engl. J. Med.*, **314**, 1226-1232

15. Bailar, J.C. & Smith, E.M. (1986) Progress against cancer? *N. Engl. J. Med.*, **315**, 968

16. Balvert-Locht, H.R., Coebergh, J.W., Hop, W.C.J., Brölmann, H.A.M., Crommelin, M., van Wijck, D.J.A. & Verhagen-Teulings, M.T. (1991) Improved prognosis of ovarian cancer in the Netherlands during the period 1975-1985: a registry-based study. *Gynecologic Oncology*, **42**, 3-8

17. Bang, K.M., White, J.E., Gause, B.L. & Leffall, L.D. (1988) Evaluation of recent trends in cancer mortality and incidence among blacks. *Cancer*, **61**, 1255-1261

18. Barnes, N., Cartwright, R.A., O'Brien, C., Richards, I.D.G., Roberts, B. & Bird, C.C. (1986) Rising incidence of lymphoid malignancies - true or false? *Br. J. Cancer*, **53**, 393-398

19. Bell, J. (1992) Temporal trends in the incidence of childhood leukaemia and in radiation exposure of parents. *J. Radiol. Prot.*, **12**, 3-8

20. Bennett, J.M., Catovsky, D., Daniel, M.-T., Flandrin, G., Galton, D.A.G., Gralnick, H.R. & Sultan, C. (1976) Proposals for the classification of the acute leukaemias. French-American-British (FAB) Co-operative Group. *Br. J. Haem.*, **33**, 451-458

21. Beral, V. & Booth, M. (1986) Predictions of cervical cancer incidence and mortality in England and Wales. *Lancet*, **i**, 495

22. Berzuini, C., Clayton, D.G. & Bernardinelli, L. (1993) Bayesian inference on the Lexis diagram. *Bull. Int. Statist. Inst.*, (in press)

23. Birch, J.M. & Blair, V. (1988) Increase in childhood carcinomas in north-west England. *Lancet*, **i**, 833

24. Bitran, J.D. (1986) Progress against cancer? *N. Engl. J. Med.*, **315**, 963

25. Bjarnason, O., Day, N.E., Smaedal, G. & Tulinius, H. (1977) The effect of year of birth on the breast cancer age incidence curve in Iceland. *Int. J. Cancer*, **13**, 689-696

26. Black, R.J., Clarke, J.A. & Warner, J.M. (1991) Malignant melanoma in Scotland: trends in incidence and survival, 1968-87. A review prepared by the CSA Information and Statistics Division for the Health Monitoring Group. *Health Bull. (Edinb.)*, **49**, 97-105

27. Black, R.J., Sharp, L. & Kendrick, S.W. (1993) *Trends in Cancer Survival in Scotland, 1968-1990*, Information and Statistics Division, Edinburgh

28. Blot, W.J., Devesa, S.S. & Fraumeni, J.F. (1987) Declining breast cancer mortality among young American women. *J. Natl. Cancer Inst.*, **78**, 451-454

29. Blot, W.J., Devesa, S.S., Kneller, R.W. & Fraumeni, J.F. (1991) Rising incidence of adenocarcinoma of the esophagus and gastric cardia. *J. Am. Med. Assoc.*, **265**, 1287-1289

30. Blyth, F. & Beral, V. (1991) Monitoring cancer trends. *Br. J. Cancer*, **63**, 479-480

31. Bolumar, F., Vioque, J. & Cayuela, A. (1991) Changing mortality patterns for major cancers in Spain, 1951-1985. *Int. J. Epidemiol.*, **20**, 20-25

32. Boring, C.C., Byrnes, R.K., Chan, W.C., Causey, N., Gregory, H.R., Nadel, M.R. & Greenberg, R.S. (1985) Increase in high-grade lymphomas in young men. *Lancet*, **i**, 857-858

33. Bosch, F.X., Muñoz, N., de Sanjosé, S., Izarzugaza, I., Gili, M., Viladiu, P., Tormo, M.J., Moreo, P., Ascunce, N., Gonzalez, L.C., Tafur, L., Kaldor, J., Guerrero, E., Aristizabal, N., Santamaria, M., Alonso de Ruiz, P. & Shah, K. (1992) Risk factors for cervical cancer in Colombia and Spain. *Int. J. Cancer*, **52**, 750-758

34. Bouchardy, C., Fioretta, G., Raymond, L. & Vassilakos, P. (1990) Age differentials in trends of uterine cervical cancer incidence from 1970 to 1987 in Geneva. *Rev. Epidémiol. Santé Publique*, **38**, 261-262

35. Brancker, A. (1990) Lung cancer and smoking prevalence in Canada. *Health Rep.*, **2**, 67-83

36. Braverman, A.S. (1986) Progress against cancer? *N. Engl. J. Med.*, **315**, 967

37. Brenner, H., Stegmaier, C. & Ziegler, H. (1990) Magnitude and time trends of the life-time risk of developing cancer in Saarland, Germany. *Eur. J. Cancer*, **26**, 978-982

38. Breslow, L. & Cumberland, W.G. (1988) Progress and objectives in cancer control. *J. Am. Med. Assoc.*, **259**, 1690-1694

39. Breslow, N.E. & Clayton, D.G. (1993) Approximate inference in generalized linear mixed models. *J. Amer. Stat. Assoc.*, **88**, 9-25

40. Brinton, L.A. & Fraumeni, J.F. (1986) Epidemiology of uterine cervical cancer. *J. Chronic Dis.*, **39**, 1051-1065

41. Brinton, L.A., Huggins, G.R., Lehman, H.F., Mallin, K., Savitz, D., Trapido, E., Rosenthal, J. & Hoover, R.N. (1986) Long-term use of oral contraceptives and risk of invasive cervical cancer. *Int. J. Cancer*, **38**, 339-344

42. Brooks, S.E. & Wolff, C. (1991) 30-year cancer trends in Jamaica: Kingston & St. Andrew (1958-1987). *West Indian Med. J.*, **40**, 134-138

43. Buffler, P.A., Cooper, S.P. & Carr, D.T. (1988) Lung cancer trends and prospects for prevention: Texas and United States. *Tex. Med.*, **84**, 48-50

44. Byers, R.L., Lantz, P.M., Remington, P.L. & Phillips, J.L. (1991) Malignant melanoma: trends in Wisconsin, 1980-1989. *Wis. Med. J.*, **90**, 305, 307

45. Cairns, J. (1985) The treatment of diseases and the war against cancer. *Sci. Amer.*, **253**, 31-39

46. Cancer Research Campaign. (1982) *Trends in Cancer Survival in Great Britain: Cases Registered between 1960 and 1974*, CRC, London

47. Capocaccia, R., Verdecchia, A., Micheli, A., Sant, M., Gatta, G. & Berrino, F. (1990) Breast cancer incidence and prevalence estimated from survival and mortality. *Cancer Causes and Control*, **1**, 23-29

48. Carr, T.W. (1993) Natural history of prostate cancer. *Lancet*, **341**, 91-92

49. Caygill, C.P. & Hill, M.J. (1991) Trends in European breast cancer incidence and possible etiology. *Tumori*, **77**, 126-129

50. Cayuela, A., Lacalle, J.R. & Gili, M. (1989) Analysis of cohort mortality from prostatic cancer in Spain, 1951-1983. *J. Epidemiol. Community Health*, **43**, 249-252

51. Cayuela, A., Vioque, J. & Bolumar, F. (1991) Oesophageal cancer mortality: relationship with alcohol intake and cigarette smoking in Spain. *J. Epidemiol. Community Health*, **45**, 273-276

52. Chen, J.K., Katz, R.V., Krutchkoff, D.J. & Eisenberg, E. (1992) Lip cancer: incidence trends in Connecticut, 1935-1985. *Cancer*, **70**, 2025-2030

53. Cheng, K.K., Day, N.E. & Davies, T.W. (1992) Oesophageal cancer mortality in Europe: paradoxical time trend in relation to smoking and drinking. *Br. J. Cancer*, **65**, 613-617

54. Chow, W.H., Devesa, S.S. & Blot, W.J. (1991) Colon cancer incidence: recent trends in the United States. *Cancer Causes and Control*, **2**, 419-425

55. Clayton, D.G. & Schifflers, E. (1987) Models for temporal variation in cancer rates. I: age-period and age-cohort models. *Stat. Med.*, **6**, 449-467

56. Clayton, D.G. & Schifflers, E. (1987) Models for temporal variation in cancer rates. II: age-period-cohort models. *Stat. Med.*, **6**, 469-481

57. Coebergh, J.W., Neumann, H.A., Vrints, L.W., van der Heijden, L., Meijer, W.J. & Verhagen-Teulings, M.T. (1991) Trends in the incidence of non-melanoma skin cancer in the SE Netherlands 1975-1988: a registry-based study. *Br. J. Dermatol.*, **125**, 353-359

58. Craft, A.W., Amineddine, J.E.S. & Wagget, J. (1987) The Northern region children's malignant disease registry 1968-82: incidence and survival. *Br. J. Cancer*, **56**, 853-858

59. Cuzick, J. (1990) International time trends for multiple myeloma. *Ann. N. Y. Acad. Sci.*, **609**, 205-214

60. Damiecki, P., Estève, J. & Coleman, M.P. (1993) *Trends in Cancer Incidence and Mortality: Detailed Tables by Country and Region*, (IARC Technical Report No. 17), IARC, Lyon

61. Davis, D.L. & Hoel, D.G. (1990) *Trends in Cancer Mortality in Industrial Countries. Report of an International Workshop. Carpi, Italy, October 21-22, 1989*, New York Academy of Sciences, New York

62. Davis, D.L., Hoel, D.G., Fox, J. & Lopez, A.D. (1990) International trends in cancer mortality in France, West Germany, Italy, Japan, England and Wales, and the USA. *Lancet*, **336**, 474-481

63. Davis, D.L., Hoel, D.G., Fox, J. & Lopez, A.D. (1990) Trends in cancer mortality. *Lancet*, **336**, 1264-1265

64. Davis, D.L., Hoel, D.G., Fox, J. & Lopez, A.D. (1990) International trends in cancer mortality in France, West Germany, Italy, Japan, England and Wales, and the United States. *Ann. N. Y. Acad. Sci.*, **609**, 5-48

65. Davis, D.L., Lilienfeld, A.D., Gittelsohn, A. & Scheckenbach, M.E. (1986) Increasing trends in some cancers in older Americans: fact or artifact? *Toxicol. Ind. Health*, **2**, 127-144

66. Davis, D.L. & Schwartz, J. (1988) Trends in cancer mortality: US white males and females, 1968-83. *Lancet*, **i**, 633-636

67. Davis, S. & Severson, R.K. (1987) Increasing incidence of cancer of the tongue in the United States among young adults. *Lancet*, **ii**, 910-911

68. Day, N.E. (1987) Cumulative rate and cumulative risk. In: Muir, C.S., Waterhouse, J.A.H., Mack, T., Powell, J. & Whelan, S., eds., *Cancer Incidence in Five Continents, Volume V*, (IARC Scientific Publications No. 88), IARC, Lyon, pp. 787-789

69. de Schryver, A. (1989) Does screening for cervical cancer affect incidence and mortality trends? The Belgian experience. *Eur. J. Cancer Clin. Oncol.*, **25**, 395-399

70. de Souza, C.M. (1991) An empirical Bayes formulation of cohort models in cancer epidemiology. *Stat. Med.*, **10**, 1241-1256

71. del Junco, D.J. & Annegers, J.F. (1986) Progress against cancer? *N. Engl. J. Med.*, **315**, 964-965

72. Depue, R.H. (1986) Rising mortality from cancer of the tongue in young white males. *N. Engl. J. Med.*, **315**, 647

73. Devesa, S.S., Blot, W.J. & Fraumeni, J.F. (1989) Declining lung cancer rates among young men and women in the United States: a cohort analysis. *J. Natl. Cancer Inst.*, **81**, 1568-1571

74. Devesa, S.S., Blot, W.J. & Fraumeni, J.F. (1990) Cohort trends in mortality from oral, esophageal, and laryngeal cancers in the United States. *Epidemiology*, **1**, 116-121

75. Devesa, S.S., Blot, W.J. & Fraumeni, J.F. (1991) The authors reply: (To: Cohort trends in mortality from oral, esophageal, and laryngeal cancer. Epidemiology 2 (3) 1991). *Epidemiology*, **2**, 236-237

76. Devesa, S.S., Pollack, E.S. & Young, J.L. (1984) Assessing the validity of observed cancer incidence trends. *Am. J. Epidemiol.*, **119**, 274-291

77. Devesa, S.S., Silverman, D.T., Young, J.L., Pollack, E.S., Brown, C.C., Horm, J.W., Percy, C.L., Myers, M.H., McKay, F.W. & Fraumeni, J.F. (1987) Cancer incidence and mortality trends among whites in the United States, 1947-84. *J. Natl. Cancer Inst.*, **79**, 701-770

78. Devesa, S.S., Young, J.L., Brinton, L.A. & Fraumeni, J.F. (1989) Recent trends in cervix uteri cancer. *Cancer*, **64**, 2184-2190

79. DeVita, V.T. (1986) Progress against cancer? *N. Engl. J. Med.*, **315**, 964

80. Dimitrova, E., Pleško, I., Somogyi, J. & Kiss, J. (1989) Trends and patterns in cancer incidence in Czechoslovakia, 1968-1985. *Neoplasma*, **36**, 245-255

81. Dockerty, J.D., Marshall, S., Fraser, J. & Pearce, N. (1991) Stomach cancer in New Zealand: time trends, ethnic group differences and a cancer registry-based case-control study. *Int. J. Epidemiol.*, **20**, 45-53

82. Doll, R. (1982) Underlining concepts of cancer control in the future. In: Aoki, K., Tominagi, S., Hirayama, T. & Hirota, Y., eds., *Cancer Prevention in Developing Countries*, University of Nagoya Press, Nagoya, Japan, pp. 587-594

83. Doll, R. (1989) Progress against cancer: are we winning the war? *Acta Oncol.*, **28**, 611-621

84. Doll, R. (1991) Progress against cancer: an epidemiologic assessment. *Am. J. Epidemiol.*, **134**, 675-688

85. Doll, R. (1992) The lessons of life: keynote address to the nutrition and cancer conference. *Cancer Res.*, **52**, 2024s-2029s

86. Doll, R., Muir, C.S. & Waterhouse, J.A.H., eds. (1970) *Cancer Incidence in Five Continents, Volume II*, UICC, Geneva

87. Doll, R., Payne, P. & Waterhouse, J.A.H., eds. (1968) *Cancer Incidence in Five Continents: A Technical Report*, UICC, Geneva

88. Doll, R. & Peto, R. (1981) The causes of cancer. *J. Natl. Cancer Inst.*, **66**, 1191-1308

89. dos Santos Silva, I. & Swerdlow, A.J. (1993) Thyroid cancer epidemiology in England and Wales: time trends and geographical distribution. *Br. J. Cancer*, **67**, 330-340

90. Dubrow, R., Flannery, J.T. & Liu, W.L. (1991) Time trends in malignant melanoma of the upper limb in Connecticut. *Cancer*, **68**, 1854-1858

91. Dugan, W.M. & Mortenson, L.E. (1986) Progress against cancer? *N. Engl. J. Med.*, **315**, 967

92. Eby, N.L., Grufferman, S., Flannelly, C.M., Schold, S.C., Vogel, F.S. & Burger, P.C. (1988) Increasing incidence of primary brain lymphoma in the US. *Cancer*, **62**, 2461-2465

93. Eide, T.J. (1987) Cancer of the uterine cervix in Norway by histologic type, 1970-84. *J. Natl. Cancer Inst.*, **79**, 199-205

94. Estève, J. (1990) International study of time trends. Some methodological considerations. *Ann. N. Y. Acad. Sci.*, **609**, 77-84

95. Estève, J., Benhamou, E. & Raymond, L. (1993) *Méthodes Statistiques en Épidémiologie Descriptive. Statistiques de Santé*, INSERM, Paris

96. Estève, J. & Tuyns, A. (1988) Models for combined action of alcohol and tobacco on risk of cancer: what do we really know from epidemiological studies? In: Feo, F., Pani, P., Columbano, A. & Garcea, R., eds., *Chemical Carcinogenesis*, Plenum Press, New York, pp. 649-655

97. Ewertz, M. & Carstensen, B. (1988) Trends in breast cancer incidence and mortality in Denmark, 1943-1982. *Int. J. Cancer*, **41**, 46-51

98. Ewertz, M., Duffy, S.W., Adami, H.-O., Kvale, G., Lund, E., Meirik, O., Mellemgaard, A., Soini, I. & Tulinius, H. (1990) Age at first birth, parity and risk of breast cancer: a meta-analysis of 8 studies from the Nordic countries. *Int. J. Cancer*, **46**, 597-603

99. Ewertz, M. & Kjaer, S.K. (1988) Ovarian cancer incidence and mortality in Denmark, 1943-1982. *Int. J. Cancer*, **42**, 690-696

100. Extramural Committee to Assess Measures of Progress Against Cancer. (1990) Measurement of progress against cancer. *J. Natl. Cancer Inst.*, **82**, 825-835

101. Faivre, J. & Hill, M.J. (1987) *Causation and Prevention of Colorectal Cancer*, Excerpta Medica, Amsterdam

102. Ferlay, J. (1993) Processing of data. In: Parkin, D.M., Muir, C.S., Whelan, S., Gao, Y.-T., Ferlay, J. & Powell, J., eds., *Cancer Incidence in Five Continents, Volume VI*, (IARC Scientific Publications No. 120), IARC, Lyon, pp. 39-44

103. Fraumeni, J.F. & Boice, J.D. (1982) Bone. In: Schottenfeld, D. & Fraumeni, J.F., eds., *Cancer Epidemiology and Prevention*, Saunders, Philadelphia, pp. 814-836

104. Freni, S.C. (1990) Trends in cancer mortality. *Lancet*, **336**, 1263-1264

105. Freni, S.C. & Gaylor, D.W. (1992) International trends in the incidence of bone cancer are not related to drinking water fluoridation. *Cancer*, **70**, 611-618

106. Gallagher, R.P., Elwood, M.J. & Yang, C.P. (1989) Is chronic sunlight exposure important in accounting for increases in melanoma incidence? *Int. J. Cancer*, **44**, 813-815

107. Gallagher, R.P., Ma, B., McLean, D.I., Yang, C.P., Ho, V., Carruthers, J.A. & Warshawski, L.M. (1990) Trends in basal cell carcinoma, squamous cell carcinoma, and melanoma of the skin from 1973 through 1987. *J. Am. Acad. Dermatol.*, **23**, 413-421

108. Gao, Y.-T., Blot, W.J., Zheng, W., Fraumeni, J.F. & Hsu, C.W. (1988) Lung cancer and smoking in Shanghai. *Int. J. Epidemiol.*, **17**, 277-280

109. Gillis, C.R., Hole, D., Lamont, D.W., Graham, A.C. & Ramage, S. (1992) The incidences of lung cancer and breast cancer in women in Glasgow. *Br. Med. J.*, **305**, 1331

110. Glass, A.G. & Hoover, R.N. (1989) The emerging epidemic of melanoma and squamous cell skin cancer. *J. Am. Med. Assoc.*, **262**, 2097-2100

111. Glattre, E., Akslen, L.A., Thoresen, S.O. & Haldoren, T. (1990) Geographic patterns and trends in the incidence of thyroid cancer in Norway 1970-1986. *Cancer Detect. Prev.*, **14**, 625-631

112. Goodman, M.T., Yoshizawa, C.N. & Kolonel, L.N. (1989) Incidence trends and ethnic patterns for childhood leukemia in Hawaii: 1960-1984. *Br. J. Cancer*, **60**, 93-97

113. Greenspan, E.M. (1986) Progress against cancer? *N. Engl. J. Med.*, **315**, 963

114. Hahn, R.A. & Moolgavkar, S.H. (1989) Nulliparity, decade of first birth, and breast cancer in Connecticut cohorts, 1855 to 1945: an ecological study. *Am. J. Public Health*, **79**, 1503-1507

115. Hakama, M., Miller, A.B. & Day, N.E., eds. (1986) *Screening for Cancer of the Uterine Cervix*, (IARC Scientific Publications No. 76), IARC, Lyon

116. Hakulinen, T., Andersen, A., Malker, B., Pukkala, E., Schou, G. & Tulinius, H. (1986) *Trends in Cancer Incidence in the Nordic countries: A Collaborative Study of the Five Nordic Cancer Registries*, The Nordic Cancer Registries, Helsinki

117. Hakulinen, T. & Hakama, M. (1991) Predictions of epidemiology and the evaluation of cancer control measures and the setting of policy priorities. *Soc. Sci. Med.*, **33**, 1379-1383

118. Hakulinen, T., Kenward, M., Luostarinen, T., Oksanen, H., Pukkala, E., Soderman, B. & Teppo, L. (1989) *Cancer in Finland in 1954-2008: Incidence, Mortality and Prevalence by Region*, Cancer Society of Finland, Helsinki

119. Halme, A., Kellokumpu Lehtinen, P. & Lehtonen, T. (1989) Trends in incidence and results of treatment of testicular germ cell tumours in Finland 1972-1983. *Acta Oncol.*, **28**, 777-783

120. Hamada, G.S., Bos, A.J., Kasuga, H. & Hirayama, T. (1991) Comparative epidemiology of oral cancer in Brazil and India. *Tokai J. Exp. Clin. Med.*, **16**, 63-72

121. Hannaford, P.C., Villard Mackintosh, L., Vessey, M.P. & Kay, C.R. (1991) Oral contraceptives and malignant melanoma. *Br. J. Cancer*, **63**, 430-433

122. Hansson, L.-E., Bergström, R., Sparén, P. & Adami, H.-O. (1991) The decline in the incidence of stomach cancer in Sweden 1960-1984: a birth cohort phenomenon. *Int. J. Cancer*, **47**, 499-503

123. Harnly, M.E., Swan, S.H., Holly, E.A., Kelter, A. & Padian, N. (1988) Temporal trends in the incidence of non-Hodgkin's lymphoma and selected malignancies in a population with a high incidence of acquired immunodeficiency syndrome (AIDS). *Am. J. Epidemiol.*, **128**, 261-267

124. Harris, J.R., Lippman, M.E., Veronesi, U. & Willett, W.C. (1992) Breast cancer (first of three parts). *N. Engl. J. Med.*, **327**, 319-328

125. Heasman, M.A. & Lipworth, L. (1966) *Accuracy of Certification of Cause of Death* (Studies on Medical and Population Subjects No. 20), HMSO, London

126. Hemminki, E., Hayden, C.L. & Janerich, D.T. (1989) Recent endometrial cancer trends in Connecticut and prescriptions for estrogen replacement therapy. *Int. J. Cancer*, **44**, 952-953

127. Hill, C., Benhamou, E. & Doyon, F. (1990) Trends in cancer mortality. *Lancet*, **336**, 1262-1263

128. Hill, C., Benhamou, E. & Doyon, F. (1991) Trends in cancer mortality, France 1950-1985. *Br. J. Cancer*, **63**, 587-590

129. Hoel, D.G., Davis, D.L., Miller, A.B., Sondik, E.J. & Swerdlow, A.J. (1992) Trends in cancer mortality in 15 industrialized countries, 1969-1986. *J. Natl. Cancer Inst.*, **84**, 313-320

130. Holford, T.R. (1983) The estimation of age, period and cohort effects for vital rates. *Biometrics*, **39**, 311-324

131. Holford, T.R. (1991) Understanding the effects of age, period, and cohort on incidence and mortality rates. *Ann. Rev. Public Health*, **12**, 425-457

132. Holford, T.R., Roush, G.C. & McKay, L.A. (1991) Trends in female breast cancer in Connecticut and the United States. *J. Clin. Epidemiol.*, **44**, 29-39

133. Horn-Ross, P.L., Holly, E.A., Brown, S.R. & Aston, D.A. (1991) Temporal trends in the incidence of cutaneous malignant melanoma among Caucasians in the San Francisco-Oakland MSA. *Cancer Causes and Control*, **2**, 299-305

134. Howson, C.P., Hiyama, T. & Wynder, E.L. (1986) The decline in gastric cancer: epidemiology of an unplanned triumph. *Epidemiol. Rev.*, **8**, 1-27

135. Jablon, S., Thompson, D., McConney, M. & Mabuchi, K. (1990) Accuracy of cause-of-death certification in Hiroshima and Nagasaki, Japan. *Ann. N. Y. Acad. Sci.*, **609**, 100-109

136. Jayant, K. & Yeole, B.B. (1987) Cancers of the upper alimentary and respiratory tracts in Bombay, India: a study of incidence over two decades. *Br. J. Cancer*, **56**, 847-852

137. Jensen, O.M., Estève, J., Møller, H. & Renard, H. (1990) Cancer in the European Community and its member states. *Eur. J. Cancer*, **26**, 1167-1256

138. Kampschoer, G.H., Nakajima, T. & van de Velde, C.J. (1989) Changing patterns in gastric adeno-carcinoma. *Br. J. Surg.*, **76**, 914-916

139. Kee, F., Patterson, C.C. & Collins, B. (1990) Colorectal cancer in the north and south of Ireland 1950-1984. *J. Epidemiol. Community Health*, **44**, 220-223

140. Key, T.J.A., Darby, S.C. & Pike, M.C. (1987) Trends in breast cancer mortality and diet in England and Wales from 1911 to 1980. *Nutr. Cancer*, **10**, 1-9

141. Kirn, V.P., Kovacic, J. & Primic Zakelj, M. (1992) Epidemiological evaluation of cervical cancer screening in Slovenia up to 1986. *Eur. J. Gynaecol. Oncol.*, **13**, 75-82

142. Kizer, K.W. & Dumbauld, S. (1988) Recent trends in lung and breast cancer mortality in California women. *West. J. Med.*, **149**, 466-467

143. La Vecchia, C. & Decarli, A. (1988) Decline of childhood cancer mortality in Italy, 1955-1980. *Oncology*, **45**, 93-97

144. La Vecchia, C., Lucchini, F., Negri, E., Boyle, P. & Levi, F. (1992) Trends in cancer mortality in the Americas, 1955-1989. *Eur. J. Cancer*, **29**, 431-470

145. La Vecchia, C., Lucchini, F., Negri, E., Boyle, P., Maisonneuve, P. & Levi, F. (1992) Trends of cancer mortality in Europe, 1955-1989: I, Digestive sites. *Eur. J. Cancer*, **28**, 132-235

146. La Vecchia, C., Lucchini, F., Negri, E., Boyle, P., Maisonneuve, P. & Levi, F. (1992) Trends of cancer mortality in Europe, 1955-1989: II, Respiratory tract, bone, connective and soft tissue sarcomas, and skin. *Eur. J. Cancer*, **28**, 514-599

147. La Vecchia, C., Lucchini, F., Negri, E., Boyle, P., Maisonneuve, P. & Levi, F. (1992) Trends of cancer mortality in Europe, 1955-1989: III, Breast and genital sites. *Eur. J. Cancer*, **28**, 927-998

148. La Vecchia, C., Lucchini, F., Negri, E., Boyle, P., Maisonneuve, P. & Levi, F. (1992) Trends of cancer mortality in Europe, 1955-1989: IV, Urinary tract, eye, brain and nerves, and thyroid. *Eur. J. Cancer*, **28**, 1210-1281

149. La Vecchia, C., Lucchini, F., Negri, E., Boyle, P., Maisonneuve, P. & Levi, F. (1992) Trends of cancer mortality in Europe, 1955-1989: V, Lympho-haemopoietic cancers and all cancers. *Eur. J. Cancer*, **28**, 1509-1581

150. Larsen, P.M., Vetner, M., Hansen, K. & Fey, S.J. (1988) Future trends in cervical cancer. *Cancer Lett.*, **41**, 123-137

151. Läärä, E., Day, N.E. & Hakama, M. (1987) Trends in mortality from cervical cancer in the Nordic countries: association with organised screening programmes. *Lancet*, **i**, 1247

152. Lee, H.P. (1990) Monitoring cancer incidence and risk factors in Singapore. *Ann. Acad. Med. Singapore*, **19**, 133-138

153. Lee, H.P., Day, N.E. & Shanmugaratnam, K. (1988) *Trends in Cancer Incidence in Singapore 1968-1982*, (IARC Scientific Publications No. 91), IARC, Lyon

154. Lee, H.P., Duffy, S.W., Day, N.E. & Shanmugaratnam, K. (1988) Recent trends in cancer incidence among Singapore Chinese. *Int. J. Cancer*, **42**, 159-166

155. Lee, H.P., Gourley, L., Duffy, S.W., Estève, J., Lee, J. & Day, N.E. (1991) Dietary effects on breast cancer risk in Singapore. *Lancet*, **337**, 197-200

156. Lee, N.C., Wingo, P.A., Gwinn, M.L., Rubin, G.L., Kendrick, J.S., Webster, L.A. & Ory, H.W. (1987) The reduction in risk of ovarian cancer associated with oral contraceptive use. *N. Engl. J. Med.*, **316**, 650-655

157. Lee, P.N., Fry, J.S. & Forey, B.A. (1990) Trends in lung cancer, chronic obstructive lung disease, and emphysema death rates for England and Wales 1941-85 and their relation to trends in cigarette smoking. *Thorax*, **45**, 657-665

158. Lee, W.C. & Lin, R.S. (1990) Age-period-cohort analysis of pancreatic cancer mortality in Taiwan, 1971-1986. *Int. J. Epidemiol.*, **19**, 839-847

159. Lenner, P., Jonsson, H. & Gardfjell, O. (1991) Trends in cancer incidence, survival and mortality in northern Sweden 1960-1986. *Med. Oncol. Tumor Pharmacother.*, **8**, 105-112

160. Levi, F., Decarli, A. & La Vecchia, C. (1988) Trends in cancer mortality in Switzerland, 1951-1984. *Rev. Epidémiol. Santé Publique*, **36**, 15-25

161. Levi, F. & La Vecchia, C. (1990) Trends in multiple myeloma. *Int. J. Cancer*, **46**, 755-756

162. Levi, F., Te, V.C. & La Vecchia, C. (1990) Changes in cancer incidence in the Swiss Canton of Vaud, 1978-87. *Ann. Oncol.*, **1**, 293-297

163. Levi, F., Te, V.C. & La Vecchia, C. (1990) Testicular cancer trends in the Canton of Vaud, Switzerland, 1974-1987. *Br. J. Cancer*, **62**, 871-873

164. Levi, F., Te, V.C., Randimbison, L. & La Vecchia, C. (1991) Cancer incidence registration and trends in the Canton of Vaud, Switzerland. *Eur. J. Cancer*, **27**, 207-209

165. Liff, J.M., Sung, J.F., Chow, W.H., Greenberg, R.S. & Flanders, W.D. (1991) Does increased detection account for the rising incidence of breast cancer? *Am. J. Public Health*, **81**, 462-465

166. London, S.J., Thomas, D.C., Bowman, J.D., Sobel, E., Cheng, T.C. & Peters, J.M. (1991) Exposure to residential electric and magnetic fields and risk of childhood leukemia. *Am. J. Epidemiol.*, **134**, 923-937

167. Lopez, A.D. (1990) Competing causes of death. A review of recent trends in mortality in industrialized countries with special reference to cancer. *Ann. N. Y. Acad. Sci.*, **609**, 58-74

168. Louhivuori, K. (1991) Effect of a mass screening program on the risk of cervical cancer. *Cancer Detect. Prev.*, **15**, 471-475

169. Lu, J.B., Yang, W.X., Zu, S.K., Chang, Q.L., Sun, X.B., Lu, W.Q., Quan, P.L. & Qin, Y.M. (1988) Cancer mortality and mortality trends in Henan, China, 1974-1985. *Cancer Detect. Prev.*, **13**, 167-173

170. Lund, E. (1990) Childbearing in marriage and mortality from breast cancer in Norway. *Int. J. Epidemiol.*, **19**, 527-531

171. Lundegårdh, G., Lindgren, A., Rohul, A., Nyrén, O., Hansson, L.-E., Bergström, R. & Adami, H.-O. (1991) Intestinal and diffuse types of gastric cancer: secular trends in Sweden since 1951. *Br. J. Cancer*, **64**, 1182-1186

172. Macfarlane, G.J., Boyle, P. & Scully, C. (1987) Rising mortality from cancer of the tongue in young Scottish males. *Lancet*, **ii**, 912

173. MacKie, R., Hunter, J.A., Aitchison, T.C., Hole, D., McLaren, K., Rankin, R., Blessing, K., Evans, A.T., Hutcheon, A.W., Jones, D.H., Soutar, D.S., Watson, A.C.H., Cornbleet, M.A. & Smyth, J.F. (1992) Cutaneous malignant melanoma, Scotland, 1979-89. The Scottish Melanoma Group. *Lancet*, **339**, 971-975

174. Mahoney, M.C., Nasca, P.C., Burnett, W.S. & Melius, J.M. (1991) Bone cancer incidence rates in New York State: time trends and fluoridated drinking water. *Am. J. Public Health*, **81**, 475-479

175. Mann, D.A. (1986) Progress against cancer? *N. Engl. J. Med.*, **315**, 966

176. Manzoor Zaidi, S.H. (1986) Cancer trends in Pakistan. In: Khogali, M., Omar, Y.T., Gjorgov, A. & Ismail, A.S., eds., *Cancer Prevention in Developing Countries*, Pergamon Press, Oxford, pp. 69-73

177. Marrett, L.D., Meigs, J.W. & Flannery, J.T. (1982) Trends in the incidence of cancer of the corpus uteri in Connecticut, 1964-1979, in relation to consumption of exogenous estrogens. *Am. J. Epidemiol.*, **116**, 57-67

178. Marrett, L.D., Weir, H.K., Clarke, E.A. & Magee, C.J. (1986) Rates of death from testicular cancer in Ontario in 1964-82: analysis by major histologic subgroups. *Can. Med. Assoc. J.*, **135**, 999-1002

179. Marshall, E. (1993) Search for a killer: focus shifts from fat to hormones. Special report: the politics of breast cancer. *Science*, **259**, 618-621

180. Mauldin, W.P. & Segal, S.J. (1986) *Prevalence of Contraceptive Use in Developing Countries*, The Rockefeller Foundation, New York

181. McCredie, M., Coates, M.S. & Ford, J.M. (1989) Trends in invasive cancer of the cervix uteri in New South Wales, 1973-1982. *Aust. N. Z. J. Obstet. Gynaecol.*, **29**, 335-339

182. McLaughlin, J.R., Kreiger, N., Marrett, L.D. & Holowaty, E.J. (1991) Cancer incidence registration and trends in Ontario. *Eur. J. Cancer*, **27**, 1520-1524

183. McMichael, A.J. & Puzio, A. (1988) Time trends in upper alimentary tract cancer rates and alcohol and tobacco consumption in Australia. *Community Health Stud.*, **12**, 289-295

184. McWhirter, W.R. & Petroeschevsky, A.L. (1991) Incidence trends in childhood cancer in Queensland, 1973-1988. *Med. J. Aust.*, **154**, 453-455

185. McWhorter, W.P. & Eyre, H.J. (1990) Impact of mammographic screening on breast cancer diagnosis. *J. Natl. Cancer Inst.*, **82**, 153-154

186. Meirik, O., Mygren, K.G. & Smedby, B. (1979) Demographic techniques in describing contraceptive use applied on the situation in Sweden. *Acta Obstet. Gynecol. Scand. Suppl.*, **88**, 61-64

187. Miller, A.B., Chamberlain, J., Day, N.E., Hakama, M. & Prorok, P.C. (1990) Report on a workshop of the UICC project on evaluation of screening for cancer. *Int. J. Cancer*, **46**, 761-769

188. Miller, B.A., Feuer, E.J. & Hankey, B.F. (1991) The increasing incidence of breast cancer since 1982: relevance of early detection. *Cancer Causes and Control*, **2**, 67-74

189. Møller, H., Boyle, P., Maisonneuve, P., La Vecchia, C. & Jensen, O.M. (1990) Changing mortality from esophageal cancer in males in Denmark and other European countries, in relation to changing levels of alcohol consumption. *Cancer Causes and Control*, **1**, 181-188

190. Møller, H., Mellemgaard, A. & Jensen, O.M. (1988) Measuring progress against cancer. *J. Cancer Res. Clin. Oncol.*, **114**, 613-617

191. Morales Suárez-Varela, M., Llopis-González, A., Lacasaña-Navarro, M. & Ferrandiz-Ferragud, J. (1990) Trends in malignant skin melanoma and other skin cancers in Spain, 1975-1983, and their relation to solar radiation intensity. *J. Environ. Pathol. Toxicol. Oncol.*, **10**, 245-253

192. Morris Brown, L., Pottern, L.M. & Hoover, R.N. (1987) Testicular cancer in young men: the search for causes of the epidemic increase in the United States. *J. Epidemiol. Community Health*, **41**, 349-354

193. Morris Brown, L., Pottern, L.M., Hoover, R.N., Devesa, S.S., Aselton, P. & Flannery, J.T. (1986) Testicular cancer in the United States: trends in incidence and mortality. *Int. J. Epidemiol.*, **15**, 164-170

194. Mosso, M.L., Colombo, R., Giordano, L., Pastore, G., Terracini, B. & Magnani, C. (1992) Childhood cancer registry of the Province of Torino, Italy. Survival, incidence, and mortality over 20 years. *Cancer*, **69**, 1300-1306

195. Muir, C.S. (1982) Time trends as indicators of etiology. In: Magnus, K., ed., *Trends in Cancer Incidence: Causes and Practical Implications*, Hemisphere, Washington, pp. 89-102

196. Muir, C.S. (1987) Classification. In: Muir, C.S., Waterhouse, J.A.H., Mack, T., Powell, J. & Whelan, S., eds., *Cancer Incidence in Five Continents, Volume V*, (IARC Scientific Publications No. 88), IARC, Lyon, pp. 19-25

197. Muir, C.S. (1990) Epidemiology, basic science, and the prevention of cancer: implications for the future. *Cancer Res.*, **50**, 6441-6448

198. Muir, C.S., Choi, N.W. & Schifflers, E. (1981) Time trends in cancer mortality in some countries - their possible causes and significance. In: Bostrom, H. & Ljungstedt, N., eds., *Medical Aspects of Mortality Statistics*, Almqvist & Wiksell, Stockholm, pp. 269-309

199. Muir, C.S. & Malhotra, A. (1987) Changing patterns of cancer incidence in five continents. *Gann. Monogr. Cancer Res.*, **33**, 3-23

200. Muir, C.S. & Nectoux, J. (1982) Time trends in malignant melanoma of the skin. In: Magnus, K., ed., *Trends in Cancer Incidence: Causes and Practical Implications*, Hemisphere, Washington, pp. 365-385

201. Muir, C.S. & Waterhouse, J.A.H. (1982) Comparability of data and reliability of registration. In: Waterhouse, J.A.H., Muir, C.S., Shanmugaratnam, K. & Powell, J., eds., *Cancer Incidence in Five Continents, Volume IV*, (IARC Scientific Publications No. 42), IARC, Lyon, pp. 55-165

202. Muir, C.S., Waterhouse, J.A.H., Mack, T., Powell, J. & Whelan, S., eds. (1987) *Cancer Incidence in Five Continents, Volume V*, (IARC Scientific Publications No. 88), IARC, Lyon

203. Muñoz, N., Bosch, F.X. & de Sanjosé, S. (1993) Risk factors for CIN III in Spain and Colombia. *Cancer Epid. Biomarkers Prev.*, (in press)

204. Muñoz, N. & Day, N.E. (1993) Oesophagus. In: Schottenfeld, D. & Fraumeni, J.F., eds., 2nd edition, Oxford University Press, Oxford (in press)

205. Murphy, M., Campbell, M.J. & Goldblatt, P. (1988) Twenty years screening for cancer of the uterine cervix in Great Britain, 1964-84: further evidence for its ineffectiveness. *J. Epidemiol. Community Health*, **42**, 49-53

206. Murphy, M. & Milne, R. (1991) Trends in cervical cancer mortality. *Lancet*, **338**, 1081-1082

207. Murphy, M. & Osmond, C. (1992) Predicting mortality from cancer of the uterine cervix from 1991-2001. *J. Epidemiol. Community Health*, **46**, 271-273

208. Nandakumar, A., Thimmasetty, K.T., Sreeramareddy, N.M., Venugopal, T.C., Rajanna, Vinutha, A.T., Srinivas, & Bhargava, M.K. (1990) A population-based case-control investigation on cancers of the oral cavity in Bangalore, India. *Br. J. Cancer*, **62**, 847-851

209. Neumann, G. (1988) Malignant neoplasms of the lip, mouth, pharynx, nose, ear and larynx. A descriptive-epidemiologic study. *HNO*, **36**, 345-354

210. Newell, G.R., Mills, P.K. & Johnson, D.E. (1984) Epidemiologic comparison of cancer of the testis and Hodgkin's disease among young males. *Cancer*, **54**, 1117-1123

211. OPCS. (1983) *Mortality Statistics: Comparison of 8th and 9th Revisions of the International Classification of Diseases (ICD), incorporating Shortlist Bridge-coding, 1978 (sample) for England and Wales. Series DH1 no. 10*, HMSO, London

212. Osmond, C., Gardner, M.J. & Acheson, E.D. (1982) Analysis of trends in cancer mortality in England and Wales during 1951-80 separating changes associated with period of birth and period of death. *Br. Med. J.*, **284**, 1005-1008

213. Osmond, C., Gardner, M.J., Acheson, E.D. & Adelstein, A.M. (1983) *Trends in Cancer Mortality 1951-1980: Analyses by Period of Birth and Period of Death*, HMSO, London

214. Østerlind, A., Engholm, G. & Jensen, O.M. (1988) Trends in cutaneous malignant melanoma in Denmark 1943-1982 by anatomic site. *Acta Pathol. Microbiol. Immunol. Scand.*, **96**, 953-963

215. Østerlind, A., Hou-Jensen, K. & Jensen, O.M. (1988) Incidence of cutaneous malignant melanoma in Denmark 1978-1982: anatomic site distribution, histologic types and comparisons with non-melanoma skin cancer. *Br. J. Cancer*, **58**, 385-391

216. Østerlind, A. & Jensen, O.M. (1987) Increasing incidence of trunk melanoma in young Danish women. *Br. J. Cancer*, **55**, 467

217. Palmeiro, R., Senra, A., Garcia Blanco, P. & Millan, J. (1988) Changing patterns of gastric cancer mortality in Spain. *Cancer Lett.*, **42**, 99-102

218. Pannonian Tumor Epidemiology Study Group. (1989) Comparative study on cancer incidence in neighboring regions of Hungary, Austria, Yugoslavia and Czechoslovakia in 1969-1980. *Neoplasma*, **36**, 377-386

219. Parkin, D.M., Läärä, E. & Muir, C.S. (1988) Estimates of the worldwide frequency of sixteen major cancers in 1980. *Int. J. Cancer*, **41**, 184-197

220. Parkin, D.M. & Muir, C.S. (1993) Comparability and quality of data. In: Parkin, D.M., Muir, C.S., Whelan, S., Gao, Y.-T., Ferlay, J. & Powell, J., eds., *Cancer Incidence in Five Continents, Volume VI*, (IARC Scientific Publications No. 120), IARC, Lyon, pp. 45-173

221. Parkin, D.M., Muir, C.S., Whelan, S., Gao, Y.-T., Ferlay, J. & Powell, J., eds. (1993) *Cancer Incidence in Five Continents, Volume VI*, (IARC Scientific Publications No. 120), IARC, Lyon

222. Parkin, D.M., Nguyen-Dinh, X. & Day, N.E. (1985) The impact of screening on the incidence of cervical cancer in England and Wales. *Br. J. Obstet. Gynaecol.*, **92**, 150-157

223. Parkin, D.M., Stiller, C.A., Draper, G.J., Bieber, C.A., Terracini, B. & Young, J.L. (1988) *International Incidence of Childhood Cancer*, (IARC Scientific Publications No. 87), IARC, Lyon

224. Patterson, C.C. & Kee, F. (1991) Geographical variations and recent trends in cancer mortality in Northern Ireland (1979-88). *Ulster Med. J.*, **60**, 136-149

225. Pawlega, J., Staneczek, W., Rahu, M., Pleško, I., Mehnert, W.H., Dimitrova, E., Witek, J. & Somogyi, J. (1988) Trends and patterns in lung cancer incidence in four cities of Eastern Europe, 1971-1980. *Neoplasma*, **35**, 635-641

226. Pearce, N., Sheppard, R.A., Howard, J.K., Fraser, J. & Lilley, B.M. (1987) Time trends and occupational differences in cancer of the testis in New Zealand. *Cancer*, **59**, 1677-1682

227. Percy, C. & Dolman, A.B. (1978) Comparison of the coding of death certificates related to cancer in seven countries. *Publ. Hlth. Rep.*, **93**, 335-350

228. Percy, C., Garfinkel, L., Krueger, D.E & Dolman, A.B. (1974) Apparent changes in cancer mortality, 1968: a study of the effects of the introduction of the eighth revision International Classification of Diseases. *Publ. Hlth. Rep.*, **89**, 418-428

229. Percy, C.L., Miller, B.A. & Gloeckler Ries, L.A. (1990) Effect of changes in cancer classification and the accuracy of cancer death certificates on trends in cancer mortality. *Ann. N. Y. Acad. Sci.*, **609**, 87-97

230. Persky, V., Davis, F., Barrett, R., Ruby, E., Sailer, C. & Levy, P. (1990) Recent time trends in uterine cancer. *Am. J. Public Health*, **80**, 935-939

231. Persson, I., Schmidt, M., Adami, H.-O., Bergström, R., Pettersson, B. & Sparén, P. (1990) Trends in endometrial cancer incidence and mortality in Sweden, 1960-84. *Cancer Causes and Control*, **1**, 201-208

232. Peters, R.K., Chao, A., Mack, T., Thomas, D., Bernstein, L. & Henderson, B.E. (1986) Increased frequency of adenocarcinoma of the uterine cervix in young women in Los Angeles County. *J. Natl. Cancer Inst.*, **76**, 423-428

233. Peters, R.K. & Henderson, B.E. (1988) Trends in cervical cancer rates in Norway. *J. Natl. Cancer Inst.*, **80**, 288-289

234. Peto, R., Lopez, A.D., Boreham, J., Thun, M. & Heath, C. (1992) Mortality from tobacco in developed countries: indirect estimation from national vital statistics. *Lancet*, **339**, 1268-1278

235. Pettersson, B., Adami, H.-O., Wilander, E. & Coleman, M.P. (1991) Trends in thyroid cancer incidence in Sweden, 1958-1981, by histopathologic type. *Int. J. Cancer*, **48**, 28-33

236. Pillon, D., Boutron, M.-C., Arveux, P., Milan, C., Bedenne, L., Hillon, P. & Faivre, J. (1989) Evolution de l'incidence du cancer colo-rectal dans le département de la Côte-d'Or entre 1976 et 1985. *Gastroenterol. Clin. Biol.*, **13**, 860-864

237. Pleško, I., Kramárová, E., Vlasák, V. & Obšitníková, A. (1991) Development of registration and cancer incidence rates and trends in Slovakia. *Eur. J. Cancer*, **27**, 1049-1052

238. Pollán, M., López-Abente, G. & Plá-Mestre, R. (1993) Time trends in mortality for multiple myeloma in Spain, 1957-1986. *Int. J. Epidemiol.*, **22**, 45-49

239. Pontén, J., Adami, H.-O. & Sparén, P. (1991) Trends in cancer survival and mortality rates. *Med. Oncol. Tumor Pharmacother.*, **8**, 147-153

240. Popescu, N.A., Beard, C.M., Treacy, P.J., Winkelmann, R.K., O'Brien, P.C. & Kurland, L.T. (1990) Cutaneous malignant melanoma in Rochester, Minnesota: trends in incidence and survivorship, 1950 through 1985. *Mayo Clin. Proc.*, **65**, 1293-1302

241. Potosky, A.L., Kessler, L., Gridley, G., Brown, C.C. & Horm, J.W. (1990) Rise in prostatic cancer incidence associated with increased use of transurethral resection. *J. Natl. Cancer Inst.*, **82**, 1624-1628

242. Pottern, L.M., Stone, B.J., Day, N.E., Pickle, L.W. & Fraumeni, J.F. (1980) Thyroid cancer in Connecticut, 1935-1975: an analysis by cell type. *Am. J. Epidemiol.*, **112**, 764-774

243. Powell, J. & McConkey, C.C. (1990) Increasing incidence of adenocarcinoma of the gastric cardia and adjacent sites. *Br. J. Cancer*, **62**, 440-443

244. Pratt, J.A., Velez, R., Brender, J.D. & Manton, K.G. (1988) Racial differences in acute lymphocytic leukemia mortality and incidence trends. *J. Clin. Epidemiol.*, **41**, 367-371

245. Prentice, R.L. & Sheppard, L. (1990) Dietary fat and cancer: rejoinder and discussion of research strategies. *Cancer Causes and Control*, **2**, 53-58

246. Prentice, R.L. & Sheppard, L. (1990) Dietary fat and cancer: consistency of the epidemiologic data, and disease prevention that may follow from a practical reduction in fat consumption. *Cancer Causes and Control*, **1**, 81-97

247. Puffer, R.R. & Griffith, G.W. (1967) Cancer. In: *Patterns of Urban Mortality. Report of the Inter-American Investigation of Mortality*, (PAHO Scientific Publications No. 151), PAHO, Washington, pp. 88-132

248. Rabkin, C.S., Biggar, R.J. & Horm, J.W. (1991) Increasing incidence of cancers associated with the human immunodeficiency virus epidemic. *Int. J. Cancer*, **47**, 692-696

249. Ranstam, J., Janzon, L. & Olsson, H. (1990) Rising incidence of breast cancer among young women in Sweden. *Br. J. Cancer*, **61**, 120-122

250. Ratkin, G.A. (1986) Progress against cancer? *N. Engl. J. Med.*, **315**, 964

251. Raymond, L., Enderlin, F., Levi, F., Leyvraz, S., Pellaux, S., Schüler, G., Torhorst, J. & Tuyns, A. (1987) Données épidémiologiques récentes sur les cancers testiculaires controlatéraux en Suisse. *Bull. Suisse du Cancer*, **7**, 17-20

252. Roush, G.C., Schymura, M.J., Holford, T.R., White, C. & Flannery, J.T. (1985) Time period compared to birth cohort in Connecticut incidence rates for twenty-five malignant neoplasms. *J. Natl. Cancer Inst.*, **74**, 779-788

253. Rutqvist, L.E., Mattsson, B. & Signomklao, T. (1989) Cancer mortality trends in Sweden 1960-1986. *Acta Oncol.*, **28**, 771-775

254. Rybolt, A.H. & Waterbury, L. (1989) Breast cancer in older women: trends in diagnosis. *Geriatrics*, **44**, 69-77

255. Sandstadt, B. (1982) Predictions of cancer incidence based on cohort analysis. In: Magnus, K., ed., *Trends in Cancer Incidence: Causes and Practical Implications*, Hemisphere, Washington, pp. 103-110

256. Sasieni, P. (1991) Trends in cervical cancer mortality. *Lancet*, **338**, 818-819

257. Schaapveld, K. & Cleton, F.J. (1989) Cancer in the Netherlands: from scenarios to health policy. *Eur. J. Cancer Clin. Oncol.*, **25**, 767-771

258. Schifflers, E., Smans, M. & Muir, C.S. (1985) Birth cohort analysis using irregular cross-sectional data: a technical note. *Stat. Med.*, **4**, 63-75

259. Schottenfeld, D. & Fraumeni, J.F., eds. (1982) *Cancer Epidemiology and Prevention*, Saunders, Philadelphia

260. Schraub, S., Bourgeois, P. & Mercier, M. (1992) Cancer incidence registration and trends in the department of Doubs, France. *Eur. J. Cancer*, **28**, 1759-1760

261. Scotto, J., Pitcher, H. & Lee, J.A. (1991) Indications of future decreasing trends in skin-melanoma mortality among whites in the United States. *Int. J. Cancer*, **49**, 490-497

262. Severson, R.K. (1990) Have transurethral resections contributed to the increasing incidence of prostatic cancer? *J. Natl. Cancer Inst.*, **82**, 1597-1598

263. Shanmugaratnam, K., Lee, H.P. & Day, N.E. (1983) *Cancer Incidence in Singapore, 1968-1977*, (IARC Scientific Publications No. 47), IARC, Lyon

264. Shanmugaratnam, K. & Powell, J. (1982) Special study on histomorphological types of cancer. In: Waterhouse, J.A.H., Muir, C.S., Shanmugaratnam, K. & Powell, J., eds., *Cancer Incidence in Five Continents, Volume IV*, (IARC Scientific Publications No. 42), IARC, Lyon, pp. 166-206

265. Shemen, L.J., Klotz, J., Schottenfeld, D. & Strong, E.W. (1984) Increase of tongue cancer in young men. *J. Am. Med. Assoc.*, **252**, 1857

266. Shimkin, M.B. (1986) Progress against cancer? *N. Engl. J. Med.*, **315**, 965

267. Simon, M.S., Schwartz, A.G., Martino, S. & Swanson, G.M. (1992) Trends in the diagnosis of in situ breast cancer in the Detroit metropolitan area, 1973 to 1987. *Cancer*, **69**, 466-469

268. Skov, T., Sprøgel, P., Engholm, G. & Frølund, C. (1991) Cancer of the lung and urinary bladder in Denmark, 1943-87: a cohort analysis. *Cancer Causes and Control*, **2**, 365-369

269. Smans, M., Muir, C.S. & Boyle, P., eds. (1992) *Atlas of Cancer Mortality in the European Economic Community*, (IARC Scientific Publications No. 107), IARC, Lyon

270. Smith, P. (1987) Comparison between registries: age-standardised rates. In: Muir, C.S., Waterhouse, J.A.H., Mack, T., Powell, J. & Whelan, S., eds., *Cancer Incidence in Five Continents, Volume V*, (IARC Scientific Publications No. 88), IARC, Lyon, pp. 790-795

271. Soskolne, C.L. (1991) Cohort trends in mortality from oral, esophageal, and laryngeal cancer. *Epidemiology*, **2**, 236-237

272. Staehelin, J., Blumthaler, M., Ambach, W. & Torhorst, J. (1990) Skin cancer and the ozone shield. *Lancet*, **336**, 502

273. Stanley, K., Stjernswärd, J. & Koroltchouk, V. (1988) Cancers of the stomach, lung and breast: mortality trends and control strategies. *World Health Stat. Q.*, **41**, 107-114

274. Staszewski, J., Muir, C.S. & Smans, M. (1986) *Rank Orders, Sex Ratios and Other Numerical and Descriptive Data, Based on Volume IV of Cancer Incidence in Five Continents*, (IARC Internal Technical Report 86/005), IARC, Lyon

275. Stiller, C.A. & Bunch, K.J. (1990) Trends in survival for childhood cancer in Britain diagnosed 1971-85. *Br. J. Cancer*, **62**, 806-815

276. Stjernswärd, J., Stanley, K., Hansluwka, H. & Lopez, A.D. (1986) Progress against cancer? *N. Engl. J. Med.*, **315**, 965

277. Swanson, G.M., Satariano, E.R., Satariano, W.A. & Threatt, B.A. (1990) Racial differences in the early detection of breast cancer in metropolitan Detroit, 1978 to 1987. *Cancer*, **66**, 1297-1301

278. Swerdlow, A.J. (1990) International trends in cutaneous melanoma. *Ann. N. Y. Acad. Sci.*, **609**, 235-251

279. Tarone, R.E. & Chu, K.C. (1992) Implications of birth cohort patterns in interpreting trends in breast cancer rates. *J. Natl. Cancer Inst.*, **84**, 1402-1410

280. Temple, N.J. & Burkitt, D.P. (1991) The war on cancer - failure of therapy and research: discussion paper. *J. Roy. Soc. Med.*, **84**, 95-98

281. Thomas, D.B. (1993) Oral contraceptives and breast cancer. *J. Natl. Cancer Inst.*, **85**, 359-364

282. Thornhill, J.A., Conroy, R.M., Kelly, D.G., Walsh, A., Fennelly, J.J. & Fitzpatrick, J.M. (1986) Recent trends in mortality due to testicular cancer in Ireland: a comparison with England and Wales. *J. Epidemiol. Community Health*, **40**, 218-222

283. Thörn, M., Adami, H.-O., Bergström, R., Ringborg, U. & Krusemo, U.B. (1989) Trends in survival from malignant melanoma: remarkable improvement in 23 years. *J. Natl. Cancer Inst.*, **81**, 611-617

284. Thörn, M., Bergström, R., Adami, H.-O. & Ringborg, U. (1990) Trends in the incidence of malignant melanoma in Sweden, by anatomic site, 1960-1984. *Am. J. Epidemiol.*, **132**, 1066-1077

285. Thörn, M., Sparén, P., Bergström, R. & Adami, H.-O. (1992) Trends in mortality rates from malignant melanoma in Sweden 1953-1987 and forecasts up to 2007. *Br. J. Cancer*, **66**, 563-567

286. Tomatis, L., Aitio, A., Day, N.E., Heseltine, E., Kaldor, J., Miller, A.B., Parkin, D.M. & Riboli, E., eds. (1990) *Cancer: Causes, Occurrence and Control*, (IARC Scientific Publications No. 100), IARC, Lyon

287. Tominaga, S. & Kato, I. (1990) Changing patterns of cancer and diet in Japan. *Prog. Clin. Biol. Res.*, **346**, 1-10

288. Tuyns, A. & Audigier, J.C. (1976) Double wave cohort increase for oesophageal and laryngeal cancer in France in relation to reduced alcohol consumption during the Second World War. *Digestion*, **14**, 197-208

289. Tuyns, A., Estève, J., Raymond, L., Berrino, F., Benhamou, E., Blanchet, F., Boffetta, P., Crosignani, P., del Moral, A., Lehmann, W., Merletti, F., Péquignot, G., Riboli, E., Sancho-Garnier, H., Terracini, B., Zubiri, A. & Zubiri, L. (1988) Cancer of the larynx/hypopharynx, tobacco and alcohol: IARC international case-control study in Turin and Varese (Italy), Zaragoza and Navarra (Spain), Geneva (Switzerland) and Calvados (France). *Int. J. Cancer*, **41**, 483-491

290. van der Esch, E.P., Muir, C.S., Nectoux, J., Macfarlane, G.J., Maisonneuve, P., Bharucha, H., Briggs, J., Cooke, R.A., Dempster, A.G., Essex, W.B., Hofer, P.A., Hood, A.F., Ironside, P., Larsen, T.E., Little, J.H., Philipp, R., Pfau, R.S., Prade, M., Pozharisski, K.M., Rilke, F. & Schafler, K. (1991) Temporal change in diagnostic criteria as a cause of the increase of malignant melanoma over time is unlikely. *Int. J. Cancer*, **47**, 483-490

291. van der Graaf, Y., Zielhuis, G.A. & Vooijs, G.P. (1988) Cervical cancer mortality in the Netherlands. *Int. J. Epidemiol.*, **17**, 270-276

292. van Eys, J. (1986) Progress against cancer? *N. Engl. J. Med.*, **315**, 966

293. van Hoff, J., Schymura, M.J. & Curnen, M.G. (1988) Trends in the incidence of childhood and adolescent cancer in Connecticut, 1935-1979. *Med. Pediatr. Oncol.*, **16**, 78-87

294. Villard Mackintosh, L. & Murphy, M. (1990) Endometrial cancer trends in England and Wales: a possible protective effect of oral contraception. *Int. J. Epidemiol.*, **19**, 255-258

295. Villard Mackintosh, L., Murphy, M. & Vessey, M.P. (1989) Cervical cancer deaths in young women. *Lancet*, **i**, 377

296. Villard Mackintosh, L., Vessey, M.P. & Jones, L. (1989) The effects of oral contraceptives and parity on ovarian cancer trends in women under 55 years of age. *Br. J. Obstet. Gynaecol.*, **96**, 783-788

297. Vlasák, V., Pleško, I., Dimitrova, E. & Hudáková, G. (1991) Recent trends in uterine cervix cancer in Slovakia, 1968-1987. *Neoplasma*, **38**, 533-540

298. Waterhouse, J.A.H., Muir, C.S., Correa, P. & Powell, J., eds. (1976) *Cancer Incidence in Five Continents, Volume III*, (IARC Scientific Publications No. 15), IARC, Lyon

299. Waterhouse, J.A.H., Muir, C.S., Shanmugaratnam, K. & Powell, J., eds. (1982) *Cancer Incidence in Five Continents, Volume IV*, (IARC Scientific Publications No. 42), IARC, Lyon

300. Whelan, S., Parkin, D.M. & Masuyer, E., eds. (1990) *Patterns of Cancer in Five Continents*, (IARC Scientific Publications No. 102), IARC, Lyon

301. White, E. (1987) Projected changes in breast cancer incidence due to the trend toward delayed childbearing. *Am. J. Public Health*, **77**, 495-497

302. White, E., Lee, C.Y. & Kristal, A.R. (1990) Evaluation of the increase in breast cancer incidence in relation to mammography use. *J. Natl. Cancer Inst.*, **82**, 1546-1552

303. Willett, W.C., Stampfer, M.J., Colditz, G.A., Rosner, B.A. & Speizer, F.E. (1990) Relation of meat, fat, and fiber intake to the risk of colon cancer in a prospective study among women. *N. Engl. J. Med.*, **323**, 1664-1672

304. Williams, F.L. & Lloyd, O. (1991) Trends in lung cancer mortality in Scotland and their relation to cigarette smoking and social class. *Scott. Med. J.*, **36**, 175-178

305. Wise, R.P. (1986) Progress against cancer? *N. Engl. J. Med.*, **315**, 967-968

306. World Health Organisation. (1986) Female lung cancer increases in the developed countries/Le cancer du poumon chez les femmes en augmentation dans les pays développés. *Wkly. Epidemiol. Rec.*, **39**, 297-299

307. Yatani, R., Shiraishi, T., Nakakuki, K., Kusano, I., Takanari, H., Hayashi, T. & Stemmermann, G.N. (1988) Trends in frequency of latent prostate carcinoma in Japan from 1965-1979 to 1982-1986. *J. Natl. Cancer Inst.*, **80**, 683-687

308. Yeole, B.B., Jayant, K. & Jussawalla, D.J. (1989) Declining trend in cervical cancer incidence in Bombay, India (1964-1985). *J. Surg. Oncol.*, **42**, 267-271

309. Yeole, B.B., Jayant, K. & Jussawalla, D.J. (1990) Trends in breast cancer incidence in greater Bombay: an epidemiological assessment. *Bull. World Health Organ.*, **68**, 245-249

310. Zaridze, D.G. & Basieva, T.H. (1990) Incidence of cancer of the lung, stomach, breast, and cervix in the USSR: pattern and trends. *Cancer Causes and Control*, **1**, 39-49

PUBLICATIONS OF THE
INTERNATIONAL AGENCY FOR RESEARCH ON CANCER
Scientific Publications Series

(Available from Oxford University Press through local bookshops)

No. 1 **Liver Cancer**
1971; 176 pages (*out of print*)

No. 2 **Oncogenesis and Herpesviruses**
Edited by P.M. Biggs, G. de-Thé and L.N. Payne
1972; 515 pages (*out of print*)

No. 3 *N*-**Nitroso Compounds: Analysis and Formation**
Edited by P. Bogovski, R. Preussman and E.A. Walker
1972; 140 pages (*out of print*)

No. 4 **Transplacental Carcinogenesis**
Edited by L. Tomatis and U. Mohr
1973; 181 pages (*out of print*)

No. 5/6 **Pathology of Tumours in Laboratory Animals, Volume 1, Tumours of the Rat**
Edited by V.S. Turusov
1973/1976; 533 pages (*out of print*)

No. 7 **Host Environment Interactions in the Etiology of Cancer in Man**
Edited by R. Doll and I. Vodopija
1973; 464 pages (*out of print*)

No. 8 **Biological Effects of Asbestos**
Edited by P. Bogovski, J.C. Gilson, V. Timbrell and J.C. Wagner
1973; 346 pages (*out of print*)

No. 9 *N*-**Nitroso Compounds in the Environment**
Edited by P. Bogovski and E.A. Walker
1974; 243 pages (*out of print*)

No. 10 **Chemical Carcinogenesis Essays**
Edited by R. Montesano and L. Tomatis
1974; 230 pages (*out of print*)

No. 11 **Oncogenesis and Herpesviruses II**
Edited by G. de-Thé, M.A. Epstein and H. zur Hausen
1975; Part I: 511 pages
Part II: 403 pages (*out of print*)

No. 12 **Screening Tests in Chemical Carcinogenesis**
Edited by R. Montesano, H. Bartsch and L. Tomatis
1976; 666 pages (*out of print*)

No. 13 **Environmental Pollution and Carcinogenic Risks**
Edited by C. Rosenfeld and W. Davis
1975; 441 pages (*out of print*)

No. 14 **Environmental *N*-Nitroso Compounds. Analysis and Formation**
Edited by E.A. Walker, P. Bogovski and L. Griciute
1976; 512 pages (*out of print*)

No. 15 **Cancer Incidence in Five Continents, Volume III**
Edited by J.A.H. Waterhouse, C. Muir, P. Correa and J. Powell
1976; 584 pages (*out of print*)

No. 16 **Air Pollution and Cancer in Man**
Edited by U. Mohr, D. Schmähl and L. Tomatis
1977; 328 pages (*out of print*)

No. 17 **Directory of On-going Research in Cancer Epidemiology 1977**
Edited by C.S. Muir and G. Wagner
1977; 599 pages (*out of print*)

No. 18 **Environmental Carcinogens. Selected Methods of Analysis. Volume 1: Analysis of Volatile Nitrosamines in Food**
Editor-in-Chief: H. Egan
1978; 212 pages (*out of print*)

No. 19 **Environmental Aspects of *N*-Nitroso Compounds**
Edited by E.A. Walker, M. Castegnaro, L. Griciute and R.E. Lyle
1978; 561 pages (*out of print*)

No. 20 **Nasopharyngeal Carcinoma: Etiology and Control**
Edited by G. de-Thé and Y. Ito
1978; 606 pages (*out of print*)

No. 21 **Cancer Registration and its Techniques**
Edited by R. MacLennan, C. Muir, R. Steinitz and A. Winkler
1978; 235 pages (*out of print*)

No. 22 **Environmental Carcinogens. Selected Methods of Analysis. Volume 2: Methods for the Measurement of Vinyl Chloride in Poly(vinyl chloride), Air, Water and Foodstuffs**
Editor-in-Chief: H. Egan
1978; 142 pages (*out of print*)

No. 23 **Pathology of Tumours in Laboratory Animals. Volume II: Tumours of the Mouse**
Editor-in-Chief: V.S. Turusov
1979; 669 pages (*out of print*)

No. 24 **Oncogenesis and Herpesviruses III**
Edited by G. de-Thé, W. Henle and F. Rapp
1978; Part I: 580 pages, Part II: 512 pages (*out of print*)

Prices, valid for March 1993, are subject to change without notice

No. 25 Carcinogenic Risk. Strategies for Intervention
Edited by W. Davis and
C. Rosenfeld
1979; 280 pages (*out of print*)

No. 26 Directory of On-going Research in Cancer Epidemiology 1978
Edited by C.S. Muir and G. Wagner
1978; 550 pages (*out of print*)

No. 27 Molecular and Cellular Aspects of Carcinogen Screening Tests
Edited by R. Montesano,
H. Bartsch and L. Tomatis
1980; 372 pages £30.00

No. 28 Directory of On-going Research in Cancer Epidemiology 1979
Edited by C.S. Muir and G. Wagner
1979; 672 pages (*out of print*)

No. 29 Environmental Carcinogens. Selected Methods of Analysis. Volume 3: Analysis of Polycyclic Aromatic Hydrocarbons in Environmental Samples
Editor-in-Chief: H. Egan
1979; 240 pages (*out of print*)

No. 30 Biological Effects of Mineral Fibres
Editor-in-Chief: J.C. Wagner
1980; **Volume 1:** 494 pages **Volume 2:** 513 pages (*out of print*)

No. 31 *N*-Nitroso Compounds: Analysis, Formation and Occurrence
Edited by E.A. Walker, L. Griciute,
M. Castegnaro and M. Börzsönyi
1980; 835 pages (*out of print*)

No. 32 Statistical Methods in Cancer Research. Volume 1. The Analysis of Case-control Studies
By N.E. Breslow and N.E. Day
1980; 338 pages £18.00

No. 33 Handling Chemical Carcinogens in the Laboratory
Edited by R. Montesano *et al.*
1979; 32 pages (*out of print*)

No. 34 Pathology of Tumours in Laboratory Animals. Volume III. Tumours of the Hamster
Editor-in-Chief: V.S. Turusov
1982; 461 pages (*out of print*)

No. 35 Directory of On-going Research in Cancer Epidemiology 1980
Edited by C.S. Muir and G. Wagner
1980; 660 pages (*out of print*)

No. 36 Cancer Mortality by Occupation and Social Class 1851-1971
Edited by W.P.D. Logan
1982; 253 pages (*out of print*)

No. 37 Laboratory Decontamination and Destruction of Aflatoxins B_1, B_2, G_1, G_2 in Laboratory Wastes
Edited by M. Castegnaro *et al.*
1980; 56 pages (*out of print*)

No. 38 Directory of On-going Research in Cancer Epidemiology 1981
Edited by C.S. Muir and G. Wagner
1981; 696 pages (*out of print*)

No. 39 Host Factors in Human Carcinogenesis
Edited by H. Bartsch and
B. Armstrong
1982; 583 pages (*out of print*)

No. 40 Environmental Carcinogens. Selected Methods of Analysis. Volume 4: Some Aromatic Amines and Azo Dyes in the General and Industrial Environment
Edited by L. Fishbein,
M. Castegnaro, I.K. O'Neill and
H. Bartsch
1981; 347 pages (*out of print*)

No. 41 *N*-Nitroso Compounds: Occurrence and Biological Effects
Edited by H. Bartsch, I.K. O'Neill,
M. Castegnaro and M. Okada
1982; 755 pages £50.00

No. 42 Cancer Incidence in Five Continents, Volume IV
Edited by J. Waterhouse, C. Muir,
K. Shanmugaratnam and J. Powell
1982; 811 pages (*out of print*)

No. 43 Laboratory Decontamination and Destruction of Carcinogens in Laboratory Wastes: Some *N*-Nitrosamines
Edited by M. Castegnaro *et al.*
1982; 73 pages £7.50

No. 44 Environmental Carcinogens. Selected Methods of Analysis. Volume 5: Some Mycotoxins
Edited by L. Stoloff, M. Castegnaro,
P. Scott, I.K. O'Neill and H. Bartsch
1983; 455 pages £32.50

No. 45 Environmental Carcinogens. Selected Methods of Analysis. Volume 6: *N*-Nitroso Compounds
Edited by R. Preussmann, I.K.
O'Neill, G. Eisenbrand, B.
Spiegelhalder and H. Bartsch
1983; 508 pages £32.50

No. 46 Directory of On-going Research in Cancer Epidemiology 1982
Edited by C.S. Muir and G. Wagner
1982; 722 pages (*out of print*)

No. 47 Cancer Incidence in Singapore 1968-1977
Edited by K. Shanmugaratnam,
H.P. Lee and N.E. Day
1983; 171 pages (*out of print*)

No. 48 Cancer Incidence in the USSR (2nd Revised Edition)
Edited by N.P. Napalkov,
G.F. Tserkovny, V.M. Merabishvili,
D.M. Parkin, M. Smans and
C.S. Muir
1983; 75 pages (*out of print*)

No. 49 Laboratory Decontamination and Destruction of Carcinogens in Laboratory Wastes: Some Polycyclic Aromatic Hydrocarbons
Edited by M. Castegnaro *et al.*
1983; 87 pages (*out of print*)

No. 50 Directory of On-going Research in Cancer Epidemiology 1983
Edited by C.S. Muir and G. Wagner
1983; 731 pages (*out of print*)

No. 51 Modulators of Experimental Carcinogenesis
Edited by V. Turusov and R.
Montesano
1983; 307 pages (*out of print*)

No. 52 **Second Cancers in Relation to Radiation Treatment for Cervical Cancer: Results of a Cancer Registry Collaboration**
Edited by N.E. Day and J.C. Boice, Jr
1984; 207 pages (*out of print*)

No. 53 **Nickel in the Human Environment**
Editor-in-Chief: F.W. Sunderman, Jr
1984; 529 pages (*out of print*)

No. 54 **Laboratory Decontamination and Destruction of Carcinogens in Laboratory Wastes: Some Hydrazines**
Edited by M. Castegnaro *et al.*
1983; 87 pages (*out of print*)

No. 55 **Laboratory Decontamination and Destruction of Carcinogens in Laboratory Wastes: Some N-Nitrosamides**
Edited by M. Castegnaro *et al.*
1984; 66 pages (*out of print*)

No. 56 **Models, Mechanisms and Etiology of Tumour Promotion**
Edited by M. Börzsönyi, N.E. Day, K. Lapis and H. Yamasaki
1984; 532 pages (*out of print*)

No. 57 **N-Nitroso Compounds: Occurrence, Biological Effects and Relevance to Human Cancer**
Edited by I.K. O'Neill, R.C. von Borstel, C.T. Miller, J. Long and H. Bartsch
1984; 1013 pages (*out of print*)

No. 58 **Age-related Factors in Carcinogenesis**
Edited by A. Likhachev, V. Anisimov and R. Montesano
1985; 288 pages (*out of print*)

No. 59 **Monitoring Human Exposure to Carcinogenic and Mutagenic Agents**
Edited by A. Berlin, M. Draper, K. Hemminki and H. Vainio
1984; 457 pages (*out of print*)

No. 60 **Burkitt's Lymphoma: A Human Cancer Model**
Edited by G. Lenoir, G. O'Conor and C.L.M. Olweny
1985; 484 pages (*out of print*)

No. 61 **Laboratory Decontamination and Destruction of Carcinogens in Laboratory Wastes: Some Haloethers**
Edited by M. Castegnaro *et al.*
1985; 55 pages (*out of print*)

No. 62 **Directory of On-going Research in Cancer Epidemiology 1984**
Edited by C.S. Muir and G. Wagner
1984; 717 pages (*out of print*)

No. 63 **Virus-associated Cancers in Africa**
Edited by A.O. Williams, G.T. O'Conor, G.B. de-Thé and C.A. Johnson
1984; 773 pages (*out of print*)

No. 64 **Laboratory Decontamination and Destruction of Carcinogens in Laboratory Wastes: Some Aromatic Amines and 4-Nitrobiphenyl**
Edited by M. Castegnaro *et al.*
1985; 84 pages (*out of print*)

No. 65 **Interpretation of Negative Epidemiological Evidence for Carcinogenicity**
Edited by N.J. Wald and R. Doll
1985; 232 pages (*out of print*)

No. 66 **The Role of the Registry in Cancer Control**
Edited by D.M. Parkin, G. Wagner and C.S. Muir
1985; 152 pages £10.00

No. 67 **Transformation Assay of Established Cell Lines: Mechanisms and Application**
Edited by T. Kakunaga and H. Yamasaki
1985; 225 pages (*out of print*)

No. 68 **Environmental Carcinogens. Selected Methods of Analysis. Volume 7. Some Volatile Halogenated Hydrocarbons**
Edited by L. Fishbein and I.K. O'Neill
1985; 479 pages (*out of print*)

No. 69 **Directory of On-going Research in Cancer Epidemiology 1985**
Edited by C.S. Muir and G. Wagner
1985; 745 pages (*out of print*)

No. 70 **The Role of Cyclic Nucleic Acid Adducts in Carcinogenesis and Mutagenesis**
Edited by B. Singer and H. Bartsch
1986; 467 pages (*out of print*)

No. 71 **Environmental Carcinogens. Selected Methods of Analysis. Volume 8: Some Metals: As, Be, Cd, Cr, Ni, Pb, Se, Zn**
Edited by I.K. O'Neill, P. Schuller and L. Fishbein
1986; 485 pages (*out of print*)

No. 72 **Atlas of Cancer in Scotland, 1975–1980. Incidence and Epidemiological Perspective**
Edited by I. Kemp, P. Boyle, M. Smans and C.S. Muir
1985; 285 pages (*out of print*)

No. 73 **Laboratory Decontamination and Destruction of Carcinogens in Laboratory Wastes: Some Antineoplastic Agents**
Edited by M. Castegnaro *et al.*
1985; 163 pages £12.50

No. 74 **Tobacco: A Major International Health Hazard**
Edited by D. Zaridze and R. Peto
1986; 324 pages £22.50

No. 75 **Cancer Occurrence in Developing Countries**
Edited by D.M. Parkin
1986; 339 pages £22.50

No. 76 **Screening for Cancer of the Uterine Cervix**
Edited by M. Hakama, A.B. Miller and N.E. Day
1986; 315 pages £30.00

No. 77 **Hexachlorobenzene: Proceedings of an International Symposium**
Edited by C.R. Morris and J.R.P. Cabral
1986; 668 pages (*out of print*)

No. 78 **Carcinogenicity of Alkylating Cytostatic Drugs**
Edited by D. Schmähl and J.M. Kaldor
1986; 337 pages (*out of print*)

No. 79 **Statistical Methods in Cancer Research. Volume III: The Design and Analysis of Long-term Animal Experiments**
By J.J. Gart, D. Krewski, P.N. Lee, R.E. Tarone and J. Wahrendorf
1986; 213 pages £22.00

No. 80 **Directory of On-going Research in Cancer Epidemiology 1986**
Edited by C.S. Muir and G. Wagner
1986; 805 pages (*out of print*)

No. 81 **Environmental Carcinogens: Methods of Analysis and Exposure Measurement. Volume 9: Passive Smoking**
Edited by I.K. O'Neill, K.D. Brunnemann, B. Dodet and D. Hoffmann
1987; 383 pages £35.00

No. 82 **Statistical Methods in Cancer Research. Volume II: The Design and Analysis of Cohort Studies**
By N.E. Breslow and N.E. Day
1987; 404 pages £35.00

No. 83 **Long-term and Short-term Assays for Carcinogens: A Critical Appraisal**
Edited by R. Montesano, H. Bartsch, H. Vainio, J. Wilbourn and H. Yamasaki
1986; 575 pages £35.00

No. 84 **The Relevance of *N*-Nitroso Compounds to Human Cancer: Exposure and Mechanisms**
Edited by H. Bartsch, I.K. O'Neill and R. Schulte-Hermann
1987; 671 pages (*out of print*)

No. 85 **Environmental Carcinogens: Methods of Analysis and Exposure Measurement. Volume 10: Benzene and Alkylated Benzenes**
Edited by L. Fishbein and I.K. O'Neill
1988; 327 pages £40.00

No. 86 **Directory of On-going Research in Cancer Epidemiology 1987**
Edited by D.M. Parkin and J. Wahrendorf
1987; 676 pages (*out of print*)

No. 87 **International Incidence of Childhood Cancer**
Edited by D.M. Parkin, C.A. Stiller, C.A. Bieber, G.J. Draper, B. Terracini and J.L. Young
1988; 401 pages £35.00

No. 88 **Cancer Incidence in Five Continents Volume V**
Edited by C. Muir, J. Waterhouse, T. Mack, J. Powell and S. Whelan
1987; 1004 pages £55.00

No. 89 **Method for Detecting DNA Damaging Agents in Humans: Applications in Cancer Epidemiology and Prevention**
Edited by H. Bartsch, K. Hemminki and I.K. O'Neill
1988; 518 pages £50.00

No. 90 **Non-occupational Exposure to Mineral Fibres**
Edited by J. Bignon, J. Peto and R. Saracci
1989; 500 pages £50.00

No. 91 **Trends in Cancer Incidence in Singapore 1968–1982**
Edited by H.P. Lee , N.E. Day and K. Shanmugaratnam
1988; 160 pages (*out of print*)

No. 92 **Cell Differentiation, Genes and Cancer**
Edited by T. Kakunaga, T. Sugimura, L. Tomatis and H. Yamasaki
1988; 204 pages £27.50

No. 93 **Directory of On-going Research in Cancer Epidemiology 1988**
Edited by M. Coleman and J. Wahrendorf
1988; 662 pages (*out of print*)

No. 94 **Human Papillomavirus and Cervical Cancer**
Edited by N. Muñoz, F.X. Bosch and O.M. Jensen
1989; 154 pages £22.50

No. 95 **Cancer Registration: Principles and Methods**
Edited by O.M. Jensen, D.M. Parkin, R. MacLennan, C.S. Muir and R. Skeet
1991; 288 pages £28.00

No. 96 **Perinatal and Multigeneration Carcinogenesis**
Edited by N.P. Napalkov, J.M. Rice, L. Tomatis and H. Yamasaki
1989; 436 pages £50.00

No. 97 **Occupational Exposure to Silica and Cancer Risk**
Edited by L. Simonato, A.C. Fletcher, R. Saracci and T. Thomas
1990; 124 pages £22.50

No. 98 **Cancer Incidence in Jewish Migrants to Israel, 1961–1981**
Edited by R. Steinitz, D.M. Parkin, J.L. Young, C.A. Bieber and L. Katz
1989; 320 pages £35.00

No. 99 **Pathology of Tumours in Laboratory Animals, Second Edition, Volume 1, Tumours of the Rat**
Edited by V.S. Turusov and U. Mohr
740 pages £85.00

No. 100 **Cancer: Causes, Occurrence and Control**
Editor-in-Chief L. Tomatis
1990; 352 pages £24.00

No. 101 **Directory of On-going Research in Cancer Epidemiology 1989/90**
Edited by M. Coleman and J. Wahrendorf
1989; 818 pages £36.00

No. 102 **Patterns of Cancer in Five Continents**
Edited by S.L. Whelan, D.M. Parkin & E. Masuyer
1990; 162 pages £25.00

No. 103 **Evaluating Effectiveness of Primary Prevention of Cancer**
Edited by M. Hakama, V. Beral, J.W. Cullen and D.M. Parkin
1990; 250 pages £32.00

No. 104 **Complex Mixtures and Cancer Risk**
Edited by H. Vainio, M. Sorsa and A.J. McMichael
1990; 442 pages £38.00

No. 105 **Relevance to Human Cancer of *N*-Nitroso Compounds, Tobacco Smoke and Mycotoxins**
Edited by I.K. O'Neill, J. Chen and H. Bartsch
1991; 614 pages £70.00

No. 106 **Atlas of Cancer Incidence in the Former German Democratic Republic**
Edited by W.H. Mehnert, M. Smans, C.S. Muir, M. Möhner & D. Schön
1992; 384 pages £55.00

No. 107 **Atlas of Cancer Mortality in the European Economic Community**
Edited by M. Smans, C.S. Muir and P. Boyle
1992; 280 pages £35.00

No. 108 **Environmental Carcinogens: Methods of Analysis and Exposure Measurement. Volume 11: Polychlorinated Dioxins and Dibenzofurans**
Edited by C. Rappe, H.R. Buser, B. Dodet and I.K. O'Neill
1991; 426 pages £45.00

No. 109 **Environmental Carcinogens: Methods of Analysis and Exposure Measurement. Volume 12: Indoor Air Contaminants**
Edited by B. Seifert, H. van de Wiel, B. Dodet and I.K. O'Neill
1993; 384 pages £45.00

No. 110 **Directory of On-going Research in Cancer Epidemiology 1991**
Edited by M. Coleman and J. Wahrendorf
1991; 753 pages £38.00

No. 111 **Pathology of Tumours in Laboratory Animals, Second Edition, Volume 2, Tumours of the Mouse**
Edited by V.S. Turusov and U. Mohr
Publ. due 1993; approx. 700 pages

No. 112 **Autopsy in Epidemiology and Medical Research**
Edited by E. Riboli and M. Delendi
1991; 288 pages £25.00

No. 113 **Laboratory Decontamination and Destruction of Carcinogens in Laboratory Wastes: Some Mycotoxins**
Edited by M. Castegnaro, J. Barek, J.-M. Frémy, M. Lafontaine, M. Miraglia, E.B. Sansone and G.M. Telling
1991; 64 pages £11.00

No. 114 **Laboratory Decontamination and Destruction of Carcinogens in Laboratory Wastes: Some Polycyclic Heterocyclic Hydrocarbons**
Edited by M. Castegnaro, J. Barek J. Jacob, U. Kirso, M. Lafontaine, E.B. Sansone, G.M. Telling and T. Vu Duc
1991; 50 pages £8.00

No. 115 **Mycotoxins, Endemic Nephropathy and Urinary Tract Tumours**
Edited by M. Castegnaro, R. Plestina, G. Dirheimer, I.N. Chernozemsky and H Bartsch
1991; 340 pages £45.00

No. 116 **Mechanisms of Carcinogenesis in Risk Identification**
Edited by H. Vainio, P.N. Magee, D.B. McGregor & A.J. McMichael
1992; 616 pages £65.00

No. 117 **Directory of On-going Research in Cancer Epidemiology 1992**
Edited by M. Coleman, J. Wahrendorf & E. Démaret
1992; 773 pages £42.00

No. 118 **Cadmium in the Human Environment: Toxicity and Carcinogenicity**
Edited by G.F. Nordberg, R.F.M. Herber & L. Alessio
1992; 470 pages £60.00

No. 119 **The Epidemiology of Cervical Cancer and Human Papillomavirus**
Edited by N. Muñoz, F.X. Bosch, K.V. Shah & A. Meheus
1992; 288 pages £28.00

No. 120 **Cancer Incidence in Five Continents, Volume VI**
Edited by D.M. Parkin, C.S. Muir, S.L. Whelan, Y.T. Gao, J. Ferlay & J.Powell
1992; 1080 pages £120.00

No. 121 **Trends in Cancer Incidence and Mortality**
Edited by M. Coleman, J. Estève and P. Damiecki
1993; 806 pages, £120.00

No. 122 **International Classification of Rodent Tumours. Part 1. The Rat**
Editor-in-Chief: U. Möhr
1992/93; 10 fascicles of 60–100 pages, £120.00

No. 123 **Cancer in Italian Migrant Populations**
Edited by M. Geddes, D.M. Parkin, M. Khlat, D. Balzi and E. Buiatti
1993; 292 pages, £40.00

No. 124 **Postlabelling Methods for Detection of DNA Adducts**
Edited by D.H. Phillips, M. Castegnaro and H. Bartsch
1993; 392 pages; £46.00

IARC MONOGRAPHS ON THE EVALUATION OF CARCINOGENIC RISKS TO HUMANS

(Available from booksellers through the network of WHO Sales Agents)

Volume 1 **Some Inorganic Substances, Chlorinated Hydrocarbons, Aromatic Amines, N-Nitroso Compounds, and Natural Products**
1972; 184 pages (*out of print*)

Volume 2 **Some Inorganic and Organometallic Compounds**
1973; 181 pages (*out of print*)

Volume 3 **Certain Polycyclic Aromatic Hydrocarbons and Heterocyclic Compounds**
1973; 271 pages (*out of print*)

Volume 4 **Some Aromatic Amines, Hydrazine and Related Substances, N-Nitroso Compounds and Miscellaneous Alkylating Agents**
1974; 286 pages Sw. fr. 18.-

Volume 5 **Some Organochlorine Pesticides**
1974; 241 pages (*out of print*)

Volume 6 **Sex Hormones**
1974; 243 pages (*out of print*)

Volume 7 **Some Anti-Thyroid and Related Substances, Nitrofurans and Industrial Chemicals**
1974; 326 pages (*out of print*)

Volume 8 **Some Aromatic Azo Compounds**
1975; 357 pages Sw. fr. 36.-

Volume 9 **Some Aziridines, N-, S- and O-Mustards and Selenium**
1975; 268 pages Sw.fr. 27.-

Volume 10 **Some Naturally Occurring Substances**
1976; 353 pages (*out of print*)

Volume 11 **Cadmium, Nickel, Some Epoxides, Miscellaneous Industrial Chemicals and General Considerations on Volatile Anaesthetics**
1976; 306 pages (*out of print*)

Volume 12 **Some Carbamates, Thiocarbamates and Carbazides**
1976; 282 pages Sw. fr. 34.-

Volume 13 **Some Miscellaneous Pharmaceutical Substances**
1977; 255 pages Sw. fr. 30.-

Volume 14 **Asbestos**
1977; 106 pages (*out of print*)

Volume 15 **Some Fumigants, The Herbicides 2,4-D and 2,4,5-T, Chlorinated Dibenzodioxins and Miscellaneous Industrial Chemicals**
1977; 354 pages Sw. fr. 50.-

Volume 16 **Some Aromatic Amines and Related Nitro Compounds - Hair Dyes, Colouring Agents and Miscellaneous Industrial Chemicals**
1978; 400 pages Sw. fr. 50.-

Volume 17 **Some N-Nitroso Compounds**
1978; 365 pages Sw. fr. 50.-

Volume 18 **Polychlorinated Biphenyls and Polybrominated Biphenyls**
1978; 140 pages Sw. fr. 20.-

Volume 19 **Some Monomers, Plastics and Synthetic Elastomers, and Acrolein**
1979; 513 pages (*out of print*)

Volume 20 **Some Halogenated Hydrocarbons**
1979; 609 pages (*out of print*)

Volume 21 **Sex Hormones (II)**
1979; 583 pages Sw. fr. 60.-

Volume 22 **Some Non-Nutritive Sweetening Agents**
1980; 208 pages Sw. fr. 25.-

Volume 23 **Some Metals and Metallic Compounds**
1980; 438 pages (*out of print*)

Volume 24 **Some Pharmaceutical Drugs**
1980; 337 pages Sw. fr. 40.-

Volume 25 **Wood, Leather and Some Associated Industries**
1981; 412 pages Sw. fr. 60.-

Volume 26 **Some Antineoplastic and Immunosuppressive Agents**
1981; 411 pages Sw. fr. 62.-

Volume 27 **Some Aromatic Amines, Anthraquinones and Nitroso Compounds, and Inorganic Fluorides Used in Drinking Water and Dental Preparations**
1982; 341 pages Sw. fr. 40.-

Volume 28 **The Rubber Industry**
1982; 486 pages Sw. fr. 70.-

Volume 29 **Some Industrial Chemicals and Dyestuffs**
1982; 416 pages Sw. fr. 60.-

Volume 30 **Miscellaneous Pesticides**
1983; 424 pages Sw. fr. 60.-

Volume 31 **Some Food Additives, Feed Additives and Naturally Occurring Substances**
1983; 314 pages Sw. fr. 60.-

Volume 32 **Polynuclear Aromatic Compounds, Part 1: Chemical, Environmental and Experimental Data**
1983; 477 pages Sw. fr. 60.-

Volume 33 **Polynuclear Aromatic Compounds, Part 2: Carbon Blacks, Mineral Oils and Some Nitroarenes**
1984; 245 pages Sw. fr. 50.-

Volume 34 **Polynuclear Aromatic Compounds, Part 3: Industrial Exposures in Aluminium Production, Coal Gasification, Coke Production, and Iron and Steel Founding**
1984; 219 pages Sw. fr. 48.-

Volume 35 **Polynuclear Aromatic Compounds, Part 4: Bitumens, Coal-tars and Derived Products, Shale-oils and Soots**
1985; 271 pages Sw. fr. 70.-

Volume 36 **Allyl Compounds, Aldehydes, Epoxides and Peroxides**
1985; 369 pages Sw. fr. 70.–

Volume 37 **Tobacco Habits Other than Smoking: Betel-quid and Areca-nut Chewing; and some Related Nitrosamines**
1985; 291 pages Sw. fr. 70.–

Volume 38 **Tobacco Smoking**
1986; 421 pages Sw. fr. 75.–

Volume 39 **Some Chemicals Used in Plastics and Elastomers**
1986; 403 pages Sw. fr. 60.–

Volume 40 **Some Naturally Occurring and Synthetic Food Components, Furocoumarins and Ultraviolet Radiation**
1986; 444 pages Sw. fr. 65.–

Volume 41 **Some Halogenated Hydrocarbons and Pesticide Exposures**
1986; 434 pages Sw. fr. 65.–

Volume 42 **Silica and Some Silicates**
1987; 289 pages Sw. fr. 65.

Volume 43 **Man-Made Mineral Fibres and Radon**
1988; 300 pages Sw. fr. 65.–

Volume 44 **Alcohol Drinking**
1988; 416 pages Sw. fr. 65.

Volume 45 **Occupational Exposures in Petroleum Refining; Crude Oil and Major Petroleum Fuels**
1989; 322 pages Sw. fr. 65.–

Volume 46 **Diesel and Gasoline Engine Exhausts and Some Nitroarenes**
1989; 458 pages Sw. fr. 65.–

Volume 47 **Some Organic Solvents, Resin Monomers and Related Compounds, Pigments and Occupational Exposures in Paint Manufacture and Painting**
1989; 536 pages Sw. fr. 85.–

Volume 48 **Some Flame Retardants and Textile Chemicals, and Exposures in the Textile Manufacturing Industry**
1990; 345 pages Sw. fr. 65.–

Volume 49 **Chromium, Nickel and Welding**
1990; 677 pages Sw. fr. 95.–

Volume 50 **Pharmaceutical Drugs**
1990; 415 pages Sw. fr. 65.–

Volume 51 **Coffee, Tea, Mate, Methylxanthines and Methylglyoxal**
1991; 513 pages Sw. fr. 80.–

Volume 52 **Chlorinated Drinking-water; Chlorination By-products; Some Other Halogenated Compounds; Cobalt and Cobalt Compounds**
1991; 544 pages Sw. fr. 80.–

Volume 53 **Occupational Exposures in Insecticide Application and some Pesticides**
1991; 612 pages Sw. fr. 95.–

Volume 54 **Occupational Exposures to Mists and Vapours from Strong Inorganic Acids; and Other Industrial Chemicals**
1992; 336 pages Sw. fr. 65.–

Volume 55 **Solar and Ultraviolet Radiation**
1992; 316 pages Sw. fr. 65.–

Volume 56 Some Naturally Occurring Substances: Food Items and Constituents, Heterocyclic Aromatic Amines and Mycotoxins
1993; 600 pages Sw. fr. 95.–

Volume 56 Some Naturally Occurring Substances: Food Items and Constituents, Heterocyclic Aromatic Amines and Mycotoxins
1993; 600 pages Sw. fr. 95.–

Volume 57 **Occupational Exposures of Hairdressers and Barbers and Personal Use of Hair Colourants; Some Hair Dyes, Cosmetic Colourants, Industrial Dyestuffs and Aromatic Amines**
1993; 428 pages Sw. fr. 75.–

Supplement No. 1
Chemicals and Industrial Processes Associated with Cancer in Humans (IARC Monographs, Volumes 1 to 20)
1979; 71 pages (*out of print*)

Supplement No. 2
Long-term and Short-term Screening Assays for Carcinogens: A Critical Appraisal
1980; 426 pages Sw. fr. 40.–

Supplement No. 3
Cross Index of Synonyms and Trade Names in Volumes 1 to 26
1982; 199 pages (*out of print*)

Supplement No. 4
Chemicals, Industrial Processes and Industries Associated with Cancer in Humans (IARC Monographs, Volumes 1 to 29)
1982; 292 pages (*out of print*)

Supplement No. 5
Cross Index of Synonyms and Trade Names in Volumes 1 to 36
1985; 259 pages (*out of print*)

Supplement No. 6
Genetic and Related Effects: An Updating of Selected IARC Monographs from Volumes 1 to 42
1987; 729 pages Sw. fr. 80.–

Supplement No. 7
Overall Evaluations of Carcinogenicity: An Updating of IARC Monographs Volumes 1-42
1987; 440 pages Sw. fr. 65.–

Supplement No. 8
Cross Index of Synonyms and Trade Names in Volumes 1 to 46
1990; 346 pages Sw. fr. 60.–

IARC TECHNICAL REPORTS*

No. 1 Cancer in Costa Rica
Edited by R. Sierra,
R. Barrantes, G. Muñoz Leiva, D.M.
Parkin, C.A. Bieber and
N. Muñoz Calero
1988; 124 pages Sw. fr. 30.-

No. 2 SEARCH: A Computer Package to Assist the Statistical Analysis of Case-control Studies
Edited by G.J. Macfarlane,
P. Boyle and P. Maisonneuve
1991; 80 pages (out of print)

No. 3 Cancer Registration in the European Economic Community
Edited by M.P. Coleman and
E. Démaret
1988; 188 pages Sw. fr. 30.-

No. 4 Diet, Hormones and Cancer: Methodological Issues for Prospective Studies
Edited by E. Riboli and
R. Saracci
1988; 156 pages Sw. fr. 30.-

No. 5 Cancer in the Philippines
Edited by A.V. Laudico,
D. Esteban and D.M. Parkin
1989; 186 pages Sw. fr. 30.-

No. 6 La genèse du Centre International de Recherche sur le Cancer
Par R. Sohier et A.G.B. Sutherland
1990; 104 pages Sw. fr. 30.-

No. 7 Epidémiologie du cancer dans les pays de langue latine
1990; 310 pages Sw. fr. 30.-

No. 8 Comparative Study of Anti-smoking Legislation in Countries of the European Economic Community
Edited by A. Sasco, P. Dalla Vorgia and P. Van der Elst
1992; 82 pages Sw. fr. 30.-

No. 9 Epidemiologie du cancer dans les pays de langue latine
1991; 346 pages Sw. fr. 30.-

No. 11 Nitroso Compounds: Biological Mechanisms, Exposures and Cancer Etiology
Edited by I.K. O'Neill & H. Bartsch
1992; 149 pages Sw. fr. 30.-

No. 12 Epidémiologie du cancer dans les pays de langue latine
1992; 375 pages Sw. fr. 30.-

No. 13 Health, Solar UV Radiation and Environmental Change
Edited by A. Kricker, B.K. Armstrong, M.E. Jones and R.C. Burton
1993; 216 pages Sw.fr. 30.-

**No. 14
Epidémiologie du cancer dans les pays de langue latine**
1993; 385 pages Sw. fr. 30.-

DIRECTORY OF AGENTS BEING TESTED FOR CARCINOGENICITY (Until Vol. 13 Information Bulletin on the Survey of Chemicals Being Tested for Carcinogenicity)*

No. 8 Edited by M.-J. Ghess,
H. Bartsch and L. Tomatis
1979; 604 pages Sw. fr. 40.-

No. 9 Edited by M.-J. Ghess,
J.D. Wilbourn, H. Bartsch and
L. Tomatis
1981; 294 pages Sw. fr. 41.-

No. 10 Edited by M.-J. Ghess,
J.D. Wilbourn and H. Bartsch
1982; 362 pages Sw. fr. 42.-

No. 11 Edited by M.-J. Ghess,
J.D. Wilbourn, H. Vainio and
H. Bartsch
1984; 362 pages Sw. fr. 50.-

No. 12 Edited by M.-J. Ghess,
J.D. Wilbourn, A. Tossavainen and
H. Vainio
1986; 385 pages Sw. fr. 50.-

No. 13 Edited by M.-J. Ghess,
J.D. Wilbourn and A. Aitio 1988;
404 pages Sw. fr. 43.-

No. 14 Edited by M.-J. Ghess,
J.D. Wilbourn and H. Vainio
1990; 370 pages Sw. fr. 45.-

No. 15 Edited by M.-J. Ghess, J.D.
Wilbourn and H. Vainio
1992; 318 pages Sw. fr. 45.-

NON-SERIAL PUBLICATIONS †

Alcool et Cancer
By A. Tuyns (in French only)
1978; 42 pages Fr. fr. 35.-

Cancer Morbidity and Causes of Death Among Danish Brewery Workers
By O.M. Jensen
1980; 143 pages Fr. fr. 75.-

Directory of Computer Systems Used in Cancer Registries
By H.R. Menck and D.M. Parkin
1986; 236 pages Fr. fr. 50.-

* Available from booksellers through the network of WHO Sales agents.

† Available directly from IARC

Achevé d'imprimer sur les presses
de l'imprimerie Darantiere à Dijon-Quetigny
en septembre 1993

N° d'impression : 406
Dépôt légal : 3ᵉ trimestre 1993